Psychiatry Test Preparation and Review Manual

Content Strategist: Lotta Kryhl
Content Development Specialist: Rachael Harrison/Sharon Nash
Project Manager: Srividhya Shankar
Design: Christian Bilbow
Marketing Manager (UK/USA): Gaynor Jones/Carla Holloway

Psychiatry Test Preparation and Review Manual

Second Edition

J. Clive Spiegel, MD

Clinical Assistant Professor
Department of Psychiatry and Behavioral Sciences
Montefiore Medical Center
Albert Einstein College of Medicine
Bronx, NY, USA

John M. Kenny, MD

Assistant Professor
Department of Psychiatry and Behavioral Sciences
Montefiore Medical Center
Albert Einstein College of Medicine
Bronx, NY, USA

For additional online content visit
expertconsult website

Expert|CONSULT

SAUNDERS   London, New York, Oxford, St Louis, Sydney, Toronto

ELSEVIER
SAUNDERS

SAUNDERS is an imprint of Elsevier Inc.

© 2013, Elsevier Inc. All rights reserved.

First edition 2007

Notices

British Library Cataloguing-in-Publication Data
A catalogue record for this book is held in the British Library

ISBN: 9780323088695

eBook ISBN: 9781455775750

Printed in China

Last digit is the print number: 9 8 7 6 5 4 3 2 1

CONTENTS

Test Number Six

Vignettes

Topic Index

vi

Preface

It has been five years since the first edition of this book hit the shelves and rapidly became a best seller in the field of psychiatric test preparation. We have been overwhelmed with the positive response our book received. We sought to write a question and answer book that presented comprehensive answer explanations to save the reader time and effort by having all of the information they need for exam preparation in one volume. We sought to emphasize high yield information for standardized exams and to present it in a format that would allow students to practice test-taking technique and timing in addition to bolstering their knowledge base. By all measures we succeeded, and we are delighted to present you with our newest edition.

We have expanded and revised this book by adding two more tests of 150 questions each, bringing the total to 900 questions. Now that the new format for the ABPN certification examination contains case vignettes and video cases, we have responded by adding a set of twenty vignettes on a wide variety of topics that have an additional 160 questions with explanations attached. This new volume also features a subject index which will help the reader locate questions that fall into the same category, something many readers of the first edition have strongly recommended. We have improved the electronic version of the book for those who would rather do the questions on computer, as this is how the ABPN exams are now given. We hope that you will find this new version an invaluable asset in your test preparation, whether you are studying for the ABPN certification exam, ABPN maintenance of certification exam, PRITE, or USMLE. We have worked very hard to keep this book up to date with the latest information likely to show up on standardized exams. Keep in mind that each test closely mimics the balance of material found on the psychiatry board exam and that all of the answer choices are valuable opportunities to learn. Even wrong answer choices can form the basis of questions on the board exam which is why we spend so much effort on them in the answer explanations. Each answer explanation is also followed by a "K&S" or "B&D" reference. These refer to *Kaplan and Sadock's Synopsis of Psychiatry* and Daroff et al *Bradley's Neurology in Clinical Practice*. We believe these authoritative texts in psychiatry and neurology are the gold standard and candidates need only refer to the chapter corresponding to a particular question to gain a more in depth coverage of the subject involved. And don't forget, to test your timing for the actual exam, take each test in one sitting giving yourself two and a half hours for a 150 question test. When timing yourself on vignettes allow yourself one minute per question and an extra 3 minutes to read the vignette.

We would like to thank you, our many readers, for your support. To those of you who took the time to email us with questions, concerns, corrections, critiques and comments, we extend our sincere thanks. We listened to your feedback, and it has made this edition better than the first. We owe a big debt of gratitude to the many psychiatry training directors who have endorsed our book and encouraged their trainees to use this volume as a primary study guide for the ABPN psychiatry certification examination. We hope your trust in us has been rewarded by many happy trainees who are now board certified psychiatrists. And lastly, we would like to thank Charlotta Kryhl and all those at Elsevier whose hard work has been essential in bringing this book to the shelves.

J. Clive Spiegel, MD
Manhasset, New York

John M. Kenny, MD
Scarsdale, New York

References

Sadock, B.J., Kaplan, V.A. (Eds.), 2007. *Kaplan & Sadock's Synopsis of Psychiatry: Behavioral Sciences/Clinical Psychiatry*, 10th edn. Lippincott Williams & Wilkins, Philadelphia.

Daroff, R.B., Fenichel, G.M., Jankovic, J., Mazziotta, J. (Eds.), 2012. *Bradley's Neurology in Clinical Practice*, 6th edn. Elsevier Saunders, Philadelphia.

Figure Credits

All figures in this book are reproduced from Daroff, R.B., Fenichel, G.M., Jankovic, J., Mazziotta, J. (Eds.), 2012. *Bradley's Neurology in Clinical Practice*, 6th edn. Elsevier Saunders, Philadelphia, with permission, and Bradley, W.G., Daroff, R.B., Fenichel, G.M., Jankovic, J. (Eds.), 2003. *Neurology in Clinical Practice*, 4th edn. Elsevier Butterworth-Heinemann, Philadelphia, with permission.

Dedication

We would like to dedicate this book to our wives,

Jacqueline Hattem-Spiegel
and
Jennifer Halstead-Kenny

without whose love, support, and understanding
this book would never have seen the light of day.

Test Number One

1. A 16-year-old male suffers from irritable mood, increased energy, decreased need for sleep, and pressured speech. He was recently started on medication by his psychiatrist to control these symptoms. He comes into your office complaining of a significant worsening of his acne since starting this new medication. What drug was he started on?

    A. *Oxcarbazepine*

    B. *Lorazepam*

    C. *Risperidone*

    D. *Lithium*

    E. *Lamotrigine*

2. Which one of the following is not true regarding bonding and attachment?

    A. *Attachment lasts for life*

    B. *Attachment is the emotional dependence of an infant on his mother*

    C. *Bonding is the emotional attachment of a mother to her child*

    D. *Bonding is anchored by resources and security*

    E. *Poor attachments may lead to personality disorders*

3. What is the best test for diagnosing Huntington's disease?

    A. *Karyotype of chromosomes*

    B. *Serum ceruloplasmin*

    C. *Urine porphobilinogens*

    D. *Serum polymerase chain reaction (PCR)*

    E. *Cerebrospinal fluid (CSF) assay for 14-3-3 proteinase inhibitor protein*

4. Lesions in the orbitofrontal region of the brain will present as a patient who is:

    A. *Profane, irritable, and irresponsible*

    B. *Manic*

    C. *Depressed*

    D. *Apathetic*

    E. *Psychotic*

 Full test available online - see inside front cover for details.

1

5. A 65-year-old woman with schizophrenia believes that she is pregnant with God's child. She has been convinced of this for the past 5 years. When you confront her on this she tells you that she is certain that she is pregnant and that God is the father. She will not agree that this is not true. Her thinking is an example of which one of the following?

    A. *Egomania*
    B. *Coprolalia*
    C. *Delusion*
    D. *Ailurophobia*
    E. *Obsession*

6. A group of patients are looked at with regard to a risk factor for heart disease. They are divided into those who have the risk factor and those who do not. These groups are then followed for a number of years to see who does and who does not develop heart disease. This is an example of a:

    A. *Cohort study*
    B. *Case–control study*
    C. *Clinical trial*
    D. *Cross-sectional survey*
    E. *Crossover study*

7. Who developed the theory of "good enough mothering"?

    A. *Piaget*
    B. *Freud*
    C. *Mahler*
    D. *Winnicott*
    E. *Erikson*

8. A 47-year-old man presents to the emergency room in an acute state of disorientation, with tachycardia, ophthalmoparesis, diaphoresis, and ataxia. He dies in the hospital 48 hours later. Brain autopsy of this patient would reveal:

    A. *Frontal and temporal lobe atrophy*
    B. *Substantia nigra depigmentation*
    C. *Hemorrhages in the ependyma of the third ventricle and superior vermis*
    D. *Diffuse Lewy bodies in cortex*
    E. *Subcortical white matter lesions perpendicular to the ventricles*

9. Which one of the following statements is true concerning monoamine oxidase inhibitors (MAOIs)?

    A. *MAOIs are not likely to cause orthostatic hypotension*
    B. *To switch between an MAOI and a selective serotonin reuptake inhibitor (SSRI) you need a 3-day washout period*
    C. *Giving meperidine with an MAOI is contraindicated*
    D. *Lithium is contraindicated with MAOIs*
    E. *All MAOIs require adherence to a tyramine free diet*

10. You are called to consult on an agitated patient on the medical unit. The patient is elderly, confused and pulling out her lines. You decide that she must be tranquilized for her own safety. Which one of the following drugs would be the best choice?

    A. *Lorazepam*

    B. *Lithium*

    C. *Diazepam*

    D. *Aripiprazole*

    E. *Haloperidol*

11. You are talking to one of your colleagues from surgery. He tells you about a postoperative patient that he is covering who keeps complaining of pain. He tells you that the patient was originally on intramuscular meperidine and was switched to the same dose of oral meperidine just yesterday. The patient has been complaining constantly and is getting the nursing staff upset. What do you think is responsible for this situation?

    A. *The patient has low pain tolerance*

    B. *The patient has borderline personality disorder and is splitting the staff*

    C. *The patient has an intractable pain disorder*

    D. *The analgesic potency of oral meperidine is less than intramuscular meperidine*

    E. *The patient has a conversion disorder*

12. A therapist gets assigned a new patient in his clinic. While looking at the materials the patient filled out in the waiting area he finds out that the patient has a substance abuse history. He immediately says "Stupid drug addicts, they're so annoying. They're such a waste of time. They never want to get better." This is an example of:

    A. *Projection*

    B. *Transference*

    C. *Countertransference*

    D. *Resistance*

    E. *Confrontation*

13. What is the likelihood of a patient acquiring Huntington's disease if his father is a carrier and has the illness?

    A. *25%*

    B. *50%*

    C. *75%*

    D. *90%*

    E. *100%*

14. Which one of the following is not a developmental task of middle adulthood?

    A. *Taking stock of accomplishments*

    B. *Reassessing commitments to family, work and marriage*

    C. *Using accumulated power ethically*

    D. *Engaging in risk-taking behavior*

    E. *Dealing with parental illness and death*

15. A chronic schizophrenic has been taking medication for 20 years. Every morning he goes to his pill bottle and takes the pills his doctor prescribes. This is an example of:

    A. *Primary prevention*

    B. *Secondary prevention*

    C. *Tertiary prevention*

    D. *Malingering*

    E. *Noncompliance*

16. A patient with metastatic carcinoma of the lung presents with generalized muscle weakness and is found to have improved muscle strength with minimal exercise. The most likely diagnosis is:

    A. *Myasthenia gravis*

    B. *Multiple sclerosis*

    C. *Guillain–Barré syndrome*

    D. *Polymyositis*

    E. *Lambert–Eaton myasthenic syndrome*

17. Which one of the following tests does NOT detect psychotic thought processes?

    A. *Draw a person test*

    B. *Minnesota multiphasic personality inventory (MMPI)*

    C. *Sentence completion test*

    D. *Thematic apperception test (TAT)*

    E. *Rorschach test*

18. A patient presents with slowly progressive muscle weakness, fasciculations of arm muscles and tongue, difficulty swallowing and becomes wheelchair-bound. The diagnosis is amyotrophic lateral sclerosis. Postmortem studies of this patient's central nervous system would reveal:

    A. *Nigrostriatal depigmentation and atrophy*

    B. *Frontal and temporal lobe atrophy*

    C. *Anterior horn cell degeneration*

    D. *Corpus callosum thinning and atrophy*

    E. *Dorsal column volume loss*

19. Which one of the following is not part of the ethical code of the American Psychiatric Association?

    A. *It is unethical to accept a commission for patient referrals*

    B. *It is unethical to have sexual relations with patients*

    C. *It is a psychiatrist's obligation to report other psychiatrist's unethical behavior*

    D. *Retiring psychiatrists must provide patients with sufficient notice of their retirement and make every reasonable effort to find follow up care for their patients*

    E. *Psychiatrists have an obligation to participate in executions*

20. You are called by the medicine team to do a psychiatric consultation on a 90-year-old female with sepsis who is agitated, confused, disoriented and pulling out her lines. The medical team tells you that her mentation has been waxing and waning throughout the day. Your first consideration in approaching the case is:

    A. *Determining capacity to refuse treatment*
    B. *Speaking to the patient's family*
    C. *Examining the patient's medication regimen*
    D. *Developing a therapeutic relationship with the patient*
    E. *Protecting the patient from unintended harm*

21. Positive reinforcement, negative reinforcement, the operant, and the reinforcing stimulus are integral parts of what theory?

    A. *Operant conditioning developed by Skinner*
    B. *Operant conditioning developed by Bandura*
    C. *Attribution theory developed by Hull*
    D. *Learned helplessness developed by Kandel*
    E. *Habituation theory developed by Pavlov*

22. A 7-year-old girl with staring spells and 3-per-second spike and wave activity on electroencephalogram (EEG) fails therapy with ethosuximide and has breakthrough spells. The next best medication of choice to treat this patient is:

    A. *Phenytoin*
    B. *Divalproex sodium*
    C. *Phenobarbital*
    D. *Diazepam*
    E. *Carbamazepine*

23. Episodes of sudden sleep onset, with sudden loss of muscle tone, followed by quick entry into rapid eye movement (REM) sleep are characteristic of which one of the following?

    A. *Sleep changes associated with depression*
    B. *Sleep apnea*
    C. *Primary insomnia*
    D. *Narcolepsy*
    E. *Shift-work sleep disorder*

24. Which one of the following neurotransmitters is not associated with the inhibition of aggressive behavior?

    A. *Dopamine*
    B. *Norepinephrine*
    C. *Serotonin*
    D. *GABA*
    E. *Glycine*

25. Which one of the following anticonvulsant agents needs rapid dosage increases early in therapy due to autoinduction of its own metabolism?

    A. *Carbamazepine*
    B. *Divalproex sodium*
    C. *Phenytoin*
    D. *Phenobarbital*
    E. *Diazepam*

26. Giving positive reinforcement intermittently at a variable schedule is the best way to prevent:

    A. *Discrimination*

    B. *Generalization*

    C. *Extinction*

    D. *Respondent conditioning*

    E. *Transference*

27. A young woman presents to the emergency room with a history of intractable seizures and mental retardation. You discover she has severe acne, skin depigmentation on her back and blotchy patches on her retinal surface on funduscopic examination. The most likely diagnosis is:

    A. *Down's syndrome*

    B. *Rett's disorder*

    C. *Neurofibromatosis*

    D. *Tuberous sclerosis*

    E. *Williams' syndrome*

28. Which one of the following drugs does not work by blocking the catabolism of acetylcholine?

    A. *Donepezil*

    B. *Memantine*

    C. *Tacrine*

    D. *Rivastigmine*

    E. *Galantamine*

29. Which one of the following tests would be best used for testing executive function?

    A. *Thematic apperception test*

    B. *Halstead–Reitan neuropsychological battery*

    C. *Minnesota multiphasic personality inventory (MMPI)*

    D. *Brief psychiatric rating scale (BPRS)*

    E. *Trail-making tests*

30. You are asked as a psychiatrist to determine if a patient has the capacity to make a will. In order to make the will which one of the following does the patient not have to prove to you?

    A. *He knows that he is making a will*

    B. *He knows how the will distributes his property*

    C. *He knows the nature of the property to be distributed*

    D. *He knows who will inherit the property*

    E. *He understands court procedure*

31. Which one of the following is not correct regarding the onset of puberty?

    A. *Onset of puberty is triggered by the maturation of the hypothalamic–pituitary–adrenal–gonadal axis*

    B. *Primary sex characteristics are those directly involved in coitus and reproduction*

    C. *The average age of onset of puberty is 11 years of age for boys and 13 years of age for girls*

    D. *Increases in height and weight occur earlier in girls than in boys*

    E. *In adolescent boys testosterone levels correlate with libido*

32. Sumatriptan (Imitrex) is contraindicated in patients with:

    A. *Ischemic heart disease*

    B. *Kidney disease*

    C. *Obstructive pulmonary disease*

    D. *Inflammatory bowel disease*

    E. *Carcinoma*

33. Which one of the following does not increase tricyclic antidepressant concentrations?

    A. *Clozapine*

    B. *Haloperidol*

    C. *Risperidone*

    D. *Cigarette smoking*

    E. *Methylphenidate*

34. Which one of the following is true regarding suicide?

    A. *Completed suicide is most frequently related to bipolar disorder*

    B. *Adolescents most frequently succeed in committing suicide by hanging*

    C. *In recent years the suicide rate has increased dramatically among middle-aged adults*

    D. *Previous suicidal behavior is the best predictor of risk for future suicide*

    E. *Women successfully commit suicide more often than men*

35. Which one of the following symptoms is not part of the classic stroke condition known as Gerstmann's syndrome

    A. *Acalculia*

    B. *Right and left confusion*

    C. *Finger agnosia*

    D. *Alexia without agraphia*

    E. *Pure agraphia*

36. Which one of the following is most appropriate for treatment with dialectical behavioral therapy

    A. *Histrionic personality disorder*

    B. *Borderline personality disorder*

    C. *Dependant personality disorder*

    D. *Schizoid personality disorder*

    E. *Obsessive–compulsive personality disorder*

37. A 45-year-old woman with bipolar disorder complains of amenorrhea, galactorrhea, decreased libido and anorgasmia. She presents to the emergency room with an elevated serum prolactin level and is on risperidone 4 mg daily for bipolar disorder. On neurologic examination you discover decreased vision in both lateral visual fields. The most likely diagnosis is:

    A. *Acute right parietal stroke*

    B. *Thalamic hemorrhage*

    C. *Pituitary macroadenoma*

    D. *Acute left parietal stroke*

    E. *Midbrain infarct*

38. Which one of the following is not true regarding the mental status examination?

    A. *Racing thoughts are considered part of thought process*

    B. *Blunted is a term used to describe affect*

    C. *Hallucinations are part of thought content*

    D. *Delusions are part of thought content*

    E. *Circumstantiality is part of thought form*

39. A Malaysian man was brought into the emergency room after trying to commit suicide. The family describes an unusual course of events preceding the suicide attempt. The patient was depressed, preoccupied and brooding. He suddenly had an unprovoked outburst of rage in which he went around the neighborhood and indiscriminately maimed two people and three dogs. Two of the dogs died. Afterwards he had no memory of the episode and was exhausted. He then went into the kitchen of his home, picked up a knife and slit his wrists. The most appropriate diagnosis is:

    A. *Koro*

    B. *Amok*

    C. *Piblokto*

    D. *Wihtigo*

    E. *Mal de ojo*

40. An 80-year-old man with known vascular dementia presents to your emergency room with care givers complaining of new onset right hemiparesis and mutism. Which one of the following signs is not compatible with this clinical presentation?

    A. *Meyerson's sign*

    B. *Right-sided Hoffman's sign*

    C. *Right-sided Babinski sign*

    D. *A positive palmomental reflex*

    E. *Complete loss of the gag reflex*

41. Glutamate is not:

    A. *One of the two major amino acid neurotransmitters*

    B. *An inhibitory neurotransmitter*

    C. *Involved in learning and memory*

    D. *The primary neurotransmitter in cerebellar granule cells*

    E. *A precursor of gamma aminobutyric acid (GABA)*

42. Down's syndrome is associated with defects in chromosome 21. This is a feature also shared by:

    A. *Turner's syndrome*

    B. *Klinefelter's syndrome*

    C. *Huntington's disease*

    D. *Alzheimer's disease*

    E. *Parkinson's disease*

43. Which one of the following is not compatible with the diagnosis of brain death?

    A. *Eyes fully open*

    B. *Absence of corneal reflexes*

    C. *Presence of oculovestibular reflexes*

    D. *Spontaneous activity seen on EEG*

    E. *Large, fixed pupils*

44. Patients with compromised liver function should not use which one of the following drugs?

    A. *Temazepam*

    B. *Diazepam*

    C. *Oxazepam*

    D. *Lorazepam*

    E. *Chlorazepate*

45. Which one of the following is not an appropriate part of family therapy?

    A. *Exploring family members' beliefs about the meanings of their behaviors*

    B. *Reframing problematic behaviors positively*

    C. *Focusing most of the session on the most dysfunctional member of the family*

    D. *Encouraging family members to interact differently and observe the effects*

    E. *Giving the family members things to think about and work on outside of sessions*

46. Which one of the following statements is true regarding neurotransmitters and anxiety?

    A. *GABA has nothing to do with anxiety*

    B. *GABA, norepinephrine, and serotonin are associated with anxiety in some way*

    C. *Dopamine, glutamate, and histamine are associated with anxiety in some way*

    D. *Only acetylcholine is associated with anxiety*

    E. *Anxiety can be treated with injection of epinephrine*

47. Which one of the following is not used in treating myasthenia gravis?

    A. *Pyridostigmine*

    B. *Edrophonium chloride*

    C. *Plasmapheresis*

    D. *Intravenous immunoglobulin administration*

    E. *Thymectomy*

48. You are called to evaluate a potentially delirious patient on a medical unit. As part of your workup you order an EEG. What do you expect to find on EEG if this is truly a delirium?

    A. *3-per-second spike and wave pattern*

    B. *Frontocentral beta activity*

    C. *Posterior alpha rhythm*

    D. *Generalized slow-wave activity consisting of theta and delta waves, with some focal areas of hyperactivity*

    E. *Right temporal spikes*

49. Gower's maneuver or sign is typically seen in which one of the following neurologic conditions?

    A. *Myasthenia gravis*

    B. *Multiple sclerosis*

    C. *Huntington's disease*

    D. *Duchenne's muscular dystrophy*

    E. *Myotonic dystrophy*

50. Which one of the following antidepressants does not have strong sedative effects?

    A. *Trazodone*

    B. *Paroxetine*

    C. *Doxepin*

    D. *Clomipramine*

    E. *Mirtazapine*

51. One of your patients of the opposite sex begins to act seductively and proceeds to ask you out for dinner. Which one of the following would be an appropriate response?

    A. *Ignore the patient's advances*

    B. *Compliment the patient on the way she is dressed*

    C. *Tell the patient that you are seeing someone and therefore can't accept the offer*

    D. *Examine your own countertransference and explore the meaning of the patient's behavior*

    E. *Have sex with the patient and then make the patient find a new doctor*

52. While on call one night in the emergency room, you are asked to evaluate a distraught couple that has been brought in by the police following a fight that started after the wife found out that her husband was wearing her panties to work. It turns out that he has been wearing women's undergarments for over a year because he finds this very sexually arousing. He has developed several fantasies imagining himself in women's undergarments. The most appropriate diagnosis for the husband is:

    A. *Exhibitionism*

    B. *Fetishism*

    C. *Frotteurism*

    D. *Voyeurism*

    E. *Transvestic fetishism*

53. A 48-year-old woman presents to your office with complaints of lancinating, brief, sharp pain to the left side of her face. The pain is short-lived and recurrent. It is triggered frequently by cold air touching her face. The pharmacologic treatment of choice for this condition would be:

    A. *Divalproex sodium*

    B. *Clonazepam*

    C. *Carbamazepine*

    D. *Tiagabine*

    E. *Risperidone*

54. A 75-year-old man presents to the emergency room with new onset headache, fever, vague joint pains and complaints of recent diminished vision. The first test of choice in this case is:

    A. *Head CT scan*

    B. *MRI brain with diffusion-weighted imaging*

    C. *Lumbar puncture looking for CSF xanthochromia*

    D. *Serum sedimentation rate*

    E. *Carotid ultrasound looking for dissection*

55. The concept that different mental disorders have different outcomes was pioneered by:

    A. *Freud*

    B. *Bleuler*

    C. *Winnicott*

    D. *Kraepelin*

    E. *Kohut*

56. A patient comes into your practice after referral from his primary care physician. He is convinced that he has cancer. He thinks that it hasn't been found yet, but is convinced that it is there. He remains convinced despite a full workup with negative results. Despite further reassurance by his doctors, he remains convinced that he has cancer. Which is the most appropriate diagnosis?

    A. *Conversion disorder*

    B. *Hypochondriasis*

    C. *Body dysmorphic disorder*

    D. *Somatization disorder*

    E. *Briquet's syndrome*

57. Which one of the following is not characteristic of cluster headaches?

    A. *Attacks of short duration of 3 hours or less.*

    B. *Daytime attacks*

    C. *Male predominance*

    D. *Sharp, severe, retro-orbital pain*

    E. *Cyclical pattern of occurrence mainly in spring and fall seasons*

58. Which one of the following is not a contraindication to bupropion?

    A. *Seizure*

    B. *Anorexia*

    C. *Use of a MAOI in the past 14 days*

    D. *Head trauma*

    E. *Hypertension*

59. Which one of the following is it safe to combine with MAOIs?

    A. *Meperidine*

    B. *Lithium*

    C. *Levodopa*

    D. *SSRIs*

    E. *Spinal anesthetic containing epinephrine*

60. Which one of the following will not result in an acquired peripheral neuropathy?

    A. *Systemic lupus erythematosus (SLE)*

    B. *Toluene intoxication*

    C. *Acetaminophen overdose*

    D. *Vincristine therapy*

    E. *Epstein–Barr virus infection*

61. Which one of the following is false regarding tricyclic antidepressants (TCAs)?

    A. *Cigarette smoking decreases TCA levels*

    B. *Clozapine will increase TCA levels*

    C. *Methylphenidate will decrease TCA levels*

    D. *TCAs can have adverse cardiac effects*

    E. *TCAs have strong anticholinergic effects*

62. Which one of the following antidepressants has the longest half-life?

    A. *Fluvoxamine*

    B. *Paroxetine*

    C. *Citalopram*

    D. *Fluoxetine*

    E. *Sertraline*

63. Self-mutilation is most common in which one of the following personality disorders?

    A. *Borderline*

    B. *Narcissistic*

    C. *Histrionic*

    D. *Dependent*

    E. *Schizoid*

64. A young man is admitted to the hospital with progressive proximal muscle weakness, generalized fatigue and a red non-pruritic rash to the face and body, especially around the knees and elbows. His workup should include screening for:

    A. *Carcinoma*

    B. *Heart disease*

    C. *Intestinal bleeding*

    D. *Fibrotic lung disease*

    E. *Stroke*

65. You are on call and get paged to go see a schizophrenic patient on the inpatient unit. The patient has a tremor, is ataxic and is restless. During the interview the patient vomits. The nurse tells you he has been having diarrhea and has been urinating very frequently. What question would be most useful to ask the patient?

    A. *Can you count from 100 backwards by sevens?*

    B. *Where are you right now?*

    C. *Who is the current president?*

    D. *How much water have you been drinking recently?*

    E. *Are you HIV positive?*

66. In what kind of schizophrenia is the onset late, the thought process more linear, and the outcome usually better?

    A. *Paranoid*

    B. *Disorganized*

    C. *Catatonic*

    D. *Residual*

    E. *Undifferentiated*

67. Which one of the following is not associated with good outcomes in schizophrenia?

    A. *High premorbid functioning*

    B. *Little prodrome*

    C. *Early age at onset*

    D. *Acute onset*

    E. *Absence of family history of schizophrenia*

68. During a workup you send a patient for an EEG. The results reveal shortened latency of rapid eye movement (REM) sleep, decreased stage IV sleep and increased REM density. These findings are most consistent with:

    A. *Tumor*

    B. *Petit mal epilepsy*

    C. *Hepatic encephalopathy*

    D. *Delirium*

    E. *Depression*

69. Homozygosity for which one of the following is believed to predispose patients to Alzheimer-type dementia?

    A. *Tau*

    B. *Apolipoprotein E4*

    C. *Amyloid precursor protein*

    D. *Trisomy 21*

    E. *Presenelin*

70. Which one of the following is not characteristic of narcissistic personality disorder?

    A. *Grandiosity*

    B. *Need for admiration*

    C. *Showing self-dramatization, theatricality, and exaggerated expression of emotion*

    D. *Preoccupation with fantasies of unlimited success, power and brilliance*

    E. *Interpersonally exploitative*

71. Which one of the following is not a criterion of post-traumatic stress disorder?

    A. *Re-experiencing the event*

    B. *Increased arousal*

    C. *Avoidance of stimuli associated with the trauma*

    D. *The duration of the disturbance is more than two months*

    E. *The person's response to the trauma involved intense fear or horror*

72. After her mother died, Sarah felt extreme sadness, cried, blamed God, felt guilty, and became convinced that she was worthless and eventually tried to hang herself. Her diagnosis is:

    A. *Normal bereavement*

    B. *Bipolar disorder*

    C. *Delusional disorder*

    D. *Anticipatory grief*

    E. *Pathological grief*

73. The brains of patients with schizophrenia often reveal enlargement of the:

    A. *Hippocampus*

    B. *Caudate*

    C. *Ventricles*

    D. *Corpus callosum*

    E. *Cerebellum*

74. A 20-year-old patient comes into the emergency room while you are on call. She is 5 feet (152 cm) tall and has difficulty maintaining her body weight above 67 pounds (30 kg). She has lost weight in the past by dieting and was encouraged by her progress. She continued to decrease food intake and increase exercising until her weight dropped below 63 pounds (28 kg). At this time she is no longer having her menstrual periods. She comes to the emergency room with symptoms of peptic ulcer disease. Which one of the following would be considered the most important and urgent part of her initial medical workup?

    A. *Bone scan*

    B. *Head CT scan*

    C. *Gastric emptying study*

    D. *Cholesterol level*

    E. *Serum potassium level*

75. Which one of the following is not true of delusional disorder?

    A. *It involves nonbizarre delusions that could happen in real life*

    B. *It may involve tactile hallucinations*

    C. *The erotomanic type involves another person of higher social standing being in love with the patient*

    D. *Daily functioning is markedly impaired*

    E. *The person's behavior is not markedly odd or bizarre*

76. Which one of the following is false regarding female orgasmic disorder?

    A. *Female orgasmic disorder is the persistent absence of orgasm following a normal sexual excitement phase*

    B. *The incidence of orgasm in women increases with age*

    C. *Fears of impregnation or damage to the vagina as well as guilt are psychological factors involved in this disorder*

    D. *Female orgasmic disorder can be either life long or acquired*

    E. *Criteria include involuntary spasm of the vaginal musculature that interferes with intercourse*

77. A patient presents to your office with a complaint of intense fear of going to social functions at her child's school. On further examination you note that she has fears that she will act in a way that will be humiliating or embarrassing. She is also made anxious by having to meet new people that she does not know. Your differential diagnosis of this patient should include which one of the following Axis II disorders?

    A. *Borderline personality disorder*

    B. *Obsessive–compulsive personality disorder*

    C. *Narcissistic personality disorder*

    D. *Avoidant personality disorder*

    E. *Dependent personality disorder*

78. Which one of the following anticonvulsant agents is known to cause hirsutism, facial changes and hypertrophy of the gingiva?

   A. *Carbamazepine*

   B. *Valproate*

   C. *Phenobarbital*

   D. *Levetiracetam*

   E. *Phenytoin*

79. A 52-year-old man is brought to the emergency room after being found by police prone on the edge of the sidewalk outside. He is moderately intoxicated with alcohol and unable to give an adequate history. Upon neurologic examination you discover that his right wrist and fingers are limp and he cannot lift them. He is also weak when he tries to extend his arm from a bent to straight position. He also has trouble turning his forearm over when it is placed palm down on a flat surface. The lesion in question here is most likely a(n):

   A. *Radial nerve entrapment*

   B. *Ulnar nerve entrapment*

   C. *Median nerve entrapment*

   D. *Musculocutaneous nerve entrapment*

   E. *Suprascapular nerve entrapment*

80. A patient comes into the emergency room complaining that twice during the past week he experienced a sudden loss of muscle tone. The first time occurred when he was told that his mother was diagnosed with cancer. The second came during a track meet while he was warming up before his turn to run. These episodes are most likely to be associated with which one of the following diagnoses:

   A. *Sleep apnea*

   B. *Primary insomnia*

   C. *Primary hypersomnia*

   D. *Narcolepsy*

   E. *Circadian rhythm sleep disorder*

81. Which one of the following is true regarding conversion disorder?

   A. *It is intentionally produced*

   B. *It consists of complaints in multiple organ systems*

   C. *It involves neurologic symptoms*

   D. *It can be limited to pain*

   E. *It can be limited to sexual dysfunction*

82. Which one of the following drugs is contraindicated in conjunction with therapy with levodopa/carbidopa in Parkinson's disease patients?

   A. *Amitriptyline*

   B. *Fluoxetine*

   C. *Gabapentin*

   D. *Tranylcypromine*

   E. *Sertraline*

83. Piaget's stage of concrete operations includes which one of the following?

    A. *Identity versus role confusion*

    B. *Good enough mothering*

    C. *Conservation*

    D. *Inductive reasoning*

    E. *Object permanence*

84. A 10-year-old child engages in sex play. This should be viewed as:

    A. *A sign of homosexuality*

    B. *A sign of hormonal imbalance*

    C. *The result of excessive television viewing*

    D. *Normal development*

    E. *Premature development*

85. You see a child in the clinic who has fragile X syndrome. Which one of the following would you not expect him to have?

    A. *Mental retardation*

    B. *Long ears*

    C. *Narrow face*

    D. *Arched palate*

    E. *Short palpebral fissures*

86. What would you expect from 18-month-old children with secure attachments after their parents leave them alone with you in a room?

    A. *They would try to bring the parents back into the room*

    B. *They would immediately run to you and sit on your lap*

    C. *They would become more inquisitive*

    D. *They would not notice the parents' absence*

    E. *They would become aggressive and violent*

87. Which one of the following agents is a potent cytochrome P-450 inhibitor and can dangerously increase levels of lamotrigine in patients?

    A. *Phenytoin*

    B. *Diazepam*

    C. *Valproate*

    D. *Phenobarbital*

    E. *Gabapentin*

88. You are introduced to a child with a physical deformity. When would you predict that the deformity would have the greatest psychological impact on the child?

    A. *Infancy*

    B. *Preschool*

    C. *Elementary school age*

    D. *Early adolescence*

    E. *Adulthood*

89. Which one of the following is a specific inhibitor of monoamine oxidase type B (MAOI-B)?

    A. *Moclobemide*

    B. *Phenelzine*

    C. *Tranylcypromine*

    D. *Selegiline*

    E. *Befloxatone*

90. Which one of the following will produce a hypodopaminergic state when used chronically?

    A. *Heroin*

    B. *PCP*

    C. *Alcohol*

    D. *Amphetamines*

    E. *Cocaine*

91. The anticonvulsant agent valproic acid can cause which one of the following problems in the fetus of pregnant patients?

    A. *Spina bifida*

    B. *Macrocephaly*

    C. *Hypertelorism*

    D. *Oligohydramnios*

    E. *Intrauterine growth retardation*

92. Which one of the following agents is a dopamine agonist?

    A. *Haloperidol*

    B. *Pergolide*

    C. *Quetiapine*

    D. *Buspirone*

    E. *Fluphenazine*

93. A 25-year-old man is brought to see you because of change in personality following a boating accident. He fell off of his boat and landed head first on the dock. He was previously friendly, happy, and high functioning. Now his speech is pressured and his mood is labile. He has been irresponsible at work and has been fired from his job. His memory is intact. Which one of the following brain areas did he damage?

    A. *Temporal lobe*

    B. *Occipital lobe*

    C. *Basal ganglia*

    D. *Substantia nigra*

    E. *Frontal lobe*

94. Which one of the following inhibits norepinephrine reuptake?

    A. *Haloperidol*

    B. *Ziprasidone*

    C. *Chlorpromazine*

    D. *Olanzapine*

    E. *Aripiprazole*

95. Which one of the following is a partial agonist at the D2 receptor?

    A. *Haloperidol*

    B. *Ziprasidone*

    C. *Chlorpromazine*

    D. *Olanzapine*

    E. *Aripiprazole*

96. Damage to which one of the following brain areas is most likely to present with depression?

    A. *Occipital lobe*

    B. *Right prefrontal cortex*

    C. *Left prefrontal cortex*

    D. *Right parietal lobe*

    E. *Left parietal lobe*

97. Which one of the following brain areas is characteristically serotonergic?

    A. *Ventral tegmental area*

    B. *Substantia nigra*

    C. *Nucleus accumbens*

    D. *Cerebellum*

    E. *Raphe nuclei*

98. A patient presents to your office with a history of wing-flapping coarse tremor of the upper extremities, ataxia and a rapidly progressive confusional state developing over several months. The test of choice to diagnose this patient is:

    A. *Serum ACE level*

    B. *Chromosomal analysis for CAG triplet repeats*

    C. *Serum ceruloplasmin level*

    D. *Lumbar puncture and CSF titer for oligoclonal bands and myelin basic protein*

    E. *Edrophonium hydrochloride testing (Tensilon test)*

99. A patient comes into the emergency room high on cocaine. Which one of the following brain regions would you expect to be most active in terms of the reward he is experiencing from the drug?

    A. *Neocortex*

    B. *Substantia nigra*

    C. *Nucleus accumbens*

    D. *Locus ceruleus*

    E. *Raphe nuclei*

100. What is the therapeutic focus of motivational enhancement therapy?

    A. *Anger*

    B. *Depression*

    C. *Medical comorbidity*

    D. *Ambivalence*

    E. *Environment*

101. You are teaching a class to a group of first year psychiatric residents. You review some of the psychological tests with them and describe their use. One of the anal-retentive types in the front row asks which of the tests has the highest reliability. Your answer is?

    A. *Wechsler adult intelligence scale*

    B. *Thematic apperception test*

    C. *Draw a person test*

    D. *Minnesota multiphasic personality inventory*

    E. *Projective personality assessment*

102. Freud is best associated with which one of the following?

    A. *Learning theory*

    B. *Mesolimbic dopamine theory of positive psychotic symptoms*

    C. *Conflict theory*

    D. *Self psychology*

    E. *Drive theory*

103. The most common cause of intracerebral hemorrhage is:

    A. *Hypertension*

    B. *Intracranial tumors or metastases*

    C. *Disorders of coagulation (coagulopathies)*

    D. *Vascular malformations*

    E. *Trauma*

104. How would Beck describe the problem found in depression?

    A. *Learned helplessness*

    B. *Not good enough mothering*

    C. *Neurochemical imbalance*

    D. *Cognitive distortion*

    E. *Lack of social skills*

105. A Type I error occurs when:

    A. *The null hypothesis is rejected when it should have been retained*

    B. *The null hypothesis is retained when it should have been rejected*

    C. *There is false rejection of a difference that was truly significant*

    D. *The probability of an event occurring is 0*

    E. *The probability of an event occurring is 1*

106. The process by which a patient in a clinical trial has an equal likelihood of being in a control group versus an experimental group is:

    A. *Probability*

    B. *Risk*

    C. *Percentile rank*

    D. *Power*

    E. *Randomization*

107. A 32-year-old man who is HIV positive presents to the emergency room with mild fever to 101°F (38.3°C), headache, stiff neck, photophobia and lethargy. His CD4 count is zero and he has a highly elevated viral load. The most useful immediate diagnostic test for his current condition would be:

   A. Head CT scan with contrast

   B. MRI of the brain with and without gadolinium

   C. Lumbar puncture for CSF analysis and India ink staining

   D. Chest radiography and blood cultures

   E. Serum cold agglutinin assay

108. The probability of finding a true difference between two samples is:

   A. Probability

   B. Risk

   C. Percentile rank

   D. Power

   E. Randomization

109. The number of people who have a disorder at a specified point in time is:

   A. Probability

   B. Risk

   C. Point prevalence

   D. Power

   E. Randomization

110. To diagnose anorexia nervosa, the patient must be below what percentage of normal body weight?

   A. 85%

   B. 65%

   C. 93%

   D. 50%

   E. 75%

111. How long after taking PCP can it still be found in the urine?

   A. 1 day

   B. 2 days

   C. 5 days

   D. 8 days

   E. 10 days

112. Which one of the following is associated with the amyloid precursor protein?

   A. Wilson's disease

   B. Schizophrenia

   C. Alzheimer's disease

   D. Bipolar disorder

   E. Huntington's disease

113. A patient you put on carbamazepine has weakness and a rash. Which lab test would you order first?

    A. *Liver profile*

    B. *Electrolytes, BUN, creatinine, glucose (Chem-7)*

    C. *Complete blood count*

    D. *Thyroid function tests*

    E. *VDRL*

114. Which one of the following should not be part of an initial workup of a patient with anorexia nervosa?

    A. *Complete blood count*

    B. *Chem-7*

    C. *Thyroid function tests*

    D. *Electrocardiogram*

    E. *Head CT scan*

115. The test of choice to diagnose human central nervous system prion disease is:

    A. *Serum assay for 14-3-3 proteins*

    B. *CSF assay for 14-3-3 and tau proteins*

    C. *EEG*

    D. *MRI of the brain with and without gadolinium*

    E. *Head CT scan with contrast*

116. Which eye findings are common in schizophrenia?

    A. *Failure of adduction*

    B. *Failure of accommodation*

    C. *Pupillary dilatation*

    D. *Abnormal smooth pursuit saccades*

    E. *Weakness of the third cranial nerve*

117. A patient on risperidone comes into your office and reports that she intends on going to her gynecologist because she hasn't been having her menstrual periods. She has taken a pregnancy test and it was negative. Which lab test would you order?

    A. *Lumbar puncture*

    B. *Risperidone level*

    C. *Complete blood count*

    D. *Liver profile*

    E. *Prolactin level*

118. A 20-year-old man comes into the emergency room. He has superficial cuts on his arms, legs and abdomen. He reports being very depressed and feels that his neighbors are out to harm him. His most likely diagnosis is:

    A. *Dysthymic disorder*

    B. *Schizoaffective disorder*

    C. *Borderline personality disorder*

    D. *Bipolar disorder*

    E. *Adjustment disorder with mixed anxiety and depressed mood*

119. Which one of the following conditions has the highest prevalence?

    A. *Depressive disorders*

    B. *Anxiety disorders*

    C. *Schizophrenia*

    D. *Dementia*

    E. *Substance abuse*

120. Which one of the following has the greatest comorbidity with pathological gambling?

    A. *Schizophrenia*

    B. *Post-traumatic stress disorder*

    C. *Agoraphobia*

    D. *Major depressive disorder*

    E. *Intermittent explosive disorder*

121. A couple comes into the emergency room. The wife says that her husband has become convinced that she is cheating on him, and that it is not true. He has been following her, smelling her clothing, going through her purse, and making regular accusations. He does not meet criteria for a mood disorder. He denies other psychotic symptoms. Medical and substance abuse history are negative. What is his diagnosis?

    A. *Schizophrenia*

    B. *Major depressive disorder with psychotic features*

    C. *Delusional disorder*

    D. *Delirium*

    E. *Shared psychotic disorder*

122. Which one of the following disorders presents with the patient being preoccupied with having a given illness based on misinterpretation of bodily sensations?

    A. *Somatoform disorder*

    B. *Factitious disorder*

    C. *Conversion disorder*

    D. *Pain disorder*

    E. *Hypochondriasis*

123. A patient asks you about the data proving that alcoholism is hereditary. During your discussion, the patient asks you the following question: "The study of which group most strongly supports the heredity of alcoholism?" Your answer is:

    A. *Siblings*

    B. *Cousins*

    C. *Parents*

    D. *Mothers–daughters*

    E. *Adopted siblings*

124. A patient falls down on the floor of your office. He states that he has a terrible headache. He begins to hyperventilate. He has asynchronous tonic–clonic movements on both sides of his body. He is not incontinent, and is not injured. He is conscious the whole time. What is the most likely explanation for this presentation?

    A. *Complex seizure*

    B. *Simple seizure*

    C. *Psychogenic seizure*

    D. *Myoclonus*

    E. *Carpal tunnel syndrome*

125. The lesion that produces the classic signs of internuclear ophthalmoplegia in multiple sclerosis is most often found in the:

    A. *Superior colliculus*

    B. *Medial longitudinal fasciculus*

    C. *Inferior colliculus*

    D. *Nucleus of the third nerve*

    E. *Nucleus of the sixth nerve*

126. Which form of schizophrenia occurs later, and results in less decline in cognitive functioning as compared to the others?

    A. *Disorganized*

    B. *Paranoid*

    C. *Catatonic*

    D. *Undifferentiated*

    E. *Residual*

127. A middle-aged man comes to you with the complaint that he cannot stop gambling. He has wasted tens of thousands of dollars in casinos and his wife just left him. He has also been fired from his job because he misses so much work to gamble. Where would his diagnosis best fit in the following choices?

    A. *Personality disorders*

    B. *Psychotic disorders*

    C. *Anxiety disorders*

    D. *Substance abuse disorders*

    E. *Impulse control disorders*

128. An 8-year-old boy is getting beaten up at school because of his social interactions. He talks at the other children rather than to them. He is obsessed with cats. His cognitive and language development are appropriate. His diagnosis is:

    A. *Conduct disorder*

    B. *Oppositional defiant disorder*

    C. *Attention deficit–hyperactivity disorder*

    D. *Autism*

    E. *Asperger's disorder*

129. An 8-year-old boy is getting beaten up at school because of his lack of social interactions. He talks at the other children rather than to them. He is obsessed with cats. His cognitive and language development are significantly impaired. His diagnosis is:

   A.   Conduct disorder

   B.   Oppositional defiant disorder

   C.   Attention deficit–hyperactivity disorder

   D.   Autism

   E.   Asperger's disorder

130. A subjective sense that the environment is changed or unreal is:

   A.   Depersonalization

   B.   Derealization

   C.   Fugue

   D.   Amnesia

   E.   Anosognosia

131. A young patient presents to your office with dementia. He has been involved in heavy drug use. He has used heroin, PCP, LSD, amphetamines and inhalants. If you were to postulate which most likely caused his dementia, which one would you choose?

   A.   Heroin

   B.   LSD

   C.   PCP

   D.   Amphetamines

   E.   Inhalants

132. Which is the best matched pair among the following?

   A.   Family therapy – seclusion and restraint

   B.   Vocational assessment – social skills training

   C.   Assertive community treatment – psychoanalysis

   D.   ADHD – ECT

   E.   Psychiatric rehabilitation – social skills training

133. Which one of the following is not a clinical feature highly suggestive of multiple sclerosis?

   A.   Optic neuritis

   B.   Worsening with elevated body temperature

   C.   Fatigue

   D.   Steady progression from initial onset

   E.   Lhermitte's sign

134. A 20-year-old woman comes to the emergency room with hypokalemic alkalosis, enlarged parotids, hypotension and Russell's sign. What diagnosis do you suspect?

   A.   Psychosis

   B.   Major depressive disorder

   C.   Bulimia

   D.   Inhalant induced euphoria

   E.   HIV

135. While on call in the emergency room you receive a phone call from emergency medical services (EMS) to say that they are bringing in a patient who is highly intoxicated and behaviorally out of control. The patient's friend told EMS that he has been taking amphetamines. If this is true, what is the most prominent psychiatric symptom you would expect to see?

   A. *Hallucinations*

   B. *Suicidal tendencies*

   C. *Disorganized speech*

   D. *Paranoia*

   E. *Anxiety*

136. A 29-year-old woman has begun hearing voices since seeing her child hit by a car three weeks ago. She has become irritable, fearful, and is not sleeping well. The most likely diagnosis is:

   A. *Schizophrenia*

   B. *Acute stress disorder*

   C. *Dysthymic disorder*

   D. *Bipolar II disorder*

   E. *Adjustment disorder with depressed mood*

137. Children with depression often present with which one of the following?

   A. *Urinary incontinence*

   B. *Violence*

   C. *Irritability*

   D. *Hallucinations*

   E. *Delusions*

138. A patient comes into the clinic carrying a diagnosis of schizoid personality disorder. To confirm this diagnosis, you would look for which one of the following?

   A. *Bright, revealing clothing*

   B. *Grandiosity*

   C. *Paranoia*

   D. *Lack of close relationships*

   E. *Magical thinking*

139. If you apply your abilities solely for the patient's well being, and do no harm to the patient, you are said to have:

   A. *Beneficence*

   B. *Malignancy*

   C. *Justice*

   D. *Validity*

   E. *Autonomy*

140. Which one of the following is not true of Tourette's syndrome?

   A. *The course is usually not progressive*

   B. *Symptoms increase in times of stress*

   C. *Initial symptoms may decrease, increase, or persist*

   D. *Vocal tics are done to intentionally provoke others*

   E. *Medication can be helpful*

141. On your drive in to work you wonder if you will encounter any violent patients during your day. If you encounter the following types of patients today, which group of patients is the most likely to attack you?

    A. *Bipolar patients*

    B. *Schizophrenic patients*

    C. *Borderline patients*

    D. *Substance abusers*

    E. *Major depressive disorder patients*

142. What is the best indicator that a patient has the ego strength for psychodynamic psychotherapy?

    A. *Diagnosis*

    B. *Age*

    C. *Quality of relationships*

    D. *Gender*

    E. *Mental status examination*

143. T2-weighted MRI brain imaging of a patient reveals the scan pictured below. The patient is a 36-year-old woman who presented to the emergency room with recurrent episodes of unilateral arm and leg weakness and numbness with gait instability. The treatment of first choice in this case would be:

    A. *Intravenous ceftriaxone administration*

    B. *Intravenous immunoglobin therapy*

    C. *Plasmapheresis*

    D. *Sublingual aspirin and intravenous heparin therapy*

    E. *Intravenous corticosteroid therapy*

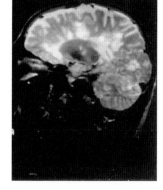

144. A patient with borderline personality disorder and past suicide attempts calls you after a fight with her boyfriend. She has been cutting herself since the fight and is hearing voices. What is the best level of care for this patient at this time?

    A. *Inpatient hospitalization*

    B. *Outpatient therapy*

    C. *Speak to her again in 5 days*

    D. *Extended inpatient stay (1+ months)*

    E. *Group therapy session*

145. A 75-year-old woman is referred to your practice by an internist for depression. On initial examination you discover that the patient has recently just recovered from a heart attack. Which one of the following medications would be the best choice for this patient?

    A. *Amitriptyline*

    B. *Doxepin*

    C. *Bupropion*

    D. *Methylphenidate*

    E. *Citalopram*

146. Which one of the following is not a classic characteristic of neurofibromatosis type 1 (von Recklinghausen's disease)?

    A. *Café au lait spots and cutaneous neurofibromas*

    B. *Bilateral acoustic schwannomas*

    C. *Optic gliomas*

    D. *Lisch nodules*

    E. *Axillary or inguinal freckling*

147. The sign that best differentiates between delirium and dementia is:

    A. *Sleep disturbance*

    B. *Hallucinations*

    C. *Disorientation to place*

    D. *Violent behavior*

    E. *Alteration of consciousness*

148. What is the first step towards treating a 23-year-old medical student who comes to your office with a complaint of insomnia?

    A. *Prescribe zolpidem*

    B. *Prescribe benzodiazepines*

    C. *Prescribe diphenhydramine*

    D. *Restrict the use of the bed to sleep and intimacy only*

    E. *Obtain a sleep study*

149. What is the American Psychiatric Association's position on therapy to change the sexual orientation of homosexuals?

    A. *This type of therapy should be encouraged*

    B. *Homosexuality is a medical disorder*

    C. *Only teens should be treated, before they become sexually active*

    D. *There is little data showing negative outcomes of such therapy*

    E. *No existing data supports doing this therapy*

150. A 20-year-old college student is brought into the emergency room after a party. He has tenting of the skin on the backs of his hands, is nauseated and vomits, acts seductively towards the nursing staff, and thinks the security guards are out to kill him. He tells you: "The one with the red hair is out to slay me." The emergency medical technician tells you the patient apparently collapsed while dancing at a "rave". What substance has he most likely taken?

    A. *Cannabis*

    B. *Ketamine*

    C. *Diacetylmorphine*

    D. *Methylenedioxyamphetamine*

    E. *Some form of volatile inhalant*

ONE

Answer Key – **Test Number One**

1.	D	26.	C	51.	D	76.	E	101.	A	126.	B
2.	D	27.	D	52.	B	77.	D	102.	E	127.	E
3.	D	28.	B	53.	C	78.	E	103.	A	128.	E
4.	A	29.	E	54.	D	79.	A	104.	D	129.	D
5.	C	30.	E	55.	D	80.	D	105.	A	130.	B
6.	A	31.	C	56.	B	81.	C	106.	E	131.	E
7.	D	32.	A	57.	B	82.	D	107.	C	132.	E
8.	C	33.	D	58.	E	83.	C	108.	D	133.	D
9.	C	34.	D	59.	B	84.	D	109.	C	134.	C
10.	E	35.	D	60.	C	85.	E	110.	A	135.	D
11.	D	36.	B	61.	C	86.	A	111.	D	136.	B
12.	C	37.	C	62.	D	87.	C	112.	C	137.	C
13.	B	38.	C	63.	A	88.	D	113.	C	138.	D
14.	D	39.	B	64.	A	89.	D	114.	E	139.	A
15.	C	40.	E	65.	D	90.	E	115.	B	140.	D
16.	E	41.	B	66.	A	91.	A	116.	D	141.	D
17.	B	42.	D	67.	C	92.	B	117.	E	142.	C
18.	C	43.	C	68.	E	93.	E	118.	C	143.	E
19.	E	44.	B	69.	B	94.	B	119.	B	144.	A
20.	E	45.	C	70.	C	95.	E	120.	D	145.	E
21.	A	46.	B	71.	D	96.	C	121.	C	146.	B
22.	B	47.	B	72.	E	97.	E	122.	E	147.	E
23.	D	48.	D	73.	C	98.	C	123.	E	148.	D
24.	A	49.	D	74.	E	99.	C	124.	C	149.	E
25.	A	50.	B	75.	D	100.	D	125.	B	150.	D

ONE

Explanations – **Test Number One**

Question 1. D. Several cutaneous side effects are possible with lithium including acne, follicular and maculopapular eruptions. Alopecia has also been reported. Major side effects of lithium include gastrointestinal complaints, tremor, diabetes insipidus, hypothyroidism, weight gain, cardiac arrhythmia and edema. Lamotrigine is an anticonvulsant that is also used for mood stabilization. Side effects can include Stevens–Johnson syndrome, anemia, thrombocytopenia, liver failure, and pancreatitis. Lorazepam is a benzodiazepine, which causes sedation, respiratory suppression, and has a high addictive potential. Risperidone is an antipsychotic that can cause extrapyramidal side effects, neuroleptic malignant syndrome, metabolic syndrome, gastrointestinal upset, increased salivation and lactation, among others. Oxcarbazepine is an anticonvulsant that may cause leukopenia, thrombocytopenia, Stevens–Johnson syndrome, and several other side effects. With the exception of lithium, the other choices do not worsen acne.

Psychopharmacology

K&S Ch. 3

Question 2. D. Attachment, which is the emotional dependence of the infant on his mother, involves resources and security, because the infant depends on the mother for these things. Attachment theory was developed by John Bowlby, and says that a secure attachment between mother and child affects the child's ability to form healthy relationships later in life. Attachment occurs when there is a warm intimate and continuous relationship between child and mother. The attachment gives the infant a feeling of security. Bonding is the mother's feelings for her infant. In bonding, the mother does not rely on her baby for food and protection. Therefore bonding does not involve resources and security. It is thought that bonding occurs with skin to skin contact between infant and mother. All other choices given are true regarding attachment theory.

Human Development

K&S Ch. 4

Question 3. D. Serum polymerase chain reaction (PCR) is the test of choice to examine the number of trinucleotide repeats (>35 in adults and >50 in children) in order to diagnose Huntington's disease (HD). The HD gene resides on the short arm of chromosome 4 at 4p16.3. A chromosomal karyotype can reveal only macroscopic defects in chromosomes such as deletions, translocations, or trisomies. Serum ceruloplasmin, when low, is diagnostic of Wilson's disease. Urine porphobilinogens and aminolevulinic acid, when detected in urine in excessive amounts, are diagnostic of acute intermittent porphyria. Creutzfeldt–Jakob disease is diagnosed by cerebrospinal fluid assay for 14-3-3 proteinase inhibitor proteins.

Neurology

B&D Ch. 71

Question 4. A. Orbitofrontal lobe lesions cause patients to appear profane, irritable, and irresponsible. When presented with cases that involve personality changes, one should suspect pathology in the frontal lobes. Also, deficits in executive functioning usually involve the frontal lobes. Medial frontal lesions cause apathy, characterized by limited spontaneous movement, gesture, and speech. Left frontal lesions can cause depression. Right frontal lobe lesions can cause mania.

Neurocognitive Disorders

K&S Ch. 3

Question 5. C. This is an example of a delusion, which is a fixed false belief that is not accepted by members of the same cultural background. Delusions may be mood congruent or mood incongruent. They may have themes that are bizarre, persecutory, paranoid, grandiose, jealous, somatic, guilty or erotic. Coprolalia is the compulsive utterance of obscene words, as seen in Tourette's disorder. Egomania is a pathological self preoccupation. Ailurophobia is a dread of cats. An obsession is the pathological persistence of an irresistible thought or feeling that cannot be eliminated from consciousness and is associated with anxiety.

Psychotic Disorders

K&S Ch. 8

Question 6. A. This is a description of a cohort study, in which a well-defined population is followed over a period of time. Cohort studies are also known as longitudinal studies. Cohort studies provide direct estimates of risk associated with a suspected causative factor. A case–control study is a retrospective study that examines persons without a particular disease. In a clinical trial, specially selected patients receive a course of treatment, and another group does not. Patients are assigned to either group on a random basis. The goal is to determine the effectiveness of the treatment. Cross-sectional surveys describe the prevalence of a disease in a population at a particular point in time. Crossover studies are a variation of the double-blind study in which the placebo and treatment groups switch at some point in the study.

Statistics

K&S Ch. 4

Question 7. D. Although all of the choices contributed to our understanding of child development, it is Winnicott who developed the concept of good enough mothering. This concept is based on the understanding that the mother plays a vital role in bringing the world to the infant and offering empathic anticipation of the infant's needs. If she does these things well enough the baby will move towards the development of a healthy sense of self. Piaget described stages of cognitive development consisting of sensorimotor, preoperational thought, concrete operations, and formal operations. Freud was the founder of psychoanalysis, giving us the oral, anal, phallic and latency stages of development. Mahler developed stages of separation–individuation to describe how children develop identity that is separate from their mothers. Her stages were normal autism, symbiosis, differentiation, practicing, rapprochement and object constancy. Erikson developed an 8-stage life cycle. The stages are trust vs mistrust, autonomy vs shame and doubt, initiative vs guilt, industry vs inferiority, identity vs role diffusion, intimacy vs self absorption, generativity vs stagnation, and integrity vs despair and isolation.

Human Development

K&S Chs 2&6

Question 8. C. The clinical picture presented is that of Wernicke's encephalopathy. Classically seen in alcoholics, the clinical triad is that of mental confusion, ophthalmoplegia and gait ataxia. The usual brain autopsy finding is that of microhemorrhages in the periventricular gray matter, particularly around the aqueduct and third and fourth ventricles. Frontal and temporal lobe atrophy is consistent with Pick's dementia. Parkinson's disease would result in depigmentation of the pars compacta of the substantia nigra in the midbrain. Diffuse Lewy bodies can be seen in both Parkinson's disease and Alzheimer's disease. Subcortical white matter lesions perpendicular to the ventricles (also called Dawson's fingers) are consistent with a demyelinating disease such as multiple sclerosis.

Neurology

B&D Ch. 57

Question 9. C. Monoamine oxidase inhibitors (MAOIs) increase levels of biogenic amine neurotransmitters (serotonin, norepinephrine, and dopamine) by preventing their degradation. There are two types of MAO enzyme, MAO-A which breaks down serotonin, norepinephrine, and dopamine, and MAO-B which breaks down dopamine. It is contraindicated to give meperidine with an MAOI. Because these drugs increase intrasynaptic levels of biogenic amine neurotransmitters they should not be given with other drugs that do the same. There have been reports of death in patients given MAOIs and meperidine simultaneously. Patients should inform each of the doctors that they are seeing that they are taking an MAOI. Lithium can be given with MAOIs. When switching a patient from a selective serotonin reuptake inhibitor to an MAOI you need to allow a 14-day washout (28 days for fluoxetine). This is because the combination of these drugs in the system at the same time can potentiate a serotonin syndrome. Orthostatic hypotension is a major side effect of the MAOIs. Other side effects include weight gain, edema, sexual dysfunction, and insomnia. Moclobemide and selegiline are reversible MAO-A inhibitors and because they only weakly potentiate the pressor effects of tyramine they do not require a tyramine free diet at low doses.

Psychopharmacology

K&S Ch. 36

Question 10. E. The best choice for tranquilizing agitated patients is haloperidol. Given that the patient in question is elderly, starting with a small dose of haloperidol would be appropriate. Benzodiazepines should be avoided in cases of suspected delirium, which based on the question stem is a concern for this patient. Hence answer choices A and C are out. A benzodiazepine given to a delirious patient can worsen the delirium and further disinhibit the patient making them more agitated. In general one should use great caution in giving benzodiazepines to the elderly, and when used, they should be given in small doses. Aripiprazole, an atypical antipsychotic, only comes in oral form, which would likely be unfeasible in an acutely agitated patient. Other atypical antipsychotic drugs that come in intramuscular injectable form such as olanzapine or ziprasidone would be appropriate choices. Lithium is not standardly used to tranquilize patients. It is a mood stabilizer used in the treatment of bipolar disorder and can only be administered orally.

Psychopharmacology

K&S Ch. 10

Question 11. D. Oral meperidine has lower analgesic potency than intramuscular meperidine; therefore the same dose of the oral agent will not cover pain as well as the same dose of the intramuscular agent. There is no reason to suspect that the patient has low pain tolerance or a pain disorder as she is only very recently postoperative and would be expected to be in pain. There is no evidence of a personality disorder given. Conversion disorder presents with neurological symptoms which are not solely limited to pain and as such this is not a conversion disorder.

Somatic Symptom Disorders

K&S Ch. 12

Question 12. C. This is an example of countertransference, which refers to the conscious and unconscious feelings the therapist has towards the patient. Transference refers to the feelings the patient has towards the therapist. Resistance is when ideas that are unacceptable to the patient are prevented from reaching awareness. The term is usually used in reference to therapy where the patient withholds relevant information, remains silent, is late, or misses appointments. Confrontation is addressing an issue that the patient does not want to accept. Projection is reacting to unacceptable inner impulses as if they were outside the self. It may often take the form of perceiving one's own feelings in another and then acting on that perception.

Psychotherapy

K&S Ch. 6

Question 13. B. Huntington's disease is transmitted by an autosomal dominant inheritance pattern. If one parent is an affected carrier, the likelihood of transmission to any given child is 50%. The protein huntingtin is coded on the short arm of chromosome 4. The gene contains an expanded trinucleotide repeat sequence of CAG (normally less than 29 repeats occur).

Neurology

B&D Ch. 71

Question 14. D. Middle adulthood spans the years between ages 40 and 65. At the end of early adulthood people review the past and decide what the future will hold for them. In their occupation they start to see differences between early aspirations and what they have actually achieved. In middle adulthood people take stock of accomplishment, reassess commitment to family, work, and marriage, use power ethically, and deal with the illness of their parents. Hence, all of the choices are life tasks faced in middle adulthood except risk-taking behavior. This takes place traditionally in adolescence. Adulthood typically begins with selecting a mate, deciding on an occupation, and achieving independence and self sufficiency.

Human Development

K&S Ch. 2

Question 15. C. This is an example of tertiary prevention. Primary prevention is when a clinician does something to prevent the onset of a disease. This is done by reducing causative agents, reducing risk factors, increasing host resistance, or interfering with the transmission of a disease. Secondary prevention is when one identifies a disease in its early stages and seeks prompt treatment. Tertiary prevention involves reducing deficits caused by an illness in order to obtain the highest possible level of functioning. The other answer choices have nothing to do with prevention. Malingering is consciously faking illness for secondary gain. Noncompliance is a term that refers to not following a doctor's instructions.

Statistics

K&S Ch. 4

Question 16. E. Lambert–Eaton myasthenic syndrome (LEMS) is a paraneoplastic abnormality of presynaptic acetylcholine release, often described in conjunction with small cell lung carcinoma. The likely mechanism is immune-mediated, directed against voltage-gated calcium channels. The clinical hallmark of the disorder is generalized weakness with initial improvement in strength after minimal exercise. The electromyogram (EMG) reveals a classic decrementing to 3 Hz stimulation in muscles of the hands or feet. Multiple sclerosis would be expected to cause numerous different deficits, motor, sensory, or both, that are diffuse in space and time. Guillain–Barré syndrome, also known as acute inflammatory demyelinating polyneuropathy (AIDP), is a rapidly occurring demyelinating disease that can present with ascending pain, paralysis, sensory loss, or any combination of these symptoms. The clinical hallmark of AIDP is a loss of deep tendon reflexes in the extremities. The test of choice is EMG and nerve conduction studies which usually reveal loss of H reflex and decreased nerve conduction velocities. Polymyositis is an inflammatory disease of the muscle.

Neurology

B&D Ch. 78

Question 17. B. This question is really asking which of the choices is not a projective test, as one of the purposes of a projective test is to detect psychosis. The only choice that is not a projective test is the Minnesota multiphasic personality inventory (MMPI), which is a self-report inventory used to assess personality and areas of psychopathologic functioning. The draw a person test consists of the patient being asked to draw a person. The level of detail is thought to correlate with intelligence and developmental level. Then the patient is asked to draw a person of the opposite sex. The patient is then questioned on what they drew. The assumption is that the drawing represents the expression of the self or the body in the environment. The sentence completion test consists of asking the patient to complete a series of incomplete sentences. The tester focuses attention on strong affect, repeated answers, humor, or unusual responses. The thematic apperception test is a series of pictures shown to a patient. The patient then generates a story to explain the pictures. The patient's most accepted and conscious traits and motives are attributed to the character closest to the patient in sex, age, and appearance. More unconscious or unacceptable traits are attributed to those characters most unlike the patient. The Rorschach test is a series of 10 inkblots that serve as inspiration for free association. The patient's responses to each card are recorded and closely interpreted.

Psychological Theory and Psychometric Testing

K&S Ch. 5

Question 18. C. Amyotrophic lateral sclerosis (ALS) is a disorder of the upper and lower motor neurons. The spinal cord lower motor neurons are also known as the anterior horn cells. These classically degenerate in ALS and can be demonstrated on autopsy. Callosal thinning and atrophy are hallmarks of multiple sclerosis. Frontotemporal atrophy can be seen in Pick's dementia. Nigrostriatal depigmentation is a result of Parkinson's disease. Dorsal column pathology can be seen in vitamin B12 deficiency polyneuropathy with loss of vibration and joint position sensation.

Neurology

B&D Ch. 74

Question 19. E.   It is considered unethical for psychiatrists to participate in executions. According to the American Psychiatric Association, it is unethical to accept commission for patient referrals. It is unethical to have romantic or sexual relationships with patients. Psychiatrists are expected to report the unethical behavior of other psychiatrists. When retiring, the psychiatrist needs to give patients sufficient notice and make an effort to find them follow-up care. The above are ethical issues often questioned on standardized exams.

Ethics

K&S Ch. 58

Question 20. E.   This patient is clearly delirious based on the description. While all of the other choices are logical steps, the first and most important is protecting the patient from harm. In this case that would involve sedating the patient before she gets harmed as a result of her own agitation. This is a good rule to keep in mind whenever dealing with an agitated patient. The first responsibility is to keep both patient and staff from getting harmed.

Management in Psychiatry

K&S Ch. 10

Question 21. A.   The use of positive and negative reinforcement is part of operant conditioning developed by Skinner. In operant conditioning the animal is active and behaves in a way that produces a reward. Learning occurs as a consequence of action. The desired behavior reaps a positive reward. An undesired behavior gets a negative reward. Bandura is a proponent of social learning theory, which says we learn through modeling others and through social interaction. Attribution theory says that people are likely to attribute their own behavior to situational causes, and the behavior of others to personality traits. This then affects their feelings and behavior. Hull did work in the neurophysiologic aspects of learning, developing a drive reduction theory of learning. Learned helplessness is a model for depression developed by Seligman, in which an organism learns that no behavioral change can influence the environment. The organism becomes depressed and apathetic because no matter what it does its environmental circumstances never change. Kandel studied habituation and sensitization in snails. Habituation theory says that an animal can learn to stop responding to a repeated stimulus. Sensitization theory says that an organism can be taught to respond more easily to a stimulus, or be made more sensitive to that stimulus. Pavlov developed classical conditioning. In classical conditioning, a neutral stimulus is paired with one that evokes a response so that eventually the neutral stimulus comes to evoke the same response. He did the classic experiments with dogs salivating when hearing their master's footsteps.

Psychological Theory and Psychometric Testing

K&S Ch. 4

Question 22. B.   Ethosuximide is the treatment of choice for uncomplicated absence seizures, the clinical presentation depicted in this question. Failing ethosuximide, the next best choice would be valproic acid, which has efficacy in partial complex, primary generalized and absence seizure types. Carbamazepine would be a very poor choice to treat absence seizures, as it is ineffective in absence seizures and may even worsen the condition. Phenobarbital is not indicated for use in absence seizures. Diazepam is useful only for emergencies such as status epilepticus and usually in rectal, intramuscular, or intravenous forms. Phenytoin is indicated for partial and generalized tonic–clonic seizures; not for absence seizures.

Neurology

B&D Ch. 67

Question 23. D.   The description in this question is that of narcolepsy. Narcolepsy consists of irresistible attacks of refreshing daytime sleep that occur daily for 3 months or more. The sudden loss of muscle tone described is known as cataplexy. One also sees increased intrusion of rapid eye movement (REM) sleep into the transition between sleep and wakefulness causing hypnopompic (while awakening) and hypnagogic (while falling asleep) hallucinations, as well as sleep paralysis. This disorder can be dangerous as it can lead to automobile or industrial accidents. Treatments can involve stimulants such as amphetamines, methylphenidate (Ritalin), or modafinil (Provigil), as well as structured napping times during the day. Modafinil is a non-stimulant medication FDA-approved for narcolepsy. Its mechanism of action is on histamine neurons in the reticular activating system in the pons. Sleep changes associated with depression include early morning awakening and difficulty falling asleep. Sleep apnea presents with daytime irritability and drowsiness with prominent snoring at night. Primary insomnia is characterized by difficulty initiating or maintaining sleep, or nonrestorative sleep for at least one month. Shift-work sleep disorder is a type of circadian rhythm sleep disorder that occurs in those that repeatedly and rapidly change their work schedules. This can lead to somnolence, insomnia, as well as somatic problems such as an increased likelihood of peptic ulcer.

Sleep Wake Disorders

K&S Ch. 24

Question 24. A.   Dopamine is associated with the induction of aggression. Serotonin is associated with decreased aggression. In particular, the cerebrospinal fluid levels of 5-HIAA, a major serotonin metabolite, have been shown to be inversely correlated with the frequency of aggression. GABA is the major inhibitory neurotransmitter of the brain and is associated with decreased aggression. Norepinephrine is associated with decreased aggression and its functions are thought to be connected to that of serotonin, particularly in mood disorders. Glycine is an inhibitory neurotransmitter, and as such is not associated with increased aggression. As a general rule, it is thought that cholinergic and catecholaminergic mechanisms seem to be involved in the induction of aggression, and serotonin and GABA seem to inhibit such behavior.

Basic Neuroscience

K&S Ch. 3&4

Question 25. A.   Carbamazepine induces its own metabolism. This effect decreases its 24-hour half-life by at least 50% during the first 3–4 weeks of therapy. Increments in dosages after the first few weeks of therapy are often necessary to maintain therapeutic serum levels. None of the other mentioned anticonvulsants have this unique pharmacokinetic profile.

Psychopharmacology

B&D Ch. 67

Question 26. C.   This question reviews aspects of both operant and classical conditioning. In classical conditioning a neutral (or conditioned) stimulus is repeatedly paired with one that evokes a response (the unconditioned stimulus), such that the neutral stimulus comes to evoke the response. In operant (Skinnerian) conditioning, a random behavior is reinforced with reward. Initially, every desirable response is rewarded which enables the behavior to be learned. Giving positive reinforcement intermittently and variably is the best way to prevent a behavior from going extinct. Extinction occurs when the conditioned stimulus is constantly repeated without the unconditioned stimulus until the response evoked by the unconditioned stimulus eventually disappears. Generalization is the transfer of a conditioned response from one stimulus to another. For example, the dog that learned to salivate to a bell now salivates to the sound of a cabinet being opened. Discrimination is recognizing and responding to differences between similar stimuli. For example, a dog can be trained to respond differently to two similar bells. Transference that takes place during psychotherapy can be thought of as a form of stimulus generalization. Respondent conditioning is just another term for classical conditioning.

Psychological Theory and Psychometric Testing

K&S Ch. 4

Question 27. D.   Tuberous sclerosis is an autosomal dominant neurocutaneous disorder with a prevalence of about 1 in 6000–9000 individuals. The classic neurologic features of the disease are seizures, mental retardation and behavioral problems. Cutaneous lesions include the ash leaf spot (hypomelanotic macule), adenoma sebaceum (facial angiofibromas) and shagreen spots (irregularly shaped, often raised or textured skin lesion on the back or flank). Retinal hamartomas can be observed in many patients. Neuropathologic lesions include subependymal nodules and cortical hamartomas. Down's syndrome, or trisomy 21, frequently results in early onset Alzheimer's type changes in the brain including neurofibrillary tangles and cholinergic deficits. Rett's disorder, a pervasive developmental disorder seen only in girls, involves deceleration of head growth from ages 5 months to 4 years, loss of purposeful hand skills and development of stereotyped hand movements between ages 5 months and 2.5 years, loss of social engagement and acquired impairment in expressive and receptive language skills. Although seizures can be observed in up to 75% of Rett's patients, there are typically no skin lesions associated with the disorder.

Neurofibromatosis has two types: NF1 and NF2. NF1 (classic von Recklinghausen's disease, with café au lait spots (6 or more to make the diagnosis), subcutaneous neurofibromas, axillary freckling, Lisch nodules (pigmented iris hamartomas), optic nerve glioma, neurofibromas and schwannomas) is caused by a mutation of the 60 exon *NF1* gene on chromosome 17q. NF2 is caused by a mutation of the *NF2* gene on chromosome 22. NF2 patients have few cutaneous lesions. The diagnostic hallmark of NF2 is bilateral vestibular (VIII nerve) schwannomas. Williams' syndrome is an autosomal dominant mental retardation syndrome that occurs by a hemizygous deletion including elastin locus chromosome 7q11-23. Patients with the disorder have short stature, unusual facial features that include depressed nasal bridge (an upturned nose), broad forehead, widely spaced teeth, elfin-like facies, as well as thyroid, renal and cardiovascular anomalies. Psychiatric symptoms include anxiety, hyperactivity, hypermusicality. Seizures and skin lesions are not observed in Williams' syndrome.

Neurology

B&D Ch. 65

Question 28. B. The mechanism described is that of the cholinesterase inhibitors used in Alzheimer's disease. By potentiating cholinergic transmission, these drugs cause modest improvement in memory and goal-directed thought. These drugs include medications such as tacrine, donepezil, galantamine and rivastigmine. All of the answer choices in this question are cholinesterase inhibitors except for memantine. Memantine is also used for Alzheimer's dementia, but works by binding to N-methyl-D-aspartate (NMDA) receptors, acting as an antagonist and thereby slowing calcium influx into cells. The slowing of calcium influx halts cell destruction.

Psychopharmacology

K&S Ch. 36

Question 29. E. Of the tests listed, the only one that tests executive function is the trail-making test. The trail-making test involves connecting letters and numbers in order, alternating between letters and numbers (i.e., connect A-1-B-2-C-3, etc.) Another acceptable answer would be the Wisconsin card sorting test, but is not an answer choice. The Wisconsin card sorting test evaluates abstract reasoning and flexibility in problem solving. The thematic apperception test is used to test normal personality and involves showing pictures and having the patient come up with stories. The patient's most accepted and conscious traits and motives are attributed to the character closest to the patient in sex, age, and appearance. More unconscious or unacceptable traits are attributed to those characters most unlike the patient. The Halstead–Reitan battery helps find the location of brain lesions as well as differentiate between those who are brain damaged and those who are neurologically intact. It consists of a series of 10 tests. The Minnesota multiphasic personality inventory (MMPI) is a personality assessment used to find areas of psychopathologic functioning. It consists of more than 500 statements to which the patient must respond "true", "false" or "cannot say". The brief psychiatric rating scale (BPRS) is used to assess the severity of psychosis in schizophrenia.

Psychological Theory and Psychometric Testing

K&S Ch. 5

Question 30. E. The first four choices are all very important pieces in determining whether a person can make a will, including whether or not the person knows he is making a will. In order to have the capacity to make a will, three things are needed. The first is the ability to understand the nature and extent of one's property. The second is that one must know that one is making a will. The third is that one must know to whom the property will be bequeathed. The last answer choice is part of the McGarry instrument which determines whether someone is competent to stand trial. It has nothing to do with making a will.

Forensic Psychiatry

K&S Ch. 57

Question 31. C. The average age of onset of puberty is 11 years for girls and 13 years for boys. All other answer choices are true. The onset of puberty is triggered by maturation of the hypothalamic–pituitary–adrenal–gonadal axis. This leads to secondary sex characteristics such as enlarged breasts and hips in girls and facial hair and lowered voice in boys. Primary sex characteristics are those involved in coitus – the external genitals and reproductive organs. Increases in height and weight occur earlier in girls than in boys. Sex hormones increase slowly through adolescence and correlate with bodily changes. Follicle-stimulating hormone (FSH) and leutinizing hormone (LH) increase through adolescence, being above normal adult values by age 17 or 18. Testosterone seems to increase around age 16 or 17 and then stabilize at adult levels in males.

Human Development

K&S Ch. 2

Question 32. A. Sumatriptan (Imitrex) is an antimigraine medication indicated for acute, abortive therapy of migraine headache. All drugs in the triptan class act as potent agonists at 5-HT 1B and 5-HT 1D receptors. Although these receptors reside principally on intracranial blood vessels, they may have an effect on the coronary arteries as well and could theoretically cause vasoconstriction, vasospasm and acute myocardial infarction. Therefore, these agents are contraindicated in patients with coronary ischemic heart disease, as well as with uncontrolled hypertension.

Neurology

B&D Ch. 69

Question 33. D. Antipsychotic drugs and methylphenidate increase tricyclic antidepressant (TCA) concentrations through their interaction with the cytochrome p450 system. Other drugs that increase TCA concentrations include acetazolamide, aspirin, cimetidine, thiazides, fluoxetine and sodium bicarbonate. Cigarette smoking decreases their concentration through its action on the 1A2 enzyme. Other drugs that decrease TCA concentrations include ascorbic acid, lithium, barbiturates, and primidone.

Psychopharmacology

K&S Ch. 36

Question 34. D. Completed suicide is most often associated with depression, not bipolar disorder. Adolescents most frequently commit suicide with guns, not by hanging. In recent years the suicide rate has gone up dramatically among adolescents, not among middle-aged adults. Previous suicide attempts are the best predictor of future risk of suicide. This is a very important factor which should be taken into account whenever taking a patient history. Men successfully commit suicide three times more often than women. Another factor contributing to completed suicides is age. For men, the highest risk period is after 45 years of age. For women, the highest risk period is after 55 years of age. Married people are less likely to commit suicide than single or widowed people. As far as religion is concerned, rates of suicide among Roman Catholics are less than those for Protestants or Jewish people. With race, whites are more likely to commit suicide than others, especially white males. Physical health may play a role. Thirty-two per cent of people who commit suicide have seen a doctor within the past 6 months. With regard to occupation, the higher a person's social status, the higher the rate of suicide. A fall in social status also increases the risk.

Depressive Disorders

K&S Ch. 34

Question 35. D. Alexia without agraphia is seen with lesions involving the splenium of the corpus callosum. Gerstmann's syndrome usually involves left parietal lobe damage. The clinical picture is the classic tetrad of acalculia, agraphia (without alexia), right and left confusion and finger agnosia (the inability to name the thumb, index, middle, ring and pinky fingers when called upon to do so). The lesion in Gerstmann's syndrome localizes to the left angular gyrus.

Neurology

B&D Ch. 51

Question 36. B. Dialectical behavioral therapy (DBT) is a form of therapy developed by Marsha Linehan for the treatment of borderline personality disorder. The therapist is supportive and directive. Specific exercises are performed to help solve problems and improve interpersonal skills. The focus of therapy is on reducing impulses to self-mutilate.

Psychotherapy

K&S Ch. 35

Question 37. C. The clinical picture portrayed in this question is that of hyperprolactinemia induced by dopamine blockade in the tuberoinfundibular system by a neuroleptic medication. Conventional neuroleptics and risperidone can increase the volume of pituitary microadenomas by blocking dopamine and increasing serum prolactin levels. When an adenoma grows beyond 1.5 cm in diameter it can encroach on the medial portion of both optic nerves outside of the sella turcica. This optic nerve involvement results in the classic clinical sign of bitemporal hemianopsia. Appropriate treatment would be the discontinuation of the offending drug and possibly administration of bromocriptine. Some adenomas require surgical intervention if they are unresponsive to medication therapy.

Psychopharmacology

B&D Ch. 52

Question 38. C. The mental status examination is the description of the patient's appearance, speech, actions, and thoughts during the interview. All of the choices are correct, with the exception of C. Content of thought includes such things as delusions, preoccupations, obsessions, compulsions, phobias, suicidality and homicidality. It is a common mistake to put hallucinations in the thought content section of the mental status exam. Hallucinations are false sensory perceptions and fall under the category of perception. The categories of the mental status examination are appearance, psychomotor activity, attitude, mood, affect, speech, perception, thought content and process, consciousness, orientation, memory, concentration, attention, reading and writing, visuospatial ability, abstract thought, information and intelligence, impulsivity, judgment and insight, and reliability.

Diagnostic and Treatment Procedures in Psychiatry

K&S Ch. 7

Question 39. B. This is a clear description of the Malaysian cultural syndrome of Amok. It consists of a sudden rampage including homicide and/or suicide, which ends in exhaustion and amnesia. Koro is an Asian delusion that the penis will disappear into the abdomen and cause death. Piblokto occurs in female Eskimos of northern Greenland. It involves anxiety, depression, confusion, depersonalization, derealization, ending in stuporous sleep and amnesia. Wihtigo is a delusional fear displayed by Native American Indians of being turned into a cannibal through possession by a supernatural monster, the Wihtigo. Mal de ojo is a syndrome found in those of Mediterranean descent involving vomiting, fever, and restless sleep. It is thought to be caused by the evil eye.

Cultural Issues in Psychiatry

K&S Ch. 14

Question 40. E. The patient has clearly suffered a left hemispheric stroke, possibly in the middle cerebral artery territory. Any hemispheric stroke that involves the corticospinal tract can result in an appearance of contralateral Babinski and Hoffman's signs. The Babinski sign is the upward motion of the big toe and fanning of the other toes when the plantar surface of the foot is stroked upwardly from bottom to top with a noxious stimulus or blunt instrument like the butt of a reflex hammer. The Hoffman's sign is positive when the adduction of the thumb is noted upon a fast downward flick being administered to the index or middle finger of the same hand. Hoffman's sign is equivalent to the Babinski sign except it is in the upper extremity. The palmomental reflex and Meyerson sign are two of the classic so-called frontal release signs. The palmomental reflex is positive when the chin muscle contracts as the thenar eminence of the palm contralateral to the brain lesion is stroked with a blunt instrument. Meyerson sign is the presence of a persistence of the glabellar reflex of blinking upon confrontation of the forehead by tapping with a finger. The blinking normally should extinguish after several taps of the forehead, but in the presence of frontal lobe damage, the response does not extinguish as rapidly. Complete loss of the gag reflex would be expected only in a devastating stroke involving the brain stem or complete brain death.

Neurology

B&D Ch. 51

Question 41. B. Glutamate is the major excitatory neurotransmitter in the brain. Glutamate is the precursor to gamma aminobutyric acid (GABA). The major inhibitory neurotransmitters are GABA and glycine. Glutamate works on the N-methyl-d-aspartate (NMDA) receptor as well as four types of non-NMDA receptors. The NMDA receptor is bound by PCP. Glutamate is thought to be very important in learning and memory. Glutamate is also important in the theory of excititoxicity, which postulates that excessive glutamate stimulation leads to excessive intracellular calcium and nitric oxide concentrations and cell death. Under stimulation of the NMDA receptor by glutamate has been found to cause psychosis, therefore glutamate is thought to play some role in schizophrenia, although the exact nature of that role is yet unclear. Locations for glutamate in the brain include cerebellar granule cells, striatum, hippocampus, pyramidal cells of the cortex, thalamocortical projections, and corticostriatal projections.

Basic Neuroscience

K&S Ch. 3

Question 42. D. Alzheimer's disease has been associated with defects in chromosome 21. The gene for amyloid precursor protein is found on the long arm of chromosome 21. This protein plays a significant role in the development of Alzheimer's disease. These defects have been shown to run in families. Some studies have shown as high as 40% of Alzheimer's patients have a positive family history for the disease. Turner's syndrome results from a missing sex chromosome XO. The result is absent or minimal development of the gonads. No sex hormones are produced. Individuals with Turner's syndrome are female, but with no secondary sex characteristics and an absence or minimal development of the gonads. Klinefelter's syndrome is the presence of an extra chromosome, making the patient XXY. They have a male habitus because of the presence of the Y chromosome, but because of the extra X chromosome they do not develop strong male characteristics. They have small underdeveloped genitals. They are infertile, and can develop breast tissue during adolescence. Huntington's disease results from the expansion of trinucleotide repeat sequences at chromosome 4p16.3. The disease typically presents with dementia and chorea. Parkinson's disease results from the loss of dopaminergic neurons from the substantia nigra. It can present with dementia as well as a clear pattern of symptoms including shuffling gait, pill-rolling tremor, and masked facies. Other than Alzheimer's the other diseases listed have nothing to do with chromosome 21.

Neurodevelopmental and Pervasive Developmental Disorders

K&S Ch. 10

Question 43. C. The diagnosis of brain death can be made only in the complete absence of the brainstem reflexes (i.e., absent gag, fixed pupils, absent oculocephalic and oculovestibular reflexes, absent corneal reflexes). The eyes may either be open or closed in the presence of brain death. The EEG pattern need not be flat line to diagnose brain death. There have been known cases of preserved cortical function and hence positive activity on EEG despite a complete lack of brainstem functioning.

Neurology

B&D Chs 5&55

Question 44. B. Of the drugs listed, diazepam is the one that needs oxidative metabolism by the liver. The other four are safe choices for patients with compromised liver function because they have no active metabolites or do not need oxidation by the liver. Patients with hepatic disease and elderly patients are at particular risk from adverse effects due to the benzodiazepines, especially if repeated high doses are given. Benzodiazepines should be used with caution in anyone with a history of substance abuse, cognitive disorders, renal disease, liver disease, central nervous system depression, or myasthenia gravis.

Psychopharmacology

K&S Ch. 36

Question 45. C. All of the answer choices are reasonable things to do with a family in family therapy, except focusing most of the attention on the most dysfunctional member. The focus of the therapy should be on the whole family as a system, in which everyone plays a role. The problems that the family are having should not be treated as one person's fault.

Psychotherapy

K&S Ch. 35

Question 46. B. The neurotransmitters associated with anxiety are norepinephrine, serotonin, and gamma aminobutyric acid (GABA). Poor regulation of norepinephrine is thought to be involved in anxiety disorders. Noradrenergic neurons are found primarily in the locus ceruleus. Stimulation of the locus ceruleus increases anxiety, and ablation of the locus ceruleus blocks anxiety responses. Serotonin is also thought to be involved in anxiety, although its role is less clear. Serotonergic drugs have shown a clear propensity to decrease anxiety. Serotonergic neurons are located primarily in the raphe nuclei in the pons. The role of GABA in anxiety is clearly supported by the strong effect that benzodiazepines have on lessening anxiety. Benzodiazepines enhance the effect of GABA at the GABA receptor, thus decreasing anxiety. Those neurotransmitters not directly associated with anxiety include dopamine, glutamate, histamine, and acetylcholine. There is no evidence as yet that these neurotransmitters play a role in the pathophysiology of anxiety. Injection of epinephrine would worsen anxiety.

Basic Neuroscience

K&S Ch. 3

Question 47. B. Myasthenia gravis (MG) is an autoimmune neurologic disorder involving the production of autoantibodies against postsynaptic nicotinic acetylcholinergic receptor sites on muscle. There is passive transfer of the offending antibodies to the fetus across the placenta. The clinical picture is that of diplopia, dysarthria, dysphagia and other signs and symptoms of bulbar palsy, fatigue and muscle weakness. Mental status and cognition are usually intact. Deep tendon reflexes are generally preserved. There is a relationship between MG and thymoma. About 10% of patients with MG have thymoma. Edrophonium chloride (Tensilon), a short-acting cholinergic agent, is used to diagnose the disorder clinically and pyridostigmine (Mestinon) is used to treat the disorder on an ongoing basis. Other diagnostic tests include electromyography (EMG) and nerve conduction studies, which reveal a classic decrementing upon rapid repetitive muscle stimulation. Serum antibody levels can also be titered. Other therapeutic modalities include steroids, plasmapheresis, intra-venous immunoglobulin (IVIG) administration, immunosuppressive agents, for example, azathioprine (Imuran).

Neurology

B&D Ch. 78

Question 48. D. Generalized slow activity consisting of theta and delta waves with focal areas of hyperactivity is the EEG pattern of delirium. An important characteristic of this pattern is that the rhythm is slowed. Choice A is the pattern for absence seizures. This is a commonly asked pattern on exams. Choice B is normal adult drowsiness. Choice C is a normal pattern seen when the eyes are closed. Upon awakening, the posterior alpha rhythm is replaced by random activity. Right temporal spikes, choice E, are significant for a seizure focus. In addition to the above information, the appearance of delta waves is considered abnormal and should raise concern regarding a structural lesion, except if the patient is asleep.

Neurology

K&S Chs 3&10

Question 49. D. Gower's maneuver or sign is a classic bedside indicator of muscular dystrophy or myopathy. Usually seen in children, the sign is present when a patient gets up from the floor or a chair by using the hands because of muscle weakness in the legs. Duchenne's is called a dystrophinopathy because it is an autosomal recessive hereditary disease of muscle due to a lack of dystrophin, a protein found in muscle membrane. Duchenne's is the most common of the childhood muscular dystrophies. Muscular weakness is usually greater proximally. Other features include diminished deep tendon reflexes (except the Achilles reflex), elevated CPK, mental retardation in about one third of cases and enlarged muscles, due to fat infiltration, particularly the calves.

Neurology

B&D Ch. 79

Question 50. B. The tricyclic antidepressants (TCAs), trazodone, and mirtazapine are all sedating drugs. Sedation is a common effect of the TCAs and can be a welcome one if the patient isn't sleeping well. The most sedating of the TCAs are amitriptyline, trimipramine and doxepin. The least sedating are desipramine and protriptyline, with other TCAs falling between these two groups in the amount of sedation they cause. Trazodone is an antidepressant that can be extremely sedating. For this reason it is sometimes used independently for insomnia. Trazodone can also cause priapism, in which case the patient should be switched to another medication. The SSRIs and SNRIs in general are not very sedating.

Psychopharmacology

K&S Ch. 36

Question 51. D.   The appropriate response to this situation is to examine your own behavior and countertransference. You should then share your observations about the patient's behavior with the patient and examine the meaning of the patient's behavior. Answer choice A is a bad idea as ignoring the problem will not make it go away. Flirting with the patient is inappropriate and having sex with the patient is a violation of ethics which is strictly forbidden for psychiatrists. Revealing personal information is also not appropriate for the therapist to do and does not address the patient's underlying motivations.

Psychotherapy

K&S Chs 35&58

Question 52. B.   This is an example of fetishism. In fetishism, a person, usually a male, obtains sexual arousal from an inanimate object such as women's undergarments, a glove, a shoe, etc. This needs to go on for at least six months to qualify for the diagnosis, and often involves sexual fantasies involving the object. Exhibitionism involves being sexually aroused by exposing one's genitals to a stranger. Frotteurism involves becoming sexually aroused by touching and rubbing against a nonconsenting person. Voyeurism is a pattern of obtaining sexual arousal from watching an unsuspecting person who is naked, disrobing, or engaged in sexual activity. Transvestic fetishism is a pattern of sexual arousal from cross-dressing, usually seen in a heterosexual male. The answer to this question is not transvestic fetishism because the patient was wearing women's under garments only under his normal male work clothes. He was not going to work in a dress with makeup and high heel shoes. It is not dressing like a woman that arouses him, but a fantasy connected with an inanimate object, namely the panties.

Paraphilias

K&S Ch. 21

Question 53. C.   The case above describes trigeminal neuralgia (*tic douloureux*). It is usually unilateral in about 90% of cases. It usually affects the upper two branches of the fifth nerve (V2 and V3). Treatments of choice are carbamazepine (Tegretol) and oxcarbazepine (Trileptal), which modulate pain centrally and peripherally. About 75% of patients respond to carbamazepine therapy. Other treatments include gabapentin (Neurontin), tricyclic antidepressants, tiagabine (Gabitril), opioid analgesics, nonsteroidal anti-inflammatory agents, lidocaine patches and benzodiazepine sedatives. Some patients opt for an invasive intervention, radiation therapy in the form of stereotactic gamma-knife treatment to alleviate the pain.

Neurology

B&D Chs 69&70

Question 54. D.   This is the classic clinical picture of temporal (also called giant-cell) arteritis, a systemic vasculitis of the medium-sized vessels. Women are affected more often than men (about 3:1). The disease occurs in the elderly, usually over 50 years of age. Clinically, the disease can present as new onset or change in headache with fever, fatigue, myalgia, night sweats, weight loss, and jaw claudication (tiredness upon chewing). About 25% of patients have polymyalgia rheumatica. The temporal artery can demonstrate tenderness to palpation with induration and diminished or absent pulse. The most feared complication is irreversible and sudden vision loss as a result of central retinal artery occlusion. The initial test of choice is the serum erythrocyte sedimentation rate (ESR), which is virtually always elevated. Temporal artery biopsy is the gold-standard diagnostic test of choice in the face of an elevated ESR. The treatment of choice is prednisone. Brain imaging would not reveal the abnormality. Lumbar puncture for cerebrospinal fluid xanthochromia is done to diagnose subarachnoid hemorrhage. Carotid dissection does not involve systemic constitutional symptoms, but usually presents with ipsilateral stroke-like deficits due to arterial embolization.

Neurology

B&D Ch. 69

Question 55. D.   The concept that mental disorders have different outcomes was pioneered by Emil Kraepelin. He was the first to differentiate between the course of chronic schizophrenia, and that of manic psychosis. He used the term *dementia praecox* borrowing it from the work of French psychiatrist Morel. Eugen Bleuler later renamed it as schizophrenia and stressed that it need not have a deteriorating course. Winnicott was one of the central figures in the school of object relations theory. He developed the concepts of the "good enough mother" and the "transitional object". Sigmund Freud is the founder of classic psychoanalysis. Heinz Kohut is best known for his writings of narcissism and self psychology.

History of Psychiatry

K&S Ch. 13

Question 56. B. This is a clear case of hypochondriasis. The patient believes that he has a specific serious disease despite a negative workup and the reassurance of his doctors. Conversion disorder is when a patient has a neurologic symptom which is attributed to psychological conflict and cannot be explained medically. Body dysmorphic disorder is preoccupation with an imagined defect in appearance. Often slight physical imperfections cause markedly excessive concern. Somatization disorder (also known as Briquet's syndrome) is a condition where a patient has multiple physical complaints involving several organ symptoms. These symptoms cannot be explained by a medical diagnosis. The symptoms are not intentionally produced. Symptoms can include pain, sexual symptoms, gastrointestinal symptoms, and pseudoneurological symptoms.

Somatic Symptom Disorders

K&S Ch. 17

Question 57. B. Cluster headache is a rare type of headache occurring in ≈0.5% of the population. Sufferers are usually males in their 20 s and 30 s. Most sufferers experience episodic cycles of 4–12 weeks' duration that are predominant in the spring and fall seasons. Attack periods can be considered chronic, that is lasting 1 year or more without remission or with remission periods of less than 2 weeks' duration. Attacks can last anywhere from 15 minutes to 3 hours in duration. They can occur as often as eight times a day, or as infrequently as once every other day. The attacks are generally nocturnal. Alcohol consumption is a common trigger. The attacks are excruciatingly painful and retro-orbital in location. Pain can radiate to the teeth, neck and temporal regions and can be accompanied by ipsilateral autonomic symptoms. Patients prefer moving their head or pacing rather than lying still. Abortive therapies include oxygen by nasal cannula at 8–10 liters per minute, sumatriptan subcutaneous injection and ergotamine. Prophylactic therapies include prednisone, verapamil, divalproex sodium, methysergide and lithium.

Neurology

B&D Ch. 75

Question 58. E. Seizure, anorexia, head trauma, and use of a MAOI in the past 14 days are all contraindications to using bupropion, because of the propensity of bupropion to lower the seizure threshold. One does not want to use this medication in a situation where the seizure threshold may already be lowered, or a seizure focus is present. The medication can also cause weight loss, so use in those who are under-weight is not a good idea. It can also lead to increased rates of seizures in patients with eating disorders. Although it can increase blood pressure in some patients, it does not cause hypertensive crises and is not contraindicated in patients with high blood pressure. Hypertension is a strong concern when using venlafaxine because of its ability to potentiate hypertensive crisis. Bupropion is also used for smoking cessation. Waiting for 14 days when switching to or from an MAOI is a hard and fast rule to prevent drug–drug interactions, which could lead to a serotonin syndrome. Bupropion is not associated with sexual side effects in the way that the selective serotonin reuptake inhibitors are.

Psychopharmacology

K&S Ch. 36

Question 59. B. Lithium and phentolamine are not contraindicated with MAOIs. Meperidine and selective serotonin reuptake inhibitors (SSRIs) cannot be given at the same time as MAOIs and this often comes up on standardized tests. There should be a 14-day washout period between giving an SSRI and an MAOI. Levodopa and spinal anesthetics containing epinephrine are also part of a long list of medications that should not be mixed with a MAOI.

Psychopharmacology

K&S Ch. 36

Question 60. C. There are numerous causes of acquired peripheral neuropathy. The more notable causes include: vincristine and INH therapies, excess B6 therapy, inhalant abuse such as toluene or nitrous oxide, heavy metal poisoning, hydrocarbon exposure, B12 deficiency, niacin deficiency, and complications of mononucleosis (Epstein–Barr virus infection). Autoimmune diseases such as lupus can also cause peripheral neuropathy. Acetaminophen overdose does not generally affect the peripheral nervous system.

Neurology

B&D Ch. 76

Question 61. C. Of all of the answer choices, the only one that is not true is C. Methylphenidate will increase tricyclic antidepressant (TCA) levels, as will some antipsychotics. Smoking decreases TCA levels. Antipsychotics and methylphenidate increase TCA concentrations through their interaction with the cytochrome p450 system. Other drugs that increase TCA concentrations include acetazolamide, aspirin, cimetidine, thiazides, fluoxetine and sodium bicarbonate. Cigarette smoking decreases their concentration through induction of the 1A2 enzyme. Drugs that decrease TCA concentrations include ascorbic acid, lithium, barbiturates, and primidone.

Psychopharmacology

K&S Ch. 36

Question 62. D. Of the selective serotonin reuptake inhibitors, fluoxetine has the longest half life, lasting 1–2 weeks, fluvoxamine has the shortest, lasting about 15 hours. All others have half lives of about 1 day.

Psychopharmacology

K&S Ch. 36

Question 63. A. Self-mutilation is most often associated with borderline personality disorder. Borderline patients often use this behavior to express anger, elicit help from others, or numb themselves to overwhelming affect. They have tumultuous interpersonal relationships and strong mood swings. They can have short lived psychotic episodes. Their behavior is often unpredictable. They can rarely tolerate being alone, and are known for splitting people into all good or all bad categories. They lack a consistent sense of identity.

Personality Disorders

K&S Ch. 7

Question 64. A. The clinical picture depicted in this question is that of dermatomyositis. Dermatomyositis is an autoimmune disease that affects skin and muscle. Skin rash appears generally with the onset of muscle weakness. The rash is classically purplish and is mainly seen on the face and eyelids. It can also appear on the neck, elbows and the knees which are often reddened and indurated. Serum CPK levels are often elevated. Needle electromyography (EMG) demonstrates myopathy and muscle irritability, with fibrillations, positive sharp waves and increased insertional activity. The hallmark finding on muscle biopsy is perifascicular atrophy and "ghost" fibers. There is a strong relationship between dermatomyositis and occult neoplasm in up to 50% of patients with the disorder. The usual neoplasm is carcinoma and can be in the lung, breast, stomach or ovary most typically. A cancer workup is essential in patients found to have dermatomyositis, including chest radiography, rectal and vaginal exams, hematologic studies and testing for occult blood in stool.

Neurology

B&D Ch. 79

Question 65. D. The case presented in this question is a common description of water intoxication. Symptoms include tremor, ataxia, restlessness, diarrhea, vomiting, polyuria, and eventual stupor. This is a problem that can be found in up to 20% of patients with chronic schizophrenia. When found, these patients need close monitoring of their electrolytes, and in many cases must be water restricted with close monitoring of their intake and output. The electrolyte disturbances that result from drinking enormous quantities of water can become serious medical issues and in some cases prompt medical hospitalization. Although the other questions could be useful in doing a thorough evaluation, the patient's symptoms and psychiatric diagnosis should suggest water intoxication.

Psychotic Disorders

K&S Ch. 13

Question 66. A. This question stem describes paranoid schizophrenia. In paranoid schizophrenia, there are delusions and hallucinations most prominently, but specific behaviors suggestive of disorganized or catatonic schizophrenia are absent. The onset is usually later than other types of the disease, and they show less regression of their mental facilities and emotional responses. Disorganized schizophrenia has early onset and poor outcome. It is marked by a regression to primitive, disinhibited, and unorganized behavior and absence of catatonic symptoms. Patients display prominent thought disorder and their contact with reality is poor. Catatonic schizophrenia consists of negativism, rigidity, posturing, and alteration between stupor and excitement. Patients often exhibit stereotypies, mannerisms, and waxy flexibility. Residual schizophrenia presents with evidence of a schizophrenic disturbance with absence of a complete set of active symptoms and an absence of adequate symptoms to qualify as one of the other types of schizophrenia. It can consist of emotional blunting, social withdrawal, eccentric behavior, illogical thinking and mild loosening of associations.

Psychotic Disorders

K&S Ch. 13

Question 67. C. All of the answer choices are associated with good outcomes except early age of onset. The older the patient is at onset, the better the prognosis. Good prognostic indicators for schizophrenia include late onset, obvious precipitating factors, acute onset, good premorbid functioning, mood disorder symptoms, being married, family history of mood disorders, good support systems, and positive symptoms. Poor prognostic factors include young onset, no precipitating factors, insidious onset, poor premorbid functioning, withdrawn or autistic-like behavior, being single, divorced or widowed, family history of schizophrenia, poor support systems, negative symptoms, neurological symptoms, history of perinatal trauma, no remissions in early years, many relapses, and history of assaultiveness.

Psychotic Disorders

K&S Ch. 13

Question 68. E. The findings given in this question are descriptors of sleep patterns one would find in depression. One might also find increased awakening during the second half of the night and increased length of the first rapid eye movement (REM) sleep episode. Electroencephalography can be used to evaluate sleep, but in clinical psychiatry, it is most often used to separate temporal lobe seizures from pseudoseizures and to distinguish dementia from pseudodementia caused by depression. The other answer choices given are clear distractors. Tumor is unrelated to sleep changes and could potentially show up on an EEG as a seizure focus, but we have no history here of either seizures or seizure focus on EEG. Petit mal epilepsy has a classic 3-per-second spike and wave pattern, which is clearly not mentioned in the question. Hepatic encephalopathy would cause a delirium, making answer choices C and D very similar. EEG patterns in delirium would show generalized slow activity, i.e. theta and delta waves, with possible areas of hyperactivity. Hepatic encephalopathy often shows on EEG as bilaterally synchronous triphasic slow waves. None of that is mentioned in the question, as we are solely talking about sleep patterns. Therefore E is the only reasonable answer.

Diagnostic and Treatment Procedures in Psychiatry

K&S Ch. 15

Question 69. B. The genetics of Alzheimer's dementia (AD) are the subject of ongoing research. A positive family history of the disorder is found in about one-quarter of cases. This type of Alzheimer's dementia is further classified as familial AD or FAD. The most significant genetic risk factor is believed to be homozygosity for the inheritance of the E4 allele of apolipoprotein E (apo E). Other less significant risks may be mutations in *Presenelin 1* (on chromosome 14) and *Presenelin 2* (on chromosome 1) proteins and amyloid precursor protein (APP). Apo E4 genotyping may be useful in patients with cognitive deficits as it points very strongly to the clinical diagnosis of AD. Neurofibrillary tangles are a neuropathologic hallmark of AD and a major component of these tangles is the microtubule-associated protein, tau. Abnormal hyperphosphorylation of tau results in the destruction of the neuronal cytoskeleton and the aggregation of tangles. Trisomy 21 (Down's syndrome) predisposes patients to early onset of Alzheimer's dementia in as many as 90% of cases. Neuropathologic findings in these cases are identical to those seen in elderly patients. The reason for the early onset of the condition in Down's patients is believed to be overexpression of the APP gene and thus increased β-amyloid deposition.

Neurocognitive Disorders

B&D Ch. 66

Question 70. C. The answer choices are all characteristics of narcissism, except C. Answer choice C describes characteristics of histrionic personality disorder. Histrionic personality disorder is marked by a pattern of excessive emotionality and attention seeking. Narcissism is marked by grandiosity, need for admiration, and lack of empathy.

Personality Disorders

K&S Ch. 27

Question 71. D. For post-traumatic stress disorder (PTSD) the duration of the disturbance must be at least one month. All other answer choices are correct. In PTSD the person was exposed to an event that involved either actual or threatened death or injury or a threat to their or others' physical integrity. Their response involves intense fear, helplessness, or horror. The event is re-experienced as flashbacks or recurring dreams. Patients may act or feel as if the event was recurring. If they perceive things that remind them of the event, they are caused by intense psychological distress and show physiological reactivity. Patients with PTSD often spend great energy avoiding stimuli that remind them of the event. They can also demonstrate a numbing of general responsiveness as shown by inability to remember certain aspects of the trauma, loss of interest in significant activities, feelings of detachment from others, restricted affect, and feelings of a foreshortened future. They also show signs of increased arousal such as problems with sleep, irritability and outbursts of anger, poor concentration, hypervigilance, and excited startle response.

Trauma and Stress Related Disorders

K&S Ch. 16

Question 72. E. Uncomplicated grief is often manifested as a state of shock, numbness or bewilderment. It may be followed by sighing or crying. This may lead to weakness, decreased appetite, weight loss, problems concentrating, and sleep disturbances. This is all considered part of normal grief. Once a person begins to manifest worthlessness, suicidality, excessive guilt, hallucinations, or psychomotor retardation the grief is no longer normal. Pathological grief can take many forms ranging from absent or delayed grief, to excessively intense or prolonged grief, to psychosis and suicidality. Anticipatory grief is expressed in advance of a loss deemed to be inevitable. This grief ends at the time when the loss occurs, regardless of what happens after. The grief may intensify as time goes on and the person moves closer and closer to the loss, and turn to acute grief when the loss occurs. Delusional disorder and bipolar disorder are unrelated to the information in the question stem.

Trauma and Stress Related Disorders

K&S Ch. 2

Question 73. C. Numerous neuropathologic abnormalities accompany schizophrenia on both a microscopic and macroscopic level. Hippocampal neurons can be atrophic. Lamina III neurons in the hippocampus can be disorganized and scattered. This is not solidly replicated in neuropathologic specimens. One of the most replicable findings is enlargement of the cerebral ventricular system, particularly the lateral ventricles. This finding has been extensively replicated over numerous neuropathologic specimens. Other affected areas include the thalamus and the dorsolateral prefrontal cortex.

Psychotic Disorders

K&S Ch. 3

Question 74. E. The patient presented in this question is a clear case of anorexia nervosa. No single laboratory test can diagnose the disease, but a battery of tests is needed to properly evaluate the patient medically. Tests to order include serum electrolytes, renal function tests, thyroid function tests, glucose, amylase, complete blood count, electrocardiogram, cholesterol, dexamethasone suppression test, and carotene. Of these, one of the most important tests is the serum potassium level. Eating-disorder patients can commonly become hypokalemic, develop a hypokalemic hypochloremic alkalosis and have cardiac complications including arrhythmias and sudden death. Osteoporosis can be found in anorexic patients, but a bone scan is not a vital initial procedure. A head CT scan is not warranted. Delayed gastric emptying can occur with eating disorders, but a study to prove such is not urgent. Cholesterol is often increased in these patients, but again, not urgent.

Feeding and Eating Disorders

K&S Ch. 23

Question 75. D. All of the answer choices regarding delusional disorder are true except D. You do not have to have impairment of daily functioning to qualify for delusional disorder. The most prominent feature of the disorder is delusions. These delusions can be paranoid, grandiose, erotic, jealous, somatic, or mixed. These patients lack significant mood symptoms and they lack the bizarre delusions found in schizophrenia. "I'm being followed by the police" is a nonbizarre delusion, because it is possible that it could be true. "I'm being tracked by aliens" is a bizarre delusion and is not possible. The primary medication treatment is with antipsychotics, in addition to individual therapy, and sometimes family therapy.

Psychotic Disorders

K&S Ch. 14

Question 76. E. Female orgasmic disorder is the persistent absence of orgasm in women following a normal excitement phase. It is based on the clinician's judgment that the women's orgasmic capacity is less than would be reasonable for her age, sexual experience, and adequacy of sexual stimulation she receives. The overall prevalence is thought to be somewhere around 30%. It is true that the incidence of orgasm increases with age, attributed to less psychological inhibition and more experience. Psychological factors, like those listed in answer choice D, may play a role. It can be either lifelong or acquired depending on whether the patient has ever had an orgasm at any point in life. Answer choice E refers to vaginismus, which is an involuntary contraction of the outer third of the vagina preventing intercourse. It can occur following rape, or in women with psychosexual conflicts.

Sexual Dysfunctions

K&S Ch. 21

Question 77. D. The case described in this question is consistent with social anxiety disorder (social phobia). It involves certain specific social situations which provoke intense anxiety because of fear of embarrassment or humiliation. An important differential to consider would be avoidant personality disorder. In this disorder there is a pervasive pattern of social inhibition, feelings of inadequacy, and hypersensitivity to negative evaluation. It leads to the avoidance of other people unless the sufferer is sure that he is going to be liked. Avoidant personality disorder leads to restraint of intimate relationships for fear of being shamed or ridiculed. These patients often view themselves as socially inept or personally unappealing. They avoid jobs with significant interpersonal contact. Very importantly, they desire the closeness and warmth of relationships but avoid them for fear of rejection. Borderline personality disorder is characterized by a pattern of instability of interpersonal relationships, self-image, and affect, as well as marked impulsivity. Obsessive–compulsive personality disorder is defined by a pervasive pattern of preoccupation with orderliness, perfectionism, and mental and interpersonal control, at the expense of flexibility, openness, and efficiency. Narcissistic personality disorder is defined by a pattern of grandiosity, need for admiration, and lack of empathy. Dependent personality disorder is defined by a pervasive need to be taken care of that leads to submissive and clinging behavior and fears of separation.

Anxiety Disorders

K&S Ch. 27

Question 78. E. Phenytoin (Dilantin sodium) is notorious for causing hirsutism in women, facial dysmorphism and gingival hypertrophy. The drug can also cause cerebellar atrophy when taken over a long period of time, resulting in cerebellar signs and symptoms, such as ataxic gait and dysmetria of the extremities. Carbamazepine has the distinction of inducing its own metabolism. It can also cause rash that can lead to Stevens–Johnson syndrome. Another side effect of carbamazepine includes hyponatremia by antidiuretic hormone-like effect. It can also cause leukopenia and toxic hepatitis. Valproate can cause leukopenia, liver failure, weight gain, hair loss, fetal neural tube defects such as spina bifida and polycystic ovary syndrome. Levetiracetam is an anticonvulsant with minimal side effects. One of the more worrisome, but infrequent side effects of levetiracetam is agitation or hyperactivity. Phenobarbital is a barbiturate anticonvulsant and shares the side effects of that class: central nervous system depression, sedation, respiratory compromise and depression. Phenobarbital can of course be deadly in overdose.

Neurology

B&D Ch. 67

Question 79. A.

The clinical picture depicted in this question is known as a "Saturday night palsy", which is synonymous for a radial nerve entrapment. Entrapment of the radial nerve at the axilla often results from prolonged armpit compression when the arm is draped over the edge of a chair or when a patient is on crutches. A radial nerve palsy of this kind results in weakness of the extensor muscles of the wrist and fingers, triceps weakness and supinator weakness. Such compression injury usually resolves in one to two months. Ulnar nerve entrapment can occur either at the elbow or at the wrist. Elbow trauma may result in ulnar nerve entrapment in the cubital tunnel. Other causes include arm compression during surgery under general anesthesia. Ulnar nerve compression results in weakness of the flexor carpi ulnaris, intrinsic hand muscles and fourth and fifth finger deep flexor weakness. Median nerve entrapment at the wrist can result in a classic carpal tunnel syndrome. This is the most common of the entrapment neuropathies. Tenosynovitis of the transverse carpal ligament places pressure on the median nerve in the tunnel resulting in nocturnal hand paresthesias of the thumb, index and middle fingers. There may be sensory loss, thenar atrophy and a positive Tinel's sign, in about 60% of cases. Tinel's sign is positive when percussion of the nerve over the wrist results in paresthesias in the median nerve territory. Flexing the hand at the wrist for about one minute or more is called the Phalen's maneuver and can result in similar paresthesias. Injury to the median nerve is sustained with use of handheld vibrating tools and repetitive forceful use of the hands and wrists compromising the carpal tunnel. The diagnostic test of choice for carpal tunnel syndrome is needle electromyography (EMG) and nerve conduction studies which reveal delayed sensory latency across the wrist in 70–90% of cases. Musculocutaneous nerve injury can occur with brachial plexus injuries such as by shoulder dislocation, compression to the shoulder during surgical anesthesia or by repetitively carrying heavy objects over the shoulder (carpet carrier's palsy). Biceps and brachialis weakness is the hallmark of musculocutaneous nerve injury. The suprascapular nerve is a pure motor nerve of the brachial plexus.

Entrapment injury can occur after repetitive forward traction at the shoulder. Diffuse aching pain in the posterior shoulder is a usual symptom. EMG demonstrates denervation of the infraspinatus and supraspinatus muscles.

Neurology

B&D Ch. 76

Question 80. D.

The case described shows loss of muscle tone in times of extreme emotion or physical exertion. This is found in association with narcolepsy. In narcolepsy, there are irresistible attacks of sleep that occur daily. They are characterized by either cataplexy, which is the loss of muscle tone described above, or the recurrent intrusions of rapid eye movement (REM) sleep into the transition between sleep and wakefulness, causing hypnopompic or hypnogogic hallucinations or sleep paralysis. Sleep apnea is a medical condition which can be either central or obstructive and leads to snoring, daytime drowsiness and irritability. It can have negative long term cardiac consequences as well. Primary insomnia is difficulty initiating or maintaining sleep, or nonrestorative sleep for at least one month. It is independent of any known physical or medical condition. It is often treated with benzodiazepines or zolpidem. Primary hypersomnia is excessive sleepiness for 1 month as demonstrated by prolonged sleep episodes at night or daily sleep episodes during the day. Treatment consists of stimulants such as amphetamines and the nonstimulant modafinil (Provigil). Sodium oxybate (Xyrem) is FDA-approved for cataplexy associated with narcolepsy. Xyrem is essentially a synthetic analog of gamma hydroxybutyrate (GHB), which is a drug of abuse notorious for being used as a date rape drug. Circadian rhythm sleep disorder is a persistent pattern of sleep disruption resulting from a mismatch between the sleep–wake cycle of the environment and the circadian sleep–wake pattern. It can be specified as delayed sleep phase type, jet lag type, or shift work type. Modafinil has a specific FDA indication in shift-work sleep disorder, as well as narcolepsy, obstructive sleep apnea and idiopathic hypersomnia.

Sleep Wake Disorders

K&S Ch. 24

Question 81. C.

Conversion disorder usually involves neurologic symptoms. Multiple organ system complaints are found in somatization disorder. If symptoms are limited to pain, it is a pain disorder, not a conversion disorder. If symptoms are limited to sexual dysfunction, it is a sexual disorder, not conversion disorder. Conversion disorder symptoms are not intentionally produced.

Somatic Symptom Disorders

K&S Ch. 17

Question 82. D. The monoamine oxidase (MAO) type A inhibitors are contraindicated with levodopa/carbidopa repletion therapy. MAOIs are postsynaptic enzymatic metabolizers of dopamine. Concomitant use of MAO-A type inhibitors and levodopa/carbidopa can result in poor response to the levodopa repletion therapy and worsening of parkinsonian symptoms. MAOIs need to be discontinued 2 weeks prior to the initiation of levodopa repletion therapy to avoid a negative interaction. The antidepressants in the selective serotonin reuptake inhibitor class (fluoxetine and sertraline, among others) are not contraindicated with levodopa repletion therapy. Tricyclic antidepressants are also safe with levodopa repletion, as is gabapentin.

Neurology

B&D Ch. 71

Question 83. C. Piaget proposed four stages of cognitive development. They were the sensorimotor stage, the stage of preoperational thought, the concrete operations stage, and the formal operations stage. During the concrete operations stage the child begins to deal with information outside of himself and to see things from other's perspectives. He also develops conservation, which is the idea that though objects may change, they can maintain characteristics that allow them to be recognized as the same (example: different leaves may be different shapes and colors but are all leaves). The concept of reversibility is also understood at this stage. It says that things can change form and shape and then go back again (example: ice to water to ice).

Human Development

K&S Ch. 4

Question 84. D. By 2–3 years of age, almost all children have a concept of being either male or female. Infants begin exploring their genitalia by 15 months of age. Children also develop interest in other's genitals leading to exploration and exhibition. Sexual curiosity and sex play increase during puberty, but are normally present before puberty. They are not a sign of anything abnormal, nor is it a result of television, homosexuality, hormonal imbalance, or premature development.

Human Development

K&S Ch. 21.

Question 85. E. Short palpebral fissures are found in children with fetal alcohol syndrome, not fragile X syndrome. Fragile X syndrome presents with mental retardation, long ears, narrow face, short stature, hyperextendable joints, arched palate, macro-orchidism, seizures and autistic features. There is a high rate of attention deficit–hyperactivity disorder, and learning disorders. It is the second most common cause of mental retardation. It results from a mutation of the X chromosome.

Neurodevelopmental and Pervasive Developmental Disorders

K&S Ch. 38

Question 86. A. In normal attachment, a child at 18 months of age would use a transitional object in the absence of the mother. There would be less anxiety at separation than in pervious stages, but it would not be completely gone. The child would try to master strange situations when the mother was nearby. There is object permanence. It is not until 25 months of age that the child would be expected to tolerate the mother's absence without distress. In the situations described in the other answer choices, the child would be scared, not violent. The child would not immediately run to you as he would have some stranger anxiety. He would not feel safe enough in the mother's absence to become more inquisitive. The child would definitely notice the mother's absence.

Human Development

K&S Ch. 4

Question 87. C. Valproate is the classic inhibitor of cytochrome P-450 3A4 which causes inhibition of enzymatic clearance of lamotrigine. Doses of lamotrigine need to be lowered and generally started at lower doses when administered concomitantly with valproic acid, to avoid lamotrigine toxicity. The other agents noted in this question do not have cyp-450 3A4 inhibitory properties in this fashion.

Psychopharmacology

K&S Ch. 36

Question 88. D. It is during adolescence that children move away from the family and the friend group provides the most important relationships. During this time, any deviation in appearance, dress, or behavior can lead to a decrease in self-esteem. For this reason the child would most likely suffer the most psychological impact from a deformity during adolescence.

Human Development

K&S Ch. 2

Question 89. D. Whereas some monoamine oxidase inhibitors (MAOIs) work on both MAO-A, and MAO-B, selegiline works solely on MAO-B. MAO-A is involved in the metabolism of serotonin and norepinephrine. MAO-B is involved in the metabolism of phenylethylamine. Both are involved in the metabolism of dopamine. MAO-A in the gastrointestinal tract is involved in the metabolism of tyramine. If you block these enzymes, tyramine is not broken down and can lead to hypertensive crisis.

Psychopharmacology

K&S Ch. 36

Question 90. E. Cocaine blocks dopamine reuptake from the synaptic cleft, leading to increased levels of dopamine. When chronically used, this disturbance of normal dopamine metabolism leads to depletion of dopamine. Cocaine has also been shown to be associated with decreased levels of cerebral blood flow. Patients recovering from cocaine addiction show a drop in neuronal activity and a decreased activity of dopamine which can persist for up to a year and a half after stopping the drug.

Substance Abuse and Addictive Disorders

K&S Ch. 12

Question 91. A. Neural tube defects are the most worrisome fetotoxic side effects of valproic acid in the pregnant patient. The classic presentation is that of fetal spina bifida. With formation of the neural tube early in gestation, spina bifida can usually be detected by fetal ultrasound in the first trimester. The other noted problems are not attributable to side effects of valproic acid.

Psychopharmacology

K&S Ch. 36

Question 92. B. Dopamine agonists are newer agents used to treat Parkinson's disease. The classic agents of this class available for use in the United States are pergolide, bromocriptine, pramipexole and ropinirole. Ropinirole is now also indicated in restless legs syndrome and is one of the treatments of choice for that disorder. Worrisome side effects of the dopamine agonists include hallucinations, sedation and orthostatic hypotension. There is a much lower incidence of dyskinesias with the dopamine agonists than with levodopa therapy. Haloperidol and fluphenazine are conventional antipsychotic agents and hence are dopamine antagonists. Quetiapine is a second-generation atypical antipsychotic that has dopamine antagonist properties as well. Buspirone is approved for generalized anxiety disorder and is a 5-HT 1A partial agonist.

Neurology

B&D Ch. 71

Question 93. E. The frontal lobes are the seat of executive functioning. They also play a large role in the personality. Damage to the orbitofrontal region can cause disinhibition, irritability, mood lability, euphoria, lack of remorse, poor judgment, and distractability. Damage to the dorsolateral frontal regions leads to extensive executive functioning deficits. Damage to the medial frontal region leads to an apathy syndrome.

Basic Neuroscience

K&S Ch. 3

Question 94. B. Ziprasidone (Geodon) stands alone as the one atypical antipsychotic that inhibits serotonin and norepinephrine reuptake. All of the atypical antipsychotics block the serotonin 2A and dopamine D2 receptors. The reuptake inhibition seen with ziprasidone however, is unique, as is its blockade of the serotonin-1A receptor.

Psychopharmacology

K&S Ch. 36

Question 95. E. Aripiprazole (Abilify) is a partial dopamine agonist at the D2 receptor. It is postulated to work on positive symptoms of schizophrenia by competing with dopamine in the mesolimbic pathway, and negative symptoms of schizophrenia by being an agonist at dopamine receptors in the prefrontal cortex. It is also a partial agonist at the 5HT1A receptor and an antagonist at the 5HT2A receptor. All of the other antipsychotics available only block dopamine receptors. This blockade of dopamine receptors in the frontal cortex theoretically leads to a worsening of negative symptoms by the medication, particularly by the typical antipsychotics.

Psychopharmacology

K&S Ch. 36

Question 96. C. The prefrontal cortices influence mood differently. If one activates the left prefrontal cortex, mood is lifted. If the right prefrontal cortex is activated, mood is depressed. Therefore a lesion to the left prefrontal cortex would cause depression, and a lesion to the right prefrontal cortex would cause euphoria and laughter. The parietal and occipital lobes are not the predominant lobes involved in emotion.

Basic Neuroscience

K&S Ch. 3

Question 97. E. The raphe nuclei of the brainstem, predominantly in the pons, are the major sites of serotonergic cell bodies. The ventral tegmental area, substantia nigra, and nucleus accumbens are all dopaminergic areas and are parts of the major neuronal pathways involved in the pathophysiology of schizophrenia. The cerebellum is a distracter.

Basic Neuroscience

K&S Ch. 3

Question 98. C. The clinical picture depicted in this vignette is that of Wilson's disease. Wilson's disease is an autosomal recessive disorder of abnormal copper metabolism. It is linked to the q14-21 (ATP7B) region of chromosome 13. Prevalence is about 1 in 30 000. The disorder results in a problem with incorporation of copper into ceruloplasmin and with diminished biliary excretion of copper. This results in excessive deposition of copper in the brain, with a predilection for the basal ganglia. The most useful laboratory test is serum ceruloplasmin which is most often decreased to less than 20 mg/dL (normal range is 24–45 mg/dL). The most frequent neurologic manifestations are parkinsonism, flapping tremor, ataxia, dystonia and bulbar signs such as dysphagia and dysarthria. Signs of liver failure are usually present. The treatment of choice is penicillamine, a copper-chelating agent, which in many cases can reverse the deficits of the disease. Serum angiotensin-converting enzyme (ACE) level would be a screening test for sarcoidosis. Chromosomal analysis for CAG triplet repeats by polymerase chain reaction (PCR) would be the test of choice for Huntington's disease. Lumbar puncture for cerebrospinal fluid oligoclonal bands and myelin basic protein would be a useful supportive test (in addition to brain and/or spinal cord MRI) for multiple sclerosis. The Tensilon test is for the diagnosis of myasthenia gravis.

Neurology

B&D Ch. 71

Question 99. C. The mesolimbic pathway of dopaminergic neurons, starting at the ventral tegmental area and projecting to the nucleus accumbens is thought to be highly involved in the sense of reward one gets from cocaine use, and is a major mediator of cocaine's effects. It is very involved in amphetamine's effects as well. The locus ceruleus of the brainstem contains a high number of adrenergic neurons, and mediates the effects of opiates and opioids.

Basic Neuroscience

K&S Ch. 12

Question 100. D. The therapeutic focus of motivational enhancement therapy is on the patient's ambivalence toward staying off of their drug of abuse. It is a type of therapy specifically used with patients addicted to drugs of abuse.

Psychotherapy

K&S Ch. 35

Question 101. A. Of the many psychological tests used today, the reliability of the Wechsler Adult Intelligence Scale (WAIS) is among the highest. Retesting of people, even at later ages, rarely reveals higher IQ scores. The scores are consistent and repeatable. As such it is the most reliable of the choices given. It also has a very high validity in identifying mental retardation and predicting future school performance. There is also a childhood version of the same test, the Wechsler Intelligence Scale for Children (WISC).

Psychological Theory and Psychometric Testing

K&S Ch. 5

Question 102. E. Freud's drive theory focused on basic instincts or drives that motivated human behavior. These drives were libido and aggression. In Freud's model, a drive has four parts. The "source" is the part of the body from which the drive comes. The "impetus" is the amount of intensity of the drive. The "aim" is any action that discharges the tension. The "object" is the target of the action. The other theories listed have nothing to do with Freud. Self psychology is the theory of Kohut. Learning theory cannot be attributed to any one individual, but has many theories and contributors. Conflict theory is a distracter, as is the mesolimbic dopamine theory.

Psychological Theory and Psychometric Testing

K&S Ch. 6

Question 103. A. Numerous studies have shown the principal cause of intracerebral hemorrhage (ICH) to be hypertension. Chronic hypertension likely causes lipohyalinosis of the small intraparenchymal arteries and microaneurysms of Charcot and Bouchard that rupture due to increased vascular pressure. ICH accounts for about 10% of all strokes. The most common area of predilection for ICH is the putamen in about one-third of cases, followed by the thalamus in about 10–15% of cases. The other choices listed in this question are all less-frequent causes of ICH.

Neurology

B&D Ch. 51

Question 104. D. Aaron Beck is the originator of cognitive behavioral therapy (CBT). In this theory, patients' assumptions affect their cognitions, which in turn affect their mood. As such, it would be cognitive distortion that Beck would most likely find as the cause of depression. The other answer choices may be things to which other theorists attribute depression, or are totally unrelated answer choices included to distract.

Psychotherapy

K&S Ch. 35

Question 105. A. A type I error occurs when the null hypothesis is rejected when it should have been retained. It is the equivalent of saying that a true difference exists between two samples when the difference is due solely to chance.

Statistics

K&S Ch. 4

Question 106. E. Randomization is the process by which each patient in a clinical trial has an equal chance to be assigned to a control group or an experimental group. This process protects against selection bias. Power is the probability of finding the difference between two samples. It is the probability of rejecting the null hypothesis when it should be rejected. Probability is the likelihood that an event will occur. A probability of 1 means it will occur, a probability of 0 means that it will not. Risk is a distracter.

Statistics

K&S Ch. 4

Question 107. C. The clinical picture here is that of cryptococcal meningitis in an AIDS patient with severe immunocompromise. About 10% of AIDS patients develop this infection by the encapsulated yeast *Cryptococcus neoformans*. CD4 count is generally less than 200/μL. Although MRI of the brain is a good test, in this case the results would be nonspecific. The scan might demonstrate meningeal enhancement with gadolinium, suggesting a subacute or chronic meningitis. There may also be multiple small abscesses seen on scan due to fungal invasion of the Virchow–Robin spaces surrounding meningeal vessels. Hydrocephalus due to obstruction of cerebrospinal fluid (CSF) flow may also be seen. In rarer cases a mass lesion, or cryptococcoma, with surrounding edema can be seen, due to consolidation of the infection. The most important immediate test is the lumbar puncture. Opening pressure should be measured and is usually elevated. CSF is most often colorless and clear. CSF analysis can reveal a leucocytosis of 50–1000 cells/mm^3 with lymphocytic predominance. CSF protein is usually elevated from 50–1000 mg/dL. India ink staining of CSF viewed under the microscope will quickly reveal an identifiable capsule and budding yeasts and requires no special laboratory machinery or testing. CSF cryptococcal antigen assay is indeed more sensitive than India ink staining and should concomitantly be done, as it is now readily available in most centers. Chest radiography would only be helpful with a suspicion of lung involvement or pulmonary symptoms. Blood cultures are generally negative in fungal infection and should only be done if concomitant bacterial infection is suspected. Amphotericin B intravenous administration is the treatment of choice for central nervous system fungal infections. The problem with Amphotericin B is a high rate of up to 80% renal toxicity as a side effect.

Neurology

B&D Ch. 53

Question 108. D. Power is the probability of finding the difference between two samples. It is the probability of rejecting the null hypothesis when it should be rejected. Randomization is the process by which each patient in a clinical trial has an equal chance to be assigned to a control group or an experimental group. This process protects against selection bias. Probability is the likelihood that an event will occur. A probability of 1 means it will occur, a probability of 0 means that it will not. Risk is a distracter.

Statistics

K&S Ch. 4

Question 109. C. The number of people who have a disorder at a specific point in time is the point prevalence. It is calculated by dividing the number of people with the disorder at that time by the total population at that time. Randomization is the process by which each patient in a clinical trial has an equal chance to be assigned to a control group or an experimental group. This process protects against selection bias. Power is the probability of finding the difference between two samples. It is the probability of rejecting the null hypothesis when it should be rejected. Probability is the likelihood that an event will occur. A probability of 1 means it will occur, a probability of 0 means that it will not. Risk is a distracter.

Statistics

K&S Ch. 4

Question 110. A. One of the main criteria for anorexia is a failure to maintain body weight at or above 85% of what would be expected for the person's height and age. Other criteria include a fear of becoming fat, even though the person is underweight, problems in the way one's body is experienced, and undue influence of body weight on self-esteem. Anorexic patients also deny the seriousness of their being underweight, and often have amenorrhea. There are two types of anorexia, the restricting type, and the binge eating/purging type.

Feeding and Eating Disorders

K&S Ch. 23

Question 111. D. PCP can be found in the urine up to 8 days after use. Some other drugs of note include: cannabis – up to 4 weeks, cocaine – up to 8 hours, and heroin – up to 72 hours.

Laboratory Tests in Psychiatry

K&S Ch. 7

Question 112. C. Amyloid precursor protein is the protein that makes up the amyloid plaques found in the brain in Alzheimer's disease. The protein is encoded by a gene found on chromosome 21. The amyloid deposits found in Alzheimer's disease are the hallmark of the disease's neuropathology. Wilson's disease is the result of abnormal copper metabolism, not amyloid. Schizophrenia, bipolar disorder, and Huntington's disease have nothing to do with amyloid.

Neurocognitive Disorders

K&S Ch. 10

Question 113. C. A complete blood count (CBC) would be the first test to order because of the risk of significant side effects on the hematopoietic system. Carbamazepine can cause decreased white blood cell count, agranulocytosis, pancytopenia, and aplastic anemia. Carbamazepine also has a vasopressin-like effect and can cause water intoxication and hyponatremia. Carbamazepine interacts significantly with the cytochrome P-450 system and as such has many interactions with many drugs. Great care should be taken when prescribing carbamazepine with other medications.

Laboratory Tests in Psychiatry

K&S Ch. 36

Question 114. E. Because the starvation associated with anorexia effects a multitude of organ systems, a battery of tests is warranted when working up the disease. These include electrolytes, renal function tests, thyroid tests, glucose, amylase, complete blood count, electrocardiogram, cholesterol, carotene level and a dexamethasone suppression test. There is not an indication for a head CT, as one would not find changes on the head CT of an anorexic patient that would differentiate it from a normal head CT.

Laboratory Tests in Psychiatry

K&S Ch. 23

Question 115. B. Creutzfeldt–Jakob disease (CJD) is one of a number of human spongiform encephalopathies and is associated with prion infection. The worldwide incidence of CJD is about 0.5 to 1 in one million per year. A new variant was thought to have developed during the later nineties resulting from consumption of meat from cattle infected with bovine spongiform encephalopathy. The clinical picture is that of a prodromal period of vegetative symptoms such as asthenia and sleep and appetite disturbances. This is followed by the onset of a rapidly progressive dementia with deficits in memory, concentration, depression, self-neglect and personality changes. The condition progresses to global dementia over time and death typically occurs from 2–7 months after onset of symptoms. The diagnostic test of choice today is lumbar puncture with cerebrospinal fluid assay of 14-3-3 and tau proteins, the specificity and sensitivity of which exceed 90%. CT scans of the brain are useless as they remain normal in a majority of cases. There may be atrophy seen on CT scan with ventricular enlargement, but this is nonspecific and diagnostically unhelpful. MRI of the brain may reveal atrophy with symmetrical increased signal intensity in the basal ganglia, which is again not particularly helpful in diagnosing CJD. Electroencephalogram is more helpful and is expected to reveal a characteristic one to two cycle-per-second triphasic sharp wave pattern superimposed on a background of electrical depression. This pattern is seen in up to 80% of cases at some point during the course of the illness.

Neurology

B&D Ch. 53

Question 116. D. Disorders of smooth visual pursuit and disinhibition of saccadic eye movements are commonly found in patients with schizophrenia. This has been proposed by some as a trait marker for schizophrenia, because it is found regardless of medication use and is also present in first degree relatives. It is thought that the eye movement disorders are the function of pathology in the frontal lobes.

Psychotic Disorders

K&S Ch. 13

Question 117. E. Many of the antipsychotic medications block dopamine in the tuberoinfundibular tract. Because of this dopamine blockade, the patient develops an elevated prolactin level. That elevated prolactin level leads to galactorrhea and amenorrhea. In the case given, the risperidone is the most likely cause of the patient's symptoms. You would want to check the serum prolactin level and adjust the risperidone dose, or consider switching the patient to another medication.

Laboratory Tests in Psychiatry

K&S Ch. 7

Question 118. C. Patients with borderline personality disorder have frequent mood swings. They can develop short-lived psychotic episodes. They often cut or mutilate themselves to elicit help from others, to express anger, or to numb themselves to strong affect. Both men and women can have borderline personality disorder, though it is more common in women. The other answer choices do not fit the case as well as borderline personality disorder. Schizoaffective disorder patients do not usually self-mutilate. Dysthymic disorder is not consistent with psychotic symptoms. There is no description of mania, so bipolar disorder is unlikely. There is no acute stressor so adjustment disorder doesn't fit well. Whenever a question involves cutting or self-mutilation, strongly consider borderline personality disorder.

Personality Disorders

K&S Ch. 27

Question 119. B. Of the choices given, the highest prevalence is for anxiety disorders. Over 30 million people in the United States have an anxiety disorder. About 17.5 million have depression. About 2 million have schizophrenia. About 5 million have dementia. About 12.8 million use illicit drugs.

Anxiety Disorders

K&S Ch. 4

Question 120. D. There is an association between pathological gambling and mood disorders, particularly major depressive disorder (MDD). There is also an association with panic, obsessive–compulsive disorder and agoraphobia, but the association with MDD is greater. Criteria for pathological gambling include preoccupation with gambling, gambling increased sums of money to obtain excitement, being unsuccessful at stopping or cutting back, gambling to escape dysphoric mood, lying to significant others about gambling, loss of important relationships over gambling, committing illegal acts in order to gamble, relying on others to pay the bills because of money lost gambling, and a desire to keep going back to break even.

Disruptive, Impulse Control Disorders, Conduct Disorders, and ADHD

K&S Ch. 25

Question 121. C. This is a case of delusional disorder. In delusional disorder the patient has nonbizarre delusions (i.e., they could be true, but are not). They do not meet criteria for schizophrenia. Their functioning in day to day life is relatively preserved. It may take various forms, such as erotomanic type, grandiose type, jealous type, persecutory type, somatic type, or mixed type. This patient does not meet criteria for schizophrenia. There are no mood symptoms, so this rules out depression. He is not confused, disoriented, and waxing and waning in consciousness, so this rules out a delirium. The wife is not a partner in the delusions, she thinks there is something wrong with him, so this rules out a shared psychotic disorder. Given all of this, the correct answer is delusional disorder.

Psychotic Disorders

K&S Ch. 14

Question 122. E. Hypochondriasis involves being convinced that one has a serious disease based on misinterpretation of bodily sensations. The preoccupation with having the illness persists despite reassurance by doctors. It causes clinically significant impairment in functioning. Somatoform disorders is a general category that includes somatization disorder, conversion disorder, hypochondriasis, body dysmorphic disorder, and pain disorder. Factitious disorder is when a patient feigns illness for primary gain (i.e., benefits of the sick role). Conversion disorder is the development of a neurological deficit as a result of psychological conflict. Pain disorder is the presence of pain as the predominant clinical focus, where the pain is thought to be substantially mediated by psychological factors.

Somatic Symptom Disorders

K&S Ch. 17

Question 123. E. There are multiple studies that all point to a genetic predisposition for alcoholism. The studies that separate environmental from genetic factors are some of the most convincing. Studies of adoptees clearly demonstrate that children whose biological parents were alcoholics are at increased risk for alcoholism, even when brought up by adopted families where neither parent has an alcohol problem. In addition, children whose biological parents do not have an alcohol problem are not more likely to become alcoholic if raised in a home with parents who have alcohol problems.

Substance Abuse and Addictive Disorders

K&S Ch. 12

Question 124. C. This is a psychogenic seizure (also called nonepileptic seizure). Keys to a psychogenic seizure, or pseudoseizure, are lack of an aura, no cyanotic skin changes, no self injury, no incontinence, no postictal confusion, asynchronous body movements, absent EEG changes, and seizure activity being affected by the suggestion of the doctor.

Neurology

K&S Ch. 10

Question 125. B. Internuclear ophthalmoplegia is a classic brainstem finding on neurologic examination of patients with demyelinating lesions of multiple sclerosis (MS). The lesion localizes to the medial longitudinal fasciculus (MLF) of the brainstem. The deficit involves abnormal horizontal ocular movements with absence or delayed adduction of the eye ipsilateral to the MLF lesion and coarse horizontal nystagmus in the abducting eye. Convergence is preserved. Bilateral internuclear ophthalmoplegia is highly suggestive of MS, but can also be seen with other brainstem lesions, particularly Arnold–Chiari malformation, Wernicke's encephalopathy, vascular lesions and brainstem gliomas.

Neurology

B&D Ch. 54

Question 126. B. Paranoid schizophrenia is characterized by delusions of persecution or grandeur, as well as auditory hallucinations. Patients usually have their first break at a later age than other schizophrenic patients. They show more preservation of cognitive function than in other types of schizophrenia. Disorganized schizophrenia is marked by primitive, disinhibited, disorganized behavior. Patients have significant impairment in cognition. Catatonic schizophrenia is characterized by stupor, negativism, rigidity and posturing. Mutism is common, and cognition and communication are impaired. Undifferentiated schizophrenic patients do not fit easily into one of the other categories. Residual schizophrenia consists of the continued presence of some symptoms of schizophrenia in a person who no longer meets full criteria for the disorder.

Psychotic Disorders

K&S Ch. 13

Question 127. E. Pathological gambling is categorized by the DSM as an impulse control disorder. Criteria for pathological gambling include preoccupation with gambling, gambling increased sums of money to obtain excitement, being unsuccessful at stopping or cutting back, gambling to escape dysphoric mood, lying to significant others about gambling, loss of important relationships over gambling, committing illegal acts in order to gamble, relying on others to pay the bills because of money lost gambling, and a desire to keep going back to break even.

Disruptive, Impulse Control Disorders, Conduct Disorders, and ADHD

K&S Ch. 25

Question 128. E. Asperger's disorder is characterized by the following clinical features. The patient has marked impairment in the use of nonverbal communication, failure to develop peer relationships, lack of desire to share experiences with others and restricted or stereotyped patterns of behavior. There can be preoccupation or obsessive focus on certain interests, rigid adherence to schedules, and stereotyped motor mannerisms. Unlike autism, there is not a delay in language or cognitive development. The child in this question clearly has Asperger's disorder. He is not breaking rules and violating social norms as one would expect with a conduct disorder. He is not fighting authority figures as one would expect of oppositional defiant disorder. He does not show irritability, impulsivity, and hyperactivity as one would find in attention deficit–hyperactivity disorder. His language and cognitive development are not delayed as would be expected in a case of autism.

Neurodevelopmental and Pervasive Developmental Disorders

K&S Ch. 42

Question 129. D. If you thought this was the same as question 128 you need to read more carefully! This is a case of autism. In autism there is marked impairment in the use of nonverbal communication, failure to develop peer relationships, lack of desire to share experiences with others, and restricted or stereotyped patterns of behavior. There can be preoccupation or obsessive focus on certain interests, rigid adherence to schedules, and stereotyped motor mannerisms. But very importantly, there is delay in, or total absence of spoken language. There is an inability to maintain conversation. There is stereotyped use of language. There is a lack of spontaneous or make believe play. Cognitive development is significantly impaired. There is a lack of social or emotional reciprocity.

Neurodevelopmental and Pervasive Developmental Disorders

K&S Ch. 42

Question 130. B. Derealization is a subjective feeling that the environment is strange or unreal. Depersonalization is a person's sense that they are unreal or unfamiliar. Fugue involves having amnesia for your identity and assuming a new identity. It usually also involves wandering to new places. Amnesia is the inability to recall past experiences. Anosognosia is an inability to recognize a neurological deficit that is occurring to oneself.

Dissociative Disorders

K&S Ch. 8

Question 131. E. Inhalants can cause a persisting dementia. It is irreversible except for the mildest cases. It may be the result of the neurotoxic effects of the inhalants, the metals they contain, or the effects of hypoxia. Inhalant use can also lead to delirium, psychosis, mood, and anxiety disorders. Signs of intoxication with inhalants include maladaptive behavior such as assaultiveness, impaired judgment, as well as neurological signs such as dizziness, slurred speech, ataxia, tremor, blurred vision, stupor, and coma. The other answer choices have various effects, but do not cause a persisting dementia.

Substance Abuse and Addictive Disorders

K&S Ch. 12

Question 132. E. Social skills training is an important part of psychiatric rehabilitation. Social skills are behaviors necessary for survival in the community. These are disrupted by severe illnesses such as schizophrenia. Social skills training has proven important in correcting deficits in patient's behaviors. Severely ill patients make slow progress, but can learn some necessary skills that enable them to engage in conversation and decrease social anxiety. Social skills training can be done both in a group and an individual format. The other answer choices in this question consist of unrelated pairs, some of which border on the ridiculous and are distracters.

Psychosocial Interventions

K&S Ch. 35

Question 133. D. Multiple sclerosis (MS) is the most common inflammatory demyelinating disease. The classic onset of the disease is between the ages of 15 and 50 years. About two-thirds of patients have the relapsing–remitting form of the disease at onset, which is the most common form of the illness. Only about 20% of patients have primary progressive disease at onset. Optic neuritis (ON) is a common sign of multiple sclerosis and is frequently the cause of initial presenting symptoms. ON usually presents with eye pain that increases with eye movement followed by central visual loss (scotoma) in the affected eye. ON patients will have a relative afferent pupillary defect (Marcus Gunn pupil). This is tested by the swinging flashlight test which demonstrates that the abnormal pupil paradoxically dilates when a light is moved away from the normal to the affected eye. Internuclear ophthalmoplegia is a common sign of MS and involves a lesion in the medial longitudinal fasciculus of the brainstem that produces a characteristic eye movement abnormality. The eye ipsilateral to the lesions cannot adduct past the midline while the contralateral eye fully abducts and displays a coarse end-gaze nystagmus. The finding can sometimes be bilateral. Fatigue is a common complaint in patients with MS. It often has little to do with the amount of physical exertion carried out by the patient. It may occur upon waking despite a good night's sleep the night before. Heat sensitivity is a well-described phenomenon in MS. Increases in core body temperature can bring on symptoms or worsen already existing symptoms. This is known as Uhthoff's phenomenon. The condition occurs due to conduction block that occurs as body temperature rises. Lhermitte's sign is a transient neurologic sign described by patients as a sensation of an electric shock that descends down the spine or the extremities upon neck flexion. It is most often suggestive of MS, but can also be seen in other conditions involving the cervical spinal cord, such as disk herniations, trauma and tumors.

Neurology

B&D Ch. 54

Question 134. C. Bulimia is categorized by a recurrent pattern of binge eating and self induced vomiting. Bulimic patients often develop a hypochloremic alkalosis, and are at risk for gastric and esophageal tears. Dehydration (hence low blood pressure) and electrolyte imbalances are likely. Many female bulimic patients have menstrual disturbances. Russell's sign is positive when cuts or scrapes to the backs of the hands are noted which are a result of sticking the fingers down the throat to induce vomiting.

Feeding and Eating Disorders

K&S Ch. 23

Question 135. D.   Amphetamine intoxication presents with euphoria, anxiety, anger, hypervigilance, and impaired judgment and functioning. The effects are similar to those of cocaine. There is a risk for an amphetamine-induced psychotic disorder as well, which is characterized by paranoia. One can also note visual hallucinations, hypersexuality, hyperactivity, confusion and incoherence.

Substance Abuse and Addictive Disorders

K&S Ch. 12

Question 136. B.   Acute stress disorder is characterized by similar symptoms to post-traumatic stress disorder, but with a different time frame. Symptoms occur for a minimum of two days, and a maximum of 4 weeks, and begin within 4 weeks of the traumatic event. The patient must have undergone a traumatic event. The patient then experiences emotional numbing, lack of awareness of surroundings, derealization, depersonalization, dissociative amnesia, flashbacks, avoidance of stimuli that remind them of the event, anxiety, irritability, increased arousal, or poor sleep.

Trauma and Stress Related Disorders

K&S Ch. 16

Question 137. C.   Children who are depressed can often present with irritability instead of, or in addition to depressed mood. Prepubertal children can report somatic complaints, psychomotor agitation, and mood-congruent hallucinations. Depressed children can also fail to make expected weight gains. Other signs of depression that children can present with include school phobia and excessive clinging to parents. Teens with depression often report poor school performance, substance abuse, promiscuity, antisocial behavior, truancy, and running away from home. They can withdraw from social activities and be grouchy and sulky.

Depressive Disorders

K&S Ch. 49

Question 138. D.   Schizoid personality disorder is characterized by a pervasive pattern of detachment from social relationships. The patient neither desires, nor enjoys close relationships. They choose solitary activities. They lack close friends or romantic relationships. They are indifferent to the opinions of others and are emotionally cold and detached. Some of the other choices in this question are references to schizotypal personality disorder. In the schizotypal patient, there are ideas of reference, magical thinking, paranoia, and excessive social anxiety which is fueled by paranoid thinking.

Personality Disorders

K&S Ch. 27

Question 139. A.   Beneficence is the duty to do no harm to the patient. Autonomy is the duty to protect a patient's freedom to choose. Autonomy theory views the relationship between patient and doctor as between two adults, not as parent and child. Justice in this context means a fair distribution and application of services. Validity is a statistical word meaning that a test measures what it claims to measure.

Ethics

K&S Ch. 58

Question 140. D.   Tourette's disorder often involves both motor and vocal tics. The onset is usually around 7 years of age, but may come as early as 2 years. Motor tics usually start in the face and head, and progress down the body. Vocal tics are not done intentionally to provoke others, but are the result of sudden, intrusive thoughts and urges that the patient cannot control. These intrusive thoughts may involve socially unacceptable subject matter or obscenity.

Disruptive, Impulse Control Disorders, Conduct Disorders, and ADHD

K&S Ch. 46

Question 141. D.   Substance abusers have the highest risk of becoming violent. Large doses of alcohol promote aggression, as do large doses of barbiturates. Paradoxical aggression can be observed with anxiolytics. Opioid dependence is associated with increased aggression. Stimulants, cocaine, hallucinogens, and sometimes cannabis can also lead to aggression. Aggressive behavior is more likely with those who have become acutely psychologically decompensated. More than half of people who commit homicide and engage in assaultive behavior are under the influence of significant amounts of alcohol at the time the crime is committed. Although many major psychiatric disorders can lead to aggression, you are more likely to face substance-induced aggression simply because of the sheer number of cases of aggression and violence that are substance-induced.

Substance Abuse and Addictive Disorders

K&S Ch. 4

Question 142. C. An ideal patient for psychodynamic psychotherapy should have the capacity for psychological mindedness, have at least one meaningful relationship, be able to tolerate affect, respond well to transference interpretation, be highly motivated, have flexible defenses and lack tendencies towards splitting, projection or denial. A useful screening tool for whether a patient has these characteristics is to understand the quality of their relationships, as the above-listed qualities often contribute to productive relationships.

Psychotherapy

K&S Ch. 35

Question 143. E. The clinical picture and scan are classic for multiple sclerosis (MS). The MRI scan reveals numerous subcortical white matter demyelinating lesions that are typical of MS. The lesions would be expected to enhance with gadolinium contrast early on during an attack and enhancement can persist up to 8 weeks following an acute attack. The treatment of an acute attack is generally with intravenous corticosteroids. The protocol is usually with intravenous methylprednisolone 500–1000 mg daily in divided doses for 3–7 days. This may or may not be followed with a 1- to 2-week oral prednisone taper. Antibiotics such as ceftriaxone have no place in MS. Intravenous immunoglobulin therapy and plasmapheresis are treatments for myasthenia gravis and Guillain–Barré syndrome and not for MS. Aspirin and heparin therapies are generally instituted in the emergency room setting for acute ischemic stroke when recombinant tissue plasminogen activator cannot be given.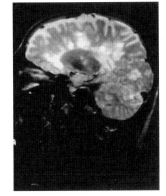

Neurology

B&D Ch. 54

Question 144. A. Borderline patients often cut, self-mutilate, and make suicide attempts. The patient in question has made past suicide attempts and past attempts are the best predictor of future attempts. She is emotionally labile following an interpersonal conflict. She is already doing harm to herself through cutting and is becoming psychotic. All of these factors add up to one very important point: this patient is highly unpredictable and could very easily kill herself. The only reasonable answer choice is hospital admission where her impulsive, self-destructive, and self mutilating impulses can be limited and her behavior observed. The other answer choices do not take her unpredictability and self-destructiveness seriously enough. The choice for extended inpatient stay is wrong because you have no way of knowing how long she is going to need to stay based on the information given. She could potentially stabilize in a few days and be safe for discharge. She could also be in the hospital for several months. There is no way to predict length of stay based on the question stem.

Management in Psychiatry

K&S Ch. 27

Question 145. E. Research in recent years has found that depression following a heart attack increases the likelihood of another heart attack. There has been evidence to suggest that there are serotonin receptors on the surface of platelets which can modify and reduce platelet aggregation and thereby reduce heart attack risk. The prescription of a selective serotonin reuptake inhibitor antidepressant following a myocardial infarction has been shown to increase the amount of serotonin in the body as a whole. This in turn modulates platelet serotonin receptors, thus decreasing platelet aggregation and making a future heart attack less likely.

Somatic Symptom Disorders

K&S Ch. 36

Question 146. B. Neurofibromatosus type 1 (NF1) is caused by a mutation in the 60 exon *NF1* gene on chromosome 17q. NF1 is the most common of the neurocutaneous illnesses occurring in about 1 in 3000 individuals. NF2 is caused by a mutation in the *NF2* gene on chromosome 22. It is less common than NF1 and appears in about 1 in 50 000 individuals. Patients with NF1 need to have any two of the following seven criteria to carry the diagnosis: six or more café au lait spots over 5 mm in diameter before puberty and over 15 mm if after puberty; axillary or inguinal freckling; optic glioma; two or more neurofibromas or one plexiform neurofibroma; a first-degree relative with NF1; two or more Lisch nodules (hamartomas of the iris); characteristic bony lesion such as thinning of long bones or sphenoid dysplasia. Patients with NF2 must have bilateral acoustic schwannomas in order to meet criteria for this condition. If the schwannoma is unilateral, the patient meets criteria only with a first-degree relative with NF2.

Neurology

B&D Ch. 65

Question 147. E. Both delirium and dementia can present with sleep problems, disorientation to place, violent behavior and hallucinations. The hallmark of delirium however is alteration of consciousness. Criteria include disturbance of consciousness with reduced ability to sustain attention, changes in cognition (memory problems, language disturbance, disorientation), and perceptual disturbances. These develop over a short period of time and can fluctuate during the course of a day. Dementia on the other hand consists of multiple cognitive deficits including memory loss, aphasia, apraxia, agnosia, and disturbance of executive function.

Neurocognitive Disorders

K&S Ch. 10

Question 148. D. The first step in treating a sleep problem is to rule out any problems in the environment that could cause insomnia and to alter the environment to make it more conducive to sleep. This approach starts with the rule that the bed is to be used for sleep and sex only. Reading in bed or watching television in bed should not be permitted. If this should fail, then pharmacologic aids can be pursued. A sleep study is not warranted by a simple complaint of insomnia. That would be overkill. Of course, a detailed history is the best tool to determine whether or not a more serious sleep disturbance is present.

Sleep Wake Disorders

K&S Ch. 24

Question 149. E. The American Psychiatric Association does not see homosexuality as a disorder. As such, there is no therapy that is warranted to change it. It is seen as a normal variant of human sexuality. There is good data to suggest that therapy to change homosexuality can be damaging to the patient. There is no evidence that supports attempting to change a patient's sexual orientation. Such therapy should not be encouraged. Neither teens nor adults should be treated for being homosexual.

Sexual Dysfunctions

K&S Ch. 21

Question 150. D. Methylenedioxyamphetamine (MDMA) is also known as ecstasy. It is in the amphetamine family and is a common drug of abuse at clubs and raves. Symptoms of intoxication with amphetamines include euphoria, changes in sociability, hypervigilance, changes in interpersonal sensitivity, anxiety, anger and impaired judgment. Amphetamines can induce a psychosis which includes paranoia, hyperactivity and hypersexuality. Physical effects include fever, headache, cyanosis, vomiting (leading to dehydration), shortness of breath, ataxia, and tremor. More serious effects can include myocardial infarction, severe hypertension, and ischemic colitis. Cannabis intoxication presents as impaired coordination, euphoria or anxiety, sense of slowed time, social withdrawal and impaired judgment. Physical signs include conjunctival injection, increased appetite, tachycardia, and dry mouth. Ketamine is a relative of PCP. Intoxication presents as belligerence, impulsivity, psychomotor agitation, and impaired judgment. Physical signs include nystagmus, hypertension, ataxia, dysarthria, or muscle rigidity. Psychosis may be present and can persist for up to two weeks after intoxication. Diacetylmorphine is heroin. Intoxication results in euphoria followed by apathy, psychomotor agitation or retardation, impaired judgment, pupillary dilation, sedation, slurred speech and impaired attention or memory. Volatile inhalant intoxication presents as belligerence, assaultiveness, apathy, impaired judgment, dizziness, nystagmus, impaired coordination, unsteady gait, lethargy, tremor, psychomotor retardation, muscle weakness, euphoria or coma. Low doses of these substances can cause feelings of euphoria. High doses can cause paranoia, fearfulness and hallucinations.

Substance Abuse and Addictive Disorders

K&S Ch. 12

TWO

Test Number Two

1. Which one of the following is false?

    A. *Carl Jung focused on the growth of the personality and individuation*

    B. *Harry Stack Sullivan saw human development as a function of social interaction*

    C. *Erik Erikson developed a model of the life cycle that spanned from childhood to old age*

    D. *Jean Piaget developed a theory of cognitive development*

    E. *The work of Freud, Jung and Erikson was a function of carefully crafted psychological and neurodevelopmental studies*

2. A 75-year-old woman presents to the emergency room with an acute onset of right hemisensory loss, mild right hemiparesis and a right-sided Babinski sign. On mental status examination, you note that she cannot repeat simple phrases, she can follow simple task instructions both verbal and on paper, she cannot write well, and she is having word-finding difficulties with multiple paraphasic errors. This clinical picture is consistent with a:

    A. *Broca's aphasia*

    B. *Wernicke's aphasia*

    C. *Transcortical sensory aphasia*

    D. *Conduction aphasia*

    E. *Transcortical motor aphasia*

3. Which one of the following statements is not true regarding receptors?

    A. *Seven-transmembrane domain receptors require G proteins to open ion channels*

    B. *In the ligand-gated ion channel receptor, the channel is built into the complex that binds the ligand*

    C. *Seven-transmembrane domain receptors have an external NH_2 terminal end and an intracellular COOH terminal end*

    D. *Nerve growth factor (NGF) and brain-derived neurotropic factor (BDNF) bind to seven-transmembrane domain receptors*

    E. *Hormones may diffuse into the cell and bind cytoplasmic receptors, which leads to influence over gene expression*

 Full test available online - see inside front cover for details.

4. Correcting hyponatremia too rapidly with hypertonic saline replacement can result in:

   A. *Guillain–Barré syndrome*

   B. *Acute thalamic hemorrhage*

   C. *Acute demyelinating encephalomyelitis (ADEM)*

   D. *Acute cerebellar syndrome*

   E. *Acute locked-in syndrome*

5. A patient comes into your office and explains away why he beat his brother with a baseball bat. He gives several examples of how his brother had mistreated him in the past and says that if he had not gotten this beating the mistreatment would have continued. Which of the following defenses does this represent?

   A. *Projection*

   B. *Blocking*

   C. *Externalization*

   D. *Rationalization*

   E. *Denial*

6. A 34-year-old obese African-American woman presents to the emergency room with a complaint of 6 weeks of intermittent bifrontal headache and vague visual obscurations. She is on oral contraceptive medication and has a history of being on tetracycline therapy for a recent sexually transmitted disease. The immediate diagnostic test of choice in the emergency room is:

   A. *Noncontrast head CT scan*

   B. *Lumbar puncture with cerebrospinal fluid opening pressure*

   C. *Brain MRI without gadolinium*

   D. *Serum sedimentation rate (ESR)*

   E. *Serum prolactin level*

7. Which of the following organizations is made up of family members of the mentally ill?

   A. *American Association for Mental Health*

   B. *National Mental Health Assembly*

   C. *National Alliance for the Mentally Ill*

   D. *Council for Mental Health Reform*

   E. *Association for the Advancement of Psychotherapy*

8. Which one of the following is not a diagnostic criterion of migraine without aura?

   A. *Headache must last 4 to 72 hours*

   B. *Pulsatile quality*

   C. *Photophobia*

   D. *Nausea and vomiting*

   E. *Mild to moderate intensity*

9. What is the lifetime prevalence of schizophrenia?

   A. *10%*

   B. *5%*

   C. *1%*

   D. *0.5%*

   E. *0.1%*

10. Which one of the following is not a contraindication to the use of recombinant tissue plasminogen activator (r-TPA) in acute ischemic stroke?

A. *Stroke occurrence 2 hours prior to r-TPA administration*

B. *Major surgery within 2 weeks of r-TPA administration*

C. *Uncontrolled hypertension*

D. *Prothrombin time > 15*

E. *Thrombocytopenia*

11. Which of the following is based on active outreach to patients in the community?

A. *Traditional social work*

B. *Assertive community treatment*

C. *Day hospitals*

D. *Psychiatric rehabilitation*

E. *Electroconvulsive therapy*

12. A 45-year-old woman presents to your office complaining of longstanding lower extremity discomfort, particularly at night prior to sleep onset. She reports shooting pains in the lower extremities that are relieved upon standing or walking. The discomfort is described as a "crawling" sensation. The treatment of choice for her condition is:

A. *Sertraline*

B. *Cyproheptadine*

C. *Ropinirole*

D. *Levetiracetam*

E. *Ziprasidone*

13. Which of the following is the best diagnostic procedure to determine if a 12-year-old boy is depressed?

A. *MMPI*

B. *Scholastic achievement test*

C. *Dexamethasone suppression test*

D. *Face to face interview with the child*

E. *Interview the child's teacher by phone*

14. A 65-year-old man presents to the emergency room with acute onset of vertigo, nausea, vomiting, dysarthria and nystagmus. On further examination, he is noted to have loss of pain and temperature sensation to the left-hand side of his face. He has right-sided loss of pain and temperature sensation to his trunk and leg. He has a left Horner's syndrome and falls to his left-hand side when you ask him to walk, and has left finger-to-nose dysmetria. You diagnose an acute stroke which is most likely localized to the:

A. *Left hemisphere*

B. *Left lateral medulla*

C. *Left pons*

D. *Right pons*

E. *Right lateral medulla*

15. Which of the following is associated with violence and aggression?

    A. *Blunted response to CRH stimulation test*

    B. *Blunted growth hormone response to hypoglycemia*

    C. *Decreased 5-HIAA in the CSF*

    D. *Decreased dopamine in the CSF*

    E. *Increased levels of norepinephrine in the CSF*

16. Metachromatic leukodystrophy is inherited by _____ pattern of inheritance and results in a deficiency in _____:

    A. *Autosomal recessive; hexosaminidase A*

    B. *Autosomal dominant; hexosaminidase A*

    C. *Autosomal dominant; arylsulfatase A*

    D. *Autosomal recessive; arylsulfatase A*

    E. *Autosomal recessive; galactocerebroside β-galactosidase*

17. Which one of the following is not true with respect to seasonal affective disorders (SAD)?

    A. *Patients are likely to respond well to light therapy*

    B. *The "with seasonal pattern" specifier can be applied to bipolar I, bipolar II, and major depressive disorders according to the DSM-IV*

    C. *It is not necessary to have full remissions of symptoms at other times of the year to make this diagnosis*

    D. *SAD involves a regular temporal relationship between the onset of symptoms and the time of year*

    E. *You must demonstrate at least two depressive episodes at the same time of year to make the diagnosis*

18. Which one of the following primitive reflexes is not generally expected to disappear by about 6 months of age?

    A. *Rooting*

    B. *Moro*

    C. *Palmar grasp*

    D. *Parachute response*

    E. *Tonic neck reflex*

19. Which of the following would fall under the heading of somatoform disorder NOS?

    A. *A patient with pain in one or more areas that is thought to be significantly mediated by psychological factors*

    B. *A patient with a persistent belief that she has cancer despite reassurance by her physician that nothing is wrong*

    C. *A patient who develops a motor deficit following significant psychological stressors*

    D. *A patient who feels that she is pregnant and presents with amenorrhea, enlarged abdomen, and breast engorgement, but a negative pregnancy test*

    E. *A patient with medical complaints involving pain, GI complaints, neurological complaints, and sexual complaints. No medical explanation can be found for these symptoms*

20. An AIDS patient presents with decreased visual acuity. The most likely offending infectious agent responsible for this presentation is:

    A. *Cytomegalovirus*

    B. *Toxoplasmosis*

    C. *Tuberculosis (Mycobacterium)*

    D. *Cryptococcus neoformans*

    E. *JC virus*

21. Which one of the following is not true regarding schizophrenia?

    A. *The disorder is chronic and usually has a prodromal phase*

    B. *Eugen Bleuler coined the term schizophrenia*

    C. *The patient's overall functioning declines or fails to reach the expected level*

    D. *The most frequent hallucinations are olfactory*

    E. *Social withdrawal and emotional disengagement are common*

22. Which one of the following is not seen in narcolepsy?

    A. *Cataplexy*

    B. *Nighttime awakening*

    C. *Excessive daytime sleepiness*

    D. *Sleep paralysis*

    E. *Hypnagogic hallucinations*

23. Uncontrollable excessive talking, as seen in mania is also known as:

    A. *Alexithymia*

    B. *Logorrhea*

    C. *Echolalia*

    D. *Flight of ideas*

    E. *Stilted speech*

24. Which one of the following is not an appropriate therapy for status epilepticus?

    A. *Rectal diazepam*

    B. *Intravenous lorazepam*

    C. *Intramuscular phenytoin*

    D. *Intravenous valproic acid*

    E. *Oxygen by nasal cannula with airway protection*

25. Which one of the following statements is true regarding atypical antipsychotics?

    A. *Ziprasidone is an agonist at the 5-HT-1A receptor, and an inhibitor of reuptake of both serotonin and norepinephrine*

    B. *Risperidone is a significantly weaker antagonist of D2 than haloperidol*

    C. *Quetiapine is known for its high incidence of extrapyramidal symptoms*

    D. *Olanzapine has been associated with weight loss in the majority of patients*

    E. *Clozapine has been shown to increase suicidality in chronically ill patients*

26. Which of the following anticonvulsant agents is most appropriate for primary generalized seizures including tonic–clonic, absence, atonic and myoclonic seizure types?

    A. *Divalproex sodium*

    B. *Phenytoin*

    C. *Oxcarbazepine*

    D. *Carbamazepine*

    E. *Ethosuximide*

27. Which of the following is not a side effect of the tricyclic antidepressants?

    A. *Tachycardia*

    B. *Prolonged PR interval*

    C. *Prolonged QRS interval*

    D. *Orthostatic hypotension*

    E. *Diarrhea*

28. The L5 motor nerve root innervates the nerves responsible for:

    A. *Foot extension*

    B. *Foot flexion*

    C. *Leg extension*

    D. *Hip flexion*

    E. *The ankle jerk reflex*

29. Which one of the following antidepressants can be used as an antipruritic agent and for the treatment of gastric ulcer because of its potent histamine blockade?

    A. *Trazodone*

    B. *Fluoxetine*

    C. *Citalopram*

    D. *Amitriptyline*

    E. *Amoxapine*

30. A patient involved in a car accident is found on MRI to have a spinal fracture and a partial crush lesion to the cervical spinal cord that effectively causes a functional hemisection of the cord. His deficits would be expected to include:

    A. *Contralateral loss of motor control and pain and temperature sensation with ipsilateral loss of proprioception and vibration sensation*

    B. *Ipsilateral loss of motor control and pain and temperature sensation with contralateral loss of proprioception and vibration sensation*

    C. *Ipsilateral loss of motor control and proprioception and vibration sensation with contralateral loss of pain and temperature sensation*

    D. *Contralateral loss of motor control and proprioception and vibration sensation with ipsilateral loss of pain and temperature sensation*

    E. *Ipsilateral loss of motor control and contralateral loss of proprioception, vibration, pain and temperature sensations*

31. A child is able to use some symbols and language. Her reasoning is intuitive. She is unable to think logically or deductively. Which of Piaget's stages does this child fit into?

    A. *Sensorimotor*

    B. *Preoperational thought*

    C. *Concrete operations*

    D. *Formal operations*

    E. *Trust vs mistrust*

32. A 72-year-old man suffers a stroke with loss of motor functioning in the left leg and, to a lesser extent, the left arm. He has abulia and his eyes and head seem preferentially deviated to the right. His left arm is apraxic. His head CT is shown below. The arterial territory involved is that of the:

A. *Right middle cerebral artery*

B. *Right posterior cerebral artery*

C. *Right vertebral artery*

D. *Right anterior cerebral artery*

E. *Right posterior communicating artery*

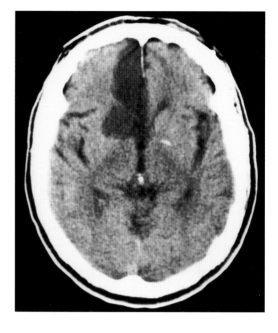

33. Which of the following is true regarding norepinephrine (NE) and/or the locus ceruleus?

A. *Norepinephrine is synthesized in the locus ceruleus*

B. *Dopamine is synthesized in the locus ceruleus, NE in the dorsal raphe nuclei*

C. *Acetylcholine is synthesized with NE in the substantia nigra*

D. *5-HT is synthesized in the locus ceruleus*

E. *The locus ceruleus is the site of the formation of serotonin*

34. Pure motor hemiparesis is most likely to result from a stroke localized to the:

A. *Midbrain*

B. *Cerebellum*

C. *Medulla*

D. *Thalamus*

E. *Internal capsule*

35. Which one of the following receptor types is associated with weight gain and sedation?

A. *5-HT-2A*

B. *Alpha 1*

C. *5-HT-1A*

D. *H1*

E. *M1*

36. The lesion causing a left-arm hemiballismus would most likely localize to the:

    A. *Right subthalamic nucleus*

    B. *Left subthalamic nucleus*

    C. *Right putamen*

    D. *Left putamen*

    E. *Right globus pallidus interna*

37. Which of the following is not a biogenic amine neurotransmitter?

    A. *Dopamine*

    B. *GABA*

    C. *Epinephrine*

    D. *Acetylcholine*

    E. *Serotonin*

38. The mechanism of action by which reserpine both improves the symptoms of adult-onset primary focal dystonia and can cause depression is:

    A. *Direct postsynaptic dopamine antagonism*

    B. *Direct postsynaptic serotonin agonism*

    C. *Direct postsynaptic serotonin antagonism*

    D. *Presynaptic dopaminergic depletion*

    E. *Direct postsynaptic cholinergic antagonism*

39. In the psychotic patient, the defense mechanism of projection takes the form of:

    A. *Feelings of persecution*

    B. *Feelings of abandonment*

    C. *Feelings of sadness*

    D. *Feelings of gratification*

    E. *Feelings of isolation*

40. The drainage of cerebrospinal fluid into the blood is a function of the:

    A. *Choroid plexus*

    B. *Virchow–Robin spaces*

    C. *Dural mitochondria*

    D. *Ventricular ependymal cells*

    E. *Arachnoid granulations*

41. Which one of the following is a method of making a prediction in order to compare the value of one variable to another?

    A. *Probability*

    B. *Point prevalence*

    C. *Incidence*

    D. *Regression analysis*

    E. *Kappa*

42. A 72-year-old woman with a history of smoking, diabetes, hypertension, hyperlipidemia and myocardial infarction presents to your emergency room by ambulance with an acute onset of obtundation with dense right hemiplegia, right hemisensory loss to light touch, pain and temperature, and mutism. You suspect a left lobar hemorrhage because of the acuity of onset of her symptoms and a blood pressure reading of 210/100 mmHg in the emergency room. Once stabilized, the best immediate diagnostic test of choice from the emergency room would be:

   A. *Lumbar puncture with opening pressure and CSF assay for xanthochromia*

   B. *Brain MRI scan without gadolinium*

   C. *Blood work for coagulation panel (PT, PTT, INR)*

   D. *Noncontrast head CT scan*

   E. *Routine bedside electroencephalogram (EEG)*

43. Which one of the following is most closely associated with prognostic outcome in psychodynamic therapy?

   A. *Length of training*

   B. *Neutrality of the therapist*

   C. *Age of the therapist*

   D. *Gender of the therapist*

   E. *Empathy and warmth*

44. Melatonin is a neuronal hormone that promotes sleep and is produced in the brain by the:

   A. *Pineal gland*

   B. *Anterior pituitary gland*

   C. *Posterior pituitary gland*

   D. *Hypothalamus*

   E. *Thalamus*

45. Which one of the following is an objective psychological test?

   A. *Rorschach*

   B. *Sentence completion test*

   C. *Thematic apperception test*

   D. *MMPI*

   E. *Draw a person test*

46. Subacute sclerosing panencephalitis is a rare late complication of which one of the following organisms:

   A. *Measles virus*

   B. *Herpes simplex virus*

   C. *Epstein–Barr virus*

   D. *Mumps virus*

   E. *JC virus*

47. Which one of the following does not describe a patient with ADHD?

   A. *The patient fails to follow through on instructions and fails to finish schoolwork*

   B. *The patient often fidgets with hands or feet or squirms in his seat*

   C. *The patient often has difficulty awaiting his turn*

   D. *The patient often seems not to listen when spoken to directly*

   E. *The patient shows impairment from symptoms at school but not at home*

48. A 13-year-old boy is brought to the emergency room from a group home because of acute agitation. On examination you note choreoathetotic movements, hyperreflexia, acute agitation, self-scratching and mutilating behavior, and a marked cognitive impairment. You peruse the group home chart and note that this young boy has an enzymatic deficiency in hypoxanthine-guanine phosphoribosyltransferase. Your keen memory brings you back to your pediatrics rotation in medical school and you realize the diagnosis is:

    A. *Tay–Sachs disease*

    B. *Metachromatic leukodystrophy*

    C. *Krabbe disease*

    D. *Gaucher's disease*

    E. *Lesch–Nyhan syndrome*

49. Which one of the following is not a DSM IV-TR criterion for schizophrenia?

    A. *Delusions*

    B. *Presence of active phase symptoms for 6 months*

    C. *Hallucinations*

    D. *Disorganized speech*

    E. *Grossly disorganized or catatonic behavior*

50. Botulinum toxin type A is not the treatment of choice for which one of the following disorders?

    A. *Hemifacial spasm*

    B. *Blepharospasm*

    C. *Cervical dystonia*

    D. *Restless legs syndrome*

    E. *Limb spasticity related to multiple sclerosis*

51. A patient presents with a delusion about being poisoned that has been present for 5 months. The patient has no hallucinations or other psychotic symptoms. There has been no major impact on the patient's daily functioning. The patient has no mood symptoms. The most likely diagnosis is:

    A. *Dementia*

    B. *Schizophrenia*

    C. *Schizoaffective disorder, bipolar type*

    D. *Delusional disorder*

    E. *Brief psychotic disorder*

52. A young woman presents to the emergency room with a complaint of a band-like, bifrontal, squeezing headache that began six hours earlier. She denies nausea, vomiting, or any other associated symptoms. She describes the pain as waxing-and-waning in intensity throughout the six-hour period. Physical examination is unremarkable. She reports suffering from similar attacks in the past. The most likely diagnosis is:

    A. *Tension-type headache*

    B. *Migraine without aura*

    C. *Migraine with aura*

    D. *Paroxysmal hemicrania*

    E. *Basilar migraine*

53. Which one of the following is not consistent with a major depressive episode?

    A. *Anhedonia*

    B. *Withdrawal from social situations*

    C. *Low frustration tolerance*

    D. *Weight loss*

    E. *Increased libido*

54. The generator of migraine headache is thought to be the:

    A. *Reticular activating system*

    B. *Trigeminal nucleus caudalis*

    C. *Dural and intracerebral blood vessels*

    D. *Suprachiasmatic nucleus*

    E. *Contraction of scalp and cranial muscles*

55. A patient comes to your clinic with complaint of hypersomnia, hyperphagia, psychomotor slowing, and depressed mood. He states that this happens yearly usually around October or November. The treatment plan for this man should include:

    A. *Risperidone*

    B. *Naloxone*

    C. *Exposure to bright artificial light for 2–6 hours per day.*

    D. *Flooding*

    E. *Alprazolam*

56. What is the mechanism of action of carbidopa in the combination agent carbidopa–levodopa that is used for the treatment of Parkinson's disease?

    A. *Postsynaptic dopamine receptor agonism*

    B. *Monoamine oxidase type B inhibition*

    C. *Dopa decarboxylase inhibition*

    D. *Catechol-O-methyltransferase inhibition*

    E. *Acetylcholine receptor antagonism*

57. A young woman presents to the emergency room with complaints of palpitations, sweating, shortness of breath, chest pain and nausea. She thinks that she is having a heart attack. EKG reveals normal sinus rhythm with no ischemic changes. Cardiac enzymes are not elevated. Given her symptoms, an alternative diagnosis would be:

    A. *Manic episode*

    B. *Myxedema madness*

    C. *Mad Hatter's syndrome*

    D. *Psychotic disorder NOS*

    E. *Panic attack*

58. The phenomenon of apoptosis refers to:

    A. *Neuronal migration*

    B. *Neuronal maturation*

    C. *Neurogenesis*

    D. *Neuronal myelination*

    E. *Neuronal programmed cell death*

59. Which of the following is not a tricyclic antidepressant?

    A. *Amitriptyline*

    B. *Amoxapine*

    C. *Doxepin*

    D. *Desipramine*

    E. *Nortriptyline*

60. A 2-year-old toddler is brought to the emergency room because of seizures, hemiparesis and apparent blindness. You immediately notice a marked reddish discoloration of the left side of the forehead and face. The parents tell you that their child has not met appropriate developmental milestones. Your most likely diagnosis is:

    A. *Tuberous sclerosis*

    B. *Sturge–Weber syndrome*

    C. *Von Hippel–Lindau disease*

    D. *Ataxia–telangiectasia*

    E. *Fabry's disease*

61. How is a doctor who agrees to take Medicare paid?

    A. *He agrees to take only what Medicare pays for the service*

    B. *He is allowed to bill the patient for the difference between what Medicare pays and what he charges*

    C. *He is paid by a third party to make up the difference between his fee for service rate and the fee allowed by Medicare*

    D. *He can sue the government if his full fee is not paid*

    E. *He is not allowed to charge copays*

62. The pain syndrome known as reflex sympathetic dystrophy does not involve which one of the following characteristics?

    A. *Hypersensitivity to painful stimuli*

    B. *Myofascial trigger points*

    C. *Cyanosis of the extremities*

    D. *Sweating and shiny skin*

    E. *Warm or hot skin on the extremities*

63. The police bring an acutely paranoid patient into the Emergency Room who was found wandering the streets. In your initial approach to this patient you should first:

    A. *Sedate the patient with haloperidol and lorazepam*

    B. *Assess the dangerousness of the patient to self or others*

    C. *Obtain an EKG*

    D. *Contact the patient's family if possible*

    E. *Obtain any old charts from medical records*

64. Carbamazepine will not lower the levels or the efficacy of which one of the following agents?

    A. *Warfarin*

    B. *Clozapine*

    C. *Alprazolam*

    D. *Propranolol*

    E. *Citalopram*

65. Which one of the following is false concerning the right to die and surrogate decision making?

    A. *Patients that believe that continuing treatment would lessen their quality of life have the right to demand that treatment be withheld or withdrawn*

    B. *Advanced directives or a living will are a way for patients to express their preferences before anything happens that would cause them to lose capacity*

    C. *If a patient leaves no clear instructions, the state will carry out a course of action to protect and preserve human life*

    D. *Surrogate decision makers can be appointed by the patient, or the courts*

    E. *The standard of substituted judgment means that the surrogate will do whatever is in the patient's best interests*

66. Patients who smoke tobacco heavily can markedly reduce levels of psychotropic medications they are taking. Which one of the following medications is not affected by tobacco smoking in this way?

    A. *Clozapine*

    B. *Olanzapine*

    C. *Haloperidol*

    D. *Risperidone*

    E. *Amitriptyline*

67. A consultation-liaison psychiatrist is called to evaluate a patient who is in denial of a major illness. The most important obligation of the psychiatrist at the first evaluation is to:

    A. *Confront the denial forcefully*

    B. *Tell the staff to "play along" with the patient's denial*

    C. *Obtain neuropsychological testing*

    D. *Meet with the patient's family*

    E. *Make sure the patient has been informed about the illness and treatment*

68. A 38-year-old delivers twins by uncomplicated cesarean section at 37 weeks. The pregnancy, her first, was unremarkable. On day three following her delivery, she experiences an acute onset of what she describes as the worst headache of her life. The neurologist is called and discovers that she has a notable bitemporal hemianopsia, neck stiffness, a positive Kernig's sign, persistent hypotension and a right third nerve palsy. The most likely diagnosis is:

    A. *Sheehan's syndrome*

    B. *Cushing's disease*

    C. *Subarachnoid hemorrhage*

    D. *Acute bacterial meningitis*

    E. *Familial hemiplegic migraine*

69. A patient describes feeling anxious about being in places or situations from which escape may be difficult or in which help may not be available should the patient begin to panic. The patient avoids various situations because of these fears. The term that best describes this patient's symptoms is:

    A. *Agonothete*

    B. *Agoniada*

    C. *Agoraphobia*

    D. *Agora*

    E. *Agouara*

70. Normal-pressure hydrocephalus presents as the triad of:

    A. *Dementia, parkinsonism, and visual hallucinations*

    B. *Dementia, ophthalmoplegia, and ataxia*

    C. *Dementia, incontinence, and gait disturbance*

    D. *Chorea, irritability, and obsessive–compulsive traits*

    E. *Dementia, axial rigidity, and vertical ophthalmoplegia*

71. Which one of the following is not true concerning cyclothymic disorder?

    A. *It is similar to bipolar disorder, but less severe*

    B. *Symptoms must be present for at least 2 years*

    C. *It is equally common in men and women*

    D. *Substance abuse is common in patients with cyclothymia*

    E. *There are often psychotic symptoms found in patients with cyclothymia*

72. Which one of the following is not a potential risk factor for ischemic stroke?

    A. *Prior cardiac disease*

    B. *Depression*

    C. *Gender*

    D. *Family history*

    E. *Obesity*

73. A patient enters your office. She is agitated, acts seductively, wears colorful clothes that are bizarre in appearance, has an excessive amount of makeup on, and vacillates between being entertaining, hyperexcited, and threatening. Based on this information, her most likely diagnosis is:

    A. *Major depressive disorder*

    B. *Brief psychotic disorder*

    C. *Body dysmorphic disorder*

    D. *Bipolar disorder*

    E. *Delusional disorder*

74. Which one of the following symptoms is not suggestive of a carotid territory transient ischemic attack or stroke?

    A. *Ataxia with vertigo*

    B. *Aphasia*

    C. *Ipsilateral monocular blindness*

    D. *Contralateral body weakness*

    E. *Contralateral homonymous visual field defects*

75. Which of the following is not commonly part of the thought process of the manic bipolar patient?

    A. *Flight of ideas*

    B. *Clang associations*

    C. *Racing thoughts*

    D. *Tangentiality*

    E. *Suicidal ideation*

76. Which one of the following agents is not potentially useful for the treatment of essential tremor?

    A. *Lorazepam*

    B. *Primidone*

    C. *Propranolol*

    D. *Desipramine*

    E. *Botulinum toxin type A*

77. To meet criteria for a major depressive disorder, a patient must have symptoms for:

    A. *1 week*

    B. *2 weeks*

    C. *1 month*

    D. *2 months*

    E. *6 weeks*

78. Which one of the following tumors is associated with myasthenia gravis?

    A. *Thyroid carcinoma*

    B. *Thymoma*

    C. *Glioblastoma multiforme*

    D. *Breast papilloma*

    E. *Non-Hodgkin's lymphoma*

79. Which one of the following is not true regarding schizophrenia?

    A. *Lifetime prevalence is about 1%*

    B. *Prevalence is greater in rural than in urban areas*

    C. *The male-to-female ratio is 1:1*

    D. *Onset is rare before age 10 years or after age 40 years*

    E. *There is a higher incidence of the disease in babies born in winter and early spring*

80. Which one of the following genetically inherited neurological disorders is not acquired by autosomal dominant heredity?

    A. *Friedrich's ataxia*

    B. *Myotonic dystrophy*

    C. *Tuberous sclerosis*

    D. *Huntington's disease*

    E. *Neurofibromatosis*

81. Which one of the following is not a characteristic of a major depressive episode?

    A. *Constipation*

    B. *Dry mouth*

    C. *Headache*

    D. *Disinhibited behavior*

    E. *Early morning awakening*

82. Migraine is most likely a hereditary disorder that maps to which chromosome:

    A. Chromosome 14

    B. Chromosome 15

    C. Chromosome 17

    D. Chromosome 18

    E. Chromosome 19

83. Which one of the following would be listed under thought content in the mental status exam?

    A. Obsessions

    B. Word salad

    C. Flight of ideas

    D. Circumstantiality

    E. Tangentiality

84. CNS cysticercosis is caused by brain parenchymal invasion by which one of the following organisms:

    A. Leishmania major

    B. Taenia solium

    C. Toxoplasma gondii

    D. Echinococcus granulosus

    E. Trichinella spiralis

85. Which of the following lab tests can be used to detect chronic alcohol abuse?

    A. RBC count

    B. WBC count

    C. GGT

    D. CPK

    E. Alkaline phosphatase

86. The most frequent neurological complication of chronic alcohol abuse is:

    A. Wernicke's encephalopathy

    B. Alcoholic cerebellar degeneration

    C. Alcoholic neuropathy

    D. Marchiafava–Bignami disease

    E. Alcoholic dementia

87. A study in which a group comes from a well-defined population and is followed over a long period of time is a:

    A. Case history study

    B. Cohort study

    C. Cross-sectional study

    D. Case–control study

    E. Retrospective study

88. The Miller–Fisher syndrome involves the classic symptom complex of:

A. *Dementia, parkinsonism, psychosis*

B. *Gait ataxia, urinary incontinence and dementia*

C. *Ataxia, areflexia, ophthalmoplegia*

D. *Alexia without agraphia*

E. *Right–left confusion, finger agnosia, acaculia*

89. Konrad Lorenz, during his work with animals demonstrated which one of the following concepts which may be used to understand early human psychological development?

A. *Sensory deprivation*

B. *Altruism*

C. *Imprinting*

D. *Stress syndromes*

E. *Episodic dyscontrol*

90. A 29-year-old woman presents to the ER by ambulance in a wheelchair. She was brought from home with a complaint of rapidly progressive bilateral leg weakness over the past 2 weeks. Her legs were also painful and she complained of numbness and tingling in the lower part of both legs. Just prior to the onset of symptoms she had a 3-day bout of bad diarrhea with fever and chills that resolved spontaneously. Which one of the following would not be a likely finding on diagnostic testing and examination of this patient?

A. *Diminished deep tendon reflexes*

B. *High cell count with absent protein in CSF*

C. *Conduction block and prolonged F-wave latencies on nerve conduction studies*

D. *Positive Campylobacter jejuni antibody serology*

E. *Complement fixing antibodies to peripheral nerve myelin on nerve biopsy*

91. Which one of the following is not a second messenger?

A. *Adenylyl cyclase*

B. *cGMP*

C. *Ca^{2+}*

D. *cAMP*

E. *IP_3*

92. Which one of the following is not more typical of a cortical dementia than of a subcortical dementia such as dementia of the Alzheimer type?

A. *Apathy and depression*

B. *Aphasia*

C. *Dyspraxia*

D. *Absence of motor abnormalities*

E. *Insidious progression of cognitive decline*

93. A child is playing in his home, and at the same time that his dog barks the doorbell also rings. The child believes that the doorbell rang because the dog barked. This child would fit best into which of Piaget's stages?

    A. Sensorimotor

    B. Preoperational thought

    C. Concrete operations

    D. Formal operations

    E. Latency

94. The sensory dermatomes of the nipples and the umbilicus are respectively located at the level of:

    A. T2 and T8

    B. T3 and T9

    C. T4 and T10

    D. T5 and T11

    E. T6 and T12

95. Which one of the following receptor subtypes is associated with the neurotransmitter glutamate?

    A. Nicotinic

    B. Muscarinic

    C. Alpha 1

    D. AMPA

    E. GABA

96. Buspirone's mechanism of action is predominantly linked to which one of the following receptors:

    A. Serotonin 2A

    B. Serotonin 1A

    C. NMDA

    D. Dopamine 2

    E. Norepinephrine

97. Which one of the following statements is true regarding excitatory neurotransmitters?

    A. They open anion channels that depolarize the cell membrane and increase the likelihood of generating an action potential

    B. They open cation channels that hyperpolarize the cell membrane and increase the likelihood of generating an action potential

    C. They open cation channels that hyperpolarize the cell membrane and decrease the likelihood of generating an action potential

    D. They open anion channels that hyperpolarize the cell membrane and decrease the likelihood of generating an action potential

    E. They open cation channels that depolarize the cell membrane and increase the likelihood of generating an action potential

98. Phencyclidine (PCP) exerts its hallucinogenic effects primarily by mediation of which of the following receptors:

    A. Serotonin 2A

    B. Serotonin 1A

    C. NMDA

    D. Dopamine 2

    E. Norepinephrine

99. Which one of the following is not an immature defense?

  A. *Hypochondriasis*

  B. *Introjection*

  C. *Sublimation*

  D. *Regression*

  E. *Passive aggression*

100. Which one of the following agents is least likely to exacerbate the extra-pyramidal symptoms of Parkinson's disease?

  A. *Amoxapine*

  B. *Perphenazine*

  C. *Thorazine*

  D. *Fluphenazine*

  E. *Phenelzine*

101. Who was the author of *The Ego and Mechanisms of Defense*, and gave us the first comprehensive study of defense mechanisms?

  A. *Sigmund Freud*

  B. *Kohut*

  C. *Erich Fromm*

  D. *Ana Freud*

  E. *Carl Jung*

102. Which one of the following is not necessary for a patient to be declared competent to stand trial?

  A. *Understanding of the nature of the charges against him*

  B. *Not having a mental illness*

  C. *Having the ability to consult a lawyer*

  D. *Helping the lawyer in his defense*

  E. *Understanding of court procedure*

103. Which one of the following is present in paranoid schizophrenia?

  A. *Flat affect*

  B. *Catatonic behavior*

  C. *Incoherence*

  D. *Preoccupation with systematized delusions*

  E. *Grossly disorganized behavior*

104. How long should a patient remain on antidepressant medication after having experienced four major depressive episodes in the last five years?

  A. *3 months*

  B. *6 months*

  C. *12 months*

  D. *2 years*

  E. *Indefinitely*

105. Which one of the following symptoms is not part of dysthymic disorder?

    A. *Poor appetite*

    B. *Low self-esteem*

    C. *Feelings of hopelessness*

    D. *Hallucinations*

    E. *Fatigue*

106. Which ruling determined that the physician–patient relationship imposes an obligation on the psychiatrist for care and safety of the patient and others?

    A. *Wyatt vs Stickney*

    B. *Durham vs the United States*

    C. *O'Connor vs Donaldson*

    D. *Tarasoff vs regents of the University of California*

    E. *Clites vs State*

107. Which one of the following tricyclic antidepressants is not considered a tertiary amine?

    A. *Imipramine*

    B. *Amitriptyline*

    C. *Desipramine*

    D. *Clomipramine*

    E. *Trimipramine*

108. Which one of the following surgical interventions can not be used for the invasive treatment of idiopathic Parkinson's disease?

    A. *Thalamotomy*

    B. *Subthalamic nucleus deep brain stimulation*

    C. *Superior colliculus deep brain stimulation*

    D. *Pallidotomy*

    E. *Pallidal deep brain stimulation*

109. The metabolite of which one of the following tricyclic antidepressants has potent dopamine blocking ability that can lead to antipsychotic-like side effects?

    A. *Amoxapine*

    B. *Clomipramine*

    C. *Desipramine*

    D. *Trimipramine*

    E. *Imipramine*

110. A patient presents with a non-dominant hemispheric stroke in the middle cerebral artery territory. Which one of the following symptoms and signs would you not find on neurologic examination?

    A. *Hemi-inattention*

    B. *Anosognosia*

    C. *Right–left disorientation*

    D. *Impaired prosody of speech*

    E. *Visual and tactile extinction*

111. Interaction with the enzyme CYP 2D6 has what bearing on the use of tricyclic antidepressants?

    A. *None. Tricyclics do not interact with CYP 2D6*

    B. *Those with decreased CYP 2D6 activity will have lower than expected plasma drug concentrations*

    C. *Giving a patient on a tricyclic a CYP 2D6 inhibitor could cause a drop in the plasma concentration of the drug*

    D. *Cimetidine can cause an increase in tricyclic levels as a result of its interaction with CYP 2D6*

    E. *Concomitant use of drugs that inhibit CYP 2D6 with tricyclics may necessitate higher than usual prescribed doses of either drug to obtain the same levels*

112. A 50-year-old man presents to the emergency room with a complaint of acute onset of right eye pain, ptosis, and diplopia. The symptoms began that morning immediately upon his awakening from sleep. Your examination reveals a normal-sized pupil that is fully reactive to light and a right eye that cannot adduct nasally with a ptotic right eyelid. The most likely cause of this condition is:

    A. *Diabetes*

    B. *Stroke*

    C. *Posterior communicating artery aneurysm*

    D. *Multiple sclerosis*

    E. *Myasthenia gravis*

113. Residual schizophrenia is characterized by:

    A. *Absence of prominent hallucinations*

    B. *Delusions*

    C. *Incoherence*

    D. *Disorganized behavior*

    E. *Posturing*

114. Which one of the following agents would not be useful for the treatment of tics in Tourette's syndrome?

    A. *Fluphenazine*

    B. *Molindone*

    C. *Botulinum toxin type A*

    D. *Haloperidol*

    E. *Protriptyline*

115. Which one of the following is not characteristic of catatonic schizophrenia?

    A. *Mutism*

    B. *Negativism*

    C. *Rigidity*

    D. *Echolalia*

    E. *Grossly inappropriate affect*

116. A right middle cerebral artery territory ischemic stroke posterior to the optic chiasm would be expected to cause:

    A. *Bitemporal hemianopsia*

    B. *Left monocular blindness*

    C. *Left homonymous hemianopsia*

    D. *Right homonymous hemianopsia*

    E. *Right upper quadrantanopsia*

117. Which one of the following statements is not true regarding chemical signaling between neurons?

   A. Neurotransmitter synthesis may be stimulated by influx of Ca^{2+}

   B. Norepinephrine-releasing neurons have presynaptic alpha receptors which are involved in a negative feedback system to stop NE release

   C. Once dopamine is released into the synaptic cleft it works until it diffuses away, or is removed by reuptake mechanisms

   D. Exocytosis is the process by which neurotransmitter storage vesicles release their contents into the synaptic cleft

   E. MAO type B metabolizes NE and serotonin

118. A 4-year-old boy presents to the ER in an acute state of agitation. Careful history-taking and examination reveal hypotonia, delayed developmental milestones, athetotic movements of the upper extremities and mental retardation. The parents explain that their son constantly bites his hands and lips to the point of bleeding. Lesch–Nyhan syndrome is the clinical diagnosis. This syndrome is caused by a deficiency of which of the following enzymes:

   A. Ornithine transcarbamylase

   B. Hypoxanthine-guanine phosphoribosyltransferase

   C. Adenylosuccinate deficiency

   D. Arginase

   E. Carbamoylphosphate synthase

119. A child is brought to your office for depression. During the course of your interview you see that the patient can think abstractly, reason deductively, and define abstract concepts. This child would fit into which of Piaget's developmental stages?

   A. Sensorimotor

   B. Preoperational thought

   C. Concrete operations

   D. Formal operations

   E. Symbiosis

120. Predisposition for dementia pugilistica is increased in carriers with defects on which one of the following chromosomes:

   A. Chromosome 16

   B. Chromosome 17

   C. Chromosome 18

   D. Chromosome 19

   E. Chromosome 20

121. Which one of the tricyclic antidepressants has the most antihistaminic activity?

   A. Amoxapine

   B. Clomipramine

   C. Desipramine

   D. Nortriptyline

   E. Doxepin

122. Which one of the following is not helpful in the treatment of obsessive–compulsive disorder?

   A. Bupropion

   B. Fluvoxamine

   C. Clomipramine

   D. Sertraline

   E. Fluoxetine

123. Which one of the following is true regarding the tricyclic antidepressants?

    A. *The downregulation of β-adrenergic receptors correlates most closely with time needed for clinical improvement in patients*

    B. *Giving tricyclics leads to an increase in β-adrenergic receptors*

    C. *Giving tricyclics leads to an increase in 5-HT receptors*

    D. *Giving tricyclics leads to an increase in β-adrenergic receptors and a decrease in 5-HT receptors*

    E. *Giving tricyclics leads to a decrease in β-adrenergic receptors and an increase in 5-HT receptors*

124. Which one of the following is not effective in treating enuresis in childhood?

    A. *Desmopressin*

    B. *Bell-and-pad conditioning*

    C. *Amitriptyline*

    D. *Imipramine*

    E. *Olanzapine*

125. Which one of the following ions uses the second ion channel to open during an action potential, acts as a second messenger once in the neuron, activates the release of neurotransmitter, and activates ion channels that allow for influx of other ions that halt the action potential?

    A. Na^+

    B. K^+

    C. Cl^-

    D. Ca^{2+}

    E. IP_3

126. Patients with which one of the following disorders may have clinically significant side effects from tricyclic antidepressant drugs?

    A. *Insomnia*

    B. *Benign prostatic hypertrophy*

    C. *Migraine*

    D. *Parkinson's disease*

    E. *Pituitary adenoma*

127. Which one of the following statements is true regarding inhibitory neurotransmitters?

    A. *They open chloride channels that depolarize the cell membrane and increase the likelihood of an action potential*

    B. *They open cation channels that depolarize the cell membrane and increase the likelihood of an action potential*

    C. *They open chloride channels that hyperpolarize the cell membrane and increase the likelihood of an action potential*

    D. *They open chloride channels that hyperpolarize the cell membrane and decrease the likelihood of an action potential*

    E. *They open potassium channels that depolarize the cell membrane and decrease the likelihood of an action potential*

128. A patient with a fear of spiders is put in a room with many spiders, and immediately a live tarantula is placed on his hand for as long as necessary until the dissipation of his anxiety. This behavioral technique is called:

    A. *Graded exposure*

    B. *Aversion therapy*

    C. *Flooding*

    D. *Assertiveness training*

    E. *Modeling*

129. Which one of the following is true regarding psychoanalytic psychotherapy?

    A. *All of the patient's remarks should be taken at face value*

    B. *Most of what the patient says is unimportant*

    C. *Disclaimers often precede emotionally charged material, and are important to note*

    D. *It's important to point out to the patient every instance in which they exhibit low self-esteem*

    E. *One should interpret the patient's resistance at each and every opportunity*

130. An 82-year-old patient in a skilled nursing facility displays confusion, restlessness, agitation, and disorganized speech only during the evening hours. Which one of the following is not an appropriate treatment approach?

    A. *Increased lighting in the room*

    B. *Low dose haloperidol at bedtime*

    C. *Having a calendar on the wall*

    D. *Flurazepam at bedtime for sleep*

    E. *Companionship and family support during the day*

131. Which one of the following is not a technique used in cognitive therapy?

    A. *Reattribution*

    B. *Role playing*

    C. *Thought recording*

    D. *Abreaction*

    E. *Developing alternatives*

132. Heroin withdrawal does not involve which one of the following symptoms?

    A. *Pinpoint pupils*

    B. *Abdominal pain*

    C. *Piloerection*

    D. *Muscle twitching*

    E. *Dysphoria*

133. Which one of the following is among the least sedating of the tricyclic anti-depressants?

    A. *Desipramine*

    B. *Amitriptyline*

    C. *Trimipramine*

    D. *Doxepin*

    E. *Imipramine*

134. Which one of the following is not an example of secondary gain?

    A. *Getting money*

    B. *Getting medical help*

    C. *Getting out of having to work*

    D. *Getting out of family responsibilities*

    E. *Getting drugs of abuse*

135. In hypothyroidism one would expect to find:

    A. *Serum free T4 is increased*

    B. *Serum total T4 concentration is increased*

    C. *Serum thyroid stimulating hormone is increased*

    D. *Serum T3 uptake is increased*

    E. *Serum T3–T4 ratio is decreased*

136. Which one of the following conditions involves increased risk in electroconvulsive shock therapy (ECT)?

    A. *Pregnancy*

    B. *Hypopituitarism*

    C. *Uncontrolled epilepsy*

    D. *Neuroleptic malignant syndrome*

    E. *Cerebral aneurysm*

137. Caution should be taken when prescribing which one of the following to a woman on oral contraception?

    A. *Risperidone*

    B. *Valproic acid*

    C. *Gabapentin*

    D. *Lithium*

    E. *Carbamazepine*

138. An 8-year-old child has a mental age of 6 years. For school placement purposes, the IQ should be reported as:

    A. *50*

    B. *75*

    C. *100*

    D. *120*

    E. *135*

139. Psychiatrist: What's on your mind?
    Patient: I've been feeling depressed.
    Psychiatrist: Can you tell me more about what's been happening?
    Patient: I haven't been eating as much as I used to.
    Psychiatrist: Could you explain to me what you've been going through.

    The psychiatrist's approach is an example of:

    A. *Closed-ended questions*

    B. *Open-ended questions*

    C. *Countertransference*

    D. *Detailed mini-mental status exam*

    E. *Negative reinforcement*

140. Violent or aggressive behavior is associated with:

    A. *Decreased levels of 5-hydroxyindoleacetic acid in spinal fluid*

    B. *Decreased growth hormone response to insulin-induced hypoglycemia*

    C. *Abnormal dexamethasone suppression test*

    D. *Decreased response to corticotrophin releasing hormone stimulation test*

    E. *Decreased response to thyrotropin releasing hormone suppression test*

141. Which one of the following is not a potential repercussion of lithium intoxication?

    A. *Seizure*

    B. *Renal toxicity*

    C. *Ataxia and coarse tremor*

    D. *Non-specific T-wave changes.*

    E. *Jaundice*

142. Obsessive–compulsive disorder is associated with abnormality of which one of the following neurotransmitters?

    A. *Norepinephrine*

    B. *Serotonin*

    C. *Melatonin*

    D. *Acetylcholine*

    E. *Dopamine*

143. Which one of the following is not true regarding use of the tricyclic antidepressants?

    A. *Due to their ability to prolong cardiac conduction time their use in patients with conduction defects is contraindicated*

    B. *These agents should be discontinued before elective surgery because they may cause hypertensive episodes during surgery*

    C. *Some patients who experience orthostatic hypotension may respond to the use of fludrocortisone*

    D. *Myoclonic twitches and tremors of the tongue and upper extremities are common in some patients on tricyclics*

    E. *Amoxapine is the least likely to cause parkinsonian symptoms of all the tricyclics*

144. Which one of the following characteristics pertaining to vascular dementia is false?

    A. *There is a stepwise decline in functioning*

    B. *Hypertension is a known risk factor*

    C. *There is abrupt onset of symptoms*

    D. *There is a good response to cholinergic therapies*

    E. *Smoking is a known risk factor*

145. Which one of the following antidepressants is the most serotonin-selective of the tricyclics?

    A. *Amoxapine*

    B. *Clomipramine*

    C. *Desipramine*

    D. *Nortriptyline*

    E. *Doxepin*

146. A team comprised of a psychiatrist, psychologist, social worker, nurse, and medical student discharge a patient because the insurance will no longer pay for her stay. She kills herself. Who will be held legally responsible for the team's actions?

    A. *The medical student*

    B. *The psychologist*

    C. *The social worker*

    D. *The nurse*

    E. *The psychiatrist*

147. Which one of the following is not a side effect of treatment with tricyclic antidepressants?

    A. *Termination of ventricular fibrillation*

    B. *Increase collateral blood supply to ischemic heart muscle*

    C. *Decreased contractility*

    D. *Tachycardia*

    E. *Hypertension*

148. The best indicator for future suicidal behavior is:

    A. *Age*

    B. *Psychosis*

    C. *Past suicidal behavior*

    D. *Substance use*

    E. *Personality disorder*

149. A patient presents to your office with obsessive–compulsive disorder (OCD). She has been tried on several SSRIs with little improvement. You decide to try a tricyclic. Which tricyclic has been shown to have significantly better efficacy in treating OCD than the others?

    A. *Desipramine*

    B. *Doxepin*

    C. *Amitriptyline*

    D. *Clomipramine*

    E. *Nortriptyline*

150. Which one of the tricyclic antidepressants is used to treat childhood enuresis?

    A. *Desipramine*

    B. *Clomipramine*

    C. *Maprotiline*

    D. *Amoxapine*

    E. *Imipramine*

TWO

Answer Key – **Test Number Two**

1.	**E**	26.	**A**	51.	**D**	76.	**D**	101.	**D**	126.	**B**
2.	**D**	27.	**E**	52.	**A**	77.	**B**	102.	**B**	127.	**D**
3.	**D**	28.	**A**	53.	**E**	78.	**B**	103.	**D**	128.	**C**
4.	**E**	29.	**D**	54.	**B**	79.	**B**	104.	**E**	129.	**C**
5.	**D**	30.	**A**	55.	**C**	80.	**A**	105.	**D**	130.	**D**
6.	**B**	31.	**B**	56.	**C**	81.	**D**	106.	**D**	131.	**D**
7.	**C**	32.	**D**	57.	**E**	82.	**E**	107.	**C**	132.	**A**
8.	**E**	33.	**A**	58.	**E**	83.	**A**	108.	**C**	133.	**A**
9.	**C**	34.	**E**	59.	**B**	84.	**B**	109.	**A**	134.	**B**
10.	**A**	35.	**D**	60.	**B**	85.	**C**	110.	**C**	135.	**C**
11.	**B**	36.	**A**	61.	**A**	86.	**C**	111.	**D**	136.	**E**
12.	**C**	37.	**B**	62.	**E**	87.	**B**	112.	**A**	137.	**E**
13.	**D**	38.	**D**	63.	**B**	88.	**C**	113.	**A**	138.	**B**
14.	**B**	39.	**A**	64.	**B**	89.	**C**	114.	**E**	139.	**B**
15.	**C**	40.	**E**	65.	**E**	90.	**B**	115.	**E**	140.	**A**
16.	**D**	41.	**D**	66.	**D**	91.	**A**	116.	**C**	141.	**E**
17.	**C**	42.	**D**	67.	**E**	92.	**A**	117.	**E**	142.	**B**
18.	**D**	43.	**E**	68.	**A**	93.	**B**	118.	**B**	143.	**E**
19.	**D**	44.	**A**	69.	**C**	94.	**C**	119.	**D**	144.	**D**
20.	**A**	45.	**D**	70.	**C**	95.	**D**	120.	**D**	145.	**B**
21.	**D**	46.	**A**	71.	**E**	96.	**B**	121.	**E**	146.	**E**
22.	**B**	47.	**E**	72.	**B**	97.	**E**	122.	**A**	147.	**E**
23.	**B**	48.	**E**	73.	**D**	98.	**C**	123.	**A**	148.	**C**
24.	**C**	49.	**B**	74.	**A**	99.	**C**	124.	**E**	149.	**D**
25.	**A**	50.	**D**	75.	**E**	100.	**E**	125.	**D**	150.	**E**

TWO

Explanations – **Test Number Two**

Question 1. E.   There are several life-cycle theorists that are important to know. Freud's theory of development involving oral, anal, and phallic stages is important. Carl Jung felt that development of the personality occurs through experiences that teach a person who they intrinsically are. For him, libido included sexual energy, but also spiritual urges and a drive to understand the meaning of life. Harry Stack Sullivan focused on social interaction. In his theory he defined each stage of life through the need to interact with certain individuals. These interactions shaped the development of the personality.

Erik Erikson developed a life cycle from childhood to adulthood. It consists of:

- Stage 1: Trust vs mistrust. Trust is shown by ease of feeding and depth of sleep, and depends on consistency of experience provided by the caretaker. If trust is strong, the child develops self-confidence. (Birth–1 year old)

- Stage 2: Autonomy vs shame and doubt. This stage includes the child learning to walk and feed himself. There is a need for outer control. Shame happens through excessive punishment, and self-doubt occurs if the child is made to feel ashamed of his actions. (Age 1–3)

- Stage 3: Initiative vs guilt. In this stage the child initiates both motor and intellectual activities. If reinforced, his intellectual curiosity is satisfied. If he is made to feel inadequate, he will develop guilt about self-initiated activities. (Age 3–5 years)

- Stage 4: Industry vs inferiority. In this stage the child is busy building, creating, and accomplishing. If he is inferior to his peers with use of tools and skills, he will have less status and develop a sense of inadequacy and inferiority. (Age 6–11 years)

- Stage 5: Ego identity vs role confusion. There is a struggle to develop a sense of inner sameness and continuity. The adolescent shows preoccupation with appearance, hero worship, and ideology. There are dangers of role confusion, and doubts about his sexual orientation and vocational identity. (Age 11 years–end of adolescence)

- Stage 6: Intimacy vs isolation. Intimacy is marked by formation of life-long attachments and self-abandonment. Separation occurs if the individual is isolates and views others as dangerous. (Age 21–40 years)

- Stage 7: Generativity vs stagnation. Generativity is marked by raising children, altruism, creativity, and guiding the next generation. Stagnation occurs if there is isolation, excessive self-concern, and an absence of intimacy. (Age 40–65 years)

- Stage 8: Ego identity vs despair. Integrity is a feeling of satisfaction that life has been worthwhile, along with an acceptance of one's place in life. Despair is the feeling of loss of hope, disgust, and fear of death. (Age 65+ years)

Piaget developed a theory of cognitive development. It consists of four stages: sensorimotor, preoperational thought, concrete operations, and formal operations. The work of Freud, Jung and Erikson was the result of observations of children, not of carefully crafted studies. Their theories are a framework to understand development, but are not intended to describe objective reality. Their work has been followed by more scientific longitudinal studies of development, and more neurobiological understandings of human behavior.

Human Development

K&S Ch. 2

Question 2. D.   The clinical picture given is that of a conduction aphasia. Conduction aphasia results from left hemispheric (dominant) lesions particularly in the inferior parietal or superior temporal regions. The area of predilection for this lesion is considered to be the arcuate fasciculus that connects Wernicke's and Broca's areas. Conduction aphasia is characterized by inability to repeat, relatively normal spontaneous speech, and the possibility of paraphasic errors and hesitancy. Naming may be impaired, but auditory comprehension is intact. Writing may or may not be impaired. Associated symptoms of a conduction aphasia may include right hemi-paresis, right hemisensory loss, right hemianopsia, and limb apraxia.

Broca's aphasia would involve a lesion of Broca's area in the left posterior inferior frontal gyrus. This results in broken, stuttering, staccato speech, with inability to repeat and phonemic and paraphasic errors. Reading is often impaired, although auditory comprehension is usually intact. Broca's aphasia is frequently associated with depression and right hemiparesis and hemisensory loss.

Wernicke's aphasia results from a lesion in the superior temporal gyrus in Wernicke's area. Speech is generally fluent, but comprehension is impaired. Speech may also be logorrheic, or overproductive. The speech displays paragrammatism, which involves neologisms, verbal paraphasic errors, and production of jargon. Repetition, naming, and auditory comprehension are impaired. Reading comprehension is impaired. Wernicke's aphasia is often accompanied by a right homonymous hemianopsia, with a marked absence of motor and sensory signs and symptoms.

Global aphasia results from large lesions involving the superior temporal, inferior frontal and parietal lobes. The region generally corresponds to the territory of the middle cerebral artery (MCA) and indeed a thrombus at the trifurcation of the MCA can produce a global aphasia. Speech is nonfluent or mute and comprehension is impaired. Naming, reading, repetition, and writing are all poor. Most patients present with a dense right hemiparesis, hemisensory loss and hemianopsia.

Transcortical aphasias involve the areas around and adjacent to Broca's and Wernicke's areas and essentially present with similar features to the two perisylvian aphasias, except that repetition is spared. Transcortical motor aphasia presents with similar features to Broca's aphasia, with telegraphic, stuttering speech, sparing of comprehension and fluent repetition. The area involved is usually anterior to Broca's area in the anterior cerebral artery territory. Transcortical sensory aphasia is the analogue of Wernicke's aphasia and presents with fluent paraphasic speech, paraphasic naming, impaired reading and auditory comprehension, and normal repetition. The lesion usually localizes to the temporo-occipital area. Transcortical mixed aphasia is a rare condition also known as isolation of the speech area. The classic presentation is that of a global aphasia with echolalic repetition only, and no propositional speech or comprehension. The patient can only repeat. The lesion localizes to large watershed areas in the left hemisphere, sparing the perisylvian areas.

Neurology

B&D Ch. 12

Question 3. D.   Major types of receptors found on neurons include the seven-transmembrane-domain receptor, which requires G proteins to open ion channels, and the ligand-gated ion channel receptor, which actually has an ion channel as part of its structure. The seven-transmembrane-domain receptor has a characteristic NH_2 terminal outside the cell, several intracytoplasmic loops, and an intracellular COOH terminal. It is the tyrosine kinase receptor which interacts with nerve growth factor (NGF) and brain derived neurotropic factor (BDNF). Through these interactions the tyrosine kinase receptor is thought to play a large role in neuronal plasticity and the remodeling of synaptic associations. It is also important to recall that hormones and steroids can diffuse into the neuron and bind to cytoplasmic receptors whose effects carry to the nucleus and regulate gene expression.

Basic Neuroscience

K&S Ch. 3

Question 4. E. The classic complication of rapid sodium replacement in hyponatremia is central pontine myelinolysis. This can result in a clinical transection of the pons and a locked-in syndrome. Locked-in syndrome is the result of a pontine lesion that is clinically devastating and produces quadriplegia, mutism and a lower cranial nerve palsy with only the ability to move the eyes up and down and blink the eyelids being preserved. Only the upper brainstem function is preserved and patients usually need to be on a respirator. Cognition and comprehension are usually grossly intact and the patient is often quite aware of the predicament. Prognosis is very poor. The locked-in syndrome is most often the result of a ventral pontine infarct as a consequence of basilar artery thrombosis, but can in certain instances result from central pontine myelinolysis, which produces a more central pontine lesion. Other possible causes of locked-in syndrome are acute inflammatory demyelinating polyneuropathy (AIDP or Guillain–Barré syndrome), myasthenia gravis, and neuromuscular blocking agents.

Neurology

B&D Ch. 5

Question 5. D. This question contains an example of rationalization. Rationalization is characterized by offering rational explanations in an attempt to justify attitudes, beliefs or behaviors that may otherwise be unacceptable. Projection is perceiving and reacting to unacceptable inner impulses as if they are outside the self. Blocking is temporarily halting thinking. It often occurs in psychosis because of hallucinations and thought disorganization. Externalization is perceiving elements of your own personality in the external world or in external objects. It is a more general term than projection. Denial is avoiding awareness of some painful aspect of reality by negating sensory data. The most primitive of the defenses are the narcissistic defenses (denial, distortion, projection). The least primitive defenses are the mature defenses (altruism, anticipation, asceticism, humor, sublimation, suppression).

Psychological Theory and Psychometric Testing

K&S Ch. 6

Question 6. B. The clinical condition depicted in this question is that of pseudotumor cerebri, also called benign intracranial hypertension. Classically a problem seen in young obese African-American women, the exact etiology is unknown. Risk factors include hypervitaminosis A, high-dose corticosteroid therapy, tetracycline therapy, oral contraceptive use and head trauma. Patients typically present with a waxing and waning headache and intermittent visual obscurations. Neurologic examination can reveal papilledema on funduscopic examination and enlargement of the blind spot on visual field testing. Brain imaging is usually normal, although some scans reveal slit-like ventricles. The diagnosis is established by lumbar puncture with measurement of the opening pressure, which is elevated over $20\,cmH_2O$. The treatment modality of choice is pharmacologic, with acetazolamide 500 mg once or twice daily or with prednisone 20–40 mg daily. In certain cases patients opt for repeated lumbar punctures to siphon off fluid to maintain normal cerebrospinal fluid pressure. Surgical options for treatment include ventriculoperitoneal shunting, or lumboperitoneal shunting if the ventricles are too small, and optic nerve sheath fenestration, which can siphon off cerebrospinal fluid. ESR would be used as a diagnostic test for temporal arteritis. Serum prolactin level is sometimes drawn following a seizure to determine if it is epileptic or nonepileptic. The prolactin level would be expected to be elevated greater than twice normal within an hour after a true epileptic seizure.

Neurology

B&D Ch. 46

Question 7. C. The National Alliance for the Mentally Ill (NAMI) is an advocacy group made up of families of the mentally ill that works at local, state, and federal levels to improve services for the mentally ill. They are involved with lawmakers, outreach and education. The other answer choices are distracters. The most important organization to know is NAMI.

Public Policy

K&S Ch. 4

Question 8. E. In 1988, the International Headache Society (IHS) established strict criteria for migraine with and without aura. The criteria for migraine without aura are as follows: at least five headache attacks lasting 4 to 72 hours (untreated or unsuccessfully treated), which have at least two out of four characteristics – unilateral location; pulsating quality; moderate or severe intensity; or aggravated by walking stairs or similar routine physical activity. During the headache at least one of the two following symptoms occur: phonophobia and photophobia; nausea and/or vomiting.

Migraine with aura involves at least two attacks with at least three of the following: one or more fully reversible aura symptoms indicating focal cerebral cortical and/or brainstem functions; At least one aura symptom develops gradually over more than 4 minutes, or two or more symptoms occur in succession; no aura symptom lasts more than 60 minutes; or headache follows aura with free interval of at least 60 minutes (it may also simultaneously begin with the aura). At least one of the following aura features establishes a diagnosis of migraine with typical aura: homonymous visual disturbance; unilateral paresthesias and/or numbness; unilateral weakness; or aphasia or unclassifiable speech difficulty.

Neurology

B&D Ch. 69

Question 9. C. The lifetime prevalence of schizophrenia is 1%. It is estimated that there are somewhere in the vicinity of 2 million patients with schizophrenia in the United States. The other answer choices are distracters.

Psychotic Disorders

K&S Ch. 4

Question 10. A. Recombinant tissue plasminogen activator (r-TPA) is FDA-approved for acute thrombolysis of ischemic cerebrovascular accident within 3 hours of the occurrence of the event. Inclusion criteria for intravenous r-TPA administration include acute ischemic stroke with a clear time of onset less than or equal to 3 hours prior to desired r-TPA administration, neurologic deficit measurable on the NIH stroke scale and CT scan of the head demonstrating an absence of intracranial hemorrhage. Exclusion criteria are: rapidly improving or minor stroke symptoms or deficits, seizure at the onset of stroke, prior intracranial hemorrhage, pretreatment blood pressure greater than 185/110 mmHg, major surgery within the previous 14 days, a prior stroke or head injury within the last 3 months, intestinal or urinary bleeding within 3 weeks prior to the stroke, subarachnoid hemorrhage, blood glucose level <50 mg/dL or >400 mg/dL, recent myocardial infarction, current use of oral anticoagulants (PT > 15 or INR > 1.7) or heparin use within the last 48 hours, a platelet count of <100 000 per mL, or arterial puncture at a noncompressible site within the last 7 days.

Neurology

B&D Ch. 51

Question 11. B. Assertive community treatment is based on the model whereby teams of psychiatrists and other mental health workers go out into the community to patients' homes to maintain contact with them, monitor their status, and encourage medication compliance. The goal is to prevent decompensation of severely mentally ill patients and catch them before they severely decompensate and require hospitalization.

Public Policy

K&S Ch. 4

Question 12. C. The condition described in this question is that of restless legs syndrome (RLS). The only FDA-approved treatment is ropinorole (Requip), a dopamine agonist, which can improve symptoms at low doses starting at 0.5 mg prior to bedtime. Other dopamine agonists, pergolide, pramipexole and bromocriptine can be useful, but are not specifically FDA approved. Other helpful agents include benzodiazepines, opiate analgesics, gabapentin and levodopa/carbidopa. Restless legs syndrome has a prevalence rate of about 5% and is most often seen in middle to older-aged patients. It is usually idiopathic, but has been associated with polyneuropathy, uremia, and iron deficiency. The classic symptoms of RLS are crawling or creeping sensations (paresthesias or dysesthesias) of the lower extremities that are worse when lying down or in bed and occur most often at the onset of sleep. There is an urge to move the legs during rest, or when lying down or sitting. The urge to move is generally relieved by movement, like walking or stretching. Symptoms are worse at night or only occur in the evening or at night. Family history can be positive in 40–50% of patients, which suggests an autosomal dominant pattern of inheritance.

Neurology

B&D Ch. 68

Question 13. D. The best method to diagnose depression is the standard psychiatric interview. Psychiatric interviews serve two functions: to find and classify symptoms, and to find psychological determinants of behavior. Interviews can either be insight or symptom oriented. The other answer choices all have major flaws. The MMPI is a self-report inventory used to assess personality traits, and as such is not appropriate to the task. The scholastic achievement test is completely unrelated to symptom identification for depression. The dexamethasone suppression test is used to demonstrate abnormal activity of the hypothalamic–pituitary–adrenal axis which can be found in 50% of major depression patients. However, the test has limited clinical usefulness because of the frequency of false positive and negative test results. Interviewing the patient's teacher is a good idea, but in no way can it replace a face-to-face meeting with the child or be the sole basis for diagnosing depression.

Diagnostic and Treatment Procedures in Psychiatry

K&S Chs 1&15

Question 14. B. This question describes a left lateral medullary syndrome (also called a Wallenberg's syndrome). The Wallenberg syndrome is a brainstem stroke syndrome usually caused by occlusion of one of the vertebral arteries, or less commonly, one of the posterior inferior cerebellar arteries. The area of infarction is the lateral medulla. The clinical syndrome involves an ipsilateral Horner's syndrome, ipsilateral loss of pain and temperature sensation in the face, cerebellar ataxia and weakness of the vocal cords, pharynx and palate. There is contralateral loss of pain and temperature sensation to the hemibody. The visual system is not affected with this syndrome.

Neurology

B&D Ch. 51

Question 15. C. Decreased levels of serotonin in the cerebrospinal fluid (CSF) have been shown to be linked to higher levels of aggression in patients. In general, dopamine seems to promote aggression, whereas norepinephrine and serotonin seem to inhibit it, as does GABA. Rapid declines in serotonin levels have been linked to irritability and aggression, and low CSF serotonin has been linked to increased frequency of suicide. Corticotropin-releasing hormone (CRH) is a hormone that may increase in major depression, anorexia, and anxiety disorders. It is produced by the hypothalamus. It has no relation to aggression. Growth hormone is also unrelated to aggression.

Basic Neuroscience

K&S Ch. 4

Question 16. D. Metachromatic leukodystrophy (MLD) is an autosomal recessive metabolic disorder of myelin that results in a deficiency in arylsulfatase A (ASA). The result is an abnormal accumulation of sulfatides in the brain and peripheral nerves. High sulfatide levels lead to progressive demyelination. The ASA gene is located on chromosome 22q13. Gait disorder with hypotonia and lower limb areflexia are early manifestations of the disease and often precedes central nervous system involvement in infantile and juvenile forms of the disease. Adult-onset MLD tends to present with progressive dementia and behavioral problems. Nerve conduction velocities (NCV) are slowed in both juvenile and adult patients. Delayed visual and somatosensory evoked potential latencies are noted more often in adult cases. The classic neuropathologic findings are segmental nerve demyelination on nerve biopsy and metachromatic inclusions within Schwann cells and macrophages. Although nerve biopsy is diagnostic of MLD, MRI of the brain combined with urine assay for increased sulfatide excretion and abnormal ASA enzyme assay in leukocytes is less invasive and the preferred diagnostic method today. Treatment by bone marrow transplantation may increase brain ASA levels sufficiently to slow or stop disease progression.

Tay–Sachs disease is the severe infantile form of the autosomal recessive gangliosidosis that results in hexosaminidase A deficiency. Hexosaminidase A codes to chromosome 15q23–q24. The classic infantile picture is that of developmental retardation, paralysis, dementia, and blindness with death in the second or third year of life. The classic finding is a "cherry-red spot" on funduscopic examination. Babies with Tay–Sachs disease have a persistent hypersensitivity to loud noise with a marked hyperreactivity of startle response.

Krabbe's disease, also called globoid cell leukodystrophy, is an autosomal recessive disease caused by a deficiency in lysosomal enzyme galactocerebrosidase β-galactosidase. The gene has been localized to chromosome 14q31. Multinucleated macrophages in central white matter are accompanied by extensive central and peripheral demyelination. Infants present with rapid deterioration in motor and intellectual development, hypertonicity, optic atrophy, opisthotonic posture, and seizures. Stem cell transplantation can improve central nervous system manifestations by providing a source of missing enzyme.

Neurology

B&D Ch. 76

Question 17. C. Seasonal affective disorder is a non-DSM term used to describe a seasonal specifier added to the diagnoses of bipolar I & II disorders, and major depressive disorder. It is associated with depressive symptoms that occur at a certain time of year, with complete remission of symptoms at other times of the year. One must show a pattern of two episodes during the same season of the previous 2 years to make the diagnosis. In addition, the seasonal depressive episodes must substantially outnumber any non-seasonally related depressive episodes during the patient's lifetime. The treatment is light therapy.

Depressive Disorders

K&S Ch. 15

Question 18. D. The parachute response can persist far longer than 6 months. The Moro reflex is elicited by startle and is usually present in the normal infant up to 6 months of age. The child extends the arms symmetrically when the head is rapidly but gently dropped a few centimeters into the examiner's hand with the baby in a supine position. The tonic neck reflex is normally present from birth to about 3 months of age. Grasp and rooting reflexes usually disappear at or about the 6 month of age mark. Any persistence of these reflexes beyond this period or recurrence later in life, would be considered abnormal. Positive grasp and rooting reflexes in the adult would be considered frontal release signs and would signal extensive frontal white matter damage or disease.

Neurology

B&D Ch. 27

Question 19. D. Answer choice D describes pseudocyesis, which is listed in the DSM under somatoform disorders NOS. It involves a false belief that one is pregnant, and can involve physical signs associated with pregnancy, such as those described. However, the patient is not pregnant and there is no endocrine disorder present to explain the findings. Other patients that fall under the heading of somatoform disorder NOS include those with other somatic symptoms that do not meet the time criteria for other diagnoses. Answer choice A describes pain disorder, in which a patient experiences pain that can not be explained by a medical condition and is thought to be significantly mediated by psychological factors. Answer choice B describes hypochondriasis, in which a patient is convinced that he has a serious disease, based on misinterpretation of bodily symptoms, and despite the reassurance of doctors. Choice C describes conversion disorder, in which the patient develops neurological symptoms with no medical explanation that are thought to be mediated by psychological factors. Choice E describes somatization disorder, in which the patient has physical complaints spanning several organ systems that have no medical explanation and are thought to be associated with psychological factors. To make the diagnosis of somatization disorder, the patient must exhibit at any time during the disturbance, four pain symptoms, two gastrointestinal symptoms, one sexual symptom, and one pseudoneurological symptom.

Somatic Symptom Disorders

K&S Ch. 17

Question 20. A. Cytomegalovirus (CMV) is the most common offending infectious agent in AIDS-related retinopathy. It accounts for 30% of cases of HIV-related retinopathy. Toxoplasmosis is less common, likely involved in about 5% of retinitis cases. Tuberculosis is a rare cause of AIDS-related retinitis. *Cryptococcus neoformans* is usually responsible for a fungal meningitis and not a retinitis in AIDS patients with low CD4 counts. JC virus is the offending agent in progressive multifocal leukoencephalopathy in AIDS patients.

Neurology

B&D Ch. 53

Question 21. D. The most common hallucinations in schizophrenia are auditory. Visual, olfactory and tactile hallucinations are also possible. Schizophrenia was first discovered by Morel who called it "démence precoce".

Later Kraepelin used "dementia praecox" to describe a group of illnesses that started in adolescence and ended in dementia. Bleuler coined the term "schizophrenia." The disorder is chronic and has a prodromal, active, and residual phase.

Psychotic Disorders

K&S Ch. 13

Question 22. B. Night-time awakening is not considered to be part of the clinical picture of narcolepsy. Narcolepsy is a lifelong sleep disorder that is believed to have a hereditary component. In the United States, the prevalence is about 3 to 6 in 10000. One to two percent of first-degree relatives of narcoleptic patients manifest the illness compared to 0.02–0.18% of the population at large. Narcolepsy is linked to the dysfunction of the hypocretin (orexin) peptide system.

The hallmark of the disease is excessive daytime sleepiness and sleep attacks. Sleep attacks manifest as the irresistible desire to fall asleep. Attacks can occur at any waking moment and last for a few minutes up to thirty minutes' duration. Performance at school, work, and in social situations usually suffers.

The second major manifestation of narcolepsy is cataplexy. Cataplexy is the sudden loss of muscle tone in the voluntary muscles, with sparing of the respiratory and ocular muscles. Attacks of cataplexy involve the patient falling to the ground following rapid complete loss of muscle tone. Consciousness is preserved during cataplexic attacks. Anywhere from 60–100% of narcoleptic patients suffer from cataplexy.

Sleep paralysis is the third major symptom of narcolepsy. It can be noted in one-quarter to one-half of narcoleptic patients. These attacks are characterized by hypnagogic or hypnopompic sudden bilateral or unilateral limb paralysis. Consciousness is preserved during these attacks, but the patient cannot move or speak.

Hypnagogic hallucination is the fourth major symptom of narcolepsy. These can occur at onset of sleep or during early morning awakening. About 20–40% of narcoleptic patients experience these hallucinations. Other major symptoms of narcolepsy include disturbance of night sleep in about 70–80% of patients and automatic behavior that can resemble a fugue-like state, which can occur in 20–40% of narcoleptic patients.

The only medications FDA-approved for narcolepsy are modafinil and sodium oxybate. Modafinil, which can be given in a single dose of 100–200 mg daily, modulates the hypocretin (orexin) neurons in the brainstem and is a non-amphetamine stimulant. Sodium oxybate (Xyrem) is a drug that was initially FDA-approved specifically for cataplexy, but now has an approval for narcolepsy as well.

Sleep Wake Disorders

B&D Ch. 68

Question 23. B. Logorrhea is uncontrollable, excessive talking. Alexithymia is a difficulty in recognizing and describing one's emotions. Echolalia is the imitative repetition of the speech of another. Flight of ideas is rapid shifting from one topic to another. Stilted speech is a formal stiff speech pattern.

Diagnostic and Treatment Procedures in Psychiatry

K&S Ch. 8

Question 24. C. Intramuscular phenytoin is a poor choice for treatment of status epilepticus because of its erratic rate of absorption. Useful status epilepticus treatments include rectal or intravenous diazepam, intravenous lorazepam, intravenous phenytoin or phosphenytoin, intravenous valproic acid, oxygen by nasal cannula and airway protection, and intravenous phenobarbital. Phenobarbital is acceptable treatment, but not the best choice because of the narrow therapeutic window and possibility of overdose leading to respiratory depression and possible death.

Neurology

B&D Ch. 67

Question 25. A. Of the statements listed, the only correct one is answer choice A. Ziprasidone is an agonist at 5-HT-1A and does inhibit reuptake of serotonin and norepinephrine. It is also an antagonist at 5-HT-1D, 2A, and 2C, as well as D2 and D3. It has low affinity for histaminic, muscarinic and alpha-2 receptors. Because of its action on serotonin and norepinephrine, it has been postulated to be of benefit not only in psychosis, but also in anxiety and depression. Risperidone is a similar blocker of D2 when compared to haldol, and as such carries one of the highest risks for EPS among the atypicals. Quetiapine is known for its low incidence of EPS, as it has only a moderate affinity for the D2 receptor. It has a high affinity for 5-HT types 2 and 6, H1, and alpha 1 and 2. It has low affinity for muscarinic receptors. Olanzapine has been associated with weight gain in many patients. It is very anticholinergic and carries with it the corresponding side effects. Clozapine has been shown to be associated with a decreased risk of suicide in schizophrenic patients. Major side effects of clozapine include seizures and agranulocytosis, among others. And while we're on the topic of anticholinergic side effects, the treatment of choice for urinary retention is urecholine (Bethanechol).

Psychopharmacology

K&S Ch. 35

Question 26. A.   Divalproex sodium (valproic acid) has the broadest spectrum of coverage and indication of all the anticonvulsant medications. It has proven efficacy in primary-generalized tonic–clonic seizures, absence seizures, and myoclonic seizures. Its likely mechanism of action is by blockade of voltage-dependent sodium channels and GABA enhancement. Phenytoin is not indicated for absence seizures and has no place in their treatment. It is indicated for treatment of partial and generalized tonic-clonic seizures. Its mechanism of action is by blockade of voltage-dependent sodium channels. Oxcarbazepine and carbamazepine are indicated for partial complex and secondary generalized seizures, but both can worsen absence seizures. Oxcarbazepine does not produce autoinduction of its own metabolism in the way that carbamazepine does. Ethosuximide is indicated only in uncomplicated absence seizures and has no place in the treatment of partial complex or secondary generalized tonic–clonic seizures. Its mechanism of action is by lowering voltage-dependent calcium conductance in thalamic neurons.

Neurology

B&D Ch. 67

Question 27. E.   Constipation is a common side effect of the tricyclic antidepressants as a result of the anticholinergic activity of these drugs. Other tricyclic side effects include dry mouth, blurry vision, sweating, orthostatic hypotension, sedation, lethargy, agitation, tremor, slowed cardiac conduction (as evidenced by prolonged PR and QRS intervals), and tachycardia.

Psychopharmacology

K&S Ch. 36

Question 28. A.   Foot flexion (also called dorsiflexion; the bending of the foot upwards) involves the tibialis anterior muscle innervated by nerves that emanate from the L5 motor nerve root. L5 also controls the extension (bending upwards) of the big toe (extensor hallucis longus). A lesion at L5 often causes a foot drop from dorsiflexor muscle weakness. Foot extension (pushing down on the gas pedal) involves the gastrocnemius (calf) and soleus muscles innervated by nerves that emanate from the S1 nerve root predominantly. Leg extension is a function of the quadriceps muscles (anterior thigh) which are innervated by nerves emanating from the L3 and L4 nerve roots. Hip flexion (raising of the knee in the air) is a function of the iliopsoas muscles which are innervated by the L1, L2 and L3 nerve roots. The Achilles or ankle jerk motor reflex is a function of the S1 motor nerve root.

Neurology

B&D Ch. 23

Question 29. D.   Amitriptyline can be used for gastric ulcer because of its strong histamine blockade. Other drugs that can also be used for this purpose include doxepin and trimipramine.

Psychopharmacology

K&S Ch. 36

Question 30. A.   The condition noted in this question is that of the classic Brown–Séquard syndrome due to a hemisection of the spinal cord. The correct combination of deficits is that of loss of motor control and posterior column function ipsilateral to and below the level of the lesion coupled with contralateral loss of pain and temperature sensation one to two dermatomal levels below the level of the lesion. Frequent causes include disk herniation, penetrating trauma, spinal fracture and radiation injury. The cervical spinal cord is most commonly affected.

Neurology

B&D Ch. 24

Question 31. B. This question focuses on Piaget's stages of cognitive development. In the sensorimotor stage children respond to stimuli in the environment, learning during the process. They eventually develop object permanence (objects exist independent of the child's awareness of their existence), and begin to understand symbols (as in the use of words to express thoughts).

During the preoperational stage there is a sense that punishment for bad deeds is unavoidable (immanent justice). There is a sense of egocentrism, and phenomenalistic causality (the thought that events that occur together cause one another). Animistic thinking (inanimate objects are given thoughts and feelings) is also seen.

In the concrete operations stage, egocentric thought changes to operational thought where another's point of view can be taken into consideration. In concrete operations children can put things in order and group objects according to common characteristics. They develop the understanding of conservation (a tall cup and a wide cup can both hold equal volumes of water) and reversibility (ice can change to water and back to ice again).

During formal operations children can think abstractly, reason deductively, and define abstract concepts. Trust vs mistrust is one of Erik Erikson's stages and is a distracter in this question.

Human Development

K&S Ch. 2

Question 32. D. The anterior cerebral artery (ACA) territory is the area affected by this stroke. The ACA irrigates the medial frontal lobes and therefore when affected causes preferential leg greater than arm and face weakness contralateral to the side of the lesion. The destruction of the nearby frontal eye fields causes loss of tonic opposition of the gaze to the opposite side so the eyes will often be noted to look toward the side of the lesion. Sphincteric incontinence is sometimes seen if the cortical bowel and bladder areas are affected. Patients often suffer from abulia, a loss of will power or the lack of ability to do things independently. Bilateral ACA territory damage can result in akinetic mutism.

Neurology

B&D Ch. 51

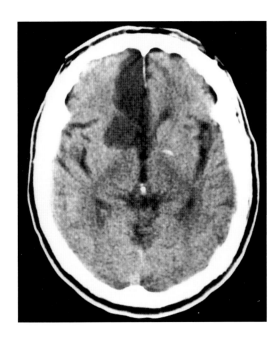

Question 33. A. Norepinephrine is made in the locus ceruleus. Serotonin is made in the dorsal raphe nuclei. Dopamine is made in the substantia nigra. Acetylcholine is made in the nucleus basalis of Meynert.

Basic Neuroscience

K&S Ch. 3

Question 34. E. Pure motor hemiparesis is one of the classic lacunar stroke syndromes and would be expected from an infarct in the area of the internal capsule, the basis pontis, or the corona radiata. Lacunar strokes are characterized as ischemic strokes resulting from small vessel lipohyalinosis that is caused by hypertension and diabetes as the two major risk factors. Lacunar infarcts by definition are small and range from 0.5 mm to 1.5 cm in diameter. Microembolism may also be a mechanism of lacunar strokes.

Other lacunar syndromes include pure sensory stroke, usually from a small lesion in the ventroposterolateral nucleus of the thalamus; sensorimotor stroke, from a stroke to the internal capsule and thalamus, or the posterior limb of the internal capsule; ataxic hemiparesis, which results from a lacunar infarct to either the basis pontis or posterior limb of the internal capsule; and the dysarthria-clumsy hand syndrome, resulting from a stroke to the deep areas of the basis pontis.

Neurology

B&D Ch. 51

Question 35. D. Of the receptors listed, it is the histamine receptor that is associated with weight gain and sedation. The M1 receptor is associated with constipation, blurred vision, dry mouth, and drowsiness. Alpha 1 receptors are associated with dizziness and decreased blood pressure. The 5-HT-1A receptor is a presynaptic autoreceptor involved in the response of neurons to the SSRIs. The 5-HT-2A receptor is one of the postsynaptic serotonin receptors involved in the neuron's response to the SSRIs. The serotonin receptors are associated with modulation of depression and anxiety, but not with weight gain or sedation.

Basic Neuroscience

K&S Ch. 3

Question 36. A. The contralateral subthalamic nucleus of Luys is most often the area where a lesion will produce hemiballismus. Hemiballismus is a dramatic, flinging movement of the proximal extremities. It can affect both the upper and lower limbs and is most often unilateral. Most frequently, the cause of hemiballismus is an acute stroke.

Neurology

B&D Ch. 71

Question 37. B. The six biogenic amine neurotransmitters are dopamine, epinephrine, norepinephrine, acetylcholine, histamine, and serotonin. Of these, dopamine, norepinephrine, and epinephrine are all synthesized from the precursor tyrosine, and are known as a group as the catecholamines. GABA is an amino acid neurotransmitter, not a biogenic amine. Of note is that cocaine works by blocking the reuptake of the biogenic amines, more specifically serotonin, norepinephrine, and dopamine.

Basic Neuroscience

K&S Ch. 3

Question 38. D. Reserpine interferes with the magnesium and ATP-dependent uptake of biogenic amines which results in the depletion of dopamine, norepinephrine and serotonin neurotransmitters. In this way, it can relieve symptoms of dystonia and can also cause depression, sedation, and a Parkinson's like syndrome.

Neurology

B&D Ch. 71

Question 39. A. Projection is perceiving and reacting to unacceptable inner impulses as though they were outside the self. On a psychotic level it takes the form of delusions about external realities that are usually persecutory in nature. One's own impulses and hostilities are projected onto another who is now assumed to have intentions to persecute you. The other answer choices are distracters that have nothing to do with projection.

Psychological Theory and Psychometric Testing

K&S Ch. 6

Question 40. E.   The arachnoid (pacchionian) granulations are the major sites for drainage of cerebrospinal fluid (CSF) into the blood. These granulations protrude through the dura into the superior sagittal sinus and act as one way valves or siphons for the CSF. Equilibrium is maintained by the arachnoid granulations, for if CSF pressure drops below a certain level, absorption stops. If the CSF pressure increases, more fluid is absorbed. The choroid plexuses that protrude into the ventricles are responsible for the majority of CSF production in humans. In humans, the rate of CSF production is about 0.35 mL/min. Drugs that can temporarily reduce production of CSF and ease increased intracranial pressure include acetazolamide and mannitol. States of hypothermia, hypocarbia, hypoxia and hyperosmolality can also temporarily decrease CSF production. Virchow–Robin spaces act as a duct for substances in the subarachnoid space to enter the brain. The other answer choices are distracters.

Neurology

B&D Ch. 59

Question 41. D.   Regression analysis is a method of predicting the value of one variable in relation to another variable based on observed data. Probability is the likelihood that an event will occur. A probability of 0 means it will not occur. A probability of 1 means it will definitely occur. Point prevalence is the number of people with a disorder at a specific point in time divided by the total population at that point in time. Incidence is the number of new cases of a disease over a given time divided by the total number of people at risk during that time. Central tendency is a central value in a distribution around which other values are arranged. Examples of central tendency are the mean, median, and mode. The mean is the average. The median is the middle value in a series of values. The mode is the value that appears most frequently in a series of measurements. Kappa is a variable used to indicate a constant value that does not change. Sensitivity is the ability of a test to detect that which is being tested for.

Statistics

K&S Ch. 4

Question 42. D.   Noncontrast head CT is the best immediate test of choice in the emergency room if a lobar hemorrhage is suspected. MRI of the brain can add precision, but in the hyperacute stage may not be able to reveal acute bleeding as well as the CT scan. The most common location of intracranial hemorrhage is from the putamen, which accounts for about 35% of cases. Lobar hemorrhage is second to putaminal hemorrhage in frequency and accounts for about one-quarter of cases. Hypertension remains the most frequent cause of intracranial hemorrhage, but arteriovenous malformations, cerebral amyloid angiopathy and sympathomimetic agents can also account for quite a number of cases.

Emergency room management of suspected intracranial hemorrhage begins with stabilization of vital signs and airway protection. Intubation is indicated if the level of consciousness drops to a Glasgow Coma Scale score of 8 or less. CT scan of the head must next be done to determine the location and size of the hemorrhage. Neurosurgical consultation may be indicated if the hemorrhage is large and increased intracranial pressure is suspected.

Blood work checking the coagulation panel is very important. If the patient is on oral or parenteral anticoagulation therapy, it is imperative to consider reversing anticoagulation by protamine sulfate for those on heparin or with parenteral vitamin K or fresh frozen plasma for those patients on warfarin therapy.

Bedside EEG is not indicated unless there is pervasive coma or seizures. Lumbar puncture is usually contraindicated if intracranial or lobar hemorrhage is suspected, because it can trigger uncal herniation and eventual death if the patient is already in a state of increased intracranial pressure. The lumbar puncture with CSF xanthochromia assay is useful only if a subarachnoid hemorrhage is suspected.

Neurology

B&D Ch. 51

Question 43. E.   Outcomes in psychodynamic therapy have been found to be closely associated with the empathy provided by the therapist. The goal is for the therapist to be in tune with the patient's internal state in an empathic way. When patients feel that therapists understand their internal world they are more likely to accept interpretations made by the therapist. The other answer choices, while important are not the most important. Some of these distracters may have impacts on the therapeutic relationship, but will not be the universally most important factor in the outcome of therapy.

Psychotherapy

K&S Ch. 35

Question 44. A.   Melatonin is believed to be released principally by the pineal gland and there is a feedback loop between the pineal gland and the suprachiasmatic nucleus in the hypothalamus that helps with sleep regulation. Melatonin is secreted predominantly at night and levels peak between 3:00 am and 5:00 am, and decrease to lower levels during the day. Melatonin is a modulator of human circadian rhythm for entrainment by the light–dark cycle.

Basic Neuroscience

B&D Ch. 68

Question 45. D.   The Minnesota Multiphasic Personality Inventory (MMPI) is an objective psychological test. It is a self report inventory used to find areas of pathological personality structure. The other tests listed are projective tests. In projective tests the patient is given a picture or incomplete piece of information and asked to fill in the details or complete the unfinished task. The answers that the patient gives reveal aspects of his personality, thought content, thought structure, and psychological makeup. In the Rorschach test the patient is shown ink blots and asked to share what they thinks the ink blots look like. In the sentence completion test the patient is asked to finish incomplete sentences. In the thematic apperception test the patient is shown a series of pictures and asked to make up stories based on the pictures. In the draw a person test the patient is asked to draw a person of the same and opposite sex. The person of the same sex is thought to represent the patient. Interpretations are made based on the details the patient puts into the drawings.

Psychological Theory and Psychometric Testing

K&S Ch. 5

Question 46. A.   Subacute sclerosing panencephalitis (SSPE) is the result of a persistent and nonproductive viral infection of the neurons and glia that is caused by the measles virus. It is a late complication of measles. Children 5 to 10 years of age are affected most often. Clinical manifestations include personality and cognitive changes, myoclonic seizures, spasticity, choreoathetoid movements, difficulty swallowing, eventually leading to coma and death. The three tests of choice are lumbar puncture for cerebrospinal fluid (CSF) assay, electroencephalogram (EEG) and brain biopsy. CSF reveals an elevated measles antibody titer, oligoclonal bands, absence of pleocytosis, normal glucose and normal to elevated protein. Brain biopsy may reveal neuronal and glial nuclear and cytoplasmic viral inclusion bodies. EEG reveals a characteristic pattern of periodic bursts of generalized slow-wave complexes. There is no specific accepted treatment, but studies have revealed that intraventricular interferon-α combined with oral isoprinosine can be helpful. Prognosis is generally poor and often death can be expected within twelve months if response to treatment is poor. There is no evidence that SSPE results from measles vaccination in children.

Neurology

B&D Ch. 53

Question 47. E.   Attention deficit–hyperactivity disorder (ADHD) is diagnosed by six or more symptoms of inattention or six or more symptoms of hyperactivity–impulsivity that persist for 6 months or more. Some symptoms that cause impairment should be present before age 7 years. Impairment must be present in more than one setting to make the diagnosis. Symptoms of inattention involve failure to pay close attention to tasks, failure to sustain attention, not listening, not following through on tasks, problems organizing tasks, forgetfulness, and being easily distracted by extraneous stimuli. Symptoms of hyperactivity–impulsivity include fidgeting, inability to remain seated when expected, running or climbing excessively, difficulty playing quietly, acting as if driven by a motor, talking excessively, blurting out answers, difficulty awaiting turn, and interrupting others.

Disruptive, Impulse Control, Conduct Disorders, and ADHD

K&S Ch. 42

Question 48. E.   Lesch–Nyhan syndrome is an X-linked recessive hereditary disorder of purine and pyrimidine metabolism. Hyperuricemia results from a deficiency in hypoxanthine-guanine phosphoribosyltransferase (HGPRT). Clinical symptoms and signs of the syndrome include choreoathetosis, hyperreflexia, hypertonia, dysarthria, behavioral disturbances, cognitive impairment and self-mutilatory behavior. Neurologic signs and symptoms are likely a result of diminished dopamine concentrations in the cerebrospinal fluid and basal ganglia.

Metachromatic leukodystrophy is an autosomal recessive disorder which is caused by arylsulfatase-A (ASA) deficiency. There is an accumulation of excess sulfatides in the nervous system which leads to progressive demyelination. The disorder localizes to chromosome 22q13.

Tay–Sachs is a recessive disorder localizing to chromosome 15q23-24. It is caused by a deficiency in hexosaminidase A. The adult form presents as progressive weakness in the proximal muscles of the upper and lower extremities. Associated symptoms may involve spasticity, dysarthria, cognitive and psychiatric impairment.

Krabbe disease, also called globoid cell leukodystrophy, is an autosomal recessive disease that localizes to chromosome 14q31. It is a result of a deficiency in lysosomal enzyme galactocerebroside β-galactosidase. Generalized central and peripheral demyelination is the hallmark of the disorder, as well as the presence of multinucleated macrophages (globoid cells) in cerebral white matter. Infantile arrest of motor and cognitive development is noted, with seizures, hypertonicity, optic atrophy and opisthotonic posturing. Stem cell transplantation may reverse the neurologic deficits by providing the missing enzyme.

Gaucher's disease is an autosomal recessive disorder resulting from β-glucosidase deficiency. It localizes to chromosome 1q21. There are three identified types. Type I presents with the characteristic findings of hematologic anomalies, hypersplenism, bone lesions, skin pigmentation and ocular pingueculae.

Neurology

B&D Chs 62&76

Question 49. B. In order to diagnose schizophrenia, active phase symptoms must be present for a 1 month period only. It may be diagnosed if other symptoms (i.e., negative) are present over a 6 month period, but at least one month of that 6 months must have contained active symptoms. All other answer choices are part of the characteristic active phase symptoms for schizophrenia. Social isolation is a bad prognostic sign for schizophrenia. Good prognostic signs include late age of onset, acute onset, and the presence of an affective component.

Psychotic Disorders

K&S Ch. 13

Question 50. D. Botulinum toxin type A is FDA-approved for the treatment of cervical dystonia, blepharospasm, hemifacial spasm, strabismus, and axillary hyperhidrosis, and cosmetically for hyperactive glabellar lines of the procerus muscles of the forehead. Although not FDA-approved for spasticity related to multiple sclerosis, it is an excellent treatment for that particular disorder. Botulinum toxin type A is also used off-label for the treatment of migraine. The mechanism of action of botulinum toxin type A is through blockade of neuromuscular transmission via blockade of presynaptic acetylcholine release. Botulinum toxin type A has no place in the treatment of restless legs syndrome.

Neurology

B&D Ch. 48

Question 51. D. This question is a clear description of a delusional disorder. In a delusional disorder, the patient usually presents with a nonbizarre delusion (i.e., something that could happen in real life). There are no other psychotic symptoms present. His ability to function in his daily life is preserved. There is not a significant mood component to the disease. The question says nothing about memory impairment, therefore dementia is not correct. The patient does not meet criteria for active phase schizophrenic symptoms, therefore schizophrenia and schizoaffective disorder are ruled out. Brief psychotic disorder lasts less than a month, and this patient has had symptoms for 5 months, so this answer choice is incorrect.

Psychotic Disorders

K&S Ch. 14

Question 52. A. The clinical presentation described in this question is that of classic tension-type or muscle contraction headache. These headaches can result from both muscular and emotional tension and stress. These headaches are not well understood and muscle tension may not fully explain their pathogenesis. The hypothalamic–mamillothalamic tract may be implicated in the generation of the pain, but studies have yet to investigate this thoroughly. Often treatment with rest, sleep, or simple analgesics is sufficient to bring relief. These headaches can begin at any age, are most often bilateral and are described as band-like around the head. Patients describe squeezing, pressure or burning types of pain. The pain can wax and wane throughout the day and can be present, if left untreated, from a period of hours to days. This headache type is usually free of any associated or autonomic symptoms, which helps to differentiate it from migraine. Treatment of tension-type headache usually begins with aspirin or acetaminophen. If headaches are more severe, combination drugs like acetaminophen-butalbital-caffeine (Fioricet) may be helpful, or non-steroidal anti-inflammatory agents such as naproxen or ibuprofen.

Migraine is differentiated from tension-type headache mainly by its stereotyped features and associated autonomic symptoms. Migraine is generally unilateral, pulsatile and is accompanied by photophobia, phonophobia, or osmophobia. Other features can include nausea and vomiting, anorexia, blurred vision, and lightheadedness. The aura that can precede a migraine involves transient visual, motor, or focal neurologic deficits or symptoms. The scintillating scotoma is the most common visual manifestation of aura. The patient can perceive a shimmering arc or zigzag pattern of light in the peripheral visual field that can gradually enlarge. Sensory aura can involve transient numbness and tingling in the extremities that can last from seconds up to a half an hour's duration. Motor aura is rare and can manifest as a transient motor weakness or hemiparesis, in much the same way as the sensory deficits. The patient may therefore misinterpret these symptoms as the onset of a stroke.

Basilar migraine usually presents with occipital headache and neurologic symptoms attributable to the brainstem. The aura can involve visual and sensory phenomena, but these are often accompanied by vertigo, dysarthria, tinnitus and speech deficits. Loss of consciousness may occur if the reticular activating system of the pons is involved. The patient will often experience severe occipital pain after awakening from the aura. These attacks resemble stroke-like symptoms in the vertebrobasilar territory.

Paroxysmal hemicrania is a special headache entity that falls into the category of indomethacin-responsive headache syndromes. This headache type begins early in life and is more common in women than in men (2:1 ratio). The hemicrania can be episodic or chronic. Pain is unilateral and brief, occurring generally in the periorbital or temporal areas. Attacks are frequent, usually five or more daily and each lasts about 20 minutes. Each attack is accompanied by autonomic features such as conjunctival injection, lacrimation, ptosis, rhinorrhea, ipsilateral to the side of the headache. Response to indomethacin 25–100 mg daily in divided doses is usually dramatic. The mechanism of indomethacin's efficacy in this headache variety is not well understood.

Neurology
B&D Ch. 69

Question 53. E.   In major depressive disorder libido is decreased. Increased libido is often found in mania.
Depressive Disorders
K&S Ch. 15

Question 54. B.   The best answer to this question is the trigeminal nucleus caudalis (TNC). Many theories exist to try to explain the pathogenesis of migraine, and unfortunately there is no perfect unified theory. It is generally believed that abnormal intracranial and extracranial vascular reactivity accounts for the pulsatile nature of migraine by the abnormal dilatation of these vessels. It is believed that the aura of migraine is caused by a phenomenon called spreading oligemia or spreading depression. This refers to a phase of oligemia that spreads over the occipital cortex at a rate of about 2–3 mm/min and causes the scintillating scotoma noted during aura. This was described by Lashley in 1941, by his analysis of his own aura. Abnormal neuronal impulses from the trigeminal nucleus caudalis in the pons send messages along the trigeminal ophthalmic branches to nerve terminals that release substance P, neurokinin A and calcitonin gene-related peptide (CGRP). These polypeptides in turn activate a cascade of sterile neurogenic perivascular inflammation in the brain. Vessels then dilate and by vascular endothelial activation, there is an extravasation of plasma proteins that triggers an inflammatory response. Ergot alkaloid medications and triptan medication effectively block neuronal firing in the TNC and can abort an attack. The reticular activating system (RAS) refers to the ascending tracts in the pons that are responsible for maintenance of wakefulness. Bilateral pontine lesions affecting the RAS can result in impairment of consciousness. The suprachiasmatic nuclei (SCN) in the hypothalamus are thought to be the generator of the human biological clock that regulates circadian rhythms. Melatonin is the neurohormone produced by the pineal gland that acts at melatonin receptor sites in the SCN by a feedback loop. The SCN has no known role in migraine. Muscular contraction of the scalp and cranial musculature is not believed to be associated with migraine, but may play a role in the manifestation of tension-type headache.

Neurology

B&D Chs 61&69

Question 55. C. This is a case of seasonal affective disorder, which is a depression that sets in during the fall and winter and resolves during the spring and summer. It is often characterized by hypersomnia, hyperphagia, and psychomotor slowing. Treatment involves exposure to bright artificial light for 2–6 hours each day during the fall and winter months. It is thought to be related to abnormal melatonin metabolism. All other answer choices given are distracters and are unrelated to the patient's primary problem.

Depressive Disorders

K&S Ch. 15

Question 56. C. Carbidopa serves a simple function: it inhibits dopa decarboxylase and thereby prevents the peripheral metabolism of levodopa to dopamine before it can cross the blood–brain barrier. The dopamine agonists such as ropinirole, pramipexole, pergolide and bromocriptine are direct postsynaptic dopamine receptor agonists indicated for Parkinson's disease treatment. Selegiline is the selective monamine oxidase type B (MAO-B) inhibitor that blocks dopamine degradation by MAO-B and can potentiate the action of levodopa in the central nervous system. Catechol-O-methyltransferase (COMT) inhibitors such as tolcapone and entacapone prevent peripheral degradation of levodopa and central metabolism of levodopa and dopamine, thereby increasing central levodopa and dopamine levels. COMT inhibitors are usually taken simultaneously with doses of levodopa-carbidopa. Anticholinergic agents such as trihexyphenidyl and benztropine can reduce tremor in Parkinson's disease by blockade of post-synaptic muscarinic receptors. These agents carry the danger of toxic side effects that include confusion, blurred vision, urinary retention, constipation and dry mouth.

Neurology

B&D Ch. 71

Question 57. E. This question includes common symptoms found in a panic attack. Others include trembling, choking sensations, dizziness, fear of losing control, fear of death, paresthesias, chills, or hot flushes. The patient in question does not present with the characteristic signs and symptoms of a manic episode. Myxedema madness is a depressed and psychotic state found in some patients with hypothyroidism. Mad Hatter's syndrome presents as manic symptoms resulting from chronic mercury intoxication. The patient describes no psychotic symptoms, so psychotic disorder NOS is clearly the wrong choice.

Anxiety Disorders

K&S Ch. 16

Question 58. E. Apoptosis refers to programmed neuronal cell death. This concept is believed to account for the pathophysiology of several neurodegenerative diseases. These diseases include spinal muscular atrophy, Parkinson's disease, amyotrophic lateral sclerosis, and Alzheimer's dementia.

Neurology

B&D Ch. 60

Question 59. B. Amoxapine and maprotiline are tetracyclic, not tricyclic antidepressants. Amoxapine has significant dopamine blocking activity, and can produce side effects similar to those found with many antipsychotics, such as tardive dyskinesia and dystonia. Maprotiline is one of the most selective inhibitors of norepinephrine reuptake. It has mild sedative and anticholinergic side effects. Notably there is an increased incidence of seizure associated with its use. It has a long half life of 43 hours.

Psychopharmacology

K&S Ch. 36

Question 60. B. Sturge–Weber syndrome is a neurocutaneous disorder that is sporadic and not genetically inherited. The hallmark is the presence of a facial cutaneous angioma (port-wine nevus) usually with a brain angioma ipsilateral to the skin lesion. Other characteristics can include contralateral hemiparesis, mental retardation and homonymous hemianopia. Glaucoma is common and if untreated can lead to blindness. Seizures develop in over 70% of Sturge–Weber patients and present most often as motor seizures or generalized tonic–clonic seizures. Treatment of seizures is achieved with anticonvulsant medication, which if proven ineffective, may lead to the consideration of surgical intervention such as hemispherectomy to excise the offending brain tissue.

Von Hippel–Lindau syndrome (VHL) is a heritable neurocutaneous disorder that is transmitted by autosomal dominant pattern of inheritance. The VHL gene is a tumor-suppressor gene on chromosome 3. Prevalence is about 1 in 40 000 to 100 000. The predominant clinical presentation is characterized by retinal and CNS hemangioblastomas and visceral cysts and tumors. Hemangioblastomas are slow-growing vascular tumors that are benign but can bleed and cause local mass effect. The most common CNS sight of this tumor type is the cerebellum in about 50% of cases. Renal cysts occur in about half of patients with VHL. Pheochromocytoma occurs in about 10–20% of patients. Frequent follow-up and screening for tumors is the management of choice for patients with VHL.

Ataxia–telangiectasia is a neurodegenerative neurocutaneous disorder that is inherited by autosomal recessive pattern of inheritance. Prevalence is about 1 in 40 000 to 100 000. The hallmark of the disorder is the development of early-onset ataxia in childhood. Ataxia tends to develop at around 12 months of age, when the child begins to walk. Children typically are wheelchair-bound by 12 years of age. Telangiectases (small dilated blood vessels) tend to develop later, from about age 3–6 years, and often affect the earlobes, nose and sclerae. There is also a higher risk of lymphoma and leukemia in patients with the disorder than in the general population at large. Abnormal eye movements are common in children with the disorder. These include nystagmus, ocular motility impairment and gaze apraxia.

Fabry's disease is an X-linked lysosomal storage disease resulting from deficiency in α-galactosidase A. Stigmata of the disease include the development of asymptomatic red or purple papules that occur around the umbilicus, hips, thighs and scrotum area. Other characteristics include corneal deposits, painful dysesthesias of the distal extremities, cerebral thrombosis or hemorrhage, and eventual vascular narrowing from deposition of glycolipids in the arterial endothelium. Renal failure is a common cause of death due to renal vascular compromise. Treatments are disappointing in Fabry's disease. Enzyme repletion does not help the clinical problems. Plasmapheresis is also not particularly effective. Renal transplantation can delay systemic complications and alleviate renal failure, but is not curative.

Tuberous sclerosis is discussed elsewhere in this volume in great detail.

Neurology

B&D Ch. 65

Question 61. A. The doctor who takes Medicare must accept Medicare's maximum fee. This fee includes any appropriate copays set forth in the patient's policy. The physician can not bill the patient or another party for the difference between what Medicare allows and what you want to charge.

Public Policy

K&S Ch. 4

Question 62. E. Reflex sympathetic dystrophy is one of the so-called complex regional pain syndromes. It is the result of regional pain and sensory changes following trauma or a noxious event. There may or may not be a diagnosable underlying nerve lesion to the problem. Soft tissue injury is the trigger in about 40% of cases and bony fracture in about 25% of cases.

There are three stages to the disorder. Stage one (acute) is associated with pain that is out of proportion to the initial injury. There is usually hypersensitivity to painful stimuli or physical contact with the extremity. Stage two (dystrophic) is associated with tissue edema and skin that is cool, cyanotic, hyperhidrotic, with livedo reticularis. Pain is constant and increases with any physical contact to the affected extremity. Stage three (atrophic) is associated with paroxysmal pain and irreversible tissue damage. The skin can become thin and shiny and the fascia can become thickened or contractured. Treatments begin with intense physical therapy which can be helpful by improving mobility of the affected extremity. Steroids may be helpful in certain cases. Phenoxybenzamine, which is a sympathetic blocking agent, can also be useful, if tolerated. Some patients require invasive anesthesia by regional block, which can be helpful in certain patients.

Neurology

B&D Ch. 29

Question 63. B.   In the situation where you are presented with an unknown psychotic or paranoid patient, the first step is to make sure that patient and staff are safe. All other options are valid, but would be taken after an initial assessment of the patient's safety has been made. When given a question such as this on an examination, maintenance of safety comes first, and diagnosis and treatment come later. You would not automatically give sedation to the patient if they were not agitated or dangerous, so answer choice A is not the correct first move. Remember that past violence is the best predictor of future violence.

Management in Psychiatry

K&S Ch. 33

Question 64. B.   Carbamazepine is an inducer of cytochrome P450 2C19 and 3A4. It can therefore induce the metabolism of any substrate of the 2C19 and 3A4 systems. The 3A4 substrates that can be induced by carbamazepine include erythromycin, clarithromycin, alprazolam, diazepam, midazolam, cyclosporine, indinavir, ritonavir, saquinavir, diltiazem, nifedipine, amlodipine, verapamil, atorvastatin, simvastatin, aripiprazole, buspirone, haloperidol, tamoxifen, trazodone, propranolol, zolpidem, zaleplon, methadone, estradiol (oral contraceptives), progesterone, testosterone, and fentanyl, to name but a few. The 2C19 substrates that can be induced by carbamazepine include amitriptyline, citalopram, clomipramine, imipramine, R-warfarin, propranolol, and primidone. Carbamazepine can lower lamotrigine levels by induction of glucuronidation enzyme 1A4. Clozapine is a substrate of cytochrome P450 1A2 and is not affected by carbamazepine.

Neurology

Psychopharmacology

B&D Chs 8,52&67

Question 65. E.   The standard of substituted judgment holds that a surrogate decision maker will make decisions based on what the patient would have wanted, and implies that the decision maker be familiar with the patient's values and attitudes. The best interest principle, which was the past, but not current standard, states that a decision maker will decide which option would be in the patient's best interests. Patients do have the right to refuse treatment that they feel would lessen their quality of life. Advanced directives and the living will are ways for patients to preserve their wishes in writing such that the correct decisions are made for them should they become incapacitated. The state will follow the course that preserves human life should a suitable surrogate decision maker not be present. Surrogate decision makers can be appointed by the patient, courts, or the hospital. In many cases this person is the patient's next of kin.

Forensic Psychiatry

K&S Ch. 56

Question 66. D.   Tobacco smoking is a potent inducer of cytochrome P450 1A2. As such it can significantly lower levels of amitriptyline, fluvoxamine, clozapine, olanzapine, haloperidol, and imipramine. Risperidone is a substrate of cytochrome P450 2D6 and its levels can be lowered by 2D6 inducers such as dexamethasone and rifampin. Risperidone levels can be significantly increased by 2D6 inhibitors such as bupropion, citalopram, clomipramine, doxepin, duloxetine, escitalopram, fluoxetine, paroxetine, sertraline, and perphenazine. Risperidone levels are not affected by tobacco smoking.

Psychopharmacology

B&D Ch. 9

Question 67. E.   One cannot treat what is assumed to be denial before actually knowing that it is denial. Often in medical settings things are not clearly explained to patients in language they can understand. As such it is first necessary to explain what is going on to the patient clearly and in language they can follow. Confronting the patient's denial forcefully, and aggressively removing his defenses against overwhelming emotion, is potentially more harmful than helpful. Playing along with the denial can lead to noncompliance and failed treatment outcomes and is a bad idea. Neuropsychological testing is not necessary if a patient is in denial. If he had a neurocognitive deficit that precluded his understanding of the material presented to him it could be considered, but those were not the circumstances described in this question. Meeting the family is important, but not more important than making sure the patient has had the situation explained properly. The patient is the primary person who has to understand. Informing the family while the patient is left in the dark is not the best approach.

Psychological Theory and Psychometric Testing

K&S Ch. 28

Question 68. A. This is a classic case of Sheehan's syndrome, which is essentially a postpartum pituitary infarction or apoplexy. The classic symptoms are those similar to a pituitary hemorrhage. The pituitary infarction can cause chiasmal compression that can lead to bitemporal hemianopsia from bilateral medial optic nerve compression. Hypotension can occur due to pre-existing adrenocorticotropic hormone deficiency. The clinical picture can resemble a subarachnoid hemorrhage due to the rupture of a berry aneurysm or an arteriovenous malformation. This would account for the severe acute headache and cranial nerve palsy. The syndrome can also result in meningeal irritation with positive Kernig's and Brudzinski's signs and a stiff neck. The diagnosis can often be confirmed by a CT or MRI scan of the brain. Treatment is generally supportive and only in certain cases is it necessary to provide corticosteroid replacement or conduct a surgical decompression.

Cushing's disease is caused by endogenous overproduction of adrenocorticotropic hormone from the anterior pituitary gland. Cushing's syndrome is the result of exposure to either excessive exogenous or endogenous corticosteroids. The clinical picture is that of hypertension, truncal obesity, impaired glucose tolerance or diabetes mellitus, menstrual irregularities, hirsutism, acne, purplish abdominal striae, osteoporosis, thin skin with excessive bruising, and proximal myopathy. The diagnostic test of choice is the dexamethasone suppression test.

Subarachnoid hemorrhage is most often the result of an intracranial arterial aneurysmal rupture. The acute presentation very often consists of a sudden explosive headache ("the worst headache of my life"), meningeal signs, nausea, vomiting, photophobia, and obtundation. Head CT scan is the imaging test of choice as it reveals acute blood better than MRI. CT scans can only reveal subarachnoid blood in about 90–95% of patients within 24 hours of the hemorrhage. This sensitivity drops to about 80% after 72 hours. A negative CT scan should therefore be followed by a lumbar puncture with centrifuging of CSF looking for characteristic xanthochromia (from lysed red blood cells). If either CT or lumbar puncture is positive for subarachnoid hemorrhage, then cerebral angiography should be performed as soon as possible to determine the location of the aneurysm and best method of intervening. The most popular interventions for intracranial aneurysms are endovascular coiling, microsurgical clipping, and balloon embolization. Saccular or berry aneurysms are the most common kind of intracranial aneurysms. Between 80 and 85% of aneurysms stem from the anterior cerebral circulation, most often arising from the anterior communicating artery, posterior communicating artery, or the trifurcation of the middle cerebral artery. Between 15 and 20% of aneurysms originate in the posterior circulation, most often from the origin of the posterior inferior cerebellar artery or at the bifurcation of the basilar artery.

Bacterial meningitis presents in adults as a febrile illness involving headache, stiff neck, and signs of cerebral dysfunction, which are present in over 85% of patients. Associated signs and symptoms include nausea, vomiting, photophobia, and myalgia. Often Kernig's and Brudzinski's signs can be elicited. Cerebral dysfunction can involve delirium, confusion, and decreased level of consciousness that ranges from lethargy to coma. Seizures can occur in about 40% of cases. Cranial nerve palsies can be seen in 10–20% of patients. Increased intracranial pressure may result in the appearance of bilateral VI nerve palsies. Lumbar puncture and blood cultures clinch the diagnosis. Cerebrospinal fluid (CSF) opening pressure is high (200–500 mmH$_2$O) and protein is also high (100–500 mg/dL, normal = 15–45 mg/dL), with decreased glucose and marked pleocytosis (100–10 000 WBC/mL, normal = <5), with 60% or more polymorphonuclear leukocytes. CSF cultures are positive in about 75% of cases. In the United States, the predominant causative organism in children ages 2 to 18 years is *N. meningitidis* and in adults, *S. pneumoniae*. Intravenous ampicillin, penicillin-G and third-generation cephalosporins (ceftriaxone, cefotaxime, ceftazidime) are the usual agents of first-line treatment.

Familial hemiplegic migraine (FHM) is a rare autosomal dominant migraine subtype in which the aura is accompanied by hemiplegia. FHM has been mapped to chromosome 19p13 that codes for the α1-subunit of brain-specific voltage-gated P/Q-type calcium channel. There is some notion that because FHM has similar symptoms to traditional migraine with aura that this implies that migraine with aura may also be genetically linked to chromosome 19.

Neurology

B&D Chs 42&53

Question 69. C. The question stem accurately describes agoraphobia. The other answer choices are distracters. Agonothete is the judge of games in ancient Greece. Agoniada is the bark of a South American shrub.

Agora is the market place in ancient Greece. Agouara is a South American wild dog or a crab-eating raccoon. Needless to say, the only one that will show up on the boards is agoraphobia.

Anxiety Disorders

K&S Ch. 16

Question 70. C. Normal-pressure hydrocephalus (NPH) presents with the triad of dementia, incontinence, and gait disturbance. The cause, in up to one-third of cases, is undetermined. NPH can be caused by trauma, infection, or subarachnoid hemorrhage. Brain CT scan or MRI reveal enlargement of the third, fourth, and lateral ventricles. NPH causes an apraxic, or magnetic gait, making it difficult for the patient to raise the legs off the ground. The dementia is considered to be subcortical, and results in slowing of verbal and motor functioning while the cortical functions remain intact. Abulia, apathy and depression are common in NPH. Urinary incontinence occurs early in the course of the illness, particularly when there is prominent gait disturbance. Lumbar puncture reveals a normal opening pressure. Serial lumbar punctures with drainage of cerebrospinal fluid can improve the symptoms and support the diagnosis of NPH. Ventriculoperitoneal shunting is the treatment of choice and is successful in up to 80% of cases. Shunts fail about one-third of the time and complications of shunting include subdural hematoma and infection.

Diffuse Lewy-body disease, or dementia with Lewy bodies is the second-most prevalent dementia after Alzheimer's disease. The symptomatic triad is that of dementia, parkinsonism, and visual hallucinations. A hallmark of the disease is extreme sensitivity to dopamine receptor antagonists which can result in severe parkinsonism when treatment with neuroleptics is undertaken. Dopaminergic therapy is generally not that helpful. Hallucinations are ideally treated with the newer antipsychotics, particularly quetiapine, clozapine, and ziprasidone. Rivastigmine and donepezil may be useful cholinergic therapy to try to improve cognition.

Wernicke's encephalopathy presents with the acute triad of mental confusion, ophthalmoplegia and gait ataxia, predominantly in alcoholic patients. On autopsy, the neuropathologic hallmark is multiple small hemorrhages in the periventricular gray matter, mainly around the aqueduct and the third and fourth ventricles. MRI of the brain often reveals abnormalities in the periaqueductal regions, bilateral mamillary bodies, and medial thalami.

Sydenham's chorea (SC) is a result of rheumatic fever. It is extremely rare these days because of the widespread availability of antistreptococcal therapy. The disorder is more frequent in girls, generally between 5 and 15 years of age. Chorea begins insidiously over a period of weeks and can last up to 6 months. Behavioral manifestations can include irritability, obsessive–compulsive traits and restlessness. Enlargement of the basal ganglia can be noted on MRI. Symptoms are generally self-limited, lasting up to about 6 months. Antibasal ganglia antibodies can be detected by Western blot testing and these antibodies seem to account for the mechanism of the disorder. Valproic acid is a useful therapy for the chorea.

Neurology

B&D Chs 66&71

Question 71. E. Cyclothymic disorder does not involve psychotic symptoms, although these symptoms may be found in bipolar disorder. Cyclothymia is a less severe form of bipolar with alternation between hypomania and moderate depression. Symptoms must exist for two years to make the diagnosis. It is equally common in men and women. Substance use often coexists. The onset is usually insidious and occurs in late adolescence or early adulthood.

Bipolar Disorders

K&S Ch. 15

Question 72. B. Depression is not considered a stroke risk factor. Common risk factors for stroke include older age, male gender, low socioeconomic status, diabetes mellitus, obesity, cigarette smoking, excessive alcohol consumption, and family history. Other important risk factors are arterial hypertension, prior stroke or transient ischemic attack, asymptomatic carotid bruit, dyslipidemia, hyperhomocysteinemia and oral contraceptive use. Hereditary blood dyscrasias also elevate stroke risk, such as protein C or S deficiency, antithrombin III deficiency and factor V Leiden deficiency.

Neurology

B&D Ch. 51

Question 73. D. This question gives a classic description of the appearance of a patient in the manic phase of bipolar disorder. They are often very bizarre, colorful, seductive and erratically behaved. A depressed patient would be apathetic and psychomotor retarded, not hyperexcited. There was no mention made in the question of psychosis or delusions so brief psychotic disorder and delusional disorder are incorrect. There is also no mention of abnormally perceived body image so body dysmorphic disorder is incorrect as well. There is an equal prevalence of bipolar disorder in women versus men. Bipolar I disorder in women most often starts with depression.

Bipolar Disorders

K&S Ch. 15

Question 74. A. Ataxia is indicative of a cerebellar lesion and the cerebellum is perfused by the vertebrobasilar arterial system. Symptoms indicative of a carotid territory transient ischemic attack or stroke would be: transient ipsilateral monocular blindness (amaurosis fugax), contralateral body weakness or sensory loss, aphasia with dominant hemisphere involvement, contralateral homonymous visual field deficits. Symptoms that suggest a vertebrobasilar territory stroke or transient ischemic attack include: bilateral, shifting, or crossed weakness or sensory loss (ipsilateral face with contralateral body), bilateral or contralateral homonymous visual field defects or binocular visual loss, two or more of vertigo, diplopia, dysphagia, dysarthria and ataxia.

Neurology

B&D Ch. 51

Question 75. E. Suicidal ideation is part of the thought content of the depressed patient. It is possible to find it in the manic bipolar patient, but is more likely during the depressed phase of the illness and is not part of the thought process.

Diagnostic and Treatment Procedures in Psychiatry

K&S Ch. 15

Question 76. D. Essential tremor (ET) is one of the most common movement disorders. It has been noted in up to 5% of patients over 60 years of age. It is defined as a postural and kinetic tremor of the forearms and hands (sometimes with other body parts) that gradually increases in amplitude over time. ET is believed to be a monosymptomatic illness, without other neurologic deficits. As many as two-thirds of patients have a positive family history of ET. The disease is likely heterogeneous with an autosomal dominant pattern of inheritance.

The mainstay of treatment is the use of β-adrenergic blocking agents and primidone. Propranolol is the β-blocker of choice and can be given in doses of 120–320 mg daily in divided doses. This helps reduce tremor amplitude in roughly half of patients. Primidone can be given as a single nighttime dose of 25 mg and subsequently titrated to a therapeutic dose of 50–350 mg daily. Benzodiazepine sedative–hypnotic agents, like clonazepam and lorazepam are also frequently used and can be helpful. Botulinum toxin type A can be injected intramuscularly for head and hand tremor and can be effective in certain cases. Desipramine and the tricyclic antidepressants are not useful in ET and may in fact worsen tremor. If oral therapy fails, surgical intervention can be contemplated if symptoms are serious. Stereotactic thalamotomy has been shown to reduce contralateral tremor by 75% in as many as 90% of cases. Thalamic deep brain stimulation has also been demonstrated to be effective in treating ET and can improve symptoms in up to 80% of cases.

Neurology

B&D Ch. 71

Question 77. B. To qualify for a diagnosis of major depressive disorder, symptoms must be present for at least two weeks. Symptoms can include depressed mood, diminished interest in activities, weight loss or gain, insomnia or hypersomnia, psychomotor retardation, fatigue, feelings of worthlessness, decreased concentration, recurrent thoughts of death, and recurrent suicidal ideation.

Depressive Disorders

K&S Ch. 15

Question 78. B. The thymus gland is believed to play a role in the pathogenesis of myasthenia gravis (MG). MG is an autoimmune disorder and the thymus gland is involved in tolerance to self-antigens. Ten per cent of patients with MG have a thymic tumor and 70% have cellular hyperplasia of the thymus indicative of an active immune response. About 20% of patients with MG who develop symptoms between ages 30 and 60 years have a thymoma. The thymus contains myoid cells that express the AChR (acetylcholine receptor) antigen, antigen presenting cells and immunocompetent T cells. The thymus is believed to produce AChR subunits that act as autoantigens in the sensitization of the patient against the AChR. Most thymomas in MG patients are benign and are amenable to easy surgical resection which may in certain cases improve symptomatology. The other tumor types mentioned above are not typically associated with MG.

Neurology

B&D Ch. 78

Question 79. B. Prevalence for schizophrenia is higher in urban than in rural areas, as are morbidity and severity of presentation. The lifetime prevalence is about 1%. The male to female ratio is 1:1. Onset is usually between 15 and 35 years, with onset before 10 years and after 40 years being rare. There is a higher incidence of cases in babies born in the winter and early spring.

Psychotic Disorders

K&S Ch. 13

Question 80. A. Friedrich's ataxia (FA) is an autosomal recessive disease that localizes to chromosome 9q13-21.1. It is the result of an unstable expansion of a trinucleotide repeat (GAA). Onset is typically noted in adolescence with gait ataxia, loss of lower extremity proprioception, and absence of deep tendon reflexes, more often in the lower extremities. There is also predominant central nervous system involvement with noted dysarthria, presence of Babinski signs and eye movement anomalies. The natural progression of the disease is towards a complete loss of ambulation ability and ultimately death due to hypertrophic cardiomyopathy in about 50% of cases. Death occurs on average by late in the fourth decade.

Myotonic dystrophy (MD) type I is an autosomal dominantly inherited disease with trinucleotide repeat expansion of CTG that codes to chromosome 19q13.3. The incidence is 1 in 8000 live births. Classic symptoms and signs include ptosis, bifacial weakness, frontal baldness, triangular drooping facies. Motor weakness is greater distally than proximally. Myotonia is a classic sign, which is the inability to relax a contracted muscle or group of muscles. For example, a patient is unable to let go after shaking hands. Percussion myotonia can also be demonstrated, particularly in the thenar and hypothenar hand muscles. This is involuntary contraction of muscles after percussion with a reflex hammer. Fibrotic or infiltrative cardiomyopathy is a frequent associated problem in myotonic dystrophy. DNA testing by serum polymerase chain reaction is the diagnostic modality of choice for MD. Electromyography reveals myopathic features and myotonic discharges ("dive-bomber" sound after muscular relaxation). Perifascicular muscle fiber atrophy is the classic histopathologic finding on muscle biopsy. Please note that the other three answer choices are explained in questions elsewhere in this volume and are all diseases inherited by autosomal dominant transmission.

Neurology

B&D Chs 72&79

Question 81. D. Disinhibited behavior is more characteristic of mania than it is of depression. All of the other symptoms are somatic or sleep complaints that are frequently associated with depression. Patients with depression have disrupted REM sleep, including shortened REM latency, increased percentage of REM sleep, and a shift in REM distribution from the last half to the first half of the night. Acetylcholine is associated with the production of REM sleep.

Depressive Disorders

K&S Ch. 15

Question 82. E. It is believed that migraine maps to several regions on chromosome 19, because of the entity FHM (familial hemiplegic migraine) that has been associated with this gene locus. FHM is thought to be a channelopathy involving a brain-specific calcium channel α-1 subunit gene that has been mapped to chromosome 19p13. Given the similarity between FHM and typical migraine, researchers believe that chromosome 19 may well be the locus that links both disorders.

Neurology

B&D Ch. 69

Question 83. A. Obsessions are part of thought content, as are delusions, ideas of reference, phobias, suicidal or homicidal thought, depersonalization, derealization, and neologisms, to name a few. Thought process would include word salad, flight of ideas, circumstantiality, tangentiality, clang associations, perseveration, and goal directed ideas.

Diagnostic and Treatment Procedures in Psychiatry

K&S Ch. 7

Question 84. B. CNS cysticercosis involves parenchymal invasion of the brain by the larval stage pork tapeworm *Taenia solium*. Cysticercosis occurs by ingestion of undercooked pork containing cysticerci. The infection occurs most frequently in Central and South America where poor hygiene and sanitation lead to unsanitary conditions. After ingestion of tainted pork, the tapeworm eggs hatch in the gastric tract, develop to larval stage and eventually penetrate the bowel to migrate to host tissue, most often in the CNS. Clinical presentation ranges from epilepsy, focal neurological deficits, hydrocephalus, cognitive decline, meningitis, or myelopathy. Diagnosis is confirmed by brain MRI demonstrating the parasites in the brain and from confirmatory serology and/or CSF enzyme-linked immunosorbent assay (ELISA) tests. ELISA on CSF is more sensitive and specific than serologic tests. Treatment is with albendazole or praziquantel oral therapy, coupled with parenteral steroids. *Trichinella spiralis* infection causes trichinosis which is also caused by ingestion of poorly cooked pork or other game meats in endemic areas. *Echinococcus granulosus* are the larval tapeworms that cause CNS echinococcosis. Humans generally acquire echinococci through contact with dogs that are infected. *E. granulosus* tends to cause solitary CNS spherical cysts without edema. Treatment can involve surgical resection of the cyst or conservative medical management with albendazole if the cysts are not resectable. *Leishmania major* is a protozoan that causes leishmaniasis. The vector is a sandfly bite. Visceral disease can be accompanied by inflammatory neuropathies that resemble Guillain–Barré syndrome. Treatment is by parenteral administration of antimony or amphotericin B. *Toxoplasma gondii* is the intracellular protozoan responsible for toxoplasmosis infection. Vectors include migratory birds and cats and so the infection can be found worldwide. Toxoplasmosis rarely occurs in immunocompetent patients, but is more often seen in AIDS patients with low CD4 counts. CNS lesions present as ring enhancing on both CT and MRI. CSF titers may contain *T. gondii* DNA detectable by PCR. Treatment is usually a combined regimen of pyrimethamine and sulfadiazine with folinic acid. Ventricular shunting may be required if lesions are space-occupying and cause hydrocephalus.

Neurology

B&D Ch. 53

Question 85. C. The effects of alcohol can be seen in several lab tests. The GGT will be elevated in 80% of alcoholic patients, while MCV is increased in 60% of alcoholic patients. Uric acid, triglycerides, AST and ALT can also be elevated. The other lab values given in the question are unrelated to alcohol abuse.

Laboratory Tests in Psychiatry

K&S Ch. 12

Question 86. C. Alcoholic neuropathy is the most common neurologic manifestation of chronic alcoholism. Up to 75% of alcoholic patients are diagnosed with this disorder. Most patients are chronic alcohol abusers between 40 and 60 years of age. This type of neuropathy is a mixed motor and sensory disorder. Symptoms usually begin gradually, symmetrically in the feet.

Alcoholic dementia refers to older patients with a lifelong history of heavy alcohol use, who experience an insidious decline in their cognitive functioning. Nearly 20% of older alcoholics have some form of dementia, but this is complicated by the presence of other comorbidities such as liver abnormalities, head trauma, malnutrition and stroke. Alcoholic dementia results in more of a predominance of fine motor control and verbal fluency deficits than is seen in patients with dementia of the Alzheimer type.

Marchiafava–Bignami disease is a rare demyelinating disease preferentially affecting the corpus callosum in chronic alcoholics. The exact etiology of the disorder is not well-understood. It may be related to nutritional factors or direct toxic effects of alcohol on the cerebral white matter, but this is unclear. The most common neurologic manifestation is that of frontal lobe damage and dementia noted on neurologic examination. The central portion of the corpus callosum is more often affected than the anterior or posterior portions. Treatment is directed at nutritional support and alcoholic rehabilitation.

Alcoholic-nutritional cerebellar degeneration is seen more often in men than in women. The disorder presents in longstanding alcoholics as unsteadiness in walking evolving over weeks to months. The most common presentation on examination is truncal ataxia, with a wide-based gait and difficulty with tandem walking. Pathologically, the disorder results from preferential atrophy of the superior and anterior cerebellar vermis, with lesser involvement of the cerebellar hemispheres. Wernicke's encephalopathy is explained extensively elsewhere in this volume.

Neurology

B&D Chs 57&76

Question 87. B.   A cohort study is when a group from a well-known population is chosen and followed over a long period of time. These studies give us estimates of risk based on suspected causative factors for a given disease. Case history studies look back on people with a given disease. Cross-sectional studies give information on prevalence of a disease in a population at a given point in time. Retrospective studies are based on past data, as opposed to prospective studies which are based on observing things as they occur.

Statistics

K&S Ch. 4

Question 88. C.   The Miller–Fisher syndrome is a variant of Guillain–Barré syndrome (GBS, acute inflammatory demyelinating polyneuropathy). The classic triad of symptoms is gait ataxia, areflexia and ophthalmoplegia. This accounts for about 5% of GBS cases. Motor strength is usually intact. Serum IgG antibodies to the ganglioside GQ1b can be detected in serum early in the course of the Miller–Fisher variant of GBS. F-wave latencies may be intact on EMG with reduced or absent SNAP amplitudes. CSF protein is elevated without pleocytosis about one week into the course of the illness. Dementia, parkinsonism and psychosis make up the triad of dementia with Lewy bodies. The clinical picture is that of dementia, extrapyramidal symptoms, fluctuations and visual hallucinations. Visual hallucinations occur in as many as 80% of cases. Neuroleptic sensitivity is another diagnostic characteristic. The classic pathologic finding is the Lewy bodies which are diffuse throughout the cortex and are eosinophilic inclusions with a core halo on hematoxylin and eosin stain. Treatment with newer atypical antipsychotics, particularly clozapine, is usually best and cholinesterase inhibitors such as donepezil may also be helpful. The triad of gait ataxia, urinary incontinence and dementia is classic for normal pressure hydrocephalus.

Neurology

B&D Ch. 76

Question 89. C.   Konrad Lorenz is known best for his work with imprinting. Imprinting is the phenomenon whereby during a critical period of early development a young animal will attach to their parent, or whatever surrogate is in the parent's place. From then on the presence of that parent or surrogate will elicit a specific behavior pattern even when the animal is much older. In Lorenz's case newborn goslings imprinted on him instead of their mother and followed him around as if he were their mother. This has correlates in psychiatry because it is evidence of the link between early experiences and later behaviors. Lorenz also studied aggression in animals and worked on the need for aggression in humans given the pressures of natural selection. All the other answer choices in this question are distracters which have nothing to do with the work of Lorenz.

Human Development

K&S Ch. 4

Question 90. B.   This case depicts a classic case of acute inflammatory demyelinating polyneuropathy (Guillain–Barré syndrome or GBS). The annual incidence is 1.8 in 100 000. About 65% of patients report a prior "insult" before the onset of symptoms. This often takes the form of a gastrointestinal infection, an upper respiratory infection, surgery, or immunization a few weeks before symptoms appear. The most commonly identified organism responsible for prodromal infection is *Campylobacter jejuni. C. jejuni* can be detected in stool cultures and serologic studies. The clinical presentation of GBS can vary from case to case. Typically patients present with symmetrical lower extremity weakness, with paresthesias and possibly with sensory symptoms. The paralysis is usually an ascending paralysis and the most worrisome outcome is paralysis of the muscles of respiration which can prove fatal in some cases. Deep tendon reflexes are usually greatly diminished or absent. Diagnostic testing reveals the classic nerve conduction abnormalities of conduction block and prolonged F-wave latencies, which are pathognomonic of GBS. CSF studies reveal cytoalbuminergic dissociation: elevated protein with an acellular fluid. In certain cases, nerve biopsy can reveal complement fixing antibodies to peripheral nerve myelin. Treatment should take place in the hospital and in an intensive care unit setting if respiratory compromise is imminent. Two treatments of choice are high dose intravenous immunoglobulin administration and plasmapheresis. These have been proven to be equally efficacious in numerous recent studies.

Neurology

B&D Ch. 76

Question 91. A. Second messengers are molecules that work within the cell to carry on the message delivered by the neurotransmitter on the cell surface. IP$_3$, cGMP, Ca^{2+}, cAMP, DAG, NO, and CO are all common second messenger molecules. Adenylyl cyclase is not a second messenger itself, but rather is the enzyme that makes cAMP from ATP. Adenylyl cyclase is turned on or off by G proteins depending on the need for cAMP. Binding cAMP to transcription factors regulates gene transcription, including the machinery to make certain neurotransmitters. Calcium plays a number of roles within the cell, and excess Ca^{2+} is linked to production of NO and cell death through excitotoxicity. One of the major functions of IP3 is to cause the release of intracellular Ca^{2+} from the endoplasmic reticulum.

Basic Neuroscience

K&S Ch. 3

Question 92. A. The cortical dementias such as Alzheimer's disease generally produce a gradual decline in cognitive function, with normal speed of cognition and the presence of aphasia, dyspraxia, and agnosia. Depression is less common in cortical dementia than in subcortical disease. Motor abnormalities are typically absent in cortical dementia, unless the disease is in the terminal stages. Subcortical dementia, as exemplified in Parkinson's disease, typically presents with dysarthria and extrapyramidal motor abnormalities. Apathy and depression are often present. Frontal memory impairment, with recall aided by cues, is often noted. Speed of cognition in subcortical dementia is slow.

Neurocognitive Disorders

B&D Ch. 66

Question 93. B. This question focuses on Piaget's stages of cognitive development. In the sensorimotor stage children respond to stimuli in the environment, and learn during this process. They eventually develop object permanence (objects exist independent of the child's awareness of their existence), and begin to understand symbols (as in the use of words to express thoughts).

During the preoperational stage there is a sense that punishment for bad deeds is unavoidable (immanent justice). There is a sense of egocentrism, and phenomenalistic causality (the thought that events that occur together cause one another). Phenomenalistic causality is the subject of this question. Animistic thinking (inanimate objects are given thoughts and feelings) is also seen.

In the concrete operations stage, egocentric thought changes to operational thought where another's point of view can be taken into consideration. In concrete operations children can put things in order and group objects according to common characteristics. They develop the understanding of conservation (a tall cup and a wide cup can both hold equal volumes of water) and reversibility (ice can change to water and back to ice again).

During formal operations children can think abstractly, reason deductively, and define abstract concepts. Latency is a distracter. It occurs in Freud's model after the genital phase and before puberty.

Human Development

K&S Ch. 2

Question 94. C. T4 is the dermatome at the level of the nipples. T10 is the dermatome at the level of the umbilicus. Other important dermatomes to remember include: C2 – back of head, C4 – above collar bone, C6 – thumb, C7 – middle fingers, C8 – little finger, L1 – groin, L2 – lateral thigh, L3 – medial thigh, L4 – medial leg, L5 – lateral leg, big toe, S1 – little toe, sole of foot, S5 – perianal area.

Neurology

B&D Ch. 24

Question 95. D. The three receptor types associated with glutamate are AMPA, kainate, and NMDA. Acetylcholine is associated with the nicotinic and muscarinic receptors. Norepinephrine is associated with the alpha 1, alpha 2, and beta receptors. Serotonin is associated with the various 5-HT receptors. GABA is associated with the GABA receptor. Opioids are associated with the mu and delta receptors. Dopamine is associated with the D1, D2 etc. receptors.

Basic Neuroscience

K&S Ch. 3

Question 96. B. Buspirone is a serotonin 1A agonist or partial agonist. It is indicated for the treatment of anxiety disorders, in particular, generalized anxiety disorder. It does have activity at the serotonin 2 and dopamine 2 receptor sites, but its significance at those sites is not well understood. It may have mild dopamine 2 agonistic and antagonistic effects, but this is not its predominant mechanism of action. Buspirone takes 2–3 weeks to exert therapeutic effects. The initial dose is 15 mg daily in two or three divided doses. Therapeutic effects are usually not seen until a dose of 30 mg or above is reached. The maximum approved daily dose is 60 mg. Buspirone can increase blood levels of haloperidol. Buspirone cannot be used with monoamine oxidase inhibitors (MAOI) and a two-week washout needs to happen after an MAOI is stopped before buspirone can be started. Buspirone levels can be increased by nefazodone, erythromycin, itraconazole and grapefruit juice by their inhibition of cytochrome P450 3A4 in the liver.

Psychopharmacology

K&S Ch. 36

Question 97. E. Excitatory neurotransmitters open cation channels that depolarize the cell membrane and increase the likelihood of generating an action potential. These neurotransmitters elicit excitatory post-synaptic potentials or EPSPs.

Basic Neuroscience

K&S Ch. 3

Question 98. C. Phencyclidine (PCP) is a potent N-methyl-D-aspartate (NMDA) receptor antagonist. The NMDA receptor is a subtype of the glutamate receptor. PCP has calcium channel binding properties and prevents the influx of calcium into neurons. PCP also has dopaminergic properties that would seem to explain the reinforcing effects of the drug.

Tolerance can occur with PCP, but it is generally held that PCP does not cause a physical dependence. There is psychological dependence to the agent and users can become dependent to its euphoric effects in this way. PCP intoxication is characterized by maladaptive behavioral changes, such as violence, impulsivity, belligerence, agitation, impaired judgment. Symptoms of intoxication include nystagmus, hypertension, decreased pain responsiveness, ataxia, dysarthria, muscle rigidity, seizures, coma, and hyperacusis. PCP can induce a delirium with agitated, bizarre, or violent behavior. It can also cause an acute psychotic disorder with delusions and hallucinations that can persist for several weeks following ingestion of the drug. PCP can remain in the blood and urine for more than a week. Treatment of the behavioral abnormalities related to PCP is best undertaken with benzodiazepines and dopamine antagonists.

Substance Abuse and Addictive Disorders

K&S Ch. 12

Question 99. C. Sublimation is one of the mature defenses. It is characterized by obtaining gratification by transforming a socially unacceptable aim or object into an acceptable one. Sublimation allows instincts to be channeled in an acceptable direction rather than blocked. All other choices are immature defenses. Hypochondriasis is exemplified by exaggerating an illness for the purpose of evasion or regression. Introjection is demonstrated by internalizing the qualities of an outside object. It is an important part of development but can also be used as an unproductive defense. The classic example is identification with an aggressor. Regression is characterized by attempting to return to an earlier libidinal phase of functioning to avoid the tension and conflict of the current level of development. Passive aggression takes the form of expressing anger towards others through passivity, masochism, and turning against the self. Manifestations can include failure and procrastination.

Psychological Theory and Psychometric Testing

K&S Ch. 6

Question 100. E. Phenelzine is a monoamine oxidase inhibitor and is not likely to worsen the movement disorder symptoms of Parkinson's disease. The other four agents are antagonists of dopamine D2 receptors and can of course worsen symptoms of Parkinson's disease and cause drug-induced parkinsonism. The pathophysiology involves D2 receptor antagonism in the caudate. Patients who are elderly and female are at greatest risk for neuroleptic-induced parkinsonism. More than half of patients exposed to neuroleptics on a long-term basis have been noted to develop this unwanted adverse effect. Amoxapine (Asendin) is a dibenzoxazepine tetracyclic antidepressant that has strong D2 antagonistic properties because it is a chemical derivative of the neuroleptic loxapine (Loxitane). Because of its unique structure and chemical properties, amoxapine can also cause akathisia, dyskinesia and infrequently, neuroleptic malignant syndrome.

Psychopharmacology

K&S Ch. 36

Question 101. D. Ana Freud wrote *The Ego and Mechanisms of Defense* and was the first to give a comprehensive study of the defense mechanisms. She maintained that all people, healthy or neurotic, use a number of defense mechanisms. Freud was the father of psychoanalysis whose work focused on the importance of libido, aggression, and the oedipal complex, among other concepts. Kohut was the father of self psychology. Fromm defined five character types common to western culture. Jung went beyond Freud's work and founded the school of analytic psychology. It focused on the growth of the personality through one's experiences.

Psychological Theory and Psychometric Testing

K&S Ch. 6

Question 102. B. In the case of Dusky vs United States, the US Supreme Court determined that, in order to have the competence to stand trial, a criminal defendant must be able to have the ability to consult his lawyer with a reasonable degree of rational understanding and he must have a reasonable and rational understanding of the proceedings against him. The McGarry instrument is a clinical guide that identifies thirteen areas of functioning that must be demonstrated by a criminal defendant in order to be declared competent to stand trial. Answer choices A, C, D, and E are included in these 13 areas, as well as the ability to plan legal strategy, the ability to appraise the roles of participants in courtroom procedure, capacity to challenge prosecution witnesses realistically, capacity to testify relevantly, ability to appraise the likely outcome, and understanding the possible penalties, among several others.

Forensic Psychiatry

K&S Ch. 57

Question 103. D. Paranoid schizophrenia is characterized by systematized delusions or frequent auditory hallucinations related to a single theme. None of the other answer choices are characteristic of paranoid schizophrenia, but may be found in other types of schizophrenia.

Psychotic Disorders

K&S Ch. 13

Question 104. E. Studies have indicated that depression tends to be a chronic, relapsing disorder. The percentage of patients who recover following repeated episodes diminishes over time. About one-quarter of patients have a recurrence within the first 6 months after initial treatment. This figure rises to about 30–50% in the first 2 years and even higher to about 50–75% within 5 years. It has been proven than ongoing antidepressant prophylaxis helps to lower relapse rates. As a patient experiences more depressive episodes over time, the time between episodes decreases and the severity of the episodes worsens.

Depressive Disorders

K&S Ch. 15

Question 105. D. Dysthymic disorder is characterized by decreased mood over a period of 2 years with poor appetite or over eating, sleep problems, fatigue, low self esteem, poor concentration, and feelings of hopelessness. Hallucinations are not considered part of dysthymia, although it is possible to have hallucinations as part of a major depressive episode.

Depressive Disorders

K&S Ch. 15

Question 106. D.   Tarasoff vs regents of the University of California is the landmark case from 1976 in which the California Supreme Court ruled that any psychotherapist who believes that a patient could injure or kill someone must notify the potential victim, the victim's relatives or friends, or the authorities. In 1982, the same court issued a second ruling that broadened Tarasoff to include the duty to protect, not only to warn the intended victim.

The Durham Rule was determined by the ruling in the case of Durham vs the United States in 1954 by Judge Bazelon. This rule stipulates that a defendant cannot be found criminally responsible if the criminal act was the product of a mental illness or defect. In 1972 the District of Columbia Court of Appeals in the ruling United States vs Brawner, discarded the Durham Rule.

In 1976 in the ruling of O'Connor vs Donaldson, the United States Supreme Court ruled that harmless mentally ill patients cannot be confined involuntarily without treatment if they can survive outside an institution.

Clites vs State was a landmark case pertaining to a ruling in favor of a patient and his family who sued for damages resulting from chronic neuroleptic exposure that resulted in tardive dyskinesia. The appellate court ruled that the defendants deviated from the usual standards of care by failing to conduct physical examinations and routine laboratory tests and failed to intervene at the first signs of tardive dyskinesia.

Forensic Psychiatry

K&S Ch. 57

Question 107. C.   All of the drugs listed are tertiary amines except desipramine, which is a secondary amine. The other tertiary amine is doxepin. The secondary amines include desipramine, nortriptyline, and protriptyline. During metabolism the tertiary amines are converted into secondary amines.

Psychopharmacology

K&S Ch. 35

Question 108. C.   Surgical approaches to Parkinson's disease include deep brain stimulation, surgical stereotactic ablation of overactive brain areas and cellular implantation of dopaminergic neuronal cells. Stereotactic thalamotomy can reduce tremor and rigidity contralaterally in about 75–85% of patients. There is little effect on bradykinesia. Bilateral thalamotomy can cause cognitive and speech deficits. Thalamic deep brain stimulation is better tolerated and results are similar to thalamotomy without the risks involved with the ablative procedure. Stereotactic posteroventral pallidotomy can improve dopa-induced dyskinesia and akinesia in about 70% of patients. Pallidal deep brain stimulation has also been shown to be almost as effective as pallidotomy. Subthalamic deep brain stimulation is the most preferred of the surgical procedures and has demonstrated 40–50% improvement in the motor fluctuations of Parkinson's disease. Human fetal substantia nigra transplantation into the putamen has been shown to be modestly effective on an experimental basis. Injection of glial-derived neurotrophic factor (GDNF) into brain parenchyma may be of future utility, but up until recently has only been studied in animal models. The superior colliculus is not an area that is targeted in neurosurgical intervention for Parkinson's disease.

Neurology

B&D Ch. 71

Question 109. A.   Amoxapine has a 7-hydroxymetabolite that has potent dopamine blocking activity. This can lead to antipsychotic-like side effects that result from the drug's use.

Psychopharmacology

K&S Ch. 35

Question 110. C.   Right–left disorientation is a result of a lesion to the dominant angular gyrus and is one of the symptoms of Gerstmann's syndrome. A large stroke in the right middle cerebral artery territory can result in hemi-neglect, visual and tactile extinction, impaired speech prosody (loss of musical and emotional inflection), anosognosia (not knowing that you have a deficit or problem), and behavioral problems such as delirium and confusion. The patient may not recognize that the affected left arm and/or hand is his own and may have limb apraxia. A contralateral homonymous hemianopia or inferior quadrantanopia can also be noted in nondominant hemispheric strokes.

Neurology

B&D Ch. 51

Question 111. D. The metabolism of tricyclic antidepressants by CYP2D6 is an important topic that has led to an FDA-recommended precaution. Tricyclics are metabolized by CYP 2D6, and as such anything that decreases the activity of CYP 2D6 will increase the plasma level of the tricyclic, even into the toxic range. Some people are naturally "poor metabolizers" who have decreased CYP 2D6 activity, and as such, higher plasma levels. Cimetidine inhibits CYP 2D6 and as such will increase tricyclic levels. The same holds true for quinidine. Several drugs are substrates for CYP 2D6 and will decrease its ability to clear tricyclics when present. These include fluoxetine, sertraline, paroxetine, carbamazepine, phenothiazines, propafenone, and flecainide.

Psychopharmacology

K&S Ch. 35

Question 112. A. This question depicts a classic diabetic third nerve palsy. The differential diagnosis of greatest importance with an isolated third nerve palsy is diabetes (benign) versus that of an internal carotid artery (ICA) aneurysm (potentially fatal). Aneurysms that most commonly affect third nerve functioning are those originating at the ICA near the origin of the posterior communicating artery. A third nerve palsy resulting from an aneurysm is usually associated with a dilated pupil and eyelid ptosis, as contrasted with a diabetic third nerve palsy that usually spares the pupillary function.

Neurology

B&D Ch. 51

Question 113. A. Residual schizophrenia is characterized by the absence of prominent hallucinations, delusions, incoherence, and disorganized behavior. Two or more of the residual symptoms may be present (i.e., negative symptoms or active phase symptoms present in a clearly attenuated form). Posturing is a characteristic symptom of catatonic schizophrenia.

Psychotic Disorders

K&S Ch. 13

Question 114. E. Severe motor tics in Tourette's syndrome are best treated by neuroleptics, in particular haloperidol and pimozide. Recently the atypical neuroleptics have come to be used more readily because of their superior safety profiles, in particular risperidone, quetiapine, olanzapine, ziprasidone and clozapine. Fluphenazine, molindone, and other conventional antipsychotics are also acceptable treatment choices. Clonidine is also a frequently used and effective treatment of tics and is particularly favored by pediatric neurologists for its excellent safety profile. Botulinum toxin type A can be effective for blepharospasm, eyelid motor tics, and is in fact FDA-approved for this indication. Protriptyline and the other antidepressants may be effective for associated obsessive–compulsive symptoms, but these agents are not useful for treatment of tics.

Disruptive, Impulse Control, Conduct Disorders, and ADHD

B&D Ch. 71

Question 115. E. Grossly inappropriate affect is a characteristic of disorganized schizophrenia, along with disorganized behavior, incoherence, and loosening of associations. In addition to the symptoms listed in the question, catatonic schizophrenia can also present with stupor, purposeless excitement, posturing, and echopraxia.

Psychotic Disorders

K&S Ch. 13

Question 116. C. The middle cerebral artery territory includes the optic radiations. A lesion of these tracts results in either a contralateral homonymous hemianopsia or a contralateral inferior quadrantanopsia ("pie on the floor"). Bitemporal hemianopsia is of course caused by invasion of the optic chiasm, often by a sellar lesion such as a pituitary macroadenoma. Left monocular blindness would result from an ipsilateral central retinal artery occlusion.

Neurology

B&D Ch. 51

Question 117. E. The process by which neurotransmitter is released into the synaptic cleft is called exocytosis. Neurotransmitters are synthesized in the presynaptic neuron, and both their synthesis and release are mediated by Ca^{2+} influx into the cell. Feedback receptors exist on the presynaptic membranes of many cells, a good example being the alpha 2 receptor on the noradrenergic neuron which participates in a negative feedback loop to stop the release of norepinephrine. Neurotransmitters such as dopamine, norepinephrine, and serotonin will remain active until they diffuse out of the cleft or are removed by reuptake mechanisms. Degradation of recycled neurotransmitters is done via monoamine oxidases (MAOs), with MAO type A degrading NE and serotonin and MAO type B degrading dopamine.

Basic Neuroscience

K&S Ch. 3

Question 118. B.   Lesch–Nyhan syndrome is an X-linked recessive disorder. Hyperuricemia results from a deficit in hypoxanthine-guanine phosphoribosyltransferase. Clinical hallmarks of the disorder include cognitive impairment, self-mutilatory behavior, hypertonia, hyperreflexia, dysarthria, developmental delay and choreoathetotic movements. Low dopamine concentrations in the basal ganglia and cerebrospinal fluid may be a cause of the movement disorder noted in Lesch–Nyhan syndrome.

Ornithine transcarbamylase deficiency is an X-linked inborn error of metabolism of the urea cycle that causes hyperammonemia, encephalopathy and respiratory alkalosis. Treatment with low-protein diet and dietary arginine supplementation can be effective.

Carbamoylphosphate synthase deficiency is an autosomal recessive inborn error of metabolism of the urea cycle that causes hyperammonemia, encephalopathy and respiratory alkalosis. There are two forms of the disorder, type I an early fatal form and type II a delayed-onset form which may only present later in childhood or early adulthood. Treatment with dietary arginine repletion may be helpful in certain cases.

Arginase deficiency results in hyperammonemia as well. The disorder is usually caused by a point-mutation or deletion on chromosome 6q23 that codes for the ARG1 gene. The incidence of the disorder is less than 1 in 100 000.

Adenylosuccinase deficiency results in autism, growth retardation, and psychomotor delay. It is believed to be an autosomal recessive cause of autism. Seizures may also arise as a result of this disorder.

Neurology

B&D Ch. 62

Question 119. D.   This question focuses on Piaget's stages of cognitive development. In the sensorimotor stage children respond to stimuli in the environment, and learn during this process. They eventually develop object permanence (objects exist independent of the child's awareness of their existence), and begin to understand symbols (as in the use of words to express thoughts).

During the preoperational stage there is a sense that punishment for bad deeds is unavoidable (immanent justice). There is a sense of egocentrism, and phenomenalistic causality (the thought that events that occur together cause one another). Animistic thinking (inanimate objects are given thoughts and feelings) is also seen.

In the concrete operations stage, egocentric thought changes to operational thought where another's point of view can be taken into consideration. In concrete operations children can put things in order and group objects according to common characteristics. They develop the understanding of conservation (a tall cup and a wide cup can both hold equal volumes of water) and reversibility (ice can change to water and back to ice again.)

During formal operations children can think abstractly, reason deductively, and define abstract concepts. Symbiosis is one of Mahler's stages of separation–individuation. It is unrelated to Piaget.

Human Development

K&S Ch. 2

Question 120. D.   Post-traumatic dementia most often results in frontotemporal cognitive dysfunction from diffuse subcortical axonal shear that disrupts cortical and subcortical circuitry. Slowing of mental processing and difficulty with executive functioning, set-shifting, organization and planning, are the most frequent cognitive deficits noted. Dementia pugilistica can occur in patients with repeated head trauma and is not simply limited to boxers. Clinical features include severe memory and attentional deficits and extrapyramidal signs. ApoE4 carriers (which resides on chromosome 19) are at increased risk of post-traumatic dementia as well as Alzheimer's disease.

Neurology

B&D Ch. 68

Question 121. E. Doxepin is the tricyclic with the most antihistaminic activity.
Psychopharmacology
K&S Ch. 35

Question 122. A. Bupropion is neither indicated nor effective in the treatment of obsessive–compulsive disorder (OCD). The selective serotonin reuptake inhibitors (SSRIs) have demonstrated proven efficacy in treating OCD. Trials of 4–6 weeks' duration are usually needed to produce results, but often trials need to be extended to 8–16 weeks to achieve maximal therapeutic benefit. The standard of care is to start either an SSRI or clomipramine which generally generate a response in 50–70% of cases. Four of the SSRIs have been FDA-approved for OCD, fluoxetine, fluvoxamine, paroxetine and sertraline. Higher doses may be needed in order to achieve a response. Clomipramine (Anafranil) is the most serotonergic of the tricyclic and tetracyclic antidepressant agents, which are more noradrenergic in their nature. Clomipramine was the first agent specifically FDA-approved for OCD. It needs to be titrated upwards gradually over several weeks in order to minimize gastrointestinal and anticholinergic side effects. The best results are achieved with a combination of drug and cognitive behavioral therapy.
Psychopharmacology
K&S Ch. 16

Question 123. A. Giving tricyclic antidepressants leads to a decrease in the number of α-adrenergic and 5-HT receptors. This downregulation of receptors is what correlates most closely with the time to clinical improvement in patients.
Psychopharmacology
K&S Ch. 35

Question 124. E. Enuresis should first be treated with the bell-and-pad behavioral conditioning method before pharmacotherapy is instituted. The principle is simple: a bell awakens the child when the mattress becomes wet. Tricyclic antidepressants, such as amitriptyline and imipramine can reduce the frequency of enuresis in about 60% of patients. Desmopressin (DDAVP) is effective in about half of patients. Tricyclic antidepressants are to be given about one hour before bedtime. The response to therapy can be as rapid as a few days. Desmopressin is administered intranasally in doses of 10–40 mg daily. Children who respond completely to any of these pharmacological agents should continue the therapy for several months to prevent relapse. Olanzapine and the antipsychotic medications are not generally used in the treatment of enuresis.
Elimination Disorders
K&S Ch. 53

Question 125. D. This question stem is referring to Ca^{2+}. During an action potential, the first ion channel to open is the Na^+ channel. This lets Na^+ flow into the neuron. Next Ca^{2+} channels open allowing more positively charged ions to enter and contribute to the action potential. Once inside, Ca^{2+} ions act as second messengers involved in protein–protein interactions and gene regulation. Calcium ions are critical to the release of neurotransmitter and also activate the opening of potassium ion channels that then put a stop to the action potential through the after-hyperpolarization of the membrane. With regard to receptors, also keep in mind that the GABA receptor is a chloride ion channel.
Basic Neuroscience
K&S Ch. 3

Question 126. B. The most worrisome side effects of the tricyclic antidepressant agents are cardiac conduction abnormalities, because of course these side effects can lead to fatal cardiac arrhythmias if the medication is taken in overdose. These agents can cause flattened T waves, tachycardia, prolonged QT intervals and depressed ST segments on electrocardiograms. The tricyclics are also noted for causing orthostatic hypotension by α-1 adrenergic blockade and they can of course cause sedation and the lowering of the seizure threshold. The tricyclics can also cause anticholinergic side effects, which consist of dry mouth, constipation, blurred vision and urinary retention. In the male patient suffering from benign prostatic hypertrophy, the anticholinergic load can lead to severe urinary retention and even anuria, which can be very problematic. Bethanechol 25–50 mg three to four times daily can reduce urinary hesitancy and retention.

Tricyclic antidepressants can actually help with migraine and neuropathic pain prophylaxis, particularly at lower dosages. These are off-label uses for these agents.

Psychopharmacology

K&S Ch. 36

Question 127. D. Inhibitory neurotransmitters open chloride channels that hyperpolarize the membrane and decrease the likelihood of an action potential being generated. They cause inhibitory post-synaptic potentials or IPSPs.

Basic Neuroscience

K&S Ch. 3

Question 128. C. This question addresses different types of behavior therapy for a simple phobia of spiders (arachnophobia). Flooding (implosion) involves exposing the patient to the feared stimulus in vivo immediately, without a gradual buildup, as would be expected in therapeutic graded exposure. The goal of flooding is immediate exposure and response prevention until the patient can tolerate the anxiety and gain a sense of mastery of the anxiety. Therapeutic graded exposure is similar to systematic desensitization, except that relaxation techniques are not involved and the technique is carried out in real situations. Progress is graded and at first the patient may be exposed to pictures of the spiders only, and then later exposed to the real spiders themselves. Participant modeling involves the patient learning a new behavior by observation first, then eventually by doing it, often accompanied by the therapist. This model can work particularly well with agoraphobia. Aversion therapy is the use of a noxious stimulus or punishment to suppress an undesired behavior. Using a bad-tasting nail polish to prevent nail-biting, or taking disulfiram to prevent alcohol use would be excellent examples of aversion therapy. Assertiveness training teaches the patient to develop social and interpersonal skills through responding appropriately in social or occupational situations, expressing opinions acceptably, and achieving personal goals. Techniques such as role modeling, positive reinforcement and desensitization can be used to develop assertiveness.

Psychotherapy

K&S Ch. 35

Question 129. C. Disclaimers such as "I know you don't agree with this but …" or "I don't know why I think this but…" often precede emotionally charged material. They serve to soften the delivery of such material and relieve anxiety on the part of the person making them. Whenever a disclaimer is made by the patient in therapy the therapist should listen closely to the material that follows as that material is often a window into how the patient truly feels. The other answer choices in this question border on the ridiculous.

Psychotherapy

K&S Ch. 35

Question 130. D. This question depicts a patient with an acute delirium. The mainstay of treatment of delirium is to treat the underlying cause if it is identifiable. The other goal of treatment is to give the patient environmental, sensory and physical support. Environmental support can be given by increasing the lighting level in the room, providing a clock and calendar in the room showing the correct time and date, and by dimming the lights and closing the blinds only at night. Physical support can be provided to patients by the presence of friends and relatives in the room, or a constant caregiver figure. This can help prevent falls and other physical accidents. Low-dose haloperidol in either oral or intramuscular form can be helpful to treat psychotic symptoms or agitation. Benzodiazepines, particularly those of high potency and short duration of action like flurazepam (Dalmane) should be avoided, as they can paradoxically agitate and further confuse the delirious patient.

Neurocognitive Disorders

K&S Ch. 10

Question 131. D. Abreaction is an emotional release after recalling a painful event. It is part of psychodynamic therapy and is a large part of what Freud thought brought about cure during psychoanalysis of conversion disorder patients during his early work. The other answer choices are part of cognitive behavioral therapy (CBT). In CBT the false belief systems that underlie maladaptive behaviors and mood disturbance are examined through techniques such as those listed in the question. Underlying assumptions that feed false belief systems are also examined. The goal of therapy is to correct the underlying thoughts and assumptions, and in so doing, change the mood and behavior.

Psychotherapy

K&S Ch. 35

Question 132. A. Pinpoint pupils are a feature of opioid intoxication or usage and not withdrawal. Opioid withdrawal consists of dysphoric mood, nausea or vomiting, muscle aches or twitches, lacrimation or rhinorrhea, papillary dilatation, piloerection, sweating, diarrhea, yawning, fever and insomnia. Associated symptoms can include hypertension, tachycardia, and temperature dysregulation such as hypothermia or hyperthermia. Other possible symptoms can include depression, irritability, weakness and tremor.

Substance Abuse and Addictive Disorders

K&S Ch. 12

Question 133. A. The least sedating tricyclic antidepressants are desipramine and protriptyline. Moderately sedating tricyclics include imipramine, amoxapine, nortriptyline and maprotiline. The most sedating include amitriptyline, trimipramine, and doxepin.

Psychopharmacology

K&S Ch. 35

Question 134. B. Secondary gain refers to tangible advantages that a patient may get as a result of being unwell. Examples of secondary gain include getting out of responsibility, getting money, drugs, or other financial entitlements, or controlling other people's behavior. Getting or seeking medical help, or enjoying playing the sick role for its own sake, would be considered a form of primary gain.

Somatic Symptom Disorders

K&S Ch. 17

Question 135. C. In hypothyroidism, one would expect to find an increased TSH and a low free T4 level. Subclinical cases of hypothyroidism will present with a high TSH and a normal T4 level. Other answer choices are distracters, and are not the most important lab values to look for when trying to diagnose hypothyroidism.

Laboratory Tests in Psychiatry

K&S Ch. 7

Question 136. E. There are no absolute contraindications to electroconvulsive shock therapy (ECT). Pregnancy is not a contraindication for ECT. Fetal monitoring is only considered important if the pregnancy is high risk or complicated. Brain tumors increase the risk of ECT, especially of brain edema and herniation after ECT. If the tumor is small, complications can be minimized by administration of dexamethasone prior to ECT and close monitoring of blood pressure during the treatment. Patients with aneurysms, vascular malformations or increased intracranial pressure are at greater risk during ECT because of increased blood flow during the induction of the seizure. This risk can be decreased by careful control of blood pressure during the seizure. Epilepsy and prior neuroleptic malignant syndrome are not problematic with the administration of ECT. Recent myocardial infarction is another risk factor, but the risk decreases markedly 2 weeks after the infarction and even further 3 months after the infarction. Hypertension, if controlled and stabilized with antihypertensive medication, does not pose an increased risk during ECT.

Diagnostic and Treatment Procedures in Psychiatry

K&S Ch. 36

Question 137. E. Carbamazepine has many drug–drug interactions because of its effects on the cytochrome P450 system. Of importance is the fact that it lowers concentrations of oral contraceptives, leading to breakthrough bleeding and uncertain protection against pregnancy. It has a long list of other drugs with which it interacts including lithium, some antipsychotics, and certain cardiac medications. It should not be combined with MAOIs. Combining clozapine with carbamazepine will increase the risk of bone marrow suppression.

Psychopharmacology

K&S Ch. 36

Question 138. B. Alfred Binet developed the idea of mental age in 1905 as the average intellectual level of a particular age. Intelligence quotient (IQ) is simply the quotient of mental age divided by chronological age multiplied by 100. An IQ of 100 is therefore considered to be the average, that is, when mental age and chronological age are equal. An IQ of 100 represents the 50th percentile in intellectual ability for the general population.

Psychological Theory and Psychometric Testing

K&S Ch. 5

Question 139. B. Open-ended questions are those that allow the patient to express what he is thinking and do not direct the patient to speak about a specific topic that the doctor chooses. Ideally an interview should begin with open ended questions and become more specific and close-ended as it continues. Closed-ended questions can often be answered in one or few words. Open-ended questions often require the patient to explain and provide information.

Psychotherapy

K&S Ch. 1

Question 140. A. The Karolinska Institute has shown in numerous studies that diminished central serotonin plays a role in suicidal behavior. This group was the first to demonstrate that low levels of cerebrospinal fluid (CSF) 5-hydroxyindoleacetic acid (5-HIAA) is associated with suicidal behavior. It has also been shown that low 5-HIAA levels predict future suicidal behavior and that low 5-HIAA levels have been shown in the CSF of adolescents who kill themselves.

Depressive Disorders

K&S Ch. 34

Question 141. E. Symptoms of lithium toxicity include ataxia, tremor, nausea, vomiting, nephrotoxicity, muscle weakness, convulsions, coma, lethargy, confusion, hyperreflexia, and nystagmus. Non-specific T-wave changes can also be seen at high lithium concentrations. Jaundice is a result of hepatic dysfunction. Lithium damages the kidneys, not the liver. Lithium induced polyuria is the result of lithium antagonism to the effects of ADH (antidiuretic hormone).

Psychopharmacology

K&S Ch. 36

Question 142. B. Obsessive–compulsive disorder (OCD) is believed to be a result of an imbalance in the serotonin system. Data show that serotonergic drugs are more effective in relieving symptoms of OCD than drugs that work on other neurotransmitter systems. Studies are unclear as to whether serotonin actually is involved in the cause of OCD. Cerebrospinal fluid (CSF) assays of 5-hydroxyindoleacetic acid (5-HIAA) have reported variable findings in patients with OCD. In one study CSF levels of 5-HIAA decreased after treatment with clomipramine, leading researchers to the conclusion that the serotonin system is involved in OCD symptom genesis.

Obsessive Compulsive and Related Disorders

K&S Ch. 16

Question 143. E. Amoxapine is the most likely of the tricyclic antidepressants to cause parkinsonian symptoms. It can also cause akathisia or dyskinesia. This is because its metabolites have dopamine blocking activity. It can even cause NMS in rare cases. Tricyclics are contraindicated in patients with cardiac conduction deficits. They should be stopped before elective surgery because of the risk of hypertension when tricyclics are given concomitantly with anesthetics. Fludrocortisone can help some patients with orthostatic hypotension. Myoclonic twitches and tremors can be seen in patients on desipramine and protriptyline.

Psychopharmacology

K&S Ch. 35

Question 144. D. Vascular dementia, formerly known as multi-infarct dementia, is generally the result of one or more cerebrovascular accidents that are the consequence of ischemic or embolic risk factors for cerebrovascular events. Vascular dementia occurs more frequently in men, particularly those with known cerebrovascular risk factors, which include smoking, hypertension and diabetes. Symptoms are generally abrupt in onset and a pattern of step-wise decline in cognition and functioning can often be noted. There is often a presence of demonstrable focal neurologic deficits. Vascular dementia is generally poorly responsive to cholinergic repletion therapy by acetylcholinesterase inhibitors.

Neurocognitive Disorders

K&S Ch. 10

Question 145. B. Clomipramine is the most serotonin-selective of the tricyclic antidepressants.

Psychopharmacology

K&S Ch. 35

Question 146. E. The psychiatrist is the member of the team who is held legally responsible for the team's decisions. It stems from the concept that the highest person in the hierarchy is responsible for the actions of those he or she supervises. The psychiatrist is considered the head of this team. As such, the attending psychiatrist is responsible for the actions of the residents he or she supervises, and is responsible for the actions of the team.

Forensic Psychiatry

K&S Ch. 57

Question 147. E. The tricyclic antidepressants have many cardiac side effects that are worsened in overdose. They act as type 1A antiarrhythmics. As such they can terminate ventricular fibrillation, and increase collateral blood supply to ischemic heart tissue. In overdose they can be highly cardiotoxic and will cause decreased myocardial contractility, tachycardia, hypotension, and increased myocardial irritability. Also important to note is that nortriptyline is unique in that it has a therapeutic window. Blood levels should be obtained and the therapeutic range is 50–150 ng/mL. Levels above 150 ng/mL may reduce its efficacy.

Psychopharmacology

K&S Ch. 35

Question 148. C. Past suicidal behavior is the best predictor of future suicidal behavior. It is a better predictor than any of the other answer choices given in this question. As such, one of the most important questions to ask a patient who has suicidal thoughts is about their history of past suicide attempts. Other risk factors for suicide are as follows: men are more likely than women, divorced or single more likely than married, elderly are less likely to attempt, but more likely to succeed when they do, whites are more likely than other ethnic groups, and the higher the social status the higher the risk.

Management in Psychiatry

K&S Ch. 34

Question 149. D. Clomipramine has been shown to be particularly useful in treating obsessive–compulsive disorder in comparison to the other tricyclics. Its efficacy when compared to the SSRIs for OCD is equal or better, depending on the study.

Obsessive Compulsive and Related Disorders

K&S Ch. 35

Question 150. E. Imipramine is often used to treat childhood enuresis. Desmopressin is also useful in 50% of patients. Improvement can range from cessation of enuresis to leaking less urine. Drugs should be given 1 hour before bedtime and results are usually evident within days. Patients who achieve full dryness should take the medication for several months to prevent relapse.

Elimination Disorders

K&S Ch. 35

THREE

Test Number Three

1. During which one of Piaget's stages of development will a child be able to understand that a tall glass and a short wide glass can contain the same volume of water despite their different shapes?

   A. *Sensorimotor stage*

   B. *Preoperational thought stage*

   C. *Concrete operations stage*

   D. *Formal thought stage*

   E. *Anal stage*

2. Which one of the following is not a characteristic of Transient global amnesia?

   A. *Loss of personal information and identity*

   B. *Reversible anterograde and retrograde memory loss*

   C. *Inability to learn newly acquired information*

   D. *Preservation of alertness without motor or sensory deficits*

   E. *Men are affected more commonly than women*

3. Which one of the following answer choices is not true regarding GABA?

   A. *GABA is thought to suppress seizure activity*

   B. *GABA is thought to exacerbate mania*

   C. *GABA is thought to decrease anxiety*

   D. *GABA-A activity is potentiated by topiramate*

   E. *Gabapentin has no activity at the GABA receptors or transporter*

4. An 8-year-old boy has been at sleep-away summer camp for 2 weeks and presents with a sudden onset of facial diplegia. The most likely infectious organism that might have caused this symptom is:

   A. *Treponema pallidum*

   B. *Borrelia burgdorferi*

   C. *Leptospira interrogans*

   D. *Rickettsia rickettsii*

   E. *Yersinia pestis*

 Full test available online - see inside front cover for details.

5. A middle-aged man has been referred to your office by a plastic surgeon. The man is seeking a face lift for his "excessively large cheeks". The surgeon has not been able to find anything abnormal about the man's face or skin, and when he comes to see you, you fail to see anything wrong either. The patient insists that his cheeks are grotesque and ruining his whole appearance. When pressed, he admits that others may not consider his cheeks to be as bad as he does. His most likely diagnosis is:

    A. Malingering
    B. Schizophrenia
    C. Somatization disorder
    D. Conversion disorder
    E. Body dysmorphic disorder

6. Tourette's syndrome often involves which one of the following psychiatric manifestations?

    A. Generalized anxiety disorder
    B. Social anxiety disorder
    C. Panic disorder
    D. Obsessive–compulsive disorder
    E. Psychotic disorder

7. A young woman comes to the emergency room with a 1 week history of pressured speech, decreased sleep, grandiosity, and loosening of associations. The patient feels that she is being monitored by a satellite and she is seen talking to herself when no one else is in the room. Which one of the following criteria must be met to diagnose this patient with schizo-affective disorder instead of bipolar disorder?

    A. Presence of mania
    B. Psychotic symptoms in the absence of mood symptoms for a 1 week period
    C. At least one prior episode of depression
    D. Presence of psychotic symptoms during a manic episode
    E. Psychotic symptoms in the absence of mood symptoms for a 2 week period

8. Which one of the following therapies would be best-suited to a bipolar patient in a manic episode during pregnancy?

    A. Haloperidol
    B. Lithium
    C. Aripiprazole
    D. Divalproex sodium
    E. Electroconvulsive shock therapy

9. You are called to evaluate a 60-year-old man with a history of depression. His family reports that he has not been himself for the past 5 days. On examination he makes poor eye contact, is inattentive, mutters incoherently, keeps rearranging pieces of paper on his bed tray with no apparent logic, and drifts off to sleep while you are talking to him. What is his most likely diagnosis?

    A. Depression
    B. Dementia
    C. Delusional disorder
    D. Delirium
    E. Obsessive–compulsive disorder

10. Which one of the following pharmacologic agents would be most likely to cause extrapyramidal side effects and possible tardive dyskinesia?

    A. Hydroxyzine

    B. Diphenhydramine

    C. Metoclopramide

    D. Ondansetron

    E. Tizanidine

11. The most common symptom seen in patients with narcolepsy is:

    A. Hypnopompic hallucinations

    B. Sleep paralysis

    C. Hypnagogic hallucinations

    D. Sleep attacks

    E. Cataplexy

12. The primary auditory cortex localizes to which one of the following brain regions?

    A. Temporal lobe

    B. Parietal lobe

    C. Frontal lobe

    D. Occipital lobe

    E. Thalamus

13. Which one of the following neurotransmitters works as an adjunctive neurotransmitter for glutamate as well as an independent neurotransmitter with its own receptors?

    A. GABA

    B. Norepinephrine

    C. Serotonin

    D. Dopamine

    E. Glycine

14. Which one of the following agents is not acceptable and useful for the treatment of postherpetic neuralgia?

    A. Gabapentin

    B. Lidoderm

    C. Pregabalin

    D. Carbamazepine

    E. Phenytoin

15. A construction worker is brought to the emergency room immediately after an accident on a job site. He was standing very near a three story scaffold that fell and missed crushing him by inches. He reports feeling anxiety, a sense of numbing, detachment, difficulty remembering the accident, and states that he feels like he is in a daze. The most likely diagnosis is:

    A. Generalized anxiety disorder

    B. Major depression

    C. Delirium

    D. Dissociative amnesia

    E. Acute stress disorder

16. Trauma to which one of the following vessels or groups of vessels commonly causes epidural hematoma?

    A. *Middle meningeal artery*

    B. *Meningeal bridging veins*

    C. *Cavernous sinus*

    D. *Basilar artery*

    E. *Transverse sinus*

17. A 26-year-old woman comes into the emergency room. She reports that she has been having mood swings that go from depressed to elated to rageful in minutes to hours. She has been having paranoid feelings and vague auditory hallucinations over the past week since breaking up with her boyfriend. On this past Monday she cut her arms with a razor, but only superficially. Her history reveals promiscuity, unstable relationships, and cocaine use. She now reports suicidal ideation. Her most likely diagnosis is:

    A. *Bipolar disorder*

    B. *Depression with psychotic features*

    C. *Schizoid personality disorder*

    D. *Borderline personality disorder*

    E. *Schizotypal personality disorder*

18. What is the characteristic electroencephalographic pattern noted in Creutzfeldt–Jakob disease?

    A. *Three-per-second spike and wave*

    B. *Periodic high-amplitude sharp wave complexes*

    C. *Temporal spikes*

    D. *Generalized background slowing*

    E. *Periodic lateralizing epileptiform discharges (PLEDS)*

19. To be diagnosed with polysubstance dependence, how many substances must a patient be found dependent on?

    A. *Six substances, including caffeine*

    B. *Two groups of substances, where dependence criteria were met for one of the groups*

    C. *Four substances, including nicotine, but excluding caffeine*

    D. *Five specific substances*

    E. *Three or more groups of substances where dependence criteria were met for the groups, but not necessarily for any one particular substance*

20. Which one of the following cerebrospinal fluid findings is indicative of aseptic meningitis?

    A. *Variably increased lymphocytes, slightly decreased glucose, very high protein*

    B. *Moderately increased lymphocytes, decreased glucose, mildly elevated protein*

    C. *Highly increased neutrophils, decreased glucose, very high protein*

    D. *Slightly increased lymphocytes, normal glucose, mildly elevated protein*

    E. *Absent or few lymphocytes, normal glucose, very high protein*

21. A small child is in the park with her mother. As the two interact, the child goes off to play for a brief time, then returns to her mother, then goes off to play, then returns to her mother. The child continues this pattern, regularly checking to see that the mother is still there. She would best fit into which one of Mahler's stages of separation–individuation?

    A. *Normal autism*

    B. *Symbiosis*

    C. *Rapprochement*

    D. *Practicing*

    E. *Object constancy*

22. What type of systemic poisoning results in the development of characteristic Mees' lines of the fingernails as in the photograph?

    A. *Mercury*

    B. *Arsenic*

    C. *Lead*

    D. *Organophosphates*

    E. *Ionizing radiation*

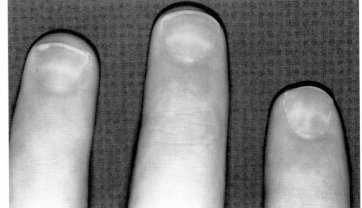

23. The assumption that there is no significant difference between two random samples of a population is called:

    A. *Correlation coefficient*

    B. *Control group*

    C. *Analysis of variance (ANOVA)*

    D. *Regression analysis*

    E. *Null hypothesis*

24. Organophosphate poisoning by pesticide exposure causes neurologic deficits by which one of the following mechanisms?

    A. *Anticholinergic toxicity*

    B. *Cholinergic toxicity*

    C. *Gamma-aminobutyric acid blockade*

    D. *Serotonergic toxicity*

    E. *Dopaminergic toxicity*

25. Emil Kraepelin used which one of the following terms in reference to schizophrenia?

    A. *Language delay*

    B. *Dementia praecox*

    C. *Split-personality*

    D. *Rebound hyperactivity*

    E. *Downward drift*

26. Which one of the following agents causes poisoning in humans that can result in a blue line at the gingival margin?

    A. *Manganese*

    B. *Thallium*

    C. *Arsenic*

    D. *Mercury*

    E. *Lead*

27. The police bring a man into the hospital who has been stealing satellite dishes off of houses and setting them up in his own yard because he feels that he has a chip in his head that allows him to talk directly to God. He states that God has instructed him to do this as preparation for the second coming. When his wife is questioned about her husband's behavior she responds that indeed God has been directly communicating with her husband, and that she has helped him steal some of the larger satellite dishes. The wife's condition can best be described as:

    A. *Schizoid personality disorder*

    B. *Delusional disorder*

    C. *Shared psychotic disorder*

    D. *Bipolar disorder*

    E. *Substance-induced psychotic disorder*

28. Truncal ataxia or instability can result most specifically from a lesion to the:

    A. *Cerebellar hemispheres*

    B. *Cerebellar vermis*

    C. *Cerebellopontine angle*

    D. *Thalamus*

    E. *Midbrain*

29. Which one of the following neurotransmitters has large numbers of receptors in the spinal cord, is synthesized primarily from serine, and has been the subject of research involving negative symptom reduction in schizophrenia?

    A. *GABA*

    B. *Glycine*

    C. *Serotonin*

    D. *Dopamine*

    E. *Glutamate*

30. Which one of the following is not a contraindication to lumbar puncture?

    A. *Thrombocytopenia*

    B. *Cerebral mass lesion*

    C. *Suspected meningitis with obtundation*

    D. *Recent head trauma*

    E. *Papilledema*

31. What is the difference between post-traumatic stress disorder and acute stress disorder?

    A. *The nature of the trauma*

    B. *The symptoms that follow the trauma*

    C. *The impairment resulting from the symptoms*

    D. *The duration of the symptoms*

    E. *The age of the patient*

32. Which chromosomal abnormality is the most common cause of mental retardation?

    A. *Trisomy 21*

    B. *Trisomy 18*

    C. *Cri-du-chat syndrome*

    D. *Fragile X syndrome*

    E. *Prader–Willi syndrome*

33. Ending up in strange places with no recollection of how one got there, or finding objects in one's possession that one doesn't recall acquiring is most characteristic of:

    A. *Anxiety*

    B. *Psychosis*

    C. *Histrionic personality*

    D. *Dissociation*

    E. *Depression*

34. Which one of the following child abuse injuries is the most likely to result in death or long-term sequelae?

    A. *Embolic stroke from multiple bone fractures*

    B. *Subdural hematoma from head trauma*

    C. *Skull fracture from head trauma*

    D. *Cerebral hypoxia from choking*

    E. *Seizures from head and brain trauma*

35. A 59-year-old man comes into your office complaining of depression. His wife of 25 years died unexpectedly 5 weeks ago. Since then he has been crying, has had little appetite but has lost no weight, and reports difficulty sleeping. He has been going out to dinner once each week with friends and says that it helps get his mind off of his wife's death. He is not suicidal. This is the first time in his life that he has had symptoms such as these. His most likely diagnosis is:

    A. *Bipolar disorder*

    B. *Major depressive disorder*

    C. *Acute stress disorder*

    D. *Bereavement*

    E. *Dysthymic disorder*

36. Which one of the following is not considered a lower motor neuron sign?

    A. *Hypotonia*

    B. *Muscle atrophy*

    C. *Fasciculations*

    D. *Babinski's sign*

    E. *Hyporeflexia*

37. Mahler's stage that is characterized by a baby considering himself a fused entity with his mother, but developing increased ability to differentiate between the inner and outer world is called:

    A. *Normal autism*

    B. *Symbiosis*

    C. *Differentiation*

    D. *Rapprochement*

    E. *Object constancy*

38. Which one of the following therapeutics can eliminate benign paroxysmal positional vertigo?

   A. *Diazepam*

   B. *Brandt–Daroff exercises*

   C. *Meclizine*

   D. *Metoclopramide*

   E. *Gabapentin*

39. Which one of the following is not a diagnostic criterion for kleptomania?

   A. *Recurrent failure to resist stealing objects*

   B. *Decreased sense of tension immediately preceding the theft*

   C. *Pleasure at the time of committing the theft*

   D. *The theft is not done to express anger*

   E. *The act is not in the context of an antisocial personality disorder*

40. The persistent vegetative state is not characterized by which one of the following?

   A. *Preserved eye opening*

   B. *Preserved response to noxious stimuli*

   C. *Preserved eye tracking*

   D. *Preserved swallowing*

   E. *Preserved sleep–wake cycles*

41. An Hispanic man comes into the emergency room complaining of headache, insomnia, fear, anger, and despair. Your differential diagnosis is most likely to include which one of the following?

   A. *Schizophrenia*

   B. *Schizoaffective disorder*

   C. *Panic disorder*

   D. *Ataque de nervios*

   E. *Myoclonic sleep disorder*

42. What is the most typical effect of depression on nocturnal sleep?

   A. *Decreased total sleep time*

   B. *Initial insomnia*

   C. *Middle insomnia*

   D. *Early morning awakening*

   E. *Sleep–wake cycle reversal*

43. Which one of the following symptoms would not be expected in a patient with pyromania?

   A. *Deliberate and purposeful fire setting*

   B. *Tension before the act*

   C. *Fascination with fire*

   D. *Pleasure when setting fires*

   E. *Setting fires for monetary gain or as an expression of political ideology*

44. Apoptosis mediated by the *N*-methyl-D-aspartate (NMDA) receptor complex is most likely caused by elevated intracellular levels of which one of the following ions?

   A. *Calcium*

   B. *Magnesium*

   C. *Sodium*

   D. *Potassium*

   E. *Chloride*

45. A patient is brought into the emergency room following a fight with police. Upon examination the psychiatrist finds that the patient has a history of several discrete assaultive acts. His aggression in these situations was out of proportion to what one would consider normal. The patient has no other psychiatric disorder and no history of substance abuse. He has no significant medical history. What is his most likely diagnosis?

   A. *Impulse control disorder NOS*

   B. *Pyromania*

   C. *Mania*

   D. *Temporal lobe epilepsy*

   E. *Intermittent explosive disorder*

46. A 45-year-old woman comes to the emergency room by ambulance unconscious and barely breathing. Paramedics found an empty bottle of 90 tablets of 2 mg clonazepam on her dresser that was filled at the pharmacy the day before. One of the first agents to administer to this patient in the acute setting is:

   A. *Naloxone*

   B. *Flumazenil*

   C. *Dimercaprol*

   D. *Atropine*

   E. *Epinephrine*

47. Which one of the following should not be considered in the differential diagnosis for intermittent explosive disorder?

   A. *Delirium*

   B. *Dementia*

   C. *Temporal lobe epilepsy*

   D. *Obsessive–compulsive disorder*

   E. *Substance intoxication*

48. The electroencephalographic pattern that most often characterizes infantile spasms is:

   A. *Three-per-second spike and wave*

   B. *Hypsarrhythmia*

   C. *Periodic lateralizing epileptiform discharges (PLEDS)*

   D. *Triphasic sharp waves*

   E. *Burst-suppression pattern*

49. Which one of the following psychiatric symptoms is not found with AIDS?

    A. *Progressive dementia*

    B. *Personality changes*

    C. *Heat intolerance*

    D. *Depression*

    E. *Loss of libido*

50. Which one of the following structures is not part of Papez' circuit?

    A. *Amygdala*

    B. *Mamillary body*

    C. *Fornix*

    D. *Cingulate gyrus*

    E. *Hippocampus*

51. A child is in the doctor's office for an evaluation. His mother is waiting outside in the waiting area. The child is aware that his mother still exists even though she is not present in the room. For this to be true, the child must have reached which one of Mahler's stages of separation–individuation?

    A. *Normal autism*

    B. *Practicing*

    C. *Differentiation*

    D. *Symbiosis*

    E. *Object constancy*

52. Which one of the following neurologic disorders is not believed to be caused by defects in the calcium channel system?

    A. *Lambert–Eaton myasthenic syndrome*

    B. *Malignant hyperthermia*

    C. *Hypokalemic periodic paralysis*

    D. *Familial hemiplegic migraine*

    E. *Benign familial neonatal convulsions*

53. A young woman comes to her psychiatrist's office for help. She feels that others are exploiting her, but has no hard evidence. She is preoccupied with the lack of loyalty that she feels all of her friends have. She reads hidden demeaning connotations into the psychiatrist's comments. She bears grudges and is unforgiving of slights. Her most likely diagnosis is:

    A. *Schizophrenia*

    B. *Schizotypal personality disorder*

    C. *Paranoid personality disorder*

    D. *Schizoid personality disorder*

    E. *Dementia*

54. Which one of the following is not a clinical feature of phenylketonuria?

    A. *Sensorineural deafness*

    B. *Infantile spasms*

    C. *Microcephaly*

    D. *A characteristic "mousy" odor*

    E. *Light hair and skin pigmentation*

55. Which one of the following dopaminergic tracts or areas is responsible for the parkinsonian side effects of antipsychotic medications?

    A. *Mesolimbic–mesocortical tract*

    B. *Tuberoinfundibular tract*

    C. *Nigrostriatal tract*

    D. *Caudate neurons*

    E. *Ventral striatum*

56. Which one of the following disorders is correctly depicted in the photomicrograph below?

    A. *Lissencephaly*

    B. *Schizencephaly*

    C. *Dandy–Walker syndrome*

    D. *Arnold–Chiari type I malformation*

    E. *Arnold–Chiari type II malformation*

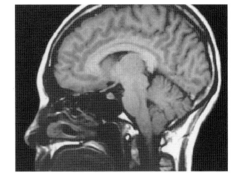

57. A schizophrenic man on an inpatient psychiatric unit develops a fever of 102.3°F (39.1°C), a high WBC count, unstable pulse and blood pressure, and rigidity in the arms and legs. The most likely diagnosis is:

    A. *Meningitis*

    B. *Serotonin-specific reuptake inhibitor withdrawal*

    C. *Lithium toxicity*

    D. *Neuroleptic malignant syndrome*

    E. *PCP use*

58. Internal carotid artery stenosis should be treated surgically by endarterectomy if the stenosis is symptomatic and above:

    A. *50%*

    B. *60%*

    C. *70%*

    D. *80%*

    E. *90%*

59. A patient comes into the clinic because his family (whom he only sees one or two times per year) keeps telling him to "go see a shrink". He has no close relationships. He participates mainly in solitary activities. He has no desire for sexual activity with others. He is indifferent to the praise or criticism of others. On examination his affect is flat. His most likely diagnosis is:

    A. *Schizoid personality disorder*

    B. *Schizotypal personality disorder*

    C. *Narcissistic personality disorder*

    D. *Major depressive disorder*

    E. *Dysthymic disorder*

60. Poor outcome in Guillain-Barré syndrome is often associated with a preceding infection by which one of the following pathogens?

    A. *Haemophilus influenzae*

    B. *Streptococcus pneumoniae*

    C. *Eescherichia coli*

    D. *Campylobacter jejuni*

    E. *Clostridium difficile*

61. Which one of the following is false regarding the Pearson correlation coefficient?

    A. *It spans from −1 to +1*

    B. *A positive value means that one variable moves the other variable in the same direction*

    C. *It can give information about cause and effect*

    D. *It indicates the degree of relationship*

    E. *A negative value means that one variable moves the other variable in the opposite direction*

62. Which one of the following solid tumors metastasizes most frequently to the brain?

    A. *Breast*

    B. *Colon*

    C. *Prostate*

    D. *Lung*

    E. *Thyroid*

63. A pervasive pattern of social inhibition, feelings of inadequacy, and hypersensitivity to negative evaluation is most characteristic of:

    A. *Obsessive–compulsive personality disorder*

    B. *Avoidant personality disorder*

    C. *Schizoid personality disorder*

    D. *Dependent personality disorder*

    E. *Passive–aggressive personality disorder*

64. The most useful treatment for intractable post-lumbar puncture headache is:

    A. *Repeat lumbar puncture with blood patch*

    B. *Bed-rest for 2 weeks*

    C. *Acetaminophen*

    D. *Hydrocodone*

    E. *Sumatriptan*

65. Which one of the following baseline lab values would be the least important to obtain on a patient starting lithium therapy:

    A. *Thyroid function tests*

    B. *Electrocardiogram*

    C. *White blood cell count*

    D. *Renal function tests*

    E. *VDRL*

66. Compression of which one of the following peripheral nerves results in meralgia paresthetica?

    A. *Sciatic*

    B. *Lateral femoral cutaneous*

    C. *Obturator*

    D. *Superior gluteal*

    E. *Common peroneal*

67. Following a long day in the hospital, you visit your best friend from college who has recently had a baby. The child has been spending more of her time asleep than awake and is not particularly aware of the environment. If your friend were to ask you which of Mahler's stages of separation–individuation the child fits into, you would confidently answer:

    A. *Normal autism*

    B. *Symbiosis*

    C. *Object constancy*

    D. *Practicing*

    E. *Differentiation*

68. The classic finding on needle electromyography (EMG) that denotes the presence of a radiculopathy is:

    A. *High-frequency, short-duration potentials*

    B. *Positive sharp waves and fibrillations*

    C. *Fasciculations*

    D. *Small, short motor unit potentials*

    E. *Myotonia*

69. Which one of the following brain structure's dopaminergic neurons have been linked with Tourette's syndrome and the development of tics?

    A. *Caudate*

    B. *Substantia nigra*

    C. *Amygdaloid body*

    D. *Frontal cortex*

    E. *Hippocampus*

70. A 35-year-old woman delivers her baby at 40 weeks gestation without complication. Seven days later she experiences an acute onset of pancephalic headache, behavioral and personality changes, irritability, intermittent seizures and diplopia. The most likely diagnosis of her problem is:

    A. *Aseptic meningitis*

    B. *Cerebral venous thrombosis*

    C. *Complicated migraine*

    D. *Bacterial meningoencephalitis*

    E. *Pseudotumor cerebri*

71. When should advanced directives be discussed with a patient?

    A. *At a time when the patient is competent*

    B. *When admitted to the hospital*

    C. *When a question of capacity arises*

    D. *When the patient is in pre-op*

    E. *When in the outpatient office*

72. The most common congenital viral infection in newborns is caused by which one of the followed pathogens?

    A. *Cytomegalovirus (CMV)*

    B. *Herpes simplex (HSV)*

    C. *Human immunodeficiency virus (HIV)*

    D. *Rubella*

    E. *Measles*

73. A pervasive and excessive need to be taken care of that leads to submissive and clinging behavior as well as fears of separation, is characteristic of which one of the following?

    A. *Obsessive–compulsive personality disorder*

    B. *Avoidant personality disorder*

    C. *Schizoid personality disorder*

    D. *Dependent personality disorder*

    E. *Passive–aggressive personality disorder*

74. The most frequent myopathy in patients over 50 years of age is:

    A. *Dermatomyositis*

    B. *Polymyositis*

    C. *Facioscapulohumeral dystrophy*

    D. *Inclusion body myositis*

    E. *Oculopharyngeal muscular dystrophy*

75. Which one of the following is a behavioral effect of opioids?

    A. *Miosis*

    B. *Increased arousal*

    C. *Euphoria*

    D. *Diarrhea*

    E. *Tachycardia*

76. Duchenne's and Becker's muscular dystrophies are both disorders linked to an absence or deficiency of which one of the following muscle membrane proteins?

    A. *Dystrophin*

    B. *Laminin*

    C. *Dystroglycan*

    D. *Spectrin*

    E. *Merosin*

77. A 60-year-old woman is 63 pounds (28 kg) overweight. She comes to her psychiatrist's office with a complaint of increased irritability, noting a fight with her husband over how much sugar he put in her coffee one morning. She is fatigued and naps several times each day. She has no history of psychiatric problems, but adds that her husband now sleeps in the living room because of her snoring. Which one of the following is the most likely cause of the patient's symptoms?

    A. *Night terrors*

    B. *Major depressive disorder*

    C. *Bipolar disorder*

    D. *Narcolepsy*

    E. *Sleep apnea*

78. The rate-limiting enzyme in the dopamine synthetic pathway is:

    A. *Dopa decarboxylase*

    B. *Tyrosine hydroxylase*

    C. *Dopamine β-hydroxylase*

    D. *Phenylethanolamine N-methyltransferase (PNMT)*

    E. *Catechol-O-methyltransferase*

79. Which one of the following is the therapeutic range for lithium?

    A. *6–12 mEq/L*

    B. *0.5–1.9 mEq/L*

    C. *0.6–1.2 mEq/L*

    D. *2–4 mEq/L*

    E. *>4 mEq/L*

80. Alcohol, benzodiazepine sedative-hypnotic agents, and barbiturates all predominantly exert their clinical effects on the brain at which one of the following receptor sites?

    A. *Cholinergic nicotinic*

    B. *N-methyl-d-aspartate (NMDA)*

    C. *Glycine*

    D. *GABA-A*

    E. *GABA-B*

81. An elderly man comes into his doctor's office with symptoms of dementia and notable loss of executive functioning. Dysfunction of which one of the following brain regions would be most closely associated with the patient's loss of executive functioning?

    A. *Caudate nucleus*

    B. *Putamen*

    C. *Globus pallidus*

    D. *Frontal lobes*

    E. *Temporal lobes*

82. A patient who is not malingering, but is believed to be producing the symptoms and signs of confusion or dementia involuntarily or unconsciously and believes that the symptoms are real is thought to have which one of the following conditions?

    A. *Conversion disorder*

    B. *Ganser's syndrome*

    C. *Capgras syndrome*

    D. *Hypochondriasis*

    E. *Folie-à-deux*

83. A child in school fails test after test. No matter how hard he studies, he fails. Over time he views himself as destined to fail and stops trying. Which one of the following theories best applies to this child's situation?

 A. *The epigenetic principle*

 B. *Industry theory*

 C. *Cognition theory*

 D. *Learned helplessness*

 E. *Sensory deprivation*

84. Entacapone and tolcapone exert their antiparkinsonian effects on which one of the following enzymes?

 A. *Catechol-O-methyltransferase*

 B. *Monamine oxidase type A*

 C. *Monoamine oxidase type B*

 D. *Dopa decarboxylase*

 E. *Dopamine β-hydroxylase*

85. Which one of the following could drastically increase lithium levels?

 A. *Citalopram*

 B. *Carbamazepine*

 C. *Sertraline*

 D. *Ibuprofen*

 E. *Acetaminophen*

86. The neurologic examination finding of Argyll Robertson pupils occurs in a majority of patients with which one of the following conditions:

 A. *Lyme disease*

 B. *Multiple sclerosis*

 C. *Tabes dorsalis*

 D. *Bubonic plague*

 E. *Intracerebral aneurysm*

87. A patient on paroxetine complains of nausea, insomnia, muscle aches, anxiety, and dizziness. Which one of the following is the most likely explanation?

 A. *He has the flu*

 B. *He has irritable bowel syndrome*

 C. *He stopped taking his antidepressant abruptly*

 D. *He is faking the symptoms*

 E. *He has multiple sclerosis*

88. A 33-year-old man with known epilepsy has a 45-second generalized tonic–clonic seizure at a bus stop outdoors. He is brought to the nearest ER and once he is arousable and awake is found to have a marked right-sided hemiparesis. What is the best explanation of this occurrence?

 A. *Postictal stroke*

 B. *Todd's paralysis*

 C. *Complicated postictal migraine*

 D. *Conversion disorder*

 E. *Transient ischemic attack (TIA)*

89. Which one of the following does not have active metabolites?

   A. *Oxazepam*

   B. *Chlordiazepoxide*

   C. *Triazolam*

   D. *Clonazepam*

   E. *Quazepam*

90. The disease known as tropical spastic paraparesis is considered to be a _____ caused by the _____ virus.

   A. *Myelopathy; HTLV-1*

   B. *Neuropathy; HTLV-1*

   C. *Myelopathy; herpes simplex*

   D. *Neuropathy; herpes simplex*

   E. *Neuropathy; HIV type 1*

91. To control aggression in a mentally retarded child, which one of the following would be most effective?

   A. *Clonazepam*

   B. *Mirtazapine*

   C. *Doxepin*

   D. *Lithium*

   E. *Naltrexone*

92. Which one of the following diseases is not associated with expansion of trinucleotide repeat sequences?

   A. *Friedrich's ataxia*

   B. *Myotonic dystrophy*

   C. *Multiple system atrophy*

   D. *Fragile X syndrome*

   E. *Huntington's disease*

93. Which one of the following dopaminergic pathways or areas is associated with the antipsychotic effects of the antipsychotic medications?

   A. *Nigrostriatal pathway*

   B. *Mesolimbic–mesocortical pathway*

   C. *Tuberoinfundibular pathway*

   D. *Caudate nucleus*

   E. *Amygdaloid body*

94. The characteristic bedside neurologic diagnostic sign known as the "battle sign" is indicative of which one of the following pathologies:

   A. *Basilar skull fracture*

   B. *Frontal lobe damage*

   C. *Increased intracranial pressure*

   D. *Hypocalcemia*

   E. *Impending transtentorial cerebral herniation*

95. Of the following combinations of medications, which one would the knowledgeable psychiatrist most want to avoid?

    A. *Fluoxetine–lithium*

    B. *Fluoxetine–phenelzine*

    C. *Citalopram–valproic acid*

    D. *Citalopram–aripiprazole*

    E. *Mirtazapine–lamotrigine*

96. Which one of the following agents is the best choice for treating attention deficit–hyperactivity disorder in a patient with Tourette's syndrome?

    A. *Bupropion*

    B. *Methylphenidate*

    C. *Dextroamphetamine*

    D. *Atomoxetine*

    E. *Clonidine*

97. A method of obtaining a prediction for the value of one variable in relation to another variable is called:

    A. *Correlation coefficient*

    B. *Control group*

    C. *Analysis of variance (ANOVA)*

    D. *Regression analysis*

    E. *Null hypothesis*

98. Which one of the following oral agents would be most beneficial in the treatment of limb spasticity related to multiple sclerosis?

    A. *Clonazepam*

    B. *Phenytoin*

    C. *Lioresal*

    D. *Phenobarbital*

    E. *Cyproheptadine*

99. A measurement of the direction and strength of the relationship between two variables is called:

    A. *Correlation coefficient*

    B. *Control group*

    C. *Analysis of variance (ANOVA)*

    D. *Regression analysis*

    E. *Null hypothesis*

100. A patient in the intensive care unit is delirious and agitated. The electroencephalogram demonstrates a characteristic pattern of triphasic waves and some generalized background slowing. What other clinical bedside sign would you be most likely to see in this patient on physical examination?

    A. *Herpetic skin vesicles*

    B. *Penile chancre*

    C. *Asterixis*

    D. *Dupuytren's contractures*

    E. *Pulmonary rales*

101. A researcher at a university hospital takes rats and randomly crowds them, shocks them, feeds them at different times, and uses bright lights and loud noise to interrupt their sleep. The rats eventually decrease their movement and exploratory behavior. What can be learned from this?

    A. This researcher has serious psychological problems and really needs a girlfriend

    B. This is evidence for Freud's theory of coercive electrocution

    C. Unpredictability and lack of environmental control play a large role in the generation of stress

    D. Rats enjoy loud noise and bright lights, especially when accompanied by electric shocks

    E. Aggression among members of the same species is common

102. Which one of the following is not a potential side effect of valproic acid?

    A. Weight gain

    B. Alopecia

    C. Hemorrhagic pancreatitis

    D. Thrombocytosis

    E. Liver failure

103. A patient is admitted to the hospital for suicidal behavior. The insurance company refuses to pay for the stay after the third day, and the patient is still suicidal. Which one of the following answer choices is the most ethical way to proceed?

    A. Send the patient home because the insurance company refuses to pay

    B. Secretly tell the patient to sign out against medical advice

    C. Make the patient pay out of pocket, and if they can't afford it, discharge them

    D. Sue the insurance company

    E. Continue to treat the patient as long as necessary, and file an appeal with the insurance company after discharge

104. The mechanism by which clonidine can help alleviate the symptoms of opioid withdrawal is through mediation of:

    A. Norepinephrine reuptake inhibition

    B. Alpha-2 adrenergic agonism

    C. Alpha-1 adrenergic antagonism

    D. Dopamine antagonism

    E. Serotonin antagonism

105. On a urine toxicology screen, how long can heroin be detected?

    A. 12 hours

    B. 48 hours

    C. 4 weeks

    D. 72 hours

    E. 8 days

106. An elderly hospitalized patient with vascular risk factors has a stroke. The patient's behavior following the stroke is noted to be unusually calm and markedly hypersexual. This presentation likely resulted from a stroke to the:

    A. Hippocampi

    B. Nucleus accumbens

    C. Hypothalamus

    D. Occipital lobes

    E. Amygdaloid bodies

107. A psychiatrist is working on an inpatient unit and one of her patients has a very resistant case of depression. She considers the option of giving the patient electroconvulsive therapy (ECT). Which one of the following should make her most concerned about giving this patient ECT?

    A. *Pregnancy*

    B. *Past seizures*

    C. *Family history of severe depression*

    D. *Psychotic symptoms*

    E. *Recent myocardial infarction*

108. A 20-year-old man comes to your office with his mother because of behavioral problems. On examination you note that he is verbally inappropriate, mildly mentally retarded, very tall and somewhat obese and has a small penis and scrotum. His condition is most likely due to which one of the following?

    A. *Absence of an X chromosome (XO)*

    B. *Presence of an extra X chromosome (XXY)*

    C. *Trisomy 21*

    D. *Deletion on the paternal chromosome 15*

    E. *Trisomy 18*

109. A psychiatrist is consulted on a medical unit because there is a patient with a substance abuse history who is in need of pain control. Which one of the following answer choices would be the best way to treat this patient's pain?

    A. *Large doses of opiates*

    B. *A mixture of opiates and benzodiazepines*

    C. *Patient-controlled analgesia*

    D. *No opiates of any kind*

    E. *PRN (as needed) buprenorphine*

110. A 35-year-old woman presents to your office with her husband. He tells you that she has experienced discrete episodes of physical and verbal aggression directed toward other people and property for the past year. Her husband states that the aggressiveness is not precipitated by any particular trigger and is completely unpredictable and intermittent. In between these bouts of aggression, the patient is otherwise fine and leads a normal life as a wife and mother. The most plausible diagnosis is:

    A. *Borderline personality disorder*

    B. *Intermittent explosive disorder*

    C. *Antisocial personality disorder*

    D. *Psychotic disorder due to temporal lobe seizures*

    E. *Bipolar I disorder, with manic and psychotic episodes*

111. While working on the ward of a state hospital, a psychiatrist comes across a patient with catatonic schizophrenia. The patient sits in one spot for extended periods of time, without changing position. This phenomenon is best described as:

    A. *Psychomotor retardation*

    B. *Catalepsy*

    C. *Cataplexy*

    D. *Catatonia*

    E. *Stereotypy*

112. Which one of the following agents has the unique mechanism of action of being a dopamine and norepinephrine reuptake inhibitor?

    A. Tiagabine

    B. Venlafaxine

    C. Duloxetine

    D. Bupropion

    E. Atomoxetine

113. Harry Harlow conducted a series of experiments with Rhesus monkeys. Some of his monkeys would stare vacantly into space, engage in self mutilation, and follow stereotyped behavior patterns. To which one of the following groups did these monkeys belong?

    A. Total isolation (no caretaker or peer bond)

    B. Mother-only reared

    C. Peer-only reared

    D. Partial isolation (can see, hear and smell other monkeys)

    E. Separation (taken from caretaker after developing bond)

114. Sildenafil, vardenafil and tadalafil all improve erectile dysfunction by which one of the following mechanisms?

    A. Phosphodiesterase 5 inhibition

    B. Calcium channel antagonism

    C. Nitric oxide antagonism

    D. Alpha 1 adrenergic antagonism

    E. Carbonic anhydrase inhibition

115. Which one of the following medications is the most likely to cause parkinsonian symptoms?

    A. Maprotiline

    B. Amoxapine

    C. Venlafaxine

    D. Doxepin

    E. Clomipramine

116. If you divide the incidence of a disease in those with risk factors by the incidence of the same disease in those without risk factors, the result is called the:

    A. Relative incidence

    B. Attributable risk

    C. Relative risk

    D. Period incidence

    E. Incidence risk

117. Cingulotomy is a treatment used for which one of the following choices?

    A. Psychosis

    B. Depression

    C. Obsessive–compulsive disorder

    D. Generalized anxiety disorder

    E. Pedophilia

118. Which one of the following causative etiologic factors is not believed to contribute to the genesis of dissociative identity disorder?

    A. A traumatic life event
    B. A vulnerability for the disorder
    C. Environmental factors
    D. Absence of external support
    E. Prior viral infection or exposure

119. Which one of the following is considered first-line treatment for a mute catatonic patient who is brought into the emergency room?

    A. Haloperidol
    B. Methylphenidate
    C. Risperidone
    D. Lorazepam
    E. Paroxetine

120. Which one of the following is not a feature of malingering?

    A. Findings are compatible with self-inflicted injuries
    B. Medical records may have been tampered with or altered
    C. Family members are able to verify the consistency of symptoms
    D. Symptoms are vague or ill defined
    E. History and examination do not yield complaints or problems

121. Which one of the following answer choices is most true concerning mutism?

    A. It is a psychiatric disorder only
    B. It is a neurological disorder only
    C. It is a function of a high-energy environment
    D. It is associated with both psychiatric and neurological conditions
    E. It is most frequently the result of head trauma

122. Therapy that is focused on the measurement of autonomic processes and teaching patients to gain voluntary control over these physiological parameters through operant conditioning is called:

    A. Stimulus-response therapy
    B. Biofeedback
    C. Relaxation training
    D. Behavior therapy
    E. Desensitization

123. A patient has overdosed on lithium following a fight with her boyfriend. Her lithium level is 2.8 mEq/L. She is exhibiting severe signs of lithium toxicity. Which one of the following answer choices is the best treatment at this time?

    A. IV fluids
    B. Celecoxib
    C. Wait and watch
    D. Hemodialysis
    E. Gastric lavage

124. The most useful long-term treatment parameter for a noncompliant patient with schizophrenia and history of violence would be:

    A. *Long-term state psychiatric hospitalization*

    B. *Partial hospitalization*

    C. *Day treatment program*

    D. *Outpatient commitment program*

    E. *Social skills training*

125. Which one of the following is a dangerous combination?

    A. *MAOI–lorazepam*

    B. *MAOI–acetaminophen*

    C. *MAOI–meperidine*

    D. *MAOI–ziprasidone*

    E. *MAOI–loxapine*

126. The psychiatrist's right to maintain a patient's secrecy in the face of a subpoena is known as:

    A. *Privilege*

    B. *Confidentiality*

    C. *Communication rights*

    D. *Private rights*

    E. *Clinical responsibility*

127. Which one of the following is not a requirement for treatment with clozapine?

    A. *Baseline white blood cell (WBC) count before starting treatment*

    B. *Two WBC counts during the first 7 days of treatment*

    C. *Weekly WBC count during the first 6 months of treatment*

    D. *WBC counts every 2 weeks after the first 6 months of treatment*

    E. *WBC count every week for 4 weeks following discontinuation of clozapine*

128. Which one of the following is not a change in sleep architecture noted in patients over age 65 years of age?

    A. *Lower percentage of stages 3 and 4 sleep*

    B. *Less total REM sleep*

    C. *Fewer REM episodes*

    D. *Increased awakening after sleep onset*

    E. *Shorter REM episodes*

129. Which one of the following will increase clozapine levels?

    A. *Red wine*

    B. *Cimetidine*

    C. *Cheese*

    D. *Acetaminophen*

    E. *Aripiprazole*

130. The most widely abused recreational substance among US high school students is:

    A. *Alcohol*

    B. *Cocaine*

    C. *Lysergic acid diethylamide (LSD)*

    D. *Inhalants*

    E. *Cannabis*

131. Beck, in the theory supporting his cognitive triad, felt that "distorted negative thoughts" lead to:

    A. *Failure of good enough mothering*

    B. *Transitional object development*

    C. *Mania*

    D. *Depression*

    E. *Aggression toward the primary caregiver*

132. The mechanism of action of the sleeping aid ramelteon involves which one of the following receptor systems?

    A. *Acetylcholine*

    B. *GABA-A*

    C. *Histamine*

    D. *Melatonin*

    E. *Norepinephrine*

133. What is alogia?

    A. *Poverty of movement*

    B. *Poverty of emotion*

    C. *Poverty of speech only*

    D. *Poverty of thought content only*

    E. *Poverty of speech and thought content*

134. The rapid-cycling specifier in bipolar I disorder applies to patients who have had _____ mood disturbance episodes over the previous _____ .

    A. *4; 6 months*

    B. *4; 12 months*

    C. *6; 24 months*

    D. *6; 12 months*

    E. *3; 12 months*

135. Which one of the following best explains pathological gambling?

    A. *Primary reinforcement*

    B. *Random reinforcement*

    C. *Poor response to dexamethasone suppression testing*

    D. *Continuous reinforcement*

    E. *Cerebellar dysfunction*

136. Late-onset schizophrenia is characterized by a more favorable prognosis and the onset of symptoms after age:

   A. *40 years*

   B. *45 years*

   C. *50 years*

   D. *55 years*

   E. *60 years*

137. A group that does not receive treatment and is the standard for comparison is called the:

   A. *Correlation coefficient*

   B. *Control group*

   C. *Analysis of variance (ANOVA)*

   D. *Regression analysis*

   E. *Null hypothesis*

138. Bowlby's stages of childhood attachment disorder, after a lengthy departure of the child's mother, do not include which one of the following?

   A. *Protest*

   B. *Despair*

   C. *Detachment*

   D. *Denial of affection*

   E. *Acceptance*

139. You have a patient whom you think has both depression and attention-deficit/hyperactivity disorder. Which one of the following medications would be the best choice for this patient?

   A. *Fluoxetine*

   B. *Paroxetine*

   C. *Bupropion*

   D. *Venlafaxine*

   E. *Imipramine*

140. Which one of the following agents is FDA approved for use in the pediatric population under 18 years of age?

   A. *Paroxetine*

   B. *Citalopram*

   C. *Sertraline*

   D. *Mirtazapine*

   E. *Venlafaxine*

141. During a session a therapist tells the patient "I know you feel terrible right now, but things are going to get better with the passage of time". This type of statement is characteristic of which type of therapy?

   A. *Supportive psychotherapy*

   B. *Psychodynamic psychotherapy*

   C. *Psychoanalysis*

   D. *Play therapy*

   E. *Cognitive behavioral therapy*

142. Which one of the following statements regarding risperidone intramuscular injection (Risperdal Consta) is false?

    A. *The formulation comes in three doses: 25, 37.5 and 50 mg*

    B. *The drug must be refrigerated before reconstitution*

    C. *The drug must be reconstituted with sterile water*

    D. *The drug must be administered only to the deltoid or the gluteus muscles*

    E. *The drug is dosed to be administered every 2 weeks*

143. A patient is brought into the emergency room unconscious with signs of respiratory depression. The patient was found unconscious on the bathroom floor and has written a suicide note saying that he wanted to die. An empty pill bottle that had contained his mother's prescription for morphine was found on the bathroom floor. Which one of the following would the knowledgeable physician use to treat this patient?

    A. *Buprenorphine*

    B. *Benztropine*

    C. *Naloxone*

    D. *Naltrexone*

    E. *Bromocriptine*

144. Which one of KüblerRoss' stages of reaction to impending death corresponds to a period when a patient goes through self-blame for his illness and asks "Why me?"

    A. *Shock and denial*

    B. *Anger*

    C. *Bargaining*

    D. *Depression*

    E. *Acceptance*

145. Asking patients if they are suicidal will:

    A. *Increase the chance that they will kill themselves*

    B. *Help them plan out their suicide*

    C. *Scare the patients*

    D. *Have no influence on whether patients will attempt suicide*

    E. *Make patients refuse to speak to their therapist any further*

146. The usual and accepted length of a period of grief following the death of a loved one can last up to:

    A. *3 months*

    B. *6 months*

    C. *9 months*

    D. *12 months*

    E. *24 months*

147. In which one of the following groups has suicide increased dramatically over the past 40+ years?

    A. *Geriatrics*

    B. *Married men*

    C. *Married women*

    D. *Adolescents*

    E. *Chronic alcoholics*

148. Which one of the following sleep-promoting agents has the longest half-life?

    A. *Ramelteon*

    B. *Zolpidem*

    C. *Zaleplon*

    D. *Eszopiclone*

    E. *Triazolam*

149. What is the therapeutic range for valproic acid?

    A. *50–150 ng/mL*

    B. *25–50 ng/mL*

    C. *200–250 ng/mL*

    D. *1000–1500 ng/mL*

    E. *0.5–0.15 ng/mL*

150. A psychiatrist interviews a Japanese immigrant who was brought to the hospital by her family for depression. In the meeting with her she does not endorse any significant symptoms. When speaking to the family, they state that she has been having many of the symptoms that she previously denied. Which one of the following is the most likely explanation for this situation?

    A. *She is lying*

    B. *She is psychotic and paranoid*

    C. *Culture*

    D. *Mental retardation*

    E. *The family is lying*

THREE

Answer Key – **Test Number Three**

1. C	26. E	51. E	76. A	101. C	126. A
2. A	27. C	52. E	77. E	102. D	127. B
3. B	28. B	53. C	78. B	103. E	128. C
4. B	29. B	54. A	79. C	104. B	129. B
5. E	30. C	55. C	80. D	105. D	130. E
6. D	31. D	56. D	81. D	106. E	131. D
7. E	32. D	57. D	82. B	107. E	132. D
8. E	33. D	58. C	83. D	108. B	133. E
9. D	34. B	59. A	84. A	109. C	134. B
10. C	35. D	60. D	85. D	110. B	135. B
11. D	36. D	61. C	86. C	111. B	136. B
12. A	37. B	62. D	87. C	112. D	137. B
13. E	38. B	63. B	88. B	113. D	138. E
14. E	39. B	64. A	89. A	114. A	139. C
15. E	40. B	65. E	90. A	115. B	140. C
16. A	41. D	66. B	91. D	116. C	141. A
17. D	42. D	67. A	92. C	117. C	142. D
18. B	43. E	68. B	93. B	118. E	143. C
19. E	44. A	69. A	94. A	119. D	144. B
20. D	45. E	70. B	95. B	120. C	145. D
21. C	46. B	71. A	96. D	121. D	146. D
22. B	47. D	72. A	97. D	122. B	147. D
23. E	48. B	73. D	98. C	123. D	148. D
24. B	49. C	74. D	99. A	124. D	149. A
25. B	50. A	75. C	100. C	125. C	150. C

THREE

Explanations – **Test Number Three**

Question 1. C. This question focuses on Piaget's stages of cognitive development. (Just in case you don't have it mastered after Test Two.) In the concrete operations stage, egocentric thought changes to operational thought where another's point of view can be taken into consideration. In concrete operations children can put things in order and group objects according to common characteristics. They develop the understanding of conservation (a tall cup and a wide cup can both hold equal volumes of water) and reversibility (ice can change to water and back to ice again).

Human Development

K&S Ch. 2

Question 2. A. Transient global amnesia (TGA) presents with a reversible anterograde and retrograde memory loss. It is accompanied by inability to learn newly acquired information and total amnesia of events occurring during the attacks. Patients remain awake and alert during attacks, without motor or sensory deficits. Patients retain their personal information and identity and can carry on personal activities as usual. The patient may ask the same question repeatedly. Affected patients are usually in their fifties or older. Men are more often affected than women. Attacks are acute in onset and can last for several hours, but rarely greater than 12 hours. The true mechanism of TGA is unknown. One potential theory is a relationship between TGA and bilateral hippocampal ischemia, possibly migrainous in nature. Other theories postulate a relationship of TGA to epilepsy, migraine, brain tumor, and cerebrovascular events or risk factors. Onset often occurs after physical exertion, sexual exertion or exposure to extremes of temperature. The prognosis of patients with TGA is generally benign. There is no noted increased risk for future ischemic attacks or stroke. Recurrence is uncommon and there is no need for extensive workup. No particular treatment is indicated.

Neurology

B&D Ch. 6

Question 3. B. GABA is the major inhibitory neurotransmitter of the CNS. It is thought to decrease seizure activity, decrease mania, and lessen anxiety. It has three receptors, GABA-A, GABA-B, and GABA-C. Topiramate works on the GABA-A receptor, potentiating its activity. Gabapentin decreases seizure activity, but does not work directly on the GABA receptors or transporter. Tiagabine is an anticonvulsant which works by blocking the GABA transporter.

Psychopharmacology

K&S Ch. 3

Question 4. B. The case described in this question is a classic presentation of Lyme disease. The offending organism in Lyme infection is the spirochete *Borrelia burgdorferi*, whose vector is the deer tick: *Ixodes dammini* in the eastern USA, *I. pacificus* in the western USA and *I. ricinus* in Europe. Lyme is the great mimicker of other neurologic conditions and it can manifest in many different ways. Early infection can appear as a meningitis, a unilateral or bilateral Bell's palsy (as in this question), a painful radiculoneuritis, optic neuritis, mononeuritis multiplex, or Guillain–Barré syndrome. After initial infection, in about two-thirds of patients a classic Lyme rash can be noted (erythema chronicum migrans), a painless expanding macular patch. Diagnosis begins with initial ELISA serologic screening, which, if positive, can be confirmed by Western blot testing. Cerebrospinal fluid lyme antibody can also be titered by polymerase chain reaction (PCR). Treatments of first choice are parenteral antibiotics: ceftriaxone or penicillin intravenously for 2–4 weeks. Tetracycline and chloramphenicol are treatment alternatives in penicillin or cephalosporin allergic patients. Cerebrospinal fluid persistence of antibody production may continue for years after successful treatment and remission and in isolation does not indicate active disease.

Rocky Mountain spotted fever is caused by the tick-borne spirochete *Rickettsia rickettsii*. Different tick species can carry this organism and the disease can be seen all over the world. The condition starts with fever, headache, muscle aches and gastrointestinal symptoms about 2–14 days after the tick bite. There is a rash that appears initially around the wrists and hands and spreads over days to the feet and forearms. Systemic symptoms can also appear and include meningoencephalitis, renal failure and pulmonary edema. Retinal vasculitis may be seen on funduscopic examination. Diagnosis is confirmed by direct immunofluorescence or immunoperoxidase skin biopsy staining. Treatment is undertaken with oral or parenteral tetracycline or chloramphenicol and a switch to oral doxycycline for a total of about 10–14 days of therapy.

Yersinia pestis is an organism causing the plague, a zoonotic infection of wild rodents, transmitted by the bites of infected fleas to human victims. Human infection can result in infectious lymphadenitis (bubonic plague), pneumonic, septicemic, or meningeal plague. Primary or secondary meningitis can occur from *Y. pestis* infection. Diagnosis is confirmed by cerebrospinal fluid Gram stain and culture. Treatment of primary infection is undertaken with intramuscular streptomycin twice daily for ten days. Meningitis is treated with intravenous chloramphenicol for at least ten days.

Leptospirosis is caused by zoonotic infection from *Leptospira interrogans*. This spirochete is transmitted to humans by contact with urine from infected rodents or farm animals or soil or water that contains the infected urine. About 15% of patients develop a meningitic picture. Severe systemic symptoms include jaundice, hemorrhage and renal failure. Diagnosis can be confirmed by organism isolation from blood or cerebrospinal fluid. Severe disease is treated with at least a week-long course of parenteral penicillin G. Less severe illness can be treated with a week-long course of oral doxycycline.

Treponema pallidum is the spirochete associated with syphilis, which is explained in depth elsewhere in this volume.

Neurology

B&D Ch. 53

Question 5. E. This is a clear case of body dysmorphic disorder. It is characterized by an imagined belief that there is a defect in part or all of the body. The belief does not approach delusional proportions. The patient complains of the defect and his perception is out of proportion to any minor physical abnormality that exists. The person's concern is grossly excessive, but when pressed he can admit that it may be excessive (this is why it is not delusional). Treatment with serotonergic drugs and therapy is usually helpful; plastic surgery is not.

Somatic Symptom Disorders

K&S Ch. 17

Question 6. D. Tourette's syndrome (TS) is a tic disorder that occurs in about 10 to 700 in 100 000 individuals. Boys are affected more often than girls. The manifestations begin between 2 and 10 years of age. Early signs include cranial motor tics, including eye blinks, stretching of the lower face and head-shaking. Vocal tics can include throat clearing, grunting, coughing, sniffing and involuntary swearing (coprolalia). Both motor and vocal tics must be present to meet criteria for the disorder. Symptoms tend to peak in severity during adolescence and often wane during adulthood. Behavioral manifestations are common in TS and can include attention-deficit/hyperactivity disorder (ADHD), obsessive–compulsive disorder, and conduct disorder. Obsessions and rituals often revolve around counting and symmetry. The diagnosis is clinical and is based on the appropriate history and physical examination.

Evidence suggests that TS is hereditary and likely follows an autosomal dominant pattern of inheritance. Concordance in monozygotic twins is greater than 85%. Exact mendelian inheritance pattern for the disorder is not yet elucidated. Positron emission tomography studies suggest increased dopaminergic activity in the ventral striatum and abnormal release and reuptake of dopamine as being probable pathophysiologic mechanisms.

Treatment of TS is symptomatic. Tics can be treated with conventional or atypical neuroleptic agents, such as haloperidol, pimozide, fluphenazine, risperidone, quetiapine, and olanzapine. Guanfacine and clonidine are useful for both tics and ADHD symptoms. Obsessive–compulsive disorder can be treated with the selective serotonin reuptake inhibitors. The stimulants methylphenidate, pemoline, and dextroamphetamine, must be used carefully as they can either alleviate or exacerbate tics. Atomoxetine, a non-stimulant ADHD medication that is a norepinephrine reuptake inhibitor, is an excellent choice for ADHD in TS because it does not exacerbate tics.

Neurology

B&D Ch. 71

Question 7. E. In order to diagnose schizoaffective disorder (as opposed to bipolar), one needs a two-week period where the patient has had psychotic symptoms in the absence of mood symptoms. The patient must also have had periods of mania or depression during which psychotic symptoms are present. A bipolar patient may have psychotic symptoms during periods of mania or depression, but these psychotic symptoms cease when the mood disturbance resolves.

Psychotic Disorders

K&S Ch. 14

Question 8. E. The safest choice of all the answers is of course electroconvulsive shock therapy (ECT). There is no real contraindication to ECT in the normal pregnancy. If the pregnancy is high-risk or complicated, fetal monitoring can be carried out during the procedure. Haloperidol would be the next best choice and is of course a butyrophenone antipsychotic agent. Haloperidol can pass into breast milk and so mothers should not breast feed if they are taking this drug. Haloperidol is a category C agent in pregnancy and it has been shown to cause teratogenicity in animals. Human studies are inadequate in this regard and the benefit needs to outweigh the risk before the drug is given to a pregnant patient. The first trimester is the most vulnerable period of pregnancy for teratogenic fetal effects. Lithium is of course contraindicated in pregnancy because of the risk of Ebstein's anomaly of the tricuspid valves. The risk of Ebstein's anomaly is 1 in 1000. Lithium is also excreted into breast milk. Lithium is a category D agent in pregnancy. Divalproex sodium is also dangerous in pregnancy because of the first trimester risk of fetal spina bifida and neural tube defects in about 1–2% of those taking the drug in their first trimester. Folic acid supplementation (1–4 mg daily) taken during the first trimester of pregnancy reduces the risk of neural tube defects with divalproex sodium. Divalproex is a category D agent in pregnancy. Aripiprazole has not been well studied in pregnancy, but is a category C agent in pregnancy. There are animal studies that have revealed fetal abnormalities as a direct result of maternal exposure to aripiprazole.

Management in Psychiatry

K&S Ch. 36

Question 9. D. This is a case of delirium. Delirium presents as confusion, impaired consciousness (often fluctuating), emotional lability, hallucinations or illusions, and irrational behavior. Its onset is rapid and its course fluctuates. Thinking is often disordered, and attention and awareness are often impaired. Causes are usually medical or organic in nature (metabolic imbalance, infection, intracranial bleed, etc.). The patient's increased age makes him more susceptible to a delirium. Dementia and depression are incorrect because the time of onset of symptoms for these disorders is over weeks to months, not days.

Neurocognitive Disorders

K&S Ch. 10

Question 10. C. Metoclopramide (Reglan) is a potent antiemetic agent that is a benzamide derivative, has phenothiazine-like properties, and can cause extrapyramidal side effects. It is a potent antagonist of dopamine type 2 (D2) receptors and blocks these receptors on the chemoreceptor trigger zone of the area postrema which prevents nausea and emesis. Because of its affinity for the D2 receptor it has been known to cause extrapyramidal side effects (EPS), especially at higher doses, and can also cause tardive dyskinesia after long-term use and discontinuation.

Ondansetron (Zofran) is a potent antiemetic like metoclopramide, but its mechanism does not involve D2 so it does not have the potential to cause EPS or tardive dyskinesia. It is a potent 5-HT3 antagonist and also works in the area postrema and likely on peripheral vagal nerve receptors.

Hydroxyzine (Atarax, Vistaril), like diphenhydramine (Benadryl) is an antihistamine that also has analgesic and antiemetic properties. Is has no effect on dopamine receptors and therefore does not cause EPS or tardive dyskinesia.

Tizanidine (Zanaflex) is a potent sedating muscle relaxant that works via α-2 adrenergic agonism. It can lower blood pressure, much like clonidine which has this same mechanism of action. It does not affect dopamine receptors and does not cause EPS or tardive dyskinesia.

Psychopharmacology

K&S Ch. 36

Question 11. D. Sleep attacks are the most common symptom of narcolepsy. Narcolepsy is also characterized by cataplexy (a sudden loss of muscle tone) and hallucinations while falling asleep and waking up. Patients with narcolepsy can have sleep paralysis where they wake up and are often unable to move. Their sleep also characteristically goes into REM cycles when sleep begins. Treatments involve taking regular naps during the day, stimulants, and antidepressants.

Sleep Wake Disorders

K&S Ch. 24

Question 12. A. The primary auditory cortex localizes to the superior temporal gyrus (Heschl's gyrus) in both temporal lobes. Cortical deafness can result from bilateral strokes to the temporal lobes destroying Heschl's gyri. The thalamus is of course the relay station for much of the sensory input to the brain. The frontal lobes are responsible for attention, concentration, set-shifting, organization and executive functioning and planning. The occipital lobes are the location of the calcarine cortex that is responsible for interpreting and processing visual input and stimuli.

Neurology

B&D Chs 11&12

Question 13. E. Glycine is a neurotransmitter synthesized from serine. It is a necessary adjunctive neurotransmitter at the NMDA receptor that binds with glutamate. It is also an independent inhibitory neurotransmitter with its own receptors that open chloride ion channels. The activity of glycine on the NMDA receptor is an area of research for schizophrenia, with some studies showing improvement in negative symptoms with the use of glycine or glycine analogues. The highest concentrations of glycine receptors have been found in the spinal cord. Mutations of this receptor lead to a rare condition called hyperekplexia where the main symptom is an exaggerated startle response.

Basic Neuroscience

K&S Ch. 3

Question 14. E. Gabapentin and pregabalin are both FDA-approved for the systemic oral treatment of postherpetic neuralgia. The lidocaine transdermal patch (Lidoderm) is FDA-approved for the topical and local treatment of postherpetic neuralgic pain. Carbamazepine and oxcarbazepine are not FDA-approved, but both have been shown to be acceptable alternatives for the treatment of trigeminal and postherpetic neuralgia. Phenytoin, an anticonvulsant agent, has no place in the treatment of postherpetic neuralgia.

Neurology

B&D Chs 44&67

Question 15. E. This is a clear case of acute stress disorder. Acute stress disorder occurs after a person is exposed to a traumatic event. The patient then feels anxiety, detachment, derealization, feelings of being "in a daze", dissociative amnesia, and numbing. Flashbacks and avoidance of stimuli can occur. The symptoms do not last longer than 4 weeks, and occur within 4 weeks of the traumatic event (as opposed to PTSD where symptoms must last more than 1 month).

Anxiety Disorders

K&S Ch. 16

Question 16. A. Epidural hematomas result most often from head trauma and skull fracture that cause a tear to the middle meningeal artery or one of its branches. They occur between the dura and the skull table and appear as a biconvex or lens-shaped hyperdensity on CT scan of the brain. Most epidural hematomas are localized to the temporal or parietal areas, but they can occur elsewhere in the brain as well.

Subdural hematoma is the most common intracranial hematoma, found in 20–25% of all traumatic brain injury patients who are comatose. The subdural hematoma is believed to result from tearing of the bridging veins over the cortical surface, or from trauma to the venous sinuses or their tributaries. Subdural hematoma is more common in patients over 60, particularly alcoholics, presumably because the dura is tightly adhered to the skull table in this population. The other answer choices are distracters.

Neurology

B&D Ch. 50

Question 17. D.   Though one could argue for bits and pieces of other diagnoses, when taking the whole picture into consideration, this patient is a case of borderline personality disorder. Borderline personality disorder is characterized by frantic efforts to avoid abandonment, unstable interpersonal relationships, disturbed self image, impulsive behavior, recurrent suicidality or self mutilation, affective instability, chronic feelings of emptiness, intense anger, and stress related paranoia or severe dissociative symptoms. The woman in the question clearly presents with many of these symptoms.

Personality Disorders

K&S Ch. 27

Question 18. B.   Electroencephalograms (EEG) of patients with Creutzfeldt–Jakob disease (CJD) classically demonstrate theta and delta waves with periodic burst-suppression pattern and periodic, rhythmic paroxysmal sharp-wave complexes. These high-amplitude sharp wave-forms are present in up to 80% of patients with CJD. This pattern can also be noted in subacute sclerosing panencephalitis, but with longer interburst intervals.

The 3-per-second spike and wave pattern is indicative of absence seizures (petit mal epilepsy). Temporal spikes would be indicative of a seizure focus in the temporal lobe, most often of the partial-complex variety. Generalized background slowing can be noted in postictal states, coma, delirium, or following anoxic brain injury. It usually indicates a decrease in the level of consciousness. Periodic lateralizing epileptiform discharges (PLEDS) are characteristic of herpes simplex encephalitis, but can also be seen in acute hemispheric stroke, tumors, abscesses and meningitis.

Neurology

B&D Chs 32&53

Question 19. E.   The criteria for polysubstance dependence state that during a 12 month period the patient repeatedly used at least three groups of substances (excluding caffeine and nicotine), but no single substance predominated. During this period, the dependence criteria need to be met for groups of substances, but not for any one particular substance.

Substance Abuse and Addictive Disorders

K&S Ch. 12

Question 20. D.   Aseptic or viral meningitis tends to produce a cerebrospinal fluid (CSF) assay with mild to moderate lymphocytic pleocytosis, normal glucose and normal to mildly elevated protein. Gram stain and cultures would be negative. A bacterial meningitis would produce a CSF as in answer choice C, with marked lymphocytosis, particularly polymorphonuclear neutrophils, markedly increased protein and decreased glucose. A fungal meningitis would produce a CSF as in answer choice B, with moderate lymphocytic pleocytosis, mildly decreased glucose and mildly increased protein. Tuberculous meningitis would produce a CSF with mild lymphocytic pleocytosis, mildly decreased glucose and markedly increased protein, as in answer choice A. Herpetic meningitis would produce a similar CSF picture to that in aseptic meningitis, but may also reveal a predominance of red blood cells in the CSF. Answer choice E is a CSF assay indicative of Guillain-Barré syndrome (acute inflammatory demyelinating polyneuropathy) which is characterized by a cytoalbuminergic dissociation with high protein (> 55 mg/dL) and an absence of significant pleocytosis.

Neurology

B&D Ch. 53

Question 21. C.   This question focuses on Mahler's stages of separation–individuation. The first stage is normal autism, lasting from birth to 2 months. In this stage the baby spends more time asleep than awake. The next stage is symbiosis, from 2 months to 5 months. In this stage the baby is developing the ability to distinguish the inner from the outer world. The child perceives himself as being part of a single entity with his mother. The following stage is differentiation, from 5 to 10 months. Here the child is drawn further into the outside world and begins to distinguish himself from his mother. Next is practicing. Practicing is from 10 to 18 months and is characterized by the baby's ability to move independently and explore the outside world. Practicing is followed by rapprochement between 18 and 24 months. In rapprochement the child's independence vacillates with his need for his mother. The child moves away from the mother, then quickly returns for reassurance. Mahler's last stage is object constancy, from 2 to 5 years. In this stage the child understands the permanence of other people, even when they are not present. It would be wise to know all of Mahler's stages well. You never know where you might see them again!

Human Development

K&S Ch. 2

Question 22. B.   Arsenic poisoning has both central and peripheral nervous system manifestations. Systemic manifestations include nausea, vomiting, diarrhea, hypotension, tachycardia, and vasomotor collapse that can lead to death. Stupor or encephalopathy may develop. Peripherally, arsenic causes a distal axonal neuropathy. Symptoms of the neuropathy may develop after two to three weeks following initial exposure. Skin manifestations

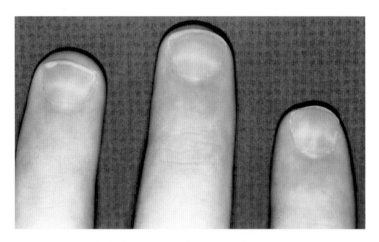

may develop with more chronic exposure, particularly keratosis, melanosis, malignancies and characteristic Mees' lines of the fingernails. Mees' lines are white transverse striations of the fingernails that occur about 3 to 6 weeks after initial arsenic exposure. Mees' lines can also be noted in thallium poisoning and from chemotherapy exposure.

Lead poisoning occurs in those who work with metal, soldering, battery manufacturing, and in smelting factories. Children tend to develop an acute encephalopathy and adults a polyneuropathy with lead poisoning. Children can get exposed to lead by ingestion of old paint that contains lead. They develop an acute gastrointestinal illness and ultimately behavioral manifestations with confusion, drowsiness, generalized seizures and intracranial hypertension. In adults, the lead neuropathy manifests predominantly as a motor neuropathy which presents as bilateral wrist drop and/or foot drop. A rare sign of lead poisoning is the appearance of a blue line at the gingival margin in patients with poor oral hygiene. Adults sometimes develop a gastrointestinal illness and a hypochromic, microcytic anemia. Lead encephalopathy is managed supportively. Systemic corticosteroids can be given to reduce brain edema and chelating agents like dimercaprol (British anti-Lewisite) are also prescribed.

Mercury poisoning can occur from mercury vapor inhalation in the making of batteries, electronics manufacturing and in the past in the hat-making industry. Clinical manifestations include personality changes ("mad as a hatter"), irritability, insomnia, drowsiness, confusion and stupor. Other systemic symptoms and signs include intention tremors ("hatter's shakes"), proteinuria, glycosuria, hyperhidrosis, and muscle weakness. Chronic exposure can lead to visual field deficits, sensory disturbances, progressive ataxia, tremor, and cognitive impairment. Treatment using chelating agents does not always increase rate or extent of recovery.

Organophosphate poisoning can occur from exposure to pesticides, herbicides, and flame retardants. Organophosphates inhibit acetylcholinesterase by phosphorylation and result in cholinergic toxicity. Clinical manifestations include salivation, lacrimation, nausea, bronchospasm, headache, weakness and in severe cases, bradycardia, tremor, diarrhea, pulmonary edema, cyanosis, and convulsions. Coma can ensue and death can result from respiratory or cardiac failure. The treatment of choice is pralidoxime and atropine. Pralidoxime helps restore acetylcholinesterase and atropine helps to counteract muscarinic adverse effects.

Ionizing radiation is a risk factor for central nervous system tumor formation, particularly meningiomas and nerve sheath tumors. Electromagnetic radiation is a likely risk factor for both leukemia and brain tumor.

Neurology

B&D Chs 52&58

Question 23. E. This question covers some of the statistical terms that could be fair game for an exam. Learn them well. A control group is a group that does not receive treatment and is a standard of comparison. Analysis of variance is a set of statistical procedures which compares two groups and determines if the differences are due to experimental influence or chance. Regression analysis is a method of using data to predict the value of one variable in relation to another. The null hypothesis is the assumption that there are no differences between two samples of a population. When the null hypothesis is rejected, differences between the groups are not attributable to chance alone. Correlation coefficient will be covered in detail in future questions.

Statistics

K&S Ch. 4

Question 24. B. Organophosphates inhibit acetylcholinesterase and cause cholinergic toxicity. Organophosphates are found predominantly in pesticides and herbicides and poisoning generally occurs in agriculture workers who are exposed following spraying in fields. Pralidoxime and atropine are the agents of choice to treat organophosphate toxicity. The other answer choices are simply distracters. For a more detailed explanation of the organophosphates, see Question 22.

Neurology

B&D Ch. 58

Question 25. B. Emil Kraepelin used the term dementia praecox to describe schizophrenia. It referred to the early onset of memory loss or decreased cognitive function often seen in patients with schizophrenia. Patients with dementia praecox were found to have a long deteriorating course with hallucinations and delusions. It was Eugen Bleuler who coined the term schizophrenia. The term schizophrenia is often misconstrued to mean split personality, which in modern times is referred to as dissociative identity disorder. Other answer choices given are unrelated distracters.

History of Psychiatry

K&S Ch. 13

Question 26. E. Lead poisoning can cause a rare appearance of a blue line at the gingival margin in patients with poor oral hygiene. Lead can also cause a microcytic, hypochromic anemia. A more detailed explanation of lead poisoning appears in Question 22 above.

Manganese classically causes neurotoxicity after months or years of exposure. Manganese miners are particularly at risk due to their prolonged inhalation of the toxin. Parkinsonism and motor symptoms can develop from manganese poisoning and usually follow initial manifestations of behavioral changes, headache and cognitive disturbances ("manganese madness"). A characteristic gait, walking on the toes with spine erect and elbows flexed, called the "cock-walk," can emerge. The condition is generally poorly-responsive to l-dopa therapy.

Thallium poisoning results in a severe neuropathy and central nervous system degeneration. A chronic, progressive sensory polyneuropathy can develop. Thallium causes potassium depletion which can result in cardiac abnormalities, such as sinus tachycardia, T-wave changes and U waves. Alopecia can develop two to four weeks after initial exposure. Treatment with intravenous potassium chloride and oral potassium ferric ferrocyanide, and hemodialysis and forced diuresis can help in recovery from acute thallium intoxication. Arsenic and mercury poisonings are discussed in more detail in Question 22.

Poisoning

B&D Ch. 58

Question 27. C.   This is a case of shared psychotic disorder (folie-à-deux). In shared psychotic disorder, a delusion develops in an individual who is in a close relationship with someone who already has an established delusion. This delusion is similar to that of the person who already has the established delusion.

Psychotic Disorders

K&S Ch. 14

Question 28. B.   Ataxia results from cerebellar lesions. Midline cerebellar vermian lesions cause truncal ataxia. Head tremor and truncal instability leading to oscillation of the head and trunk in a seated or standing posture (titubation) may result from lesions of the cerebellar vermis. In lateralized lesions to the cerebellar hemisphere, signs and symptoms occur ipsilateral to the lesion. Cerebellar hemispheric lesions would be expected to cause ipsilateral limb ataxia and/or dysmetria, either of the arm or leg, or both, depending on the location of the lesion. Dysdiadochokinesis can result from a cerebellar hemispheric lesion. This refers to a deficit in the ability to perform smooth rapid alternating movements of the hands or feet. A disturbance in both rhythm and amplitude of these alternating movements can be noted with cerebellar lesions.

Lesions arising in the cerebellopontine angle area can result in cranial neuropathy particularly to nerves V, VII and VIII. Manifestations include ipsilateral peripheral facial palsy (Bell's palsy, VII nerve palsy), ipsilateral facial numbness and weakness of masseter muscles (V nerve palsy) and ipsilateral hearing loss, tinnitus and vertigo (VIII nerve palsy).

Thalamic lesions can cause any number of deficits. Lacunar thalamic infarcts can lead to a pure sensory stroke (contralateral to the lesion), or to a sensorimotor stroke if the lesion also invades the internal capsule. Thalamic lesions can cause a rare disorder of central thalamic pain (again contralateral to the lesion and usually in the extremities and/or the face) known as the thalamic syndrome of Dejerine–Roussy.

Strokes or lesions to the midbrain can cause a variety of symptoms and syndromes. One such classic presentation is the Parinaud's syndrome which can result from a midbrain lesion arising from ischemia to the posterior cerebral artery (PCA) penetrating branches. This manifests with supranuclear paresis of eye elevation, eyelid retraction, skew deviation of the eyes, defective convergence and convergence-retraction nystagmus and light-near dissociation. Another midbrain stroke syndrome is Weber's syndrome, also arising from ischemia in the PCA territory. There is a contralateral hemiplegia of the face, arm and leg and ipsilateral oculomotor (III nerve) paresis with a dilated fixed pupil.

Neurology

B&D Chs 20&51

Question 29. B.   Here is another chance to understand glycine if you did not master it after Question 13. Glycine is a neurotransmitter synthesized from serine. It is a necessary adjunctive neurotransmitter at the NMDA receptor that binds with glutamate. It is also an independent inhibitory neurotransmitter with its own receptors that open chloride ion channels. The activity of glycine on the NMDA receptor is an area of research for schizophrenia, with some studies showing improvement in negative symptoms with the use of glycine or glycine analogs. The highest concentrations of glycine receptors have been found in the spinal cord. Mutations of this receptor lead to a rare condition called hyperekplexia where the main symptom is an exaggerated startle response.

Basic Neuroscience

K&S Ch. 3

Question 30. C.   Suspected meningitis with obtundation is not a contraindication to performing a lumbar puncture (LP). All of the other answer choices are indeed absolute or relative contraindications to LP. A localized infection at the level of the puncture would be a contraindication to performing the procedure, due to a risk of the LP needle seeding the infection into a meningitis. Thrombocytopenia may lead to excessive and uncontrollable bleeding if LP is performed. Fresh frozen plasma or platelet transfusion may need to be given prior to the procedure, if the LP is deemed to be essential to further diagnosis and management of the patient. Cerebral mass lesion is generally an absolute contraindication to LP because of the risk of cerebral or cerebellar herniation following the procedure. Transtentorial herniation can arise if a LP suddenly releases elevated cerebrospinal fluid pressure forcing the medial temporal lobe downwards causing the midbrain or the cerebellum to compress the cervicomedullary junction through the foramen magnum. Papilledema is a sign of increased intracranial pressure and a possible mass lesion. Funduscopic examination must be conducted before LP is performed. Head trauma is also a contraindication to LP, because it too may lead to a herniation syndrome because of increased intracranial pressure.

Neurology

B&D Ch. 31

Question 31. D. In case Question 15 didn't solidify acute stress disorder and post-traumatic stress disorder in your mind, take advantage of this question to clarify your understanding. Acute stress disorder occurs when a person is exposed to a traumatic event. The patient then feels anxiety, detachment, derealization, feelings of being "in a daze", dissociative amnesia, and numbing. Flashbacks and avoidance of stimuli can occur. The symptoms do not last longer than 4 weeks, and occur within 4 weeks of the traumatic event (as opposed to PTSD where symptoms must last more than 1 month).

Anxiety Disorders

K&S Ch. 16

Question 32. D. Fragile X syndrome is believed to be the most frequent cause of mental retardation (MR) in the general population. The syndrome is characterized by moderate to severe MR, macroorchidism, prominent jaw, large ears, and jocular high-pitched speech. Hyperactivity and inattention are characteristic in affected males with Fragile X syndrome. The chromosomal anomaly lies at Xq28.

Down's syndrome results generally from chromosomal nondisjunction that leads to a trisomy 21. This is most often due to advanced maternal age. Manifestations include infantile hypotonia, hyperlaxity of the joints, brachycephaly, flattened occiput, mental retardation, upslanting palpebral fissures, flattened nasal bridge, epicanthal folds, small ears, hypoplastic teeth, short neck, lenticular cataracts, speckling of the iris (Brushfield's spots), brachydactyly, simian creases and congenital cardiac anomalies (in 30–40% of cases). Down's syndrome patients acquire Alzheimer-like dementia much earlier than in the general population at large.

Trisomy 18 occurs in about 1 in 6000 live births. Fifty per cent of infants do not survive past the first week of life. Manifestations include low-set ears, small jaw, hypoplastic fingernails, mental retardation, cryptorchidism, congenital heart disease (patent ductus arteriosus, atrial septal defect, ventricular septal defect), microcephaly, and renal anomalies such as polycystic kidneys.

Cri-du-chat syndrome is a hereditary congenital mental retardation syndrome caused by a deletion at the short arm of chromosome 5p15.2. It occurs in 1 in 20000 to 50000 live births. Manifestations include severe mental retardation, microcephaly, round face, hypertelorism, micrognathia, epicanthal folds, hypotonia, and low-set ears. Newborns present with a cat-like high-pitched cry that is considered to be diagnostic of the disorder. A majority of these patients do not live past early childhood.

Prader–Willi syndrome is considered to be an autosomal dominant disorder resulting in a deletion to chromosome 15q11-13. Clinical stigmata include decreased fetal activity, obesity, mental retardation, hypotonia, short stature, hypogonadism, and small hands and feet. High caloric intake leads to diabetes and cardiac failure in many patients and many Prader–Willi syndrome patients do not survive past 25 to 30 years of age.

Neurology

B&D Ch. 61

Question 33. D. Dissociation is a disturbance in which a person fails to recall important information. There are a number of dissociative disorders including dissociative amnesia, dissociative fugue, and dissociative identity disorder. In all of these situations the patient's lack of recall is in excess of what could be explained by ordinary forgetfulness. Used as a defense mechanism, the term dissociation represents an unconscious process involving the segregation of mental or behavioral processes from the rest of the person's psychological activity. It can involve the separation of an idea from its emotional tone, as one sees in conversion disorder.

Dissociative Disorders

K&S Ch. 20

Question 34. B.   Shaken-baby syndrome from child abuse can lead to death from intracranial, subarachnoid, and sub-dural hemorrhages. These result from vascular shearing and tearing due to the violent back-and-forth movement that results in cerebral trauma. Retinal hemorrhages are often noted as well in these cases. Hemorrhages can lead to seizures and ischemic cerebral infarction due to vasospasm of intracranial vessels. Ninety-five per cent of severe intracranial injuries in children 1 year of age or younger are due to child abuse. The other answer choices are of less pathological importance in cases of child abuse.

Neurology

B&D Ch. 51

Question 35. D.   This is a case of normal bereavement. Crying, weight loss, decreased libido, withdrawal, insomnia, irritability, and poor concentration and attention can all be part of normal bereavement. Keys to normal bereavement are that suicidality is rare, it improves with social contacts, and it lacks global feelings of worthlessness. In depression, one finds anger and ambivalence towards the deceased, suicidality is common, and social contacts do not help, thus the person isolates. In addition others find the depressed person irritating or annoying, whereas the bereavement patient evokes sympathy from others. In depression the patient may feel that he or she is worthless, which is not the case in bereavement. With respect to the other answer choices, these symptoms aren't going on long enough for dysthymic disorder. There are no anxiety symptoms described to argue for acute stress disorder. There is no mania described, and the patient does not meet criteria for major depression.

Depressive Disorders

K&S Ch. 2

Question 36. D.   Lower motor neuron signs include hypotonia, muscle atrophy, fasciculations, hyporeflexia, flaccidity, muscle cramps, and marked motor weakness. These are considered to arise from lesions that are distal (i.e., peripheral) to the anterior horn cells where the upper and lower motor neurons synapse. Upper motor neuron signs include hyperreflexia, spasticity, Babinski's sign, clonus, pseudobulbar palsy, loss of dexterity, and mild motor weakness. Both upper and lower motor neuron signs can be demonstrated in amyotrophic lateral sclerosis (Lou Gehrig's disease), a disease which carries both sets of characteristics. Poliomyelitis is a classic disease of the lower motor neurons and carries the manifestations of lower motor neuron disease as noted above.

Neurology

B&D Ch. 76

Question 37. B.   Mahler's stages of separation–individuation are back again! This question describes symbiosis, which lasts from 2 months to 5 months. In this stage the baby is developing the ability to distinguish the inner from the outer world. The child perceives himself as being part of a single entity with his mother. For more details on Mahler, see Question 21.

Human Development

K&S Ch. 2

Question 38. B.   Brandt–Daroff exercises can be extremely helpful in the treatment of benign paroxysmal positional vertigo (BPPV). The exercises involve rapidly lying down on one side from a seated position and remaining there for about 30 seconds before sitting up for 30 seconds and repeating the maneuver in the opposite direction. Patients are supposed to complete 20 full repetitions twice daily. Most patients see relief within a week, but it may take three months or more to achieve complete symptom remission. Once in remission, most patients are cured of the disorder.

Benign paroxysmal positional vertigo is a vestibulopathy that is believed to be a result of sludge deposition or otoliths in the utricle of the posterior semicircular canal of the inner ear. When the patient moves his head, the movement of the material in the semicircular canal irritates the hair cells in the inner ear and triggers a severe acute onset of rotational vertigo, with nausea, possible vomiting, and characteristic rotatory nystagmus. Diagnosis is clinical and is suggested by the history. Symptoms can usually be evoked acutely by the Dix–Hallpike maneuver in which the patient's head is rapidly lowered to the bed by the examiner. The head is then turned with one ear down to the bed. The examiner notes the reproduction of vertigo and nystagmus, which are generally pathognomonic for BPPV. The fast phase of the nystagmus is noted in the direction of the lower ear (the ear with the vestibular problem) when the patient looks toward the affected side. In primary gaze, the fast rotational phase is vertical and upward, rotating toward the affected (lower) ear. Other treatments include meclizine, an antiemetic agent that helps with nausea and vomiting, but not generally with the vertigo. Metoclopramide (Reglan) is also an antiemetic agent that can help in a similar way to meclizine. Diazepam can lessen anxiety that can be associated with severe symptoms. Gabapentin is not indicated, nor is it particularly useful, in BPPV.

Neurology

B&D Ch. 37

Question 39. B. All of this question's answer choices are criteria for diagnosis of kleptomania, except that, before the theft, the patient has an increased sense of tension. Kleptomania is found within the larger heading of impulse control disorders. In kleptomania the patient engages in repeated stealing of objects that they do not need. An important part of the disorder is the sense of tension before the act and the sense of pleasure or relief afterward.

Disruptive, Impulse Control, Conduct Disorders, and ADHD

K&S Ch. 25

Question 40. B. The persistent vegetative state usually follows from a period of coma and is believed to signal the onset of severe cerebral cortical damage, often due to brain anoxia, trauma, or both. A period of one month of coma needs to elapse before the patient can be said to be in a persistent vegetative state. The condition is characterized by absence of cognitive function and absent awareness of the surrounding environment, despite a preserved sleep–wake cycle. Spontaneous movements can be noted and eye opening can be preserved, but the patient does not speak and cannot obey commands. Eye tracking and swallowing can also be preserved. There is no response to noxious stimulation in the persistent vegetative state. Permanent irreversible brain damage is believed to set in after about 12 months of a persistent vegetative state that follows brain trauma and usually after about 3 or more months following anoxic brain injury.

Neurology

B&D Ch. 5

Question 41. D. Ataque de nervios is a culture bound anxiety syndrome associated with those from Latin-American cultures. Its symptoms include headache, insomnia, anorexia, fear, anger, despair, and diarrhea.

The question says nothing about psychosis, so schizophrenia and schizoaffective disorder are incorrect. This case does not meet criteria for panic disorder. Myoclonic sleep disorder is not even remotely related to the symptoms given. Add in the fact that the patient is Hispanic, and the answer choice is clear, ataque de nervios.

Cultural Issues in Psychiatry

K&S Ch. 14

Question 42. D. Depression classically disrupts rapid eye movement (REM) sleep patterns. The most typical effect of depression on sleep however, is early morning awakening. Depression can also shorten REM latency (one hour or less). Depression can increase the total percentage of REM sleep and flip the predominance of REM from the early morning near awakening, to the beginning of the night.

Depressive Disorders

K&S Ch. 24

Question 43. E. In pyromania the patient sets fires repeatedly because of the tension before the act and the relief after. There is also a fascination with fire and its various uses. If the patient is setting fires for gain such as money or to make a political statement, then it is not a case of pyromania. One can not make the diagnosis in the presence of conduct disorder, mania, or antisocial personality disorder. Pyromania is included in the impulse control disorders.

Disruptive, Impulse Control, Conduct Disorders, and ADHD

K&S Ch. 25

Question 44. A. Apoptosis is the phenomenon of programmed cell death. Apoptosis can be triggered by exposure to antigens, exposure to corticosteroids, withdrawal of growth factors and cytokines. NMDA receptor channels, when opened, lead to calcium influx into neuronal cells and this triggers the apoptotic cascade known as hyper-excitability and excitotoxicity that leads to neuronal compromise and demise. This mechanism of cellular death is not well understood, but is believed to be implicit in the mediation of such neurologic conditions as epilepsy, stroke and neurodegenerative diseases like Alzheimer's dementia and amyotrophic lateral sclerosis.

Neurology

B&D Chs 41&60

Question 45. E. This is a case of intermittent explosive disorder. The patient has a history of violent outbursts that are out of proportion to the severity of the situation in which they occur. He has no other signs or symptoms that would suggest another axis I or II diagnosis. He has no medical history that would suggest that he could have a seizure disorder or that would otherwise explain his behavior.

Disruptive, Impulse Control, Conduct Disorders, and ADHD

K&S Ch. 25

Question 46. B. The treatment of choice for acute benzodiazepine overdose is flumazenil (Romazicon). Flumazenil is administered intravenously and has a short half-life of 7–15 minutes. The initial dosage in suspected benzodiazepine overdose is 0.2 mg IV over 30 seconds. An additional 0.3 mg can be given for more efficacy. Further doses of 0.5 mg can be given to a maximum total of 3 mg. The most common serious side effect of flumazenil administration is the onset of seizures, particularly in those patients who are dependent on benzodiazepines, or in those who have ingested large quantities of benzodiazepines.

Naloxone (Narcan) is administered in cases of acute opioid intoxication or overdose. Dimercaprol (British Anti-Lewisite) is a chelating agent that is administered in cases of acute lead poisoning and lead encephalopathy. Atropine is a potent anticholinergic agent that is administered in cases of organophosphate or herbicide poisoning. Epinephrine injection is administered in cases of allergic anaphylactic shock.

Psychopharmacology

K&S Ch. 36

Question 47. D. All of the answer choices in this question are potential considerations for the differential diagnosis of intermittent explosive disorder except obsessive–compulsive disorder (OCD). OCD patients do not have a particular likelihood to become intermittently violent and destructive. Other things to include in the differential would be personality change from a medical condition, oppositional defiant disorder, antisocial personality disorder, mania, malingering, and schizophrenia.

Disruptive, Impulse Control, Conduct Disorders, and ADHD

K&S Ch. 25

Question 48. B. The clinical triad of infantile spasms, hypsarrhythmia and psychomotor developmental arrest is known as West's syndrome. The incidence is about 1 in 5000 live births. The onset of symptoms is generally before 1 year of age. Spasms occur intermittently and involve rapid flexor/extensor movements of the body. Developmental arrest occurs prior to or at the onset of spasms. Electroencephalography reveals a characteristic interictal hypsarrhythmia pattern, which is a pattern with predominant posterior diffuse slow and sharp waves and spikes. Treatment of choice is adrenocorticotropic hormone, prednisone, or prednisolone. Prognosis is extremely poor. Only 5% of affected children achieve normal development.

The 3-per-second spike and wave pattern is characteristic of absence seizures. PLEDS are characteristic of herpes simplex virus encephalitis. Triphasic sharp waves are characteristic of Creutzfeldt–Jakob disease. Burst-suppression pattern is indicative of severe diffuse brain damage, such as in anoxic brain injury, severe drug overdose and head injury.

Neurology

B&D Ch. 67

Question 49. C. Heat intolerance is a symptom of hyperthyroidism, not AIDS. The other symptoms in this question, such as progressive dementia, personality changes, depression, and loss of libido are all worth considering in a patient with AIDS. More than 60% of AIDS patients have neuro-psychiatric symptoms. They also show impaired memory, decreased concentration, and may have seizures.

Neurocognitive Disorders

K&S Ch. 11

Question 50. A.   Papez' circuit connects the hippocampus with the thalamus, hypothalamus and cortex. The pathway includes all of the answer choices noted, plus the mammillothalamic tract and anterior nucleus of the thalamus. The amygdala is not considered part of Papez' circuit.

Neurology

B&D Ch. 6

Question 51. E.   Oh joy! Mahler's stages of separation–individuation are back again! This question focuses on Mahler's last stage of object constancy, which lasts from 2 to 5 years. In this stage the child understands the permanence of other people, even when they are not present. For more information on Mahler's stages, see Question 21.

Human Development

K&S Ch. 2

Question 52. E.   Benign familial neonatal convulsions is a rare, autosomal dominant hereditary disorder resulting from a defect in voltage-gated potassium channels. Generalized tonic–clonic seizures occur after about the third day of life and disappear spontaneously in most cases in a few weeks to months.

Lambert–Eaton myasthenic syndrome is a paraneoplastic autoimmune disorder affecting P/Q-type voltage gated calcium channels at the motor neuron terminal. Malignant hyperthermia, hypokalemic periodic paralysis and familial hemiplegic migraine are all genetic disorders involving gene mutations that result in abnormal voltage-gated calcium channels.

Neurology

B&D Ch. 64

Question 53. C.   The patient in this question has paranoid personality disorder. Symptoms not listed in this question include reluctance to confide in others for fear that the information will be used maliciously against one, perceiving attacks on one's character that others do not see, and having recurrent suspicions regarding fidelity of sexual partners. The patient in the question does not present with the usual grouping of positive and negative symptoms used to diagnose schizophrenia. Although there is a great deal of suspiciousness present she does not present with frank psychosis. There is an absence of bizarre beliefs on a number of subjects, magical thinking, and excessive social anxiety as would be expected in schizotypal personality disorder. She does not exhibit ego-syntonic social isolation, as would be expected in schizoid personality disorder. There is no suggestion of memory loss as would be noted in dementia.

Personality Disorders

K&S Ch. 27

Question 54. A.   Phenylketonuria (PKU) is an autosomal recessive heritable inborn error of metabolism resulting from a deficiency in phenylalanine hydroxylase that can cause mental retardation. The prevalence of the disorder is about 1 in 10 000 to 20 000 live births. Phenylalanine levels increase dramatically because it cannot be converted to tyrosine due to the missing enzyme. The defect localizes to chromosome 12. Classic clinical features include microcephaly, a characteristic 'mousy' odor, infantile spasms, and light hair and skin pigmentation. Sensorineural deafness is not a feature of PKU. Diagnosis can be established by measurement of blood levels of phenylalanine which are elevated. The treatment of choice is a phenylalanine free diet, which must begin during gestation in order to prevent mental retardation.

Neurology

B&D Ch. 62

Question 55. C.   The nigrostriatal tract projects from the substantia nigra to the corpus striatum. When the D2 receptors in this tract are blocked, parkinsonian side effects emerge. This tract degenerates in Parkinson's disease. Choices A, B, and C are all tracts involved in some way with antipsychotic medications. The antipsychotic medications effect both positive and negative symptoms of schizophrenia through the mesolimbic–mesocortical tract. They also lead to increased prolactin, amenorrhea, and galactorrhea through the tuberoinfundibular tract. The caudate neurons have many D2 receptors as well, and regulate motor activity. With blockade of the caudate D2 receptors bradykinesia develops. With their over stimulation tics and extraneous motor movements develop.

Neurocognitive Disorders

K&S Ch. 3

Question 56. D.

The photo depicts a classic Arnold–Chiari type I malformation. The Chiari I malformation presents as a descent of the cerebellar tonsils below the level of the foramen magnum with or without forward displacement of the medulla. This manifestation is believed to be caused by a low intracranial pressure state. The defect is often accompanied by syringomyelia, syringobulbia, and hydrocephalus. Common clinical features include headache, cranial neuropathies, and visual disturbances. Some cases present with motor and sensory complaints, particularly myelopathy with a "shawl" distribution pattern of sensory deficit over the shoulders due to the syrinx. Surgical decompression of the brainstem may be

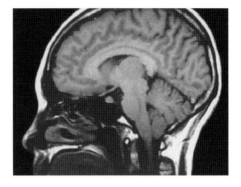

needed if the patient is highly symptomatic. Chiari type II malformation has similar features as type I, with caudal displacement of the medulla and fourth ventricle and the addition of a lumbar myelomeningocele.

Lissencephaly, also known as agyria, is a disorder of early neuroblast migration. It results from the developmental failure of the gyri of the cerebral cortex. The cortex remains smooth and lacks the convolutions that are typical of normal neuronal migration and development. Schizencephaly is a disorder associated with defective genetic expression of the *EMX2* gene. It results in clefts in the cerebral hemispheres. There are two types of schizencephaly: closed lip (the edges of the cleft are closed) and open lip (the edges of the cleft are open). Schizencephaly can be symmetrical or asymmetrical. Dandy–Walker syndrome presents as a cystic enlargement or pouching of the fourth ventricle. In addition, the posterior portion of the cerebellar vermis is hypoplastic or aplastic. Noncommunicating hydrocephalus invariably results from this anomaly. Mental retardation and spastic diplegia are frequent clinical manifestations.

Neurology

B&D Ch. 60

Question 57. D.

Neuroleptic malignant syndrome is a life-threatening condition resulting from the use of antipsychotic medications. Its symptoms are muscular rigidity, dystonia, akinesia, obtundation, or agitation. It also involves autonomic instability such as fever, sweating, unstable blood pressure, or unstable heart rate. Patients are given supportive medical treatment and medications such as dantrolene and bromocriptine may be used. Mortality is around 10–20%. The syndrome is a result of dopamine blockade, and some postulate it may be the result of a precipitous withdrawal of dopamine receptor stimulation. The other answer choices would not present with the grouping of symptoms listed, and the fact that the patient has schizophrenia and is on a psychiatric inpatient unit should point the test-taker in the direction of a side effect to antipsychotics.

Psychopharmacology

K&S Ch. 36

Question 58. C.

About 15% of ischemic strokes are caused by extracranial internal carotid artery (ICA) stenosis. Endarterectomy, surgical removal of the atherosclerotic plaque, has been deemed to be indicated and useful in symptomatic ICA stenosis of 70–99%. Symptomatic stenosis implies the prior occurrence of ipsilateral ischemic events such as transient ischemic attacks, amaurosis fugax, or completed nondisabling carotid territory stroke within the past 6 months. Asymptomatic ICA stenosis is a more difficult and controversial issue with respect to its optimal surgical management. European stroke trials and many stroke experts feel that asymptomatic ICA stenosis of 80% or greater presents a high enough risk to warrant endarterectomy only if carried out by a surgeon with morbidity statistics indicating less than a 3% complication rate.

Neurology

B&D Ch. 51

Question 59. A.

The patient in this question has schizoid personality disorder. He has a pervasive pattern of detachment from social relationships and a restricted range of emotional expression. Other symptoms include taking little to no pleasure in activities, lacking close friends or confidants, and showing emotional coldness or detachment. Schizotypal patients have odd behaviors and beliefs such as magical thinking. Narcissistic patients are grandiose, need admiration, and lack empathy. This patient is socially isolated but has none of the other criteria that one would expect to find with a major depressive disorder or dysthymic disorder, and as such they are not the correct answers.

Personality Disorders

K&S Ch. 27

Question 60. D. *Campylobacter jejuni* is the most common bacterial infection that precedes the onset of Guillain-Barré syndrome (acute inflammatory demyelinating polyneuropathy; AIDP). It accounts for about 20–40% of all cases of AIDP. *C. jejuni* causes an acute enteric and systemic illness and the onset of AIDP occurs about two to three weeks after this initial diarrheal condition. AIDP tends to follow about 1 in 1000 to 2000 cases of known *C. jejuni* infections. *C. jejuni* infection can be diagnosed by stool or blood cultures and is treated with a week-long course of oral erythromycin 250 mg four times daily.

AIDP is preceded by an upper respiratory or gastrointestinal infection, a surgical intervention, or an immunization about 1 to 4 weeks prior to the illness onset in about two-thirds of cases. *C. jejuni* infection has been linked to a worse prognosis because it tends to be associated with the more severe axonal form of AIDP.

Neurology

B&D Chs 53&76

Question 61. C. The correlation coefficient is a measurement of the direction and strength of the relationship between two variables. The Pearson correlation coefficient is on a scale from −1 to +1. A positive correlation means that one variable moves the other in the same direction. A negative value means that one moves the other in the opposite direction. A correlation close to −1 or +1 shows a strong relationship. A correlation close to 0 shows a weak relationship. Correlation coefficients indicate the degree of relationship only; they say nothing about cause and effect.

Statistics

K&S Ch. 4

Question 62. D. Brain metastases are the most common form of neurologic complication from systemic cancer and they account for about 20–40% of all central nervous system tumors. Lung cancer is the most common cause of metastases to the brain and accounts for about two-thirds of all such metastases. In particular, non-small cell lung carcinoma accounts for about two-thirds of all metastases to the brain originating from the lung. Breast cancer leads to about 15–20% of patients with brain metastases. Melanoma, gastrointestinal carcinoma and renal cell carcinoma each account for about 5–10% of metastatic brain tumors.

Neurology

B&D Ch. 52

Question 63. B. This question gives a description of avoidant personality disorder. These patients avoid interpersonal contact for fear of criticism. They are unwilling to get involved with others without assurance of being liked. They show restraint in interpersonal relationships for fear of being shamed or ridiculed. They are inhibited interpersonally because of fears of inadequacy. They see themselves as inferior to others. Of the other choices, the only one that comes close is schizoid personality disorder, but in schizoid personality disorder the person doesn't care that he is isolated, and he has a blunted affect. Passive–aggressive personality disorder is only in the DSM-IV-TR as a subject for further research. Obsessive–compulsive personality disorder (OCPD) presents as a pervasive pattern of preoccupation with orderliness, perfectionism, and control. This preoccupation comes at the expense of openness, efficiency, and flexibility. The OCPD patient's perfectionism interferes with task completion. These patients are inflexible regarding moral and ethical issues. They devote time to work at the expense of leisure activities. They are reluctant to delegate tasks to others. They are characteristically rigid and stubborn. OCPD patients often can not discard old or worn-out objects even when they have no value.

Personality Disorders

K&S Ch. 27

Question 64. A. A post-lumbar puncture (LP) headache is a frequent adverse event resulting from diagnostic or therapeutic LP. The headache is considered to be due to low cerebrospinal fluid (CSF) pressure because the needle bevel (usually a Quincke needle) leaves an open dural tear from shearing as it is pulled out of the patient. This dural tear results in a chronic CSF leak from the puncture site and an intractable headache that is noted particularly when the patient is upright. The headache is generally relieved when the patient lies recumbent. Loss of CSF results in a traction of the brain on sensory nerves and bridging veins, which causes pain.

The pain often resolves in several days if the patient lies recumbent and receives adequate hydration. A blood patch is often immediately curative of the post-LP headache and involves the gentle injection of 10 to 20 mL of the patient's own blood into the epidural space at the same site of the LP. Bed-rest for 2 weeks is far too long a period to wait before undertaking a blood patch. Acetaminophen and hydrocodone may be helpful, but are not curative therapy for post-LP headache. Sumatriptan is indicated for migraine only and not for post-LP headache.

Neurology

B&D Ch. 69

Question 65. E.   Patients starting lithium should obtain baseline thyroid function tests, electrolytes, white blood cell count, renal function tests, and a baseline electrocardiogram. Why? Because lithium can cause renal damage, hypothyroidism, increased WBC count, and ECG changes (T-wave flattening or inversion). Low sodium can lead to toxic lithium levels. VDRL is a distracter which is unrelated to starting a patient on lithium.

Laboratory Tests in Psychiatry

K&S Ch. 7

Question 66. B.   Compression of the lateral femoral cutaneous nerve as it passes beneath the inguinal ligament results in a painful sensory syndrome known as meralgia paresthetica. Predisposing factors include obesity, pregnancy and the wearing of pants that are tight at the waist or a heavy belt, such as those worn by workmen carrying heavy tools. Clinically there is pain and sensory loss (numbness) to the lateral thigh. Motor deficits are absent. Treatment is conservative and involves weight loss (if that is the cause), wearing looser clothing, or the use of tricyclic antidepressants or anticonvulsants to treat the neuropathic pain. Surgery is not generally needed in these cases. The other peripheral nerves listed as answer choices are simply distracters.

Neurology

B&D Ch. 30

Question 67. A.   Your new friend Mahler is back again! If you didn't get this right it's time to memorize her stages! Mahler's first stage is normal autism, lasting from birth to 2 months. In this stage the baby spends more time asleep than awake. For more information on Mahler's stages, see Question 21.

Human Development

K&S Ch. 2

Question 68. B.   Fibrillation potentials are the electromyographic (EMG) hallmarks of muscle denervation. Positive sharp waves are spontaneous activity emanating from groups of denervated muscle fibers. Fibrillation potentials, combined with the finding of positive sharp waves, and decreased recruitment in a segmental myotomal distribution are characteristic of a radiculopathy. Fasciculations are commonly characteristic of anterior horn cell diseases such as poliomyelitis and amyotrophic lateral sclerosis. They can also be benign and can be seen in normal healthy individuals. They represent spontaneous discharges of a single motor unit. High-frequency, short-duration potentials are seen when the EMG needle is very close to or embedded in the motor endplate. This is not a pathologic finding. Myotonia is the phenomenon of delayed muscle relaxation after needle insertion or contraction. It is the pattern noted in myotonic dystrophy and is characterized by a "dive-bomber" pattern heard on the speaker. Small, short motor unit potentials are noted in myopathies (polymyositis, muscular dystrophies). This pattern occurs from reduction in size of the muscle fibers.

Neurology

B&D Ch. 32

Question 69. A.   The caudate nucleus neurons have many D2 receptors. They regulate motor activity by determining which motor acts get carried out. With blockade of the caudate D2 receptors, bradykinesia develops from excessive dampening of motor activity. With caudate D2 receptor over-stimulation, tics and extraneous motor movements develop.

Basic Neuroscience

K&S Ch. 3

Question 70. B. Cerebral venous thrombosis (CVT) generally occurs 1 day to 4 weeks postpartum, with a peak in incidence about 7–14 days after delivery. Clinical features include puerperal headache that worsens over days, seizures, neurologic deficits, and behavior or personality changes. The condition is believed to be due to the hypercoagulable state induced by pregnancy with likely decreased protein S activity and to a possible presence of circulating antiphospholipid antibodies during the puerperal period. Brain MRI with MRI venography is the imaging modality of choice to clinch the diagnosis. Heparin anticoagulation may be helpful. Thrombolysis by either intravenous infusion or invasive venographic approach has also proved to be useful treatment, especially in severe cases where prognosis is deemed to be poor.

Meningitis and meningoencephalitis are certainly in the differential diagnosis when considering CVT, but both would be expected to be accompanied by high fever and possibly obtundation. A migraine, even when complicated, is rarely accompanied by seizures. Pseudotumor cerebri does not cause seizures and usually presents with intermittent visual obscurations and papilledema rather than diplopia.

Neurology

B&D Ch. 81

Question 71. A. Patients must make decisions regarding advanced directives at a time when they are competent to do so. At the time of admission to the hospital they may or may not be competent. If the question of capacity arises they may or may not have capacity and therefore lack competence. When immediately prior to an operation, or in the office, they may or may not be competent. Competence is a legal decision, made by the courts, that a patient has sufficient ability to manage their own affairs. Capacity is a medical decision made by a psychiatrist that says whether at a given point in time the patient is thinking clearly enough to make certain medical decisions for himself. In order to make an advanced directive one would want the patient to have both capacity and be competent at the time of the decision.

Forensic Psychiatry

K&S Ch. 57

Question 72. A. Cytomegalovirus (CMV) is the most common congenital viral infection in newborns and is the result of either primary maternal infection or from viral reactivation in the mother. Most affected newborns are asymptomatic and most develop normally. Less than 10% of patients with CMV have complications such as jaundice, hepatosplenomegaly, microcephaly, chorioretinitis, ataxia, and seizures. The mortality rate is about 20–30% in symptomatic newborns. The other neonatal infections noted in this question occur less frequently than CMV.

Neurology

B&D Ch. 80

Question 73. D. Patients with dependent personality disorder have trouble making decisions without excessive amounts of advice from others. They need others to assume responsibility for most areas of their life. They do not express disagreement with others for fear of disapproval. They feel helpless and uncomfortable when alone. They urgently seek new relationships when a prior one ends, and can be unrealistically preoccupied with fears of being left alone to care for themselves. None of the other answer choices fit these parameters. Passive–aggressive personality disorder is in the DSM as a subject for further research.

Personality Disorders

K&S Ch. 27

Question 74. D. Inclusion body myositis is the most common myopathy in those over 50 years of age and it rarely occurs in those younger than 50 years of age. Men are more frequently affected than women. The disorder affects strength in the distal muscles of the arms and legs. Wrist and finger flexors and quadriceps muscles are preferentially weak. There are no muscle pains noted in the disorder. The disorder is generally chronic, progressive and poorly responsive to corticosteroid or immunosuppressive therapies. Muscle biopsy helps confirm the diagnosis in about 80% or more cases if done properly. It classically reveals endomysial inflammation, macrophage invasion of muscle, rimmed vacuoles, and characteristic inclusion bodies in the nuclei.

Facioscapulohumeral dystrophy (FSHD) is an autosomal dominant inherited disease of muscle with a prevalence of about 1 to 2 per 100 000. The genetic anomaly localizes to 4q35 in most cases. The phenomenon of *anticipation* is noted in FSHD, which implies that as successive generations acquire the disease, the onset of the condition occurs earlier and the disease becomes more severe. Clinical features include weakness of orofacial muscles, with inability to pucker or whistle. Shoulder muscles are weak and winging of the scapula can be noted when the arms are outstretched. Biceps and triceps are often weak, as are the hip flexors and quadriceps. DNA studies establish the diagnosis. Treatment is supportive as the condition is irreversible.

Oculopharyngeal muscular dystrophy (OPMD) is an autosomal dominant inherited disease of muscle. The disorder localizes to chromosome 14q11.2-13. The disease begins in the fifth or sixth decade most often and presents initially with eye muscle weakness and ptosis. Difficulty swallowing soon follows and swallowing may become impossible. Death can occur from starvation if nutritional support is not given. DNA testing proves the diagnosis. Treatment is supportive.

Dermatomyositis and polymyositis are discussed at length in other questions in this volume.

Neurology

B&D Ch. 79

Question 75. C.   Euphoria is a behavioral effect of opioids, as are drowsiness, decreased sex drive, hypoactivity, and personality changes. Miosis is a physical effect of opioid use. Increased arousal is not an effect of opioid intoxication, drowsiness is. Diarrhea can come from withdrawal, but opioids themselves cause constipation. Bradycardia is also a physical effect of opioids, and as such tachycardia is incorrect.

Substance Abuse and Addictive Disorders

K&S Ch. 12

Question 76. A.   Duchenne's and Becker's muscular dystrophies are X-linked inherited disorders of muscle. The gene locus is Xp21 on the short arm of the X chromosome. This abnormality results in a deficiency in dystrophin, a structural muscle membrane protein located in the subsarcolemmal region of muscle fibers. These two disorders are explained in greater detail as part of other questions in this volume. The other answer choices are all muscle proteins that work together with dystrophin to stabilize the muscle membrane, but they are not implicated in the pathophysiology of the two muscular dystrophies mentioned in this question.

Neurology

B&D Ch. 79

Question 77. E.   Sleep apnea is a disorder in which there is a cessation of airflow in and out of the lungs during sleep. These stoppages of airflow must last for 10 seconds or more. In central sleep apnea, both respiratory effort and airflow stop. In obstructive sleep apnea, air stops flowing but respiratory effort increases. It is considered pathological if patients have five or more apneic episodes per hour or 30 or more episodes per night. Sleep apnea can lead to cardiovascular changes including arrhythmia and blood pressure changes. Long-standing sleep apnea can lead to pulmonary hypertension. The characteristic pattern of sleep apnea involves an older person who reports tiredness or inability to stay awake during the daytime. It can be associated with depression, irritability, and daytime sleepiness. Bed partners often report loud snoring. Patients may also awaken during the night as a result of the cessation of breathing. Patients suspected of sleep apnea should undergo sleep studies, and should be treated with a CPAP machine (continuous positive airway pressure). Losing weight helps many people, and for some surgery is the appropriate option to remove the obstruction in the airway. Now looking at the test question, the patient is not dropping into "sleep attacks" while in the middle of activities, as such narcolepsy is incorrect. There is no substantial evidence of mania given. The patient does not meet criteria for major depression. Behaviors associated with sleep terrors are not described. The snoring that drove her husband out of the bedroom should immediately point you in the direction of sleep apnea. The fact that she is overweight clinches the diagnosis.

Sleep Wake Disorders

K&S Ch. 24

Question 78. B.   Tyrosine hydroxylase is the rate-limiting enzyme in the dopamine synthetic pathway. Dopamine synthesis occurs as follows: L-tyrosine is converted to L-dopa by tyrosine hydroxylase. Dopa decarboxylase converts L-dopa to dopamine. Once dopamine is extruded into the synaptic cleft, its termination of action is carried out by monoamine oxidase, catechol-O-methyltransferase, as well as reuptake into the presynaptic bouton where it is initially synthesized. Norepinephrine synthesis occurs when dopamine β-hydroxylase converts dopamine to norepinephrine. Norepinephrine in turn is converted to epinephrine by phenylethanolamine *N*-methyltransferase (PNMT).

Neurology

B&D Ch. 71

Question 79. C. The therapeutic range for lithium is 0.6–1.2 mEq/L. Toxic levels are 2 mEq/L or higher. Lethal levels are 4.0 mEq/L or higher.

Laboratory Tests in Psychiatry

K&S Ch. 7

Question 80. D. GABA-A is a complex receptor with multiple binding sites. GABA is found throughout the central and peripheral nervous systems and is the predominant inhibitory neurotransmitter in the brain. When the GABA receptor is agonized, there is a rapid influx of negatively charged chloride ions through the postsynaptic cellular membrane. This results in fast inhibitory post-synaptic potentials. The GABA-A receptor is believed to be responsible for the clinical effects of benzodiazepines, barbiturates and alcohol. Only sodium oxybate (gamma hydroxybutyrate; GHB; Xyrem), which is a "date-rape" drug that is FDA-approved for narcolepsy and cataplexy, and Lioresal, a potent antispasticity agent, act in the central nervous system by agonism of the GABA-B receptor. The other receptor types mentioned in this question are simply distracters.

Neurology

Basic Neuroscience

B&D Ch. 71

Question 81. D. It is the frontal lobes that determine how the brain acts on information. The relatively large size of the human frontal lobes is what distinguishes our brains from those of primates. It is in the frontal lobes that executive functioning takes place, and injury of the frontal lobes leads to impairment in motivation, attention, and sequencing of actions. A "frontal lobe syndrome" exists, and consists of slowed thinking, poor judgment, decreased curiosity, social withdrawal, and irritability. Patients with frontal lobe dysfunction may have normal IQ, as IQ has been found to be mostly a parietal lobe function.

Basic Neuroscience

K&S Ch. 3

Question 82. B. Ganser's syndrome, considered to be a dissociative disorder, is the voluntary production of symptoms that involve giving approximate answers or talking past the point. This syndrome is often associated with other psychopathy such as conversion, perceptual disturbances, and dissociative symptoms like amnesia and fugue. Males and prisoners are most commonly affected. The major contributory factor is the presence of a severe personality disorder. Recovery is most often sudden and patients claim amnesia of the symptoms. It is believed to be a variant of malingering, with possible secondary gain.

Conversion disorder is a somatoform disorder characterized by the presence of one or more neurologic symptoms that are not explained by any known neurologic or medical disorder. Capgras' syndrome is a specific type of systematized delusion in which the patient feels that a familiar person is mistakenly thought to be an unfamiliar imposter. Hypochondriasis is a somatoform disorder in which the patient misinterprets bodily symptoms and functions and becomes preoccupied with the fear of contracting or having a serious disease even after reassurance to the contrary is given by a physician. Folie-à-deux is a delusional disorder, now termed a shared psychotic disorder in DSM-IV-TR. It involves the transfer of delusions from a patient to another person who has a close relationship with the patient. The associated person's delusion is similar in content to that of the patient.

Somatic Symptom Disorders

K&S Ch. 20

Question 83. D. Learned helplessness is a behavioral model for depression developed by Martin Seligman. He took dogs and gave them electric shocks from which they could not escape. Eventually they gave up and stopped trying to escape. In time this spread to other areas of functioning until they were always helpless and apathetic. This behavioral pattern has also been seen in humans with repeated setbacks or failures in their lives, as the question stem demonstrates. Industry is part of Erikson's stages and is irrelevant to the question. Cognition is the process of obtaining, learning, and using intellectual knowledge. This has some relation to the test taking but is not the explanation for the child's behavior. Sensory deprivation is removing a person or animal from external stimuli of any kind. Again, it is unrelated to the question. The epigenetic principle states that development occurs in sequential, clearly defined stages. This is clearly unrelated to the question.

Psychological Theory and Psychometric Testing

K&S Ch. 4

Question 84. A.   Entacapone (Comtan) and tolcapone (Tasmar) are catechol-O-methyl-transferase (COMT) inhibitors. COMT inhibitors block peripheral degradation of peripheral levodopa and central degradation of L-dopa and dopamine, thereby increasing L-dopa and dopamine levels centrally. The COMT inhibitor is generally given concomitantly with each dose of carbidopa-levodopa (Sinemet) throughout the day to improve parkinsonian symptoms.

Selegiline (Eldepryl) is the classic monoamine oxidase type-B (MAO-B) inhibitor. It has some potentiating effects on dopamine and prevents MAO-B dependent dopamine degradation. Phenelzine (Nardil) and tranylcypromine (Parnate) are nonspecific MAO inhibitors that affect both MAO-A and MAO-B. There are reversible MAO-A inhibitors (moclobemide and befloxatone) that are only available outside the USA. These agents do not require the strict dietary restrictions on tyramine that the nonselective MAO inhibitors require in order to avoid a hypertensive crisis. There are no specific pharmacologic agents that act upon dopa decarboxylase or dopamine β-hydroxylase. These two answer choices are simply distracters.

Neurology

B&D Ch. 71

Question 85. D.   The commonly used drug ibuprofen can drastically increase lithium levels. Many diuretics can increase lithium levels, as can ACE inhibitors and other non-steroidal anti-inflammatory drugs such as naproxen. Aspirin will not affect lithium levels. Lithium combined with anticonvulsants can increase lithium levels and worsen neurotoxic effects.

Laboratory Tests in Psychiatry

K&S Ch. 36

Question 86. C.   Argyll Robertson pupils are a characteristic of late syphilis, particularly in either general paresis or tabes dorsalis. Argyll Robertson pupils are small, irregular pupils that constrict to accommodation, but not to light. Tabes dorsalis is the spinal form of syphilis and develops about 15 to 20 years after the initial infection. The clinical triad is that of sensory ataxia, lightning pains and urinary incontinence. Lower extremity deep tendon reflexes are absent. There is impaired proprioception with a positive Romberg's sign. Ninety per cent of patients have pupillary abnormalities and about one-half have Argyll Robertson pupils. Another classic characteristic is the presence of Charcot's (neuropathic) joints.

The pupillary abnormality seen in optic neuritis or multiple sclerosis is called the Marcus Gunn pupil and is revealed when a swinging light is moved away from the affected eye. Both eyes should constrict because of consensual innervation, but the affected pupil enlarges when the flashlight is moved away to the unaffected eye. Lyme disease and bubonic plague do not present with characteristic pupillary abnormalities. Intracerebral aneurysm, particularly of the posterior communicating artery, presents with a complete third nerve palsy that involves the pupil which is fixed and slightly dilated.

Neurology

B&D Ch. 53

Question 87. C.   The symptoms given in this question are most likely the result of a serotonin withdrawal syndrome, which is possible with most serotonin-selective reuptake inhibitors (SSRIs), but which occurs particularly with paroxetine due to its shorter half-life. Symptoms include nausea, insomnia, muscle aches, anxiety and dizziness. The way to prevent this uncomfortable situation is to taper the drug off slowly. Patients on paroxetine should be warned against abruptly stopping the drug.

Psychopharmacology

K&S Ch. 36

Question 88. B. Todd's paralysis is a brief period of transient hemiparesis or hemiplegia following a seizure. The symptoms usually dissipate within 48 hours and treatment is expectant and supportive. The weakness is generally contralateral to the side of the brain with the epileptic focus. The condition may also affect speech and vision, but again the deficits are temporary. Certain studies have pointed to Todd's paralysis being the result of arteriovenous shunting that leads to transient cerebral ischemia following an ictal event. The other answer choices are distracters.

Neurology

B&D Ch. 67

Question 89. A. The 3-hydroxy benzodiazepines are directly metabolized by glucuronidation and have no active metabolites. The 3-hydroxy benzodiazepines include oxazepam, lorazepam, and temazepam. Know these three well, as they are often the subject of questions on standardized exams. Some of the longest half lives are found with the 2-keto benzodiazepines (chlordiazepoxide, diazepam, prazepam) because they have multiple active metabolites that can keep working in the body from 30 hours to over 200 hours in patients who are slow metabolizers.

Psychopharmacology

K&S Ch. 36

Question 90. A. Tropical spastic paraparesis is a chronic progressive myelopathy associated with infection by human T-lymphotropic virus type-1 (HTLV-1). The condition affects men more often than women and the onset is usually after 30 years of age. Diagnosis is confirmed by cerebrospinal fluid polymerase chain reaction and detection of HTLV-1 antibodies. Clinical features include upper motor neuron weakness, bladder disturbance and variable sensory loss. By ten years out, 60–70% of patients cannot walk. Treatment can be undertaken with corticosteroids, interferon-α, or plasmapheresis, but has proven only minimally beneficial.

Neurology

B&D Ch. 74

Question 91. D. Lithium is often used to treat aggression in patients with schizophrenia, prisoners, those with conduct disorder, and the mentally retarded. It is less useful in aggression associated with head trauma and epilepsy. Other drugs used for aggression include anticonvulsants and antipsychotics.

Psychopharmacology

K&S Ch. 36

Question 92. C. The neurodegenerative disorders that are associated with expansion of genetic trinucleotide repeat sequences are: fragile X syndrome, myotonic dystrophy, Huntington's disease, X-linked spinobulbar muscular atrophy, dentatorubral-pallidoluysian atrophy, spinocerebellar atrophies types 1, 2, 3, 6 and 7, and Friedrich's ataxia. Multiple system atrophy is a Parkinson's plus syndrome that is not associated with an expansion of trinucleotide repeat sequences.

Neurology

B&D Ch. 40

Question 93. B. The mesolimbic–mesocortical pathway projects from the ventral tegmental area (VTA) to many areas of the cortex and limbic system. This is the tract that is thought to mediate the antipsychotic effects of the antipsychotic medications. The nigrostriatal pathway is associated with parkinsonian effects of the antipsychotics. The caudate is associated with Tourette's disorder and tics (see Question 69). The tuberoinfundibular pathway is associated with prolactin increase and lactation from antipsychotics.

Basic Neuroscience

K&S Ch. 3

Question 94. A. The "battle sign" is a hematoma overlying the mastoid that results from a basilar skull fracture extending into the mastoid portion of the temporal bone. The lesion is not usually visible until 2 to 3 days after the trauma. Frontal lobe damage would be expected to yield classic frontal lobe signs on examination, such as a Meyerson's sign, rooting reflex, snout reflex, palmomental reflex, and grasp reflex. These signal extensive damage to the frontal lobe (or lobes if the sign is bilateral). Increased intracranial pressure presents with obtundation of level of consciousness, papilledema, and signs of brainstem compromise.

Hypocalcemia that is chronic may result in the clinical observation of a Chvostek's sign. The sign is positive when the cheek is tapped with the examiner's finger and the corner of the mouth involuntarily contracts. Impending cerebral herniation usually presents with all of the signs of increased intracranial pressure as noted above. Systemic hypertension and respiratory compromise are also often noted.

Neurology

B&D Chs 5&56

Question 95. B. Fluoxetine and phenelzine should not be combined because one is a serotonin-selective reuptake inhibitor (SSRI) and the other is a monoamine oxidase inhibitor (MAOI). SSRIs should not be combined with MAOIs because of the possibility of causing a fatal serotonin syndrome. Using an SSRI with selegiline, which only inhibits MAO-B, is tolerated by some patients. But the general rule to remember is: do not mix SSRIs and MAOIs. If you give one followed by the other there must be a washout period in between. It would be a good idea for the well-prepared test taker to know the symptoms of a serotonin syndrome and how to distinguish it from neuroleptic malignant syndrome. Both conditions are covered elsewhere in this volume.

Psychopharmacology

K&S Ch. 36

Question 96. D. Atomoxatine (Strattera) is FDA-approved for symptoms of attention deficit–hyperactivity disorder (ADHD) in both adults and children. Its mechanism of action is by norepinephrine reuptake inhibition. It is the most useful choice when trying to treat both tics and ADHD, as it does not worsen the tic condition and may in fact help the tic symptoms. Bupropion (Wellbutrin) is not specifically FDA-approved for ADHD and its use in the disorder has not been shown to be consistently beneficial. The amphetamine-like stimulant medications methylphenidate (Ritalin, Metadate, Concerta) and dextroamphetamine (Dexedrine), although approved, well-studied and efficacious in ADHD, have been known to worsen underlying tics in concomitant Tourette's syndrome. Clonidine (Catapres) is an alpha-2 adrenergic agonist that has little place in ADHD, although it may certainly help alleviate tics in Tourette's syndrome.

Neurology

Psychopharmacology

B&D Ch. 61

Question 97. D. More statistics! Regression analysis is a method of using data to predict the value of one variable in relation to another. The other distracters are explained elsewhere in this volume.

Statistics

K&S Ch. 4

Question 98. C. Lioresal (Baclofen) is one of the most potent of the oral muscle relaxing agents and treats spasticity highly effectively. Its full mechanism of action is not well-understood, but it is believed to have predominant effect as a GABA-B agonist. It can cause muscular weakness and difficulty with weight-bearing because of its potency. Other first-line agents to treat symptomatic spasticity include gabapentin, diazepam, clonidine, tizanidine, and dantrolene. Second-line agents include intrathecal Lioresal, Marinol, chlorpromazine, cyproheptadine, phenytoin, and phenobarbital.

Neurology

B&D Ch. 48

Question 99. A. Just in case Question 61 wasn't enough, here it is again. Correlation coefficient is a measurement of the direction and strength of the relationship between two variables. The Pearson correlation coefficient is on a scale from −1 to +1. A positive correlation means that one variable moves the other in the same direction. A negative value means that one moves the other in the opposite direction.

Statistics

K&S Ch. 4

Question 100. C. Triphasic waves on electroencephalogram are characteristic of hepatic or metabolic encephalopathy. Of course, hepatic encephalopathy is often accompanied by asterixis, particularly when the condition is severe. Asterixis is a sudden loss of postural tone and manifests as a flapping tremor of the hands. It is exhibited when the arms are fully extended. Herpetic skin vesicles would of course be expected with herpes simplex virus infections. Penile chancre can be demonstrated in cases of syphilis. Dupuytren's contractures are a form of benign progressive fibroproliferative disease of the palmar fasciae of unknown etiology. The condition is seen more often in men than women and is associated with alcoholism, hand trauma and diabetes. Pulmonary rales would be an expected sign in congestive heart failure.

Neurology

B&D Ch. 56

Question 101. C. Experiments such as the one in this question have been used to give behavioral models for depression and stress. In this situation it is the unpredictability of the insults and the animal's inability to control them that leads to a state of chronic stress. Animals put under chronic stress become restless, tense, irritable, or very inhibited. The concept of unpredictable stress is important to understand in conjunction with the theory of learned helplessness proposed by Martin Seligman. In learned helplessness experiments, animals are exposed to electric shocks from which they can not escape. They eventually become apathetic and make no attempts to escape. This can be generalized to human behavior as seen in a child who consistently fails in school and then gives up trying and becomes depressed. Learned helplessness is a proposed animal model for human depression. The other answer choices are unrelated, or are simply ridiculous.

Psychological Theory and Psychometric Testing

K&S Ch. 4

Question 102. D. Common side effects of valproic acid include weight gain, tremor, thinning of the hair, and ankle swelling. Other noted adverse effects are gastrointestinal distress, sedation, pancreatitis, bone marrow suppression (pancytopenia), and hepatotoxicity. The agent is teratogenic and the most worrisome fetotoxic effect is the neural tube defect (spina bifida) which is dangerous during neurogenesis in the first trimester of gestation.

Psychopharmacology

B&D Ch. 67

Question 103. E. It is the doctor's ethical obligation to treat the patient in question regardless of ability to pay. It is unethical to allow a suicidal patient to leave the hospital due to a dispute with the insurance company. Should the patient go and kill himself, the doctor, not the insurance company, is liable. After the patient is treated and released, the issue can be taken up more aggressively with the insurance company. As a physician, your first and most important obligation is to the patient, not to the insurance company or to your wallet.

Ethics

K&S Ch. 58

Question 104. B. Clonidine (Catapres) is a presynaptic α2-receptor agonist. It is FDA-approved as an antihypertensive agent. It acts by reducing the amount of norepinephrine that is released from the synaptic bouton. This effect decreases sympathetic tone and bodily arousal and activation. The agent diminishes the autonomic symptoms associated with opioid withdrawal, such as tachycardia, hypertension, sweating, and lacrimation. Atomoxetine (Strattera) FDA-approved for ADHD in children and adults is a norepinephrine reuptake inhibitor. The neuroleptic medications, both conventional and atypical, can cause α1 adrenergic antagonism and thereby cause orthostatic hypotension. Dopamine type 2 antagonism is the putative antipsychotic mechanism of all of the neuroleptic agents, both conventional and atypical. Serotonin antagonism is what makes an atypical antipsychotic atypical. It is in fact the ratio of D2 to 5-HT2 blockade that reduces the extrapyramidal side effects of the atypical neuroleptics.

Psychopharmacology

K&S Ch. 36

Question 105. D. Heroin can be detected on a urine toxicology screen for 36–72 hours. Alcohol can be detected for up to 12 hours. Amphetamines can be detected for up to 48 hours. Cannabis can be detected for up to 4 weeks. PCP can be detected for up to 8 days.

Substance Abuse and Addictive Disorders

K&S Ch. 7

Question 106. E.   The Klüver–Bucy syndrome results from bilateral destruction of the amygdaloid bodies and the inferior temporal cortex. Clinical features include hypersexuality, placidity and hyperorality. One of the causes of the syndrome is Pick's disease (frontotemporal dementia). Other causes include stroke and Alzheimer's dementia. Other associated features include visual agnosia (psychic blindness), hyperphagia and prosopagnosia (the inability to recognize faces). The rest of the answer choices are simply distracters.

Neurocognitive Disorders

K&S Ch. 10

Question 107. E.   Patients at high risk during electro-convulsive therapy (ECT) include the following: those with space occupying lesions in the CNS, those with increased intracranial pressure, those at risk for cerebral bleed, those who have had a recent myocardial infarction, and those with uncontrolled hypertension. There are no absolute contraindications for ECT, but patients who fall into any of the above mentioned categories should be screened carefully and decisions made on a case by case basis depending on risks, benefits, and ability to control risk factors.

Diagnostic and Treatment Procedures in Psychiatry

K&S Ch. 36

Question 108. B.   Klinefelter's syndrome results from the presence of an extra X chromosome (XXY triploidy). It is noted in about 1 in 700 men. Clinical features include small dysfunctional testes, mental retardation and pear-shaped stature. Testosterone replenishment may offset some of the stigmata of the condition. Turner's syndrome is the absence of an X chromosome in a genetic female (X0). Characteristics include short stature and lack of pubertal sexual development. Other clinical features include a webbed neck, and heart and kidney anomalies. Trisomy 21 is of course classic Down's syndrome which is explained in detail in another question in this volume. Deletion on the paternal chromosome 15 results in the Prader–Willi syndrome. The prevalence is about 1 in 12 000 to 15 000. Clinical features include profound mental retardation, hypogonadism, hypotonia, behavioral disinhibition, rapid and excessive weight gain, and facial dysmorphism. Trisomy 18 is described elsewhere in this volume.

Neurology

B&D Ch. 40

Question 109. C.   Patient controlled analgesia has proven to be an extremely good way of treating pain. Patients who control their own dosing end up using less pain medication than those who have to ask for the medication and wait for the doctor to write an order. They also have far better pain control. Some patients, particularly cancer patients may need large and escalating doses of medication to control their pain. Under these circumstances, this should not be viewed as addiction, but as a necessary part of the treatment of their illness. Cancer patients have been shown to wean themselves off of the pain medication once the pain decreases. The use of pain control in a drug addict with a painful medical illness is as important as it is in a non-addict with the same illness. They may need higher doses to control their pain, but the doctor has as much of an obligation to manage their pain as they do to manage the pain of the non-addict. The other answer choices do not address the issue of using as little medication as necessary while obtaining the best pain control. This is why patient-controlled analgesia is the best choice.

Somatic Symptom Disorders

K&S Ch. 28

Question 110. B.   This vignette points to a diagnosis of intermittent explosive disorder. Intermittent explosive disorder manifests as discrete episodes of failure to resist aggressive impulses that lead to extreme physical aggression directed towards people and/or property. The degree of aggression is completely out of proportion to any particular psychosocial stressor that may trigger such an episode.

Episodes are unpredictable and often arise without cause or particular trigger and remit as spontaneously as they begin. There are no signs or symptoms of aggressivity noted in between these discrete episodes. The disorder is more common in men than in women. Predisposing psychosocial factors include an underprivileged or tempestuous childhood, childhood abuse, and early frustration and deprivation. Biological predisposing factors are believed to be decreased cerebral serotonergic transmission, low cerebrospinal fluid (CSF) levels of 5-hydroxyindoleacetic acid (5-HIAA) and high CSF levels of testosterone in men. There is strong comorbidity with fire setting, substance use and the eating disorders.

The personality disorders such as borderline and antisocial, are distinguished from intermittent explosive disorder by a pervasive pattern of maladaptive behavior that would be expected to occur in between episodes and affect the patient's life adversely in more areas of functioning. Aggressive patients with bipolar mania would be expected to present with evidence of manic symptoms, including elevated/irritable mood, increased energy, rapid pressured speech, sleeplessness, racing thoughts, distractability, increased goal-directed behavior, and perhaps even psychosis. Temporal-lobe seizures are a remote possibility and can certainly result in aggression, most often interictally, but there is no evidence of this presented in this question.

Treatment of intermittent explosive disorder can be undertaken with mood stabilizers such as lithium, carbamazepine, divalproex sodium, and gabapentin. Selective serotonin reuptake inhibitors and tricyclic antidepressants can also be effective in reducing aggression.

Disruptive, Impulse Control, Conduct Disorders, and ADHD

K&S Ch. 25

Question 111. B.   Catalepsy is an immobile position that is constantly maintained. Cataplexy is temporary loss of muscle tone precipitated by an emotional state. Psychomotor retardation is decreased motor and cognitive activity often seen with depression. Catatonia is markedly slowed motor activity to the point of immobility and unawareness of surroundings. Stereotypy is a repetitive fixed pattern of movement or speech.

Psychotic Disorders

K&S Ch. 8

Question 112. D.   Bupropion (Wellbutrin) is the only antidepressant agent that is believed to be a dopamine and norepinephrine reuptake inhibitor. It is FDA-approved for both depression and smoking cessation. It has a unique side effect profile and is unlikely to cause the sexual dysfunction or weight gain noted with the serotonergic antidepressants. Bupropion is a noncompetitive inhibitor of nicotinic cholinergic receptors and in this way can reduce tobacco cravings in smokers. Bupropion is less likely to precipitate a bipolar manic episode than the tricyclic antidepressants. It is also less likely to induce rapid cycling in bipolar patients than other antidepressants.

Tiagabine (Gabitril) is a selective GABA reuptake inhibitor. It is FDA-approved for adjunctive therapy in partial complex seizures in adolescents and adults. Duloxetine (Cymbalta) is a serotonin and norepinephrine reuptake inhibitor. It is approved in both major depressive disorder and diabetic neuropathic pain. It works on pain modulation via the brainstem and spinal cord efferent noradrenergic tracts originating in the locus ceruleus. Venlafaxine XR is also a serotonin and norepinephrine reuptake inhibitor and is FDA-approved in major depressive disorder, generalized anxiety disorder, social anxiety disorder, and most recently obtained an indication in panic disorder. Atomoxetine (Strattera) is a norepinephrine reuptake inhibitor that is FDA-approved for the treatment of attention deficit–hyperactivity disorder in both children and adults.

Psychopharmacology

K&S Ch. 36

Question 113. D.   The description in this question is of partial isolation monkeys. Those totally isolated from other monkeys were very fearful, unable to copulate, and unable to raise young. Mother-only raised monkeys failed to copulate, didn't leave the mother to explore, and were scared of their peers. The peer-only raised monkeys were easily frightened, timid, had little playfulness, and grasped other monkeys in a clinging manner. In monkeys separated from their mothers, there was an initial protest stage followed by despair. Many of these behavior patterns can be correlated with human behaviors that are seen in our patients.

Psychological Theory and Psychometric Testing

K&S Ch. 4

Question 114. A.   Sildenafil, vardenafil and tadalafil are nonselective phosphodiesterase 5 (PDE5) inhibitors. They also have some agonistic effects on nitric oxide (NO). PDE5 blockade causes arterial smooth muscle dilatation and facilitates cavernosal blood filling which potentiates penile erection. These agents cannot be used with nitrates because the combined effect of NO agonism with nitrates can cause significant vasodilatation and precipitous lowering of the blood pressure than can result in diminished cardiac perfusion and myocardial infarction. The other answer choices are simply distracters.

Psychopharmacology

K&S Ch. 36

Question 115. B.   Amoxapine is one of the tricyclic antidepressants. What sets it apart from the others is that one of its metabolites has dopamine blocking activity. Because of this amoxapine has the potential to cause parkinsonian symptoms, akathisia, and even neuroleptic malignant syndrome. None of the other drugs listed has dopamine blocking activity.

Psychopharmacology

K&S Ch. 36

Question 116. C.   The relative risk of an illness is the ratio of the incidence of the condition in those with risk factors to the incidence of the condition in those without risk factors. Attributable risk refers to the absolute incidence of the illness in patients exposed to the condition that can be attributed to the exposure. The other answer choices are nonsense distracters and are not true biostatistical terms.

Statistics

K&S Ch. 4

Question 117. C.   Cingulotomy is a surgical treatment for obsessive–compulsive disorder. It is successful in treating about 30% of otherwise treatment resistant patients. Some patients who fail medication, and then subsequently fail surgery, will respond to medication after surgery. Complications of cingulotomy include seizures, which are then managed with anticonvulsants. The other disorders listed in this question do not have surgical treatments.

Diagnostic and Treatment Procedures in Psychiatry

K&S Ch. 16

Question 118. E.   Dissociative identity disorder (DID) also known as multiple personality disorder, is a chronic dissociative disorder. The origins of the disorder are believed to stem from early childhood trauma, most often sexual or physical. The hallmark of the disorder is the presence of two or more distinct identities or personality states that recurrently take over the person's behavior. There is also a presence of dissociative amnesia, with a noted inability to recall important personal information that is too extensive to be explained solely by forgetfulness.

The true cause of DID is unknown. Some research points to a possible connection between DID and epilepsy, with some patients having abnormal electroencephalograms. The absence of external supports, particularly from parents, siblings, relatives and significant others, seems to play a pivotal role in the genesis of the disorder. The patient's lack of stress coping mechanisms is also a likely contributory factor. The differential diagnosis includes borderline personality disorder, rapidly-cycling bipolar disorder, and schizophrenia. The disorder can start at almost any age and an early age of onset is predictive of a worse prognosis.

Treatment is focused on insight-oriented psychotherapy. Hypnotherapy may also be helpful. Antipsychotic medications are often unhelpful. Antidepressant and anxiolytic medications can be useful in addition to psychotherapy. Anticonvulsant mood stabilizers have shown some efficacy in certain studies. Viral exposure or infection has nothing to do with the etiology of DID.

Dissociative Disorders

K&S Ch. 20

Question 119. D.   The first-line therapy for the catatonic patient is intramuscular lorazepam. Many patients will respond to this treatment and will come out of their catatonic state. They can then be given subsequent treatment with antipsychotic drugs for the underlying psychotic disorder that is the most likely cause of the catatonia. Antidepressants and stimulants are not indicated for catatonia.

Psychotic Disorders

K&S Ch. 36

Question 120. C.   Malingering is diagnosed in the presence of intentional production of symptoms that are exaggerated and either physical or psychological in nature. These symptoms are motivated by secondary gain and incentives to avoid responsibility or danger, or to obtain compensation or some other benefit that is material or monetary. Symptoms are vague, ill-defined, overdramatized and do not conform to known clinical conditions. Patients seek secondary gain most often in the form of drugs, money, or the avoidance of work or jail. History and examination typically do not reveal complaints from the patient. The patient is often uncooperative and refuses to accept a good prognosis or clean bill of health. Findings can be compatible with self-inflicted injuries. Medical records may have been tampered with or altered. Family members are usually unable to verify the consistency of symptoms.

Somatic Symptom Disorders

K&S Ch. 33

Question 121. D.   Mutism refers to a patient who is voiceless without abnormalities in the structures which produce speech. Mutism is common in catatonic schizophrenia. It can be seen in conversion disorder. There is also a diagnosis known as selective mutism for children who consistently fail to speak in social situations despite speaking in other situations. Other causes of mutism include mental retardation, pervasive developmental disorder, and expressive language disorders. It can also be a component of buccofacial apraxia, locked-in syndrome, and a persistent vegetative state.

Psychotic Disorders

K&S Ch. 48

Question 122. B.   Biofeedback is a therapy in which instruments are used to measure autonomic parameters in patients who are provided with "real-time" feedback from the instrumentation about their bodily physiologic processes. This feedback enables patients to control their own physiologic functions and alter them in positive ways to alleviate symptoms using operant conditioning techniques. Feedback is provided to the patient by measuring physiologic parameters such as heart rate, blood pressure, galvanic skin response and skin temperature. The measurement is translated into a visual or auditory output signal that patients can rely on to gauge their responses. Patients can alter the tone by using guided imagery, breathing techniques, cognitive techniques and other relaxation techniques. The modality is useful for anxiety disorders, migraine, and tension-type headache in particular.

Stimulus-response therapy is a nonsense distracter, as there is no such thing. Relaxation training is a form of behavior therapy that basically encompasses techniques such as meditation and yoga to help patients to dispel anxiety by tapping into their own physiologic parameters such as heart rate and breathing rate. Guided mental imagery also helps patients to enter a relaxed state of mind. Behavior therapy is the global term used to describe different therapeutic modalities that employ either operant or classical conditioning techniques to help patients overcome their fears, phobias and anxieties. Flooding, systematic desensitization, and aversion therapy are all examples of behavior therapy. Desensitization refers to the technique that helps patients gradually overcome their fears, phobias and anxieties, by graded exposure to the very stimulus that is the source of their fears. The patient is exposed to more and more anxiety-provoking stimuli, but relaxation training helps patients to cope with their maladaptive responses and eventually ideally respond to the stimulus without it evoking anxiety.

Diagnostic and Treatment Procedures in Psychiatry

K&S Ch. 35

Question 123. D.   Lithium toxicity is a medical emergency and can result in permanent neuronal damage and death. Toxicity occurs at lithium levels above 2.5 mEq/L. Treatment includes discontinuation of lithium as well as vigorous hydration. If the level is above 4 mEq/L, or the patient shows serious signs of lithium toxicity (nephrotoxicity, convulsions, coma) the patient must have hemodialysis. Hemodialysis can be repeated every 6–10 hours until the level is no longer toxic and the patient's symptoms remit. If the patient in question was not showing serious signs of toxicity, labs to assess the situation could be sent, neurological examination done, EKG obtained, gastric lavage performed, activated charcoal given, and vigorous hydration used. The patient could then be monitored and given time to clear the lithium.

Laboratory Tests in Psychiatry

Management in Psychiatry

K&S Ch. 36

Question 124. D.   The most useful long-term treatment parameter for the noncompliant patient with schizophrenia who has a history of violence would be the use of an outpatient commitment program. Certain states have such laws in place, but others do not. Treating clinicians can petition the court to place refractory, potentially dangerous patients on this status. A judge mandates the patient's cooperativeness and the patient is compelled to report for outpatient follow-up. If the patient is noncompliant, a psychiatrist can order that the patient be picked up against his wishes and brought in for psychiatric evaluation to an emergency room where the patient can be held for a period of time. Certain states use an alternative to outpatient commitment called conservatorship. This modality involves the court appointing a conservator, often a family member, to look after the patient and make decisions on the patient's behalf, including placing the patient in involuntary hospitalization if it is deemed necessary.

Partial hospitalization is quite similar to inpatient hospitalization, except the patient sleeps at home. This modality is often a good transition between inpatient and outpatient services and patients can stay in such a program over extended periods of time if necessary. Patients have a case manager assigned to them in partial programs. The case manager helps coordinate and facilitate the patient's care and helps make the patient's transition easier to the less restrictive setting. Day treatment programs are somewhat less intense and less structured than partial hospital programs. Patients again sleep at home, but they participate in facility-based care five or more days a week. Case management and social work also play pivotal roles in the day treatment program setting.

Social skills training refers to a program that is dedicated to helping low-functioning patients, such as those with schizophrenia, to gain key skills that will enable them to function more independently in the community. The focus is on improving patients' interactions with other people in their environment.

Public Policy

K&S Chs 35&59

Question 125. C. Monoamine oxidase inhibitors (MAOIs) have several serious drug–drug interactions than must be kept in mind. Meperidine (Demerol) can *never* be given with an MAOI, as this combination has led to death in several patients (common exam question!). MAOIs should never be used with anesthetics (no spinal anesthetics, no anesthetics containing epinephrine, lidocaine is OK). MAOIs should not be combined with asthma medication or over the counter drugs that contain dextromethorphan (cold and flu medications). They can not be given with sympathomimetics (epinephrine, amphetamines, cocaine). They can not be given with SSRIs or clomipramine as this will precipitate a serotonin syndrome. There are also many food restrictions with MAOIs which will, no doubt, be the subject of another question.

Psychopharmacology

K&S Ch. 36

Question 126. A. Privilege refers to the psychiatrist's right to maintain a patient's secrecy or confidentiality even in the face of a subpoena. This implies that the right of privilege belongs to the patient, not the psychiatrist and therefore the patient can wave the right. There are many exceptions to medical privilege, and many physicians are not aware that they do not legally enjoy the same privilege that exists between husband and wife, priest and parishioner, and a client and an attorney.

Confidentiality is the professional obligation of the physician to maintain secrecy regarding all information given to him by the patient. A psychiatrist may be asked to appear in court and testify by subpoena and thereby be forced to break a patient's confidentiality. A patient may release the clinician from the obligation of confidentiality by signing a consent to release information. Each release pertains to a specific matter or piece of information and may need to be reobtained for subsequent disclosures.

Communication rights refers to the patient's right to free and open communication with the outside world by either telephone or mail, while hospitalized. Private rights refers to the patient's right to privacy. In a hospital setting, this applies to patients having private toileting and bathing space, secure storage space for personal effects, and adequate personal floor space per person. Patients also have the right to wear their own clothing and carry their own money if they desire to do so. Certain restrictions to this right may apply based on dangerousness to self or others. Clinical responsibility is not a forensic term per se, but it refers to the responsibility of the physician to the patient to provide the patient with the best care possible in any clinical setting, irrespective of the patient's financial, racial, or personal status.

Forensic Psychiatry

K&S Ch. 57

Question 127. B.   Patients being started on clozapine should have a baseline white blood cell (WBC) count with differential before treatment. A WBC count with differential is taken every week during treatment for the first 6 months, then every 2 weeks thereafter. When treatment is stopped WBC counts should be taken every week for 4 weeks. It is not a part of standard monitoring to take two WBC counts in one week. The US Food and Drug Administration recently approved monthly monitoring of WBC count after 12 months of therapy on clozapine.

Laboratory Tests in Psychiatry

K&S Ch. 7

Question 128. C.   Patients over 65 years of age undergo sleep problems that affect both rapid eye movement (REM) sleep and non-rapid eye movement (NREM) sleep. There are more REM episodes noted. REM episodes are shorter in duration. There is less total REM sleep. In NREM sleep there is a decreased amplitude of delta waves. There is a lower percentage of stages three and four sleep. There is a higher percentage of stage one and two sleep. The elderly experience increased awakening after sleep onset.

Sleep Wake Disorders

K&S Ch. 55

Question 129. B.   Clozapine has several drug–drug interactions that are noteworthy. Cimetidine, SSRIs, tricyclics, valproic acid, and erythromycin will all increase Clozaril levels. Phenytoin and carbamazepine will decrease clozapine levels. Clozapine should not be combined with any medication that can cause agranulocytosis (carbamazepine, propylthiouracil, sulfonamides, and captopril). CNS depressants (alcohol, benzodiazepines, and tricyclics) cause even more depression when combined with clozapine. The combination of lithium and Clozaril can increase neuroleptic malignant syndrome, seizures, confusion, and movement disorders. Other answer choices are distracters. The foods given should be avoided when taking MAOIs. Acetaminophen and aripiprazole have no interaction.

Psychopharmacology

K&S Ch. 36

Question 130. E.   Cannabis is the most widely abused recreational drug among US high school students. Cannabis use has been demonstrated to lead to future cocaine abuse in adolescents. About 35% of high school seniors reported using cannabis. Alcohol is also a pervasive problem among high school teens, but only in about 10–20% of students surveyed. Over 85% of high school seniors have reported that they have tried alcohol at some time. About 15% of adolescents have reported using inhalants. Fewer than 2% of high school students report having used cocaine. About 9% of high school seniors have reported trying LSD at some time.

Substance Abuse and Addictive Disorders

K&S Ch. 51

Question 131. D.   Aaron Beck is the originator of cognitive therapy. It is based on the theory that affect and behavior are determined by the way in which patients structure the world. Patients have assumptions, on which they base cognitions, which lead to affect and behavior. In depression specifically, Beck feels that there is a triad consisting of the following:

1. Depressed people see themselves as defective, inadequate, and worthless.

2. Depressed people experience the world as negative and self-defeating.

3. Depressed people have an expectation of continued hardship and failure.

It is this triad of distorted negative thoughts that Beck feels leads to depression. The goal of cognitive therapy is to help test the cognitions and develop more productive alternatives. Other answer choices given are distracters. Good enough mothering and transitional object are terms associated with the child development theory of Winnicott. Mania is not associated with Beck's cognitive triad. Aggression toward the primary caregiver has nothing to do with Beck.

Psychotherapy

K&S Ch. 35

Question 132. D.   Ramelteon (Rozerem) is a novel sleeping agent that was FDA-approved in 2005 for insomnia with sleep onset difficulties. It has a unique mechanism of action: it is a melatonin agonist. It works by stimulating melatonin type 1 and type 2 receptors in the suprachiasmatic nucleus of the hypothalamus. It has no addictive or abuse potential, because it is not a GABA-A agonist and has no activity at the benzodiazepine receptor whatsoever. It has no effects at histamine, acetylcholine, dopamine, serotonin, or norepinephrine receptors. The dosage is the same for all patients: one 8 mg tablet at bedtime. Recall that zolpidem, zaleplon and eszopiclone are all benzodiazepine receptor agonists and as such have sedative–hypnotic effects and potential for tolerance, withdrawal and abuse.

Psychopharmacology

K&S Ch. 36; also see www.rozerem.com

Question 133. E.   Alogia is a lack of speech that results from a mental deficiency or dementia. Poverty of movement is called akinesia. Poverty of emotion is described using the term "flat affect."

Diagnostic and Treatment Procedures in Psychiatry

K&S Ch. 8

Question 134. B.   To meet criteria for the rapid cycling specifier in bipolar disorder, the patient must present with at least 4 mood episodes over the past 12 months. The mood episodes must meet criteria for a major depressive, manic, mixed, or hypomanic episode. Female patients are more likely than men to have rapid cycling bipolar disorder. There is no evidence to suggest that rapid cycling is a heritable phenomenon in bipolar disorder. It is therefore likely to be a result of external factors such as stress or medication.

Bipolar Disorders

K&S Ch. 15

Question 135. B.   Random reinforcement is seen with the gambler. In random reinforcement the reward is only given a fraction of the time at random intervals. The money from a slot machine is won at random times. This keeps the gambler guessing and trying to anticipate when they will win. This is a very good way to maintain a behavior. Continuous reinforcement is when every action is rewarded, and is the best way to teach a new behavior. Primary reinforcers are independent of previous learning, for example, the need to eat is biological and not based on previous learning. Secondary reinforcers are based on previous learning, such as rewarding a child with a present when they do something well. The dexamethasone suppression test is an experimental measure associated with depression, and is unrelated to pathological gambling. Cerebellar dysfunction would lead to ataxia and gait disturbance, again, unrelated to pathological gambling.

Psychological Theory and Psychometric Testing

K&S Ch. 4

Question 136. B.   Late-onset schizophrenia is noted more often in women than in men. The prognosis seems to be more favorable when the onset is late. There is a tendency to see more paranoia in these late-onset schizophrenic patients. Schizophrenia is considered late-onset when symptoms begin after 45 years of age. It is clinically identical to schizophrenia that has normal onset.

Psychotic Disorders

K&S Ch. 13

Question 137. B.   One might think that this one was too easy, but it's just the kind of question that could show up on an exam. A control group is a group in a study that does not receive treatment and is used as a standard of comparison.

Statistics

K&S Ch. 4

Question 138. E.   Bowlby and Robertson identified three essential stages of separation response among children. The first stage is that of protest. The child protests the mother's departure by crying, calling out and searching for her. The second stage is despair and pain. The child loses faith that the mother will return. The third stage is detachment and denial of affection to the mother figure upon her return. These phases are noted universally in children who go through separation by loss of parents to death, divorce, or going off to boarding school. Acceptance is not one of Bowlby's stages of the separation response. It is the fifth and final stage of KüblerRoss' stages of reaction to impending death.

Human Development

K&S Ch. 4

Question 139. C.   Bupropion has been shown in studies to be efficacious for the treatment of attention–deficit/hyperactivity disorder (ADHD) in children and adults. It is also a very good antidepressant, which is its most common use. It has also been found very useful in patients who do not respond to a serotonin-selective reuptake inhibitor. When bupropion is added to SSRIs up to 70% of these cases improve, as both drugs together hit more neurotransmitter systems than either drug alone. The other drugs listed have no proven usefulness in ADHD.

Psychopharmacology

K&S Ch. 36

Question 140. C.   Of the agents listed in this question, only sertraline (Zoloft) is FDA-approved in the pediatric population. It is only approved for obsessive–compulsive disorder (OCD) in patients aged 6 to 17 years. It is not indicated for depression or any of the other anxiety disorders in children. Fluoxetine (Prozac) is the only SSRI that is FDA-approved for the treatment of major depressive disorder in patients age 8 years and older. Fluvoxamine (Luvox) is also FDA-approved for OCD in patients 8 years of age and older. Paroxetine and venlafaxine are FDA-approved for depression and anxiety only in the adult population 18 years of age and older. Citalopram is FDA-approved for major depressive disorder only in adults over 18 years of age. Mirtazapine is only indicated for major depressive disorder and only in the adult population over 18 years of age.

Psychopharmacology

K&S Ch. 36

Question 141. A.   This question contains a supportive statement that acknowledges how difficult things are for the patient currently, but gives her hope for the future. It is characteristic of supportive psychotherapy. In psychodynamic therapy and psychoanalysis, the therapist would wish to remain more neutral and not make statements that expressed opinion or boosted the patient's mood. The question does not involve playing with children, so play therapy is incorrect. Cognitive behavioral therapy would involve looking at the patient's assumptions and cognitions and seeing how they affect the patient's mood. That is not happening in this question stem.

Supportive psychotherapy seeks to stabilize the self and the patient's ability to cope. Defenses are strengthened. Symptom relief is sought. Neutrality is suspended. Direction by the therapist is encouraged. Free association is not part of this technique. Supportive psychotherapy can be used with those who have severe character pathology, psychosis, or are in the midst of an acute crisis or a physical illness.

Psychotherapy

K&S Ch. 35

Question 142. D.   Risperidone decanoate injection (Risperdal Consta) is one of the atypical antipsychotics currently available in long-acting injectable form. The drug is FDA-approved for schizophrenia, particularly in non-compliant and refractory cases. The formulation comes in three dosing strengths: 25 mg, 37.5 mg, and 50 mg. The recommended dosing interval is 2 weeks. The product comes prepared in a dose-pack with sterile water in a vial and a syringe for reconstituting the drug. The powdered, unreconstituted drug must be refrigerated prior to adding water. Sterile water is necessary for reconstitution. Once reconstituted, the drug must be administered within 6 hours. The drug must only be injected to the gluteus muscle. The deltoid is not a recommended injection site because it is too small a muscle to accommodate proper timed dissipation of the agent. It is advisable to keep patients on their oral medication for at least three to four weeks while initiating risperidone Consta. This prevents possible decompensation from too rapid cross titration of antipsychotic agents.

Psychopharmacology

K&S Ch. 13; also see www.risperdalconsta.com

Question 143. C.   Naloxone is an opioid antagonist. An opioid overdose is a medical emergency. Respiratory depression ensues leading to coma and shock. Naloxone is given IV and can be repeated 4–5 times in the first 30 minutes. Care must be used as the half-life is short and the patient can relapse back into coma, plus severe withdrawal can ensue from the use of an opioid antagonist.

Naltrexone is a longer acting antagonist with a half-life of 72 hours. It is a preventative measure for those with opioid addiction. It is used for blocking the euphoric effects of opioid use and thus decreases craving. Because of its long half life it is not the best choice for an emergency.

Buprenorphine is a mixed opioid agonist–antagonist. It is used in place of morphine to keep people off of heroin, and is not used in emergencies.

Benztropine is also known as Cogentin, an anticholinergic medication used to mitigate the side effects of antipsychotic drugs. It has nothing to do with opium overdose.

Bromocriptine is a mixed dopamine agonist–antagonist, which is approved in the US for treatment of Parkinson's disease.

Psychopharmacology

K&S Ch. 12

Question 144. B. Elisabeth Kübler-Ross developed a comprehensive paradigm to classify the stages of a person's reactions to impending death. Stage one is that of shock and denial. Upon learning the news that they are dying, people are initially in a state of shock and may deny that the diagnosis is correct. Stage two is that of anger. During this stage patients get frustrated, angry and irritable about their condition. They often ask: "Why me?" They typically undergo a lot of self-blame about their illness. Stage three is that of bargaining. Patients may try to negotiate or bargain with doctors, friends, family and even God to alleviate their illness in exchange for good deeds or fulfillment of certain pledges. Stage four is that of depression. During this stage patients demonstrate frank signs and symptoms of depression, including hopelessness, suicidal ideation, social withdrawal, and sleep problems. If the symptoms are severe enough to qualify as a major depressive disorder, the patient should be treated with an antidepressant. Stage five is that of acceptance. Patients acknowledge and come to terms with the inevitability of their death during this stage. Patients can begin to talk about facing the unknown without fear and with resolution.

Psychological Theory and Psychometric Testing

K&S Ch. 2

Question 145. D. Asking patients about suicide will have no effect on whether they are actually suicidal. Talking about suicide will not make patients suicidal. Most patients, when asked, are relieved to have permission to speak about something they have already thought about but were uncomfortable talking about with friends or family. The question is not frightening to them, nor will the mention of the word suicide help them plan their death.

Diagnostic and Treatment Procedures in Psychiatry

K&S Ch. 34

Question 146. D. Patients can display their grief over the death of loved ones in different ways and with different intensity. It is generally believed that a period of grief or mourning typically lasts about 6 months to 1 year. Some symptoms and signs of mourning may persist for a longer period, even up to 2 years or more. In most cases, the acute symptoms of grief improve over a period of about one to two months, after which time the individual returns to a more normal level of functioning.

Depressive Disorders

K&S Ch. 2

Question 147. D. The suicide rate for adolescents has quadrupled since 1950. Suicide accounts for 12% of deaths in the adolescent age group. The suicide rate has gone up more in this group than in any other group over the same time period.

Depressive Disorders

K&S Ch. 49

Question 148. D. Ramelteon (Rozerem) is a melatonin agonist and has a short half-life ranging from one to 2.5 hours. Ramelteon has an active metabolite, M-II, that has a half-life of about 5 hours. Zolpidem (Ambien) has a half-life of about 2.5 hours, but the duration of action can range from one to 4.5 hours. Zolpidem has no active metabolite. Zaleplon (Sonata) is a benzodiazepine receptor agonist that has the shortest half-life of all these agents at about one hour. It is therefore very useful for the treatment of middle insomnia. Eszopiclone (Lunesta) has the longest half-life of all these sleeping agents at about 6 hours. It is therefore, at least theoretically, the one most likely to cause next-day drowsiness. Triazolam (Halcion) is a benzodiazepine sedative–hypnotic agent with high potency and a short half-life ranging in duration from 2–4 hours.

Psychopharmacology

K&S Ch. 36

Question 149. A.   The therapeutic range for valproic acid is 50–150 ng/mL. At doses as high as 125 ng/mL, side effects including thrombocytopenia may occur. Liver function tests should be obtained at the start of treatment and every 6–12 months thereafter, and valproic acid levels should be checked periodically.

Laboratory Tests in Psychiatry

K&S Ch. 7

Question 150. C.   This is a question based on an understanding of the importance of culture. Different cultures view health and sickness differently. They view the medical system differently, and these differences must be taken into account when dealing with a multicultural population. In Japanese culture it is customary to minimize distress in front of an authority figure. This is the explanation for the patient's behavior in this question. If the doctor involved was unaware of cultural issues, the patient's behavior could be misinterpreted as psychosis or malingering, or the family could be seen as manipulative.

Cultural Issues in Psychiatry

K&S Ch. 4

FOUR

Test Number Four

1. Which one of the following is false regarding Freud's theories of human development?

    A. *During development, sexual energy shifts to different areas of the body that are usually associated with eroticism*
    B. *The anal phase is from age 1 year to 3 years*
    C. *Latency is marked by a sharp increase in sexual interest*
    D. *Freud thought that resolution of his stages was essential to normal adult functioning*
    E. *The phallic stage is from age 3 to 5 years*

2. Ischemia to which one of the following arterial territories is responsible for the phenomenon known as amaurosis fugax?

    A. *Carotid*
    B. *Vertebrobasilar*
    C. *Lenticulostriate*
    D. *Anterior cerebral*
    E. *Middle cerebral*

3. Which one of the following is true regarding norepinephrine (NE) and/or the locus caeruleus?

    A. *NE is synthesized in the locus caeruleus*
    B. *Dopamine is synthesized in the locus caeruleus, NE in the dorsal raphe nuclei*
    C. *Acetylcholine is synthesized with NE in the substantia nigra*
    D. *GABA is synthesized in the locus caeruleus*
    E. *The locus caeruleus is the site of formation of serotonin*

4. A 75-year-old man with a recent history of influenza vaccination presents to the emergency room with an acute onset of paraparesis and urinary incontinence. He reported that his symptoms began a week earlier with dull, progressive low back pain that soon resulted in bilateral leg weakness. The most likely diagnosis in this case is:

    A. *Spinal cord metastases*
    B. *Acute spinal cord compression*
    C. *Vacuolar myelopathy*
    D. *Transverse myelitis*
    E. *Acute disseminated encephalomyelitis*

 Full test available online – see inside front cover for details.

5. A doctor in a certain hospital makes a diagnosis for a particular patient. That diagnosis is considered reliable if:

   A. *It is accurate*

   B. *Many different doctors in different locations would agree upon the same diagnosis*

   C. *The disorder has features characteristic enough to distinguish it from other disorders*

   D. *The disorder allows doctors to predict the clinical course and treatment response*

   E. *The diagnosis is based on an understanding of the underlying pathophysiology and has biological markers*

6. Which one of the following set of symptoms and signs correctly identifies Horner's syndrome?

   A. *Ptosis, miosis, sweating*

   B. *Ptosis, mydriasis, sweating*

   C. *Ptosis, miosis, anhydrosis*

   D. *Ptosis, mydriasis, anhydrosis*

   E. *Lid-lag, miosis, anhydrosis*

7. A patient presents with the following symptoms: tremor, halitosis, dry mouth, tachycardia, hypertension, fever, euphoria, alertness, agitation, paranoia, hallucinations, and irritability. Which one of the following substances is the most likely cause?

   A. *Amphetamines*

   B. *Opioids*

   C. *Alcohol*

   D. *Barbiturates*

   E. *Benzodiazepines*

8. The inability to recognize familiar faces is known as:

   A. *Anosognosia*

   B. *Simultanagnosia*

   C. *Aprosodia*

   D. *Prosopagnosia*

   E. *Astereognosis*

9. Which one of the following is not a potential effect of PCP use?

   A. *Paranoia*

   B. *Nystagmus*

   C. *Catatonia*

   D. *Convulsions*

   E. *Hypotension*

10. A characteristic of a facial nerve (Bell's) palsy that clearly distinguishes it from a stroke-related facial paresis is:

    A. *The presence of miosis*

    B. *The involvement of the whole face*

    C. *Anhydrosis*

    D. *Rapid recovery of motor functioning*

    E. *A post-infectious onset*

11. Object permanence develops during which one of Piaget's developmental stages?

    A. *Sensorimotor*

    B. *Preoperational thought*

    C. *Concrete operations*

    D. *Formal thought*

    E. *Rapprochement*

12. Which one of the following is not a classic feature of syringomyelia?

    A. *Spasticity*

    B. *Muscular atrophy*

    C. *Fasciculations*

    D. *Loss of temperature and pain sensation*

    E. *Preservation of proprioception*

13. A patient comes into the emergency room and admits to sniffing glue daily for the past eight months. Which one of the following is not your concern as this patient's physician?

    A. *Liver damage*

    B. *Permanent brain damage*

    C. *Kidney damage*

    D. *Myocardial damage*

    E. *Urinary retention*

14. One of the most common causes of the movement disorder of opsoclonus–myoclonus in the infant is:

    A. *Neonatal seizures*

    B. *Craniopharyngioma*

    C. *Prematurity*

    D. *Neuroblastoma*

    E. *Meningioma*

15. A physician examines a patient in the emergency room who has recently been diagnosed with a social phobia. Which one of the following answer choices would most likely be the greatest fear for this patient?

    A. *Having to take responsibility for planning a dinner with her husband*

    B. *Being in a relationship with a new boyfriend*

    C. *Going to a state fair and being around thousands of people*

    D. *Being scrutinized by others*

    E. *Competing for a new position that just opened up in her company*

16. The Ramsay Hunt syndrome classically affects which one of the following pairs of cranial nerves?

    A. *III and VI*

    B. *IV and VI*

    C. *V and VII*

    D. *V and VIII*

    E. *VII and VIII*

17. Which one of the following statements is not true regarding body dysmorphic disorder?

   A. *It is a preoccupation with an imagined defect in appearance*

   B. *It is most commonly associated with a comorbid mood disorder*

   C. *The most common concerns involve facial flaws*

   D. *Treatment with surgical, medical, dental or dermatological care is usually successful*

   E. *If a slight physical anomaly is present the concern is markedly excessive*

18. Which one of the following primary brain tumors is the most common in patients over 60 years of age?

   A. *Anaplastic astrocytoma*

   B. *Glioblastoma multiforme*

   C. *Meningioma*

   D. *Ependymoma*

   E. *Acoustic neuroma*

19. Patients with obsessive–compulsive disorder are noted to have anomalies of which one of the following brain regions?

   A. *Corpus callosum*

   B. *Striatum*

   C. *Hippocampus*

   D. *Caudate nucleus*

   E. *Cerebellum*

20. Anton's syndrome results from a stroke that localizes to the:

   A. *Frontal lobes*

   B. *Temporal lobes*

   C. *Parietal lobes*

   D. *Occipital lobes*

   E. *Cerebellar hemispheres*

21. Which one of the following should not be considered a predictive factor for violence?

   A. *Alcohol intoxication*

   B. *Recent acts of violence*

   C. *Command auditory hallucinations*

   D. *High socioeconomic status*

   E. *Menacing other people*

22. Riluzole, the only agent FDA-approved in the treatment of amyotrophic lateral sclerosis, affects which one of the following neurotransmitters?

   A. *Glutamate*

   B. *GABA*

   C. *Acetylcholine*

   D. *Dopamine*

   E. *Norepinephrine*

23. A 29-year-old patient is admitted to the neurology unit for evaluation of seizures. Workup is negative and there has not been any seizure activity captured on electroencephalogram during his seizure episodes. Neurological examination is negative. The patient is noted to be very sad, and a psychiatric consult is called. Nurses have noted conflict between the patient and his wife during her visits. As the consultant, which one of the following would be the highest on your list of differential diagnoses?

    A. *Obsessive–compulsive disorder*

    B. *Conversion disorder*

    C. *Somatization disorder*

    D. *Social phobia*

    E. *Panic disorder*

24. What is the most common CNS cancer noted in patients with advanced AIDS?

    A. *Glioblastoma multiforme*

    B. *Lymphoma*

    C. *Meningioma*

    D. *High-grade brainstem glioma*

    E. *Epidermoid tumor*

25. The highest rate of synapse formation in the brain takes place during which one of the following time periods?

    A. *Adolescence*

    B. *Weeks 32 to 35 of gestation*

    C. *Weeks 13 to 26 of gestation*

    D. *Within the first 6 weeks of gestation*

    E. *As a toddler*

26. Which one of the following is not a presenting feature of AIDS dementia complex?

    A. *Poor attention and concentration*

    B. *Slowness of thinking*

    C. *Personality changes*

    D. *Apathy*

    E. *Hemiparesis*

27. Which one of the following is not a medical complication of weight loss in eating disorders?

    A. *Cachexia*

    B. *Loss of cardiac muscle*

    C. *Delayed gastric emptying*

    D. *Lanugo*

    E. *Increased bone density*

28. The most frequent opportunistic CNS infection in the AIDS patient is:

    A. *CNS toxoplasmosis*

    B. *Cryptococcal meningitis*

    C. *Herpes meningitis*

    D. *Cytomegalovirus encephalitis*

    E. *Neurosyphilis*

29. Which one of the following is not a medical complication of purging seen in eating disorders?

    A. *Electrolyte abnormalities*

    B. *Salivary gland inflammation*

    C. *Erosion of dental enamel*

    D. *Hyperkalemia*

    E. *Seizures*

30. A 45-year-old man with end-stage AIDS and CD4 count of 50/μL presents to the ER with a complaint of rapidly progressive onset of gait difficulty, spasticity, leg weakness, sphincter dysfunction and loss of proprioception to both feet and legs. The most likely diagnosis in this case is:

    A. *Progressive multifocal leukoencephalopathy*

    B. *Distal sensory polyneuropathy*

    C. *Vacuolar myelopathy*

    D. *Neurosyphilis*

    E. *HTLV-1 myelopathy*

31. Which one of the following medical conditions should not be considered when evaluating patients with anxiety disorders?

    A. *Carcinoid syndrome*

    B. *Hyperventilation syndrome*

    C. *Hypoglycemia*

    D. *Hyperthyroidism*

    E. *Central serous chorioretinopathy*

32. A 45-year-old man with end-stage AIDS and CD4 count of 0/μL presents to the ER with a complaint of progressive onset over the past few weeks of ataxia, visual field deficits, altered mental status, aphasia and fluctuating sensory deficits. T2-weighted brain MRI reveals the image to the right. The most likely diagnosis in this case is:

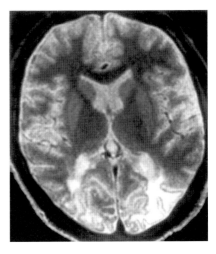

    A. *CNS toxoplasmosis*

    B. *Lymphoma*

    C. *Neurosyphilis*

    D. *AIDS dementia complex*

    E. *Progressive multifocal leukoencephalopathy*

33. When diagnosing a patient with social phobia, which axis II diagnosis is it most important for the treating psychiatrist to keep in mind?

    A. *Paranoid personality disorder*

    B. *Schizoid personality disorder*

    C. *Obsessive–compulsive personality disorder*

    D. *Avoidant personality disorder*

    E. *Borderline personality disorder*

34. Which one of the following is not a prion disease?

    A. *Kuru*
    B. *Gerstmann–Sträussler–Scheinker syndrome*
    C. *Fatal familial insomnia*
    D. *Devic's syndrome*
    E. *Creutzfeldt–Jakob disease*

35. A psychiatrist is covering the emergency room and a patient comes in who has a previous diagnosis of bipolar II disorder. Based on this diagnosis which one of the following symptoms would the knowledgeable psychiatrist expect to see in this patient over time?

    A. *Psychotic features*
    B. *Manic episodes that do not respond to treatment with mood stabilizers*
    C. *Rapid cycling between severe depression and mania*
    D. *Recurrent manic episodes in the absence of depression*
    E. *Recurrence of both depressive and hypomanic episodes*

36. The classic triad of headache, ipsilateral Horner's syndrome and contralateral hemiparesis is generally due to:

    A. *Carotid artery occlusion*
    B. *Giant cell arteritis*
    C. *Wallenberg's syndrome*
    D. *Pontine hemorrhage*
    E. *Cerebral aneurysmal rupture*

37. A set of statistical procedures designed to compare two or more groups of observations and determine whether the differences are due to chance or experimental difference is called:

    A. *Correlation coefficient*
    B. *Control group*
    C. *Analysis of variance (ANOVA)*
    D. *Regression analysis*
    E. *Null hypothesis*

38. A 55-year-old woman presents to the emergency room with a sudden and acute onset of right-sided painless complete facial paralysis, involving both the upper and lower parts of the face. The symptoms began earlier that day and were initially accompanied by a mild ache behind the ear which resolved. The organism most likely responsible for this condition is:

    A. *Borrelia burgdorferi*
    B. *Herpes simplex virus*
    C. *Epstein–Barr virus*
    D. *West Nile virus*
    E. *Varicella zoster virus*

39. A psychiatrist is asked to evaluate a child who does not make appropriate eye contact, fails to respond to the social cues of others, lacks the ability for spontaneous make-believe play, and on close examination has a delay in language development. What is this child's most likely diagnosis?

    A. *Schizophrenia*

    B. *Avoidant personality disorder*

    C. *Asperger's disorder*

    D. *Conduct disorder*

    E. *Autism*

40. A veterinary radiologist presents to the emergency room with a 4-week history of headache, vague fever, and paresthesias in the fingers and toes. His temperature is 103.5°F (39.7°C). He complains of difficulty swallowing with pharyngeal spasms for the past 3 days. The most likely diagnosis is:

    A. *West Nile virus infection*

    B. *Tetanus infection*

    C. *Acute botulism*

    D. *Rabies*

    E. *Epstein–Barr virus infection*

41. Which one of the following receptor subtypes is associated with the neurotransmitter glutamate?

    A. *Nicotinic*

    B. *Muscarinic*

    C. *Alpha 1*

    D. *AMPA*

    E. *GABA*

42. A 60-year-old woman presents to the emergency room with a progressive downward course over the past 6 months characterized by behavioral disinhibition, emotional lability, severe naming and word-finding difficulties, hyperorality, stubbornness, inability to plan, and poor judgment. Autopsy of this patient's brain would most likely reveal:

    A. *Hirano bodies*

    B. *Pick's inclusion bodies and gliosis*

    C. *Lewy bodies*

    D. *Neurofibrillary plaques and tangles*

    E. *Severe white-matter demyelination*

43. Your friend just had a baby that is 8 months old. You and she talk about the child and note its temperament. At this point in the child's development you tell your friend that the child's temperament is most likely a function of:

    A. *Biological factors*

    B. *The parent's culture*

    C. *The grandmother's influence on weekends*

    D. *The baby's birth month*

    E. *The influence of the child's siblings*

44. The neuropathological hallmark of idiopathic Parkinson's disease is:

    A. *Brainstem Lewy bodies*

    B. *Hirano bodies*

    C. *Amyloid plaques*

    D. *Mesial temporal sclerosis*

    E. *Caudate nucleus atrophy*

45. A young woman comes to a psychiatrist's office seeking help because of problems on her job. She describes nervousness talking in front of other coworkers at conferences, and difficulty at social events. She thinks that her boss knows her inner feelings and that there was wording put in everyone's contracts with her specifically in mind. Her dress is eccentric and out of date. She complains that she does not have any friends at the office. Given this picture, she most likely has which one of the following diagnoses?

    A. *Borderline personality disorder*

    B. *Dependent personality disorder*

    C. *Schizotypal personality disorder*

    D. *Histrionic personality disorder*

    E. *Schizoid personality disorder*

46. Which one of the following is not a possible symptom of fibromyalgia?

    A. *Headache*

    B. *Psychosis*

    C. *Depression*

    D. *Sleep disturbance*

    E. *Paresthesias*

47. Pancreatic cancer is most often associated with which one of the following psychiatric disorders?

    A. *Psychosis*

    B. *Anxiety*

    C. *Depression*

    D. *Impulse control disorders*

    E. *Bulimia*

48. A 75-year-old man with known history of prostate cancer presents to the emergency room with an acute onset of bilateral leg weakness, leg spasticity, sensory loss to pain and temperature below the waist, and acute bladder and bowel incontinence. The first test of choice to perform in the emergency room setting is:

    A. *Noncontrast head CT*

    B. *Brain MRI*

    C. *Screening spine MRI*

    D. *Spinal X-rays*

    E. *HTLV-1 antibody titer*

49. Which one of the following symptoms would a psychiatrist look for in a child to make the diagnosis of conduct disorder rather than depression, ADHD, or bipolar disorder?

    A. *Irritable mood*

    B. *Difficulty organizing tasks*

    C. *Excessive activity*

    D. *Starting fights with other children*

    E. *Sleep disturbance*

50. Subacute combined degeneration of the spinal cord is a result of deficiency in which one of the following:

    A. *Vitamin B12*

    B. *Vitamin B1*

    C. *Vitamin B6*

    D. *Niacin*

    E. *Folic acid*

51. When patients who have been victim to childhood incest become adults, which one of the following disorders are they most prone to develop?

    A. *Anorexia*

    B. *Bipolar disorder*

    C. *Social phobia*

    D. *Major depression*

    E. *Conversion disorder*

52. A patient presents to the emergency room with an acute onset of pure right hemiparesis that on examination is noted to affect the face, arm and leg equally. There is no sensory deficit, and no cortical signs are noted. This stroke most likely localizes to the:

    A. *Left thalamus and internal capsule*

    B. *Left internal capsule*

    C. *Right basis pontis*

    D. *Right medulla*

    E. *Left midbrain*

53. Which one of the following statements is true regarding the amino acid neurotransmitters?

    A. *Histamine is an amino acid neurotransmitter*

    B. *GABA is an excitatory amino acid neurotransmitter*

    C. *Glutamate is an inhibitory amino acid neurotransmitter*

    D. *Glutamate receptors have been found to be important in the mechanism of action for cocaine*

    E. *Benzodiazepines, barbiturates and several anticonvulsants work through mechanisms involving GABA-B*

54. Which one of the following is not a symptom or sign of Parkinson's disease?

    A. *Bradykinesia*

    B. *Loss of postural reflexes*

    C. *Tremor*

    D. *Choreoathetosis*

    E. *Rigidity*

55. A psychiatrist is asked to evaluate an 8-year-old girl. She does not want to go to school, and refuses to do her homework. Her teacher reports that she will not read out loud in class. She likes to go and spend the weekends at friends' houses or go on over-night trips with her grandparents. Her IQ is average. What diagnosis should the informed psychiatrist most strongly consider?

    A. ADHD

    B. Conduct disorder

    C. Separation-anxiety disorder

    D. Pervasive developmental disorder

    E. Reading disorder

56. Which one of the following is not a feature of botulism toxin poisoning?

    A. Myoclonus

    B. Dysphagia

    C. Diplopia

    D. Nausea

    E. Urinary retention

57. A couple brings their son in to see a psychiatrist. The child fights with his mother and father and is rude and dismissive toward them. He states that he wants to leave, and when the doctor tells him he has to stay he yells, curses, cries, and rolls around on the floor. His teacher tells the psychiatrist that his work at school is good, but that he gets very nasty with her when she tells him to do a particular task, and he often refuses to cooperate with her. The child's most likely diagnosis is:

    A. ADHD

    B. Bipolar disorder

    C. Conduct disorder

    D. Oppositional defiant disorder

    E. Separation-anxiety disorder

58. Balint's syndrome is the result of a lesion to which one of the following areas?

    A. Frontal lobe

    B. Temporal lobe

    C. Parietal lobe

    D. Occipital lobe

    E. Bilateral parietal–occipital lobes

59. A psychiatrist evaluates a 7-year-old patient who is brought in by his parents because of complaints they have been receiving from school. The child has been sexually provocative with other children, sexualizes play activities, and openly displays sexual behavior. The most likely cause of this behavior is:

    A. Normal development

    B. Early onset puberty

    C. Traumatic brain injury

    D. Sexual abuse

    E. Psychosis with sexual delusions

60. Which one of the following symptoms is a feature of Anton's syndrome?

    A. *Aphasia*

    B. *Prosopagnosia*

    C. *Apraxia*

    D. *Confabulation*

    E. *Hiccups*

61. Which one of the following personality disorders is least associated with violent behavior?

    A. *Borderline personality disorder*

    B. *Histrionic personality disorder*

    C. *Narcissistic personality disorder*

    D. *Dependent personality disorder*

    E. *Antisocial personality disorder*

62. Inhalant intoxication (sniffing glue) causes which one of the following neurologic conditions?

    A. *Myopathy*

    B. *Neuropathy*

    C. *Myelopathy*

    D. *Denervation of muscle*

    E. *Seizures*

63. A 30-year-old man presents to the emergency room with a complaint that there is a cockroach living in his rectum. He says he knows that there is a hole in the side of his rectum which was created by the roach. He has no prior psychiatric history, but states that he has felt the roach crawling around in his rectum for the past 18 months. He is a lawyer with a busy successful practice, and says he has no problems at work. During previous trips to the doctor for this complaint, he was examined and told that there was no cockroach in his rectum. He feels that they just did not examine him properly, otherwise the roach would have been found. Examination and blood work are all normal. His most likely diagnosis is:

    A. *Conversion disorder*

    B. *Schizophrenia*

    C. *Depression with psychotic features*

    D. *Delusional disorder with somatic features*

    E. *Hypochondriasis*

64. Which one of the following substances of abuse is the most likely to lower the seizure threshold during intoxication?

    A. *Morphine*

    B. *PCP*

    C. *Cocaine*

    D. *Cannabis*

    E. *Alcohol*

65. Five patients are brought into the emergency room on a Friday evening. Of the five, which one is most likely to kill themselves successfully?

    A. *Bob, who has schizophrenia*

    B. *Carol, who has alcoholism*

    C. *Dave, who is mentally retarded*

    D. *Sally, who has borderline personality disorder*

    E. *Mark, who has major depressive disorder*

66. Meige's syndrome comprises which one of the following sets of symptoms?

    A. *Hemifacial spasm and seizures*

    B. *Hemifacial spasm and cervical dystonia*

    C. *Blepharospasm and ptosis*

    D. *Blepharospasm and oromandibular dystonia*

    E. *Lid apraxia and myokymia*

67. A physician that has reason to believe a patient may kill or injure another person must notify the potential victim, authorities, or the victim's family or friends. This is the result of which one of the following answer choices?

    A. *Durham rule*

    B. *M'Naghten rule*

    C. *Ford vs Wainwright*

    D. *Tarasoff rule*

    E. *Respondeat superior*

68. The phenomenon of scanning speech results from a lesion to the:

    A. *Cerebellum*

    B. *Thalamus*

    C. *Frontal lobes*

    D. *Midbrain*

    E. *Dominant temporal lobe*

69. A friend just gave birth to a healthy baby boy 5 days ago. Now your friend is crying and irritable, and has been dysphoric over the past 2 days. Which one of the following is the most likely diagnosis based on the information given?

    A. *Postpartum depression*

    B. *Postpartum blues*

    C. *Postpartum psychosis*

    D. *Postpartum bipolar disorder*

    E. *Specific phobia of being a parent*

70. Which one of the following is a syndrome of near muteness with normal reading, writing and comprehension?

    A. *Aphasia*

    B. *Apraxia*

    C. *Agnosia*

    D. *Aphemia*

    E. *Abulia*

71. Which one of the following is not true regarding the N-methyl-D-aspartate (NMDA) receptor?

    A. *The NMDA receptor has been linked with learning and memory*

    B. *The NMDA receptor allows for the passage of potassium only*

    C. *The NMDA receptor only opens when it has bound two molecules of glutamate and one molecule of glycine*

    D. *The NMDA receptor can be blocked by physiological concentrations of magnesium*

    E. *The NMDA receptor can be blocked by PCP*

72. Which one of the following refers to a state of unresponsiveness from which arousal only occurs with vigorous and repeated stimulation?

    A. *Alertness*

    B. *Lethargy*

    C. *Stupor*

    D. *Coma*

    E. *Persistent vegetative state*

73. Of the following disorders, which one has the best prognosis?

    A. *Somatization disorder*

    B. *Body dysmorphic disorder*

    C. *Pain disorder*

    D. *Hypochondriasis*

    E. *Conversion disorder*

74. Which one of the following statements is true?

    A. *All patients with acute Guillain–Barré syndrome should be hospitalized in an intensive care unit in case of respiratory compromise*

    B. *All comatose patients require a head CT scan before a lumbar puncture is performed*

    C. *A positive grasp reflex is always a sign of frontal lobe damage*

    D. *Cerebellar hemispheric lesions produce deficits that are contralateral to the lesion*

    E. *Bell's palsy is most often caused by Borrelia burgdorferi infection*

75. Which one of the following choices is considered unethical by the American Psychiatric Association Ethics Committee?

    A. *Closing a practice and finding follow-up care for your patients*

    B. *Refusing to discuss a patient's case with her family unless she gives you permission*

    C. *Charging a colleague rent to sublet office space from you*

    D. *A patient wills you their estate after death. You accept and use the money for a new car*

    E. *You charge a fee to supervise another psychiatrist*

76. Emotional memory localizes to the:

    A. *Amygdala*

    B. *Hippocampus*

    C. *Primary auditory cortex*

    D. *Nucleus basalis of Meynert*

    E. *Pons*

77. Of the following medications, which one is the least anticholinergic?

   A. *Amitriptyline*

   B. *Imipramine*

   C. *Desipramine*

   D. *Nortriptyline*

   E. *Maprotiline*

78. By what age should a child have a six-word vocabulary, be able to self-feed, and be able to walk up steps with his hand being held?

   A. *6 months*

   B. *9 months*

   C. *12 months*

   D. *18 months*

   E. *24 months*

79. A 30-year-old male is brought to the emergency room after being arrested for exposing his genitals to women on the train. He states that he has impulses to expose himself that he can't control, and that he finds the whole experience very sexually exciting. Which one of the following medications would be an appropriate treatment for this patient?

   A. *Medroxyprogesterone acetate*

   B. *Lorazepam*

   C. *Ziprasidone*

   D. *Duloxetine*

   E. *Chlorpromazine*

80. A 45-year-old woman presents to the emergency room with an acute left hemiparesis of the arm and leg. You ask her to lift her normal right leg while you put your hand under her paretic leg. You note that while lifting her good leg, she pushes her affected leg downwards on the bed with normal strength. You suspect a hysterical or psychogenic disorder. This phenomenon is termed:

   A. *Hoffman's sign*

   B. *Hoover's sign*

   C. *Lasègue's sign*

   D. *Romberg sign*

   E. *Gegenhalten*

81. Clomipramine is not used for which one of the following?

   A. *Depression*

   B. *Obsessive–compulsive disorder*

   C. *Panic disorder*

   D. *Premature ejaculation*

   E. *Command auditory hallucinations*

82. The only true emergency in neurology that requires immediate MRI imaging and evaluation in the emergency room is:

    A. *Acute suspected early hemispheric stroke*

    B. *Acute suspected myasthenia gravis.*

    C. *Acute suspected spinal cord compression*

    D. *Acute suspected Guillain–Barré syndrome*

    E. *Acute suspected subarachnoid hemorrhage*

83. Which one of the following terms refers to the state's right to intervene and act as a surrogate parent for those who cannot care for themselves?

    A. *Actus reus*

    B. *Mens rea*

    C. *Parens patriae*

    D. *Durable power*

    E. *Respondeat superior*

84. Which one of the following medications has the unique mechanism of action of being a selective GABA reuptake inhibitor?

    A. *Gabapentin*

    B. *Tiagabine*

    C. *Pregabalin*

    D. *Vigabatrin*

    E. *Lioresal*

85. Which one of the following answer choices is measured by the trail making test?

    A. *Memory*

    B. *Language*

    C. *Social learning*

    D. *Psychosis*

    E. *Executive function*

86. The principal mechanism of action of the Alzheimer's disease agent memantine involves which one of the following receptors?

    A. *Acetylcholine*

    B. *Dopamine*

    C. *NMDA*

    D. *Glycine*

    E. *GABA*

87. Which one of the GABA receptors is thought to be the site of action of the benzodiazepines?

    A. *GABA-A*

    B. *GABA-B*

    C. *GABA-C*

    D. *GABA-D*

    E. *GABA-E*

88. Vagal nerve stimulation is FDA-approved for which one of the following indications?

    A. *Refractory epilepsy*

    B. *Bipolar mania*

    C. *Schizophrenia*

    D. *Intermittent explosive disorder*

    E. *Obsessive–compulsive disorder*

89. Which one of the following statements is true regarding carbamazepine?

    A. *Carbamazepine is approved in the US for treatment of temporal lobe epilepsy and general epilepsy, but not trigeminal neuralgia*

    B. *Carbamazepine is metabolized by the kidneys*

    C. *Carbamazepine can be associated with a transient increase in the white blood cell count*

    D. *Carbamazepine has been shown to be as effective as the benzodiazepines in some studies for management of alcohol withdrawal*

    E. *A benign pruritic rash occurs in 60–70% of patients treated with carbamazepine*

90. Auscultation of the head that reveals a bruit would likely be indicative of which one of the following?

    A. *Brain tumor*

    B. *Venous sinus thrombosis*

    C. *Temporal arteritis*

    D. *Intracranial aneurysm*

    E. *Arteriovenous malformation*

91. Which one of the following tests is considered to be projective?

    A. *Halstead–Reitan battery*

    B. *Stanford–Binet test*

    C. *Wechsler–Bellevue test*

    D. *Draw-a-Person test*

    E. *MMPI*

92. A 47 year-old man presents to the emergency with intermittent headaches, and periodic drop attacks. His brain MRI on T1 weighted imaging reveals the scan to the right. The most likely diagnosis is:

    A. *Choroid plexus papilloma*

    B. *Colloid cyst of the third ventricle*

    C. *Ependymoma*

    D. *Pineal region germinoma*

    E. *Pituitary macroadenoma*

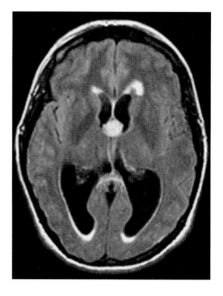

93. Which one of the following drugs is both an opioid agonist and antagonist?

    A. *Aripiprazole*

    B. *Naltrexone*

    C. *Buprenorphine*

    D. *Methadone*

    E. *Gabapentin*

94. Hallervorden–Spatz syndrome is a neurodegenerative disorder that results from lesions localizing to the:

    A. *Frontal lobes*

    B. *Parietal lobes*

    C. *Occipital lobes*

    D. *Basal ganglia*

    E. *Hippocampus*

95. A patient presents to the emergency room because of alcohol withdrawal. He and his family describe a history of alcohol-induced blackouts. Which one of the following memory problems is most consistent with alcohol induced blackouts?

    A. *Making up details of how he got to work 3 days ago*

    B. *Retrograde amnesia*

    C. *Anterograde amnesia*

    D. *Loss of memories from his daughter's birthday 5 years ago*

    E. *Inability to tell you who the current President is*

96. Strict vegetarians who ingest no meat products can suffer from deficits in proprioception and vibration sensation due to lesions that localize to the:

    A. *Posterior spinal cord*

    B. *Central spinal cord*

    C. *Anterior spinal cord*

    D. *Thalamus*

    E. *Peripheral sensory nerves*

97. A psychiatrist is treating a bipolar patient with carbamazepine. After being started on the drug he has therapeutic serum levels. Three months later the patient starts to become hypomanic and the psychiatrist decides to check a level. The level comes out below therapeutic range. Both the patient and his family reassure the psychiatrist that he has been taking the medication regularly. What should the psychiatrist do with this patient?

    A. *Confront him, because he and his family are lying*

    B. *Stop the carbamazepine and put him on divalproex sodium*

    C. *Increase the dose of carbamazepine and take follow-up serum levels*

    D. *Add a high dose of a selective serotonin reuptake inhibitor*

    E. *Hospitalize the patient*

98. Patients exposed to isoniazid (INH) for tuberculosis treatment can develop a sensory polyneuropathy as a result of a deficiency in which one of the following?

    A. *Vitamin B6*

    B. *Vitamin B12*

    C. *Niacin*

    D. *Thiamine*

    E. *Vitamin A*

99. What is the best way to handle suicidal patients with borderline personality disorder?

    A. *Take the threats seriously and take whatever steps are necessary to protect these patients*

    B. *Do not discuss suicide with them*

    C. *Isolate these patients from friends and family*

    D. *Make these patients promise not to hurt themselves (contract for safety)*

    E. *Give these patients benzodiazepine prescriptions to calm them down*

100. The West Nile virus is considered to belong to which one of the following viral families?

    A. *Arenaviruses*

    B. *Arboviruses*

    C. *Filoviruses*

    D. *Papovaviruses*

    E. *Retroviruses*

101. A patient is on lithium, risperidone, and a daily aspirin. He comes to his session confused and unsteady on his feet. He states that he has the flu, because of recent GI upset. Which one of the following should the psychiatrist do with this patient first?

    A. *Refer him to an internist*

    B. *Get a lithium level*

    C. *Review the patient's recent diet*

    D. *Send stool for ova and parasites*

    E. *Obtain a complete blood count*

102. Which one of the following neurotransmitters localizes predominantly to the basal forebrain and is responsible for memory, attention, and executive functioning?

    A. *Serotonin*

    B. *Norepinephrine*

    C. *GABA*

    D. *Glycine*

    E. *Acetylcholine*

103. Which one of the following drugs does not act by blocking the reuptake of norepinephrine into the presynaptic neuron?

    A. *Imipramine*

    B. *Venlafaxine*

    C. *Bupropion*

    D. *Nefazodone*

    E. *Mirtazapine*

104. What is the mechanism of action of the hallucinogen PCP (phencyclidine)?

    A. *Dopamine antagonism*

    B. *Serotonin antagonism*

    C. *Norepinephrine antagonism*

    D. *NMDA antagonism*

    E. *Acetylcholinesterase inhibition*

105. A physician needs to give a benzodiazepine to someone with impaired liver function. Which one of the following would be the best choice of medication in this situation?

    A. *Diazepam*

    B. *Oxazepam*

    C. *Clonazepam*

    D. *Prazepam*

    E. *Estazolam*

106. Which one of the following fungal organisms can cause vertebrobasilar strokes by invasion of vessel walls and tends to colonize in the paranasal sinuses and cause a hypersensitivity pneumonitis?

    A. *Histoplasma*

    B. *Candida albicans*

    C. *Aspergillus*

    D. *Cryptococcus neoformans*

    E. *Pseudallescheria boydii*

107. Which one of the following side effects is most likely to develop in a patient started on fluoxetine?

    A. *Loss of consciousness*

    B. *Shuffling gait*

    C. *Headache*

    D. *High blood pressure*

    E. *Blurred vision*

108. The GABA-A receptor (the most predominant GABA receptor) is which one of the following:

    A. *A sodium channel*

    B. *A chloride channel*

    C. *A calcium channel*

    D. *A potassium channel*

    E. *A magnesium channel*

109. A psychiatrist made a minor error in her last session with a patient. The patient comes to her for psychodynamic psycho-therapy. The best approach is to:

    A. *Interpret the patient's reaction*

    B. *Ignore the mistake*

    C. *Give a long but clear explanation of her reasoning*

    D. *Briefly acknowledge that she made a mistake*

    E. *Profusely apologize*

110. A failure to develop a cohesive self-awareness is known as:

    A. *Entrapment*

    B. *Climactereium*

    C. *Identity diffusion*

    D. *Activity dependent modulation*

    E. *All-or-none phenomenon*

111. What is the most important step in treating separation-anxiety disorder in an 11-year-old?

    A. *Give methylphenidate*

    B. *Give risperidone*

    C. *Rapidly send the child back to school*

    D. *Thorough psychoanalysis of the mother*

    E. *High dose benzodiazepine treatment*

112. Why do doctors use naltrexone for alcohol abuse?

    A. *It is almost 100% effective*

    B. *It blocks the effects of alcohol at the GABA receptor*

    C. *It alters dopamine levels to decrease pleasure from drinking*

    D. *It has been shown to decrease craving and decrease alcohol consumption*

    E. *It is better than behavioral modification in treating alcohol abuse*

113. A 30-year-old man on imipramine complains of difficulty urinating and impotence. What should his doctor do for him?

    A. *Increase the dose of imipramine*

    B. *Tell the patient to decrease fluid intake*

    C. *Tell the patient to stop all sexual activity*

    D. *Prescribe bethanechol*

    E. *Prescribe melatonin*

114. Which one of the following statements about mood disorders is true?

    A. *Major depression is more common in men than in women*

    B. *Bipolar disorder has equal prevalence for men and women*

    C. *Higher socioeconomic status leads to increased depression*

    D. *There is a correlation between the hyposecretion of cortisol and depression*

    E. *About 90% of those with major depressive disorder receive specific treatment*

115. A mother brings a 26-month-old child into the doctor's office. The child has not spoken any words yet. How should the doctor proceed?

    A. *Speech therapy*

    B. *Audiometry*

    C. *Sensory evoked potentials*

    D. *Tell the mother to give it more time*

    E. *Chromosomal analysis*

116. The assisted recall of information by a person in the same external environment that the information was originally acquired in is known as:

    A. *Classical conditioning*

    B. *Social learning*

    C. *Partial recovery*

    D. *Respondent conditioning*

    E. *State-dependent learning*

117. A 29-year-old man comes into the hospital with complaint of confusion, ataxia, disorientation and dysarthria. He has the smell of alcohol on his breath. Which one of the following is the best first step for the physician to take?

    A. *Phone the patient's primary care physician*

    B. *Speak with the patient's family*

    C. *Give intravenous thiamine*

    D. *Sedate the patient with haloperidol*

    E. *Give the patient an anticonvulsant*

118. Niacin deficiency (pellagra) results in which one of the following classic triads of symptoms?

    A. *Gastritis, neuropathy, stroke*

    B. *Dementia, dermatitis, diarrhea*

    C. *Neuropathy, ataxia, dementia*

    D. *Neuropathy, retinopathy, areflexia*

    E. *Neuropathy, spasticity, encephalopathy*

119. A psychiatrist is doing psychodynamic psychotherapy with a patient. The patient is usually on time, but missed a session last Tuesday. When he comes back, how should the psychiatrist approach this issue?

    A. *Do not mention the missed appointment*

    B. *Refuse to treat the patient anymore*

    C. *"You missed your appointment Tuesday. I was wondering what happened."*

    D. *"I'm glad you didn't show on Tuesday. I spent the time with a patient I like better than you."*

    E. *"I'm going to charge you twice the normal fee because you missed your appointment last Tuesday."*

120. Which one of the following is not a sign of cannabis intoxication?

    A. *Conjunctival injection*

    B. *Increased appetite*

    C. *Dry mouth*

    D. *Bradycardia*

    E. *Orthostatic hypotension*

121. A patient comes to his psychiatrist's office with complaints consistent with akathisia. Which one of the following would be the best treatment?

    A. *Bupropion*

    B. *Amoxapine*

    C. *Vitamin B6*

    D. *Captopril*

    E. *Propranolol*

122. What is the mechanism by which clonidine is effective in reducing symptoms of opiate withdrawal?

    A. *Indirect dopamine blockade*

    B. *Serotonin increase in the locus ceruleus*

    C. *Agonist activity at alpha-2 adrenergic receptors*

    D. *Generation of the metabolite trichloroethanol*

    E. *Decreased free T4*

123. Blockade of muscarinic cholinergic receptors will not lead to which one of the following?

    A. *Difficulty urinating*

    B. *Improvement in Alzheimer's symptoms*

    C. *Dry mouth*

    D. *Blurred vision*

    E. *Delirium*

124. Which one of the following lab tests is most likely to pick up alcohol abuse?

    A. *Gamma glutamyl transferase (GGT)*

    B. *Mean corpuscular volume (MCV)*

    C. *Uric acid*

    D. *Serum glutamic-oxaloacetic transaminase (SGOT)*

    E. *Serum glutamic-pyruvic transaminase (SGPT)*

125. A psychiatrist is asked by a primary care physician to treat a patient with Tourette's disorder. He is suffering from several motor tics. Which one of the following would be the best medication to give him?

    A. *Propranolol*

    B. *Pimozide*

    C. *Paroxetine*

    D. *Pindolol*

    E. *Piroxicam*

126. On which chromosome is the gene for amyloid precursor protein found?

    A. *Chromosome 19*

    B. *Chromosome 20*

    C. *Chromosome 21*

    D. *Chromosome 4*

    E. *Chromosome 13*

127. Which one of the following answer choices is central to Kohut's theories of self psychology?

    A. *The theory of oedipal conflict*

    B. *The concept of the good enough mother*

    C. *The paranoid–schizoid position*

    D. *The necessity for parental mirroring and empathic responsiveness to the child*

    E. *The importance of the depressive position*

128. A patient with bipolar disorder is on carbamazepine. He goes to his primary care physician and is placed on erythromycin. What should be expected to happen?

    A. *Carbamazepine levels will go down*

    B. *Erythromycin levels will go down*

    C. *No interaction of any kind*

    D. *Carbamazepine levels will go up*

    E. *Erythromycin levels will go up*

129. A patient with bipolar disorder gives birth to a child with spina bifida and hypospadias. What is the most likely cause for the child's defects?

    A. *Genetics*

    B. *Intrauterine infection*

    C. *Haloperidol use during pregnancy*

    D. *Valproic acid use during pregnancy*

    E. *Lithium use during pregnancy*

130. A patient presents with decreased energy, increased appetite, weight gain, increased sleep, decreased mood, lack of interest in usual activities, and social withdrawal. Which one of the following medications would be the best choice to treat him?

    A. *Citalopram*

    B. *Lithium*

    C. *Desipramine*

    D. *Phenelzine*

    E. *Venlafaxine*

131. A patient states that he was given an antidepressant in the past but does not remember the name. He does remember having his blood pressure checked regularly by the psychiatrist because of the antidepressant. Which one of the following was the patient most likely taking?

    A. *Mirtazapine*

    B. *Paroxetine*

    C. *Venlafaxine*

    D. *Citalopram*

    E. *Fluoxetine*

132. Which one of the following is the focus of interpersonal therapy?

    A. *Anxiety management*

    B. *Belief systems*

    C. *Faulty cognitions*

    D. *Social interactions*

    E. *Transference*

133. Which one of the following is not an aspect of experiments carried out by Nikolas Tinbergen?

    A. *Quantifying the power of certain stimuli in eliciting specific behavior*

    B. *Displacement activities*

    C. *Innate releasing mechanisms*

    D. *Autism*

    E. *Imprinting*

134. Which one of the following structures is most critical to the formation of memory?

    A. *Right frontal lobe*

    B. *Right parietal lobe*

    C. *Thalamus*

    D. *Cerebellum*

    E. *Hippocampus*

135. Which one of the following is not a rating scale used for mood disorders?

    A. *Beck depression inventory*

    B. *Zung self-rating scale*

    C. *Carroll rating scale*

    D. *Montgomery–Åsberg scale*

    E. *Brief psychiatric rating scale (BPRS)*

136. Which one of the following is not a characteristic of sleep terror disorder?

    A. *Awakening from sleep and screaming*

    B. *Autonomic arousal*

    C. *Recall of a detailed dream*

    D. *Sweating*

    E. *Unresponsiveness to attempts to comfort the person during the episode*

137. Thioridazine is most often associated with which one of the following side effects?

    A. *Hematuria*

    B. *Delayed orgasm*

    C. *Retrograde ejaculation*

    D. *Priapism*

    E. *Hypospadias*

138. What is the mechanism of action of donepezil?

    A. *Dopamine blockade*

    B. *Serotonin reuptake inhibition*

    C. *Acetylcholinesterase inhibition*

    D. *Increasing GABA activity*

    E. *Prevention of beta amyloid deposition*

139. Depression may present differently in different cultures. How would the knowledgeable psychiatrist predict depression would present in a 37-year-old Chinese immigrant?

    A. *Concern with mood symptoms*

    B. *Somatic complaints*

    C. *Hysteria*

    D. *Self mutilation*

    E. *Paranoia*

140. Which one of the following neurotransmitters is most involved in the effects of methylenedioxyamphetamine (ecstasy)?

    A. *Serotonin*

    B. *Norepinephrine*

    C. *GABA*

    D. *Glycine*

    E. *Acetylcholine*

141. The growth of child guidance clinics in the US in the early 1900s lead to:

    A. *The development of the first medications for ADHD*

    B. *The development of sewage systems in major US cities*

    C. *The development of child psychiatry as a profession*

    D. *Freud's three essays on the theories of sexuality*

    E. *The Ryan White Care Act*

142. The most common neurologic manifestation of neurosarcoidosis is:

    A. *Cranial neuropathy*

    B. *Cauda equina syndrome*

    C. *Peripheral neuropathy*

    D. *Meningoencephalitis*

    E. *Uveitis*

143. Trazodone is most often associated with which one of the following side effects?

    A. *Hematuria*

    B. *Delayed orgasm*

    C. *Retrograde ejaculation*

    D. *Priapism*

    E. *Hypospadias*

144. Which one of the following answer choices is true regarding aggression?

    A. *High levels of cerebrospinal fluid (CSF) serotonin are associated with increased aggression*

    B. *Serotonin is unrelated to aggression*

    C. *Low levels of CSF serotonin are associated with increased aggression*

    D. *Low levels of CSF serotonin are associated with decreased aggression*

    E. *Low levels of dopamine are associated with increased aggression*

145. How does mirtazapine work?

    A. *Serotonin reuptake inhibition*

    B. *Norepinephrine reuptake inhibition*

    C. *Alpha-2 adrenergic receptor antagonism*

    D. *Partial dopamine antagonism*

    E. *Decreasing breakdown of serotonin in the synaptic cleft*

146. Which one of the following answer choices is most consistent with sleep changes in the elderly?

    A. *Increased REM sleep only*

    B. *Increased slow wave sleep only*

    C. *Increased REM and slow wave sleep*

    D. *Decreased REM and slow wave sleep*

    E. *Decreased slow wave sleep only*

147. A score of 70 on the Global Assessment of Functioning corresponds with:

    A. *Persistent failure to maintain personal hygiene*

    B. *Major impairment in several areas*

    C. *Superior functioning in all areas*

    D. *Some difficulty functioning, but generally functioning well*

    E. *No friends, unable to keep a job*

148. Which one of the following is not an aspect of Kleine–Levin syndrome?

    A. *Irritability*

    B. *Voracious eating*

    C. *Loss of libido*

    D. *Incoherent speech*

    E. *Hypersomnia*

149. David works 17 hours per day. He does not have many friends because he feels that they interfere with his work schedule. He believes that he is a moral person and harshly criticizes those whom he finds to be unethical. He often starts projects but fails to complete them because he can not do them perfectly. His family describes him as stubborn and cheap, because he will never throw anything out. David's most likely diagnosis is:

   A. *Generalized anxiety disorder*

   B. *Obsessive–compulsive disorder*

   C. *Obsessive–compulsive personality disorder*

   D. *Schizoid personality disorder*

   E. *Avoidant personality disorder*

150. Which one of the following is an important technique of cognitive behavioral therapy?

   A. *Maintaining therapeutic neutrality*

   B. *Offering interpretations of patients' unconscious wishes*

   C. *Abreaction*

   D. *Working through unresolved conflict*

   E. *Finding and testing automatic thoughts*

FOUR

Answer Key – **Test Number Four**

1.	**C**	26.	**E**	51.	**D**	76.	**A**	101.	**B**	126.	**C**
2.	**A**	27.	**E**	52.	**B**	77.	**C**	102.	**E**	127.	**D**
3.	**A**	28.	**A**	53.	**D**	78.	**D**	103.	**E**	128.	**D**
4.	**D**	29.	**D**	54.	**D**	79.	**A**	104.	**D**	129.	**D**
5.	**B**	30.	**C**	55.	**E**	80.	**B**	105.	**B**	130.	**D**
6.	**C**	31.	**E**	56.	**A**	81.	**E**	106.	**C**	131.	**C**
7.	**A**	32.	**E**	57.	**D**	82.	**C**	107.	**C**	132.	**D**
8.	**D**	33.	**D**	58.	**E**	83.	**C**	108.	**B**	133.	**E**
9.	**E**	34.	**D**	59.	**D**	84.	**B**	109.	**D**	134.	**E**
10.	**B**	35.	**E**	60.	**D**	85.	**E**	110.	**C**	135.	**E**
11.	**A**	36.	**A**	61.	**D**	86.	**C**	111.	**C**	136.	**C**
12.	**A**	37.	**C**	62.	**B**	87.	**A**	112.	**D**	137.	**C**
13.	**E**	38.	**B**	63.	**D**	88.	**A**	113.	**D**	138.	**C**
14.	**D**	39.	**E**	64.	**C**	89.	**D**	114.	**B**	139.	**B**
15.	**D**	40.	**D**	65.	**E**	90.	**E**	115.	**B**	140.	**A**
16.	**E**	41.	**D**	66.	**D**	91.	**D**	116.	**E**	141.	**C**
17.	**D**	42.	**B**	67.	**D**	92.	**B**	117.	**C**	142.	**A**
18.	**B**	43.	**A**	68.	**A**	93.	**C**	118.	**B**	143.	**D**
19.	**D**	44.	**A**	69.	**B**	94.	**D**	119.	**C**	144.	**C**
20.	**D**	45.	**C**	70.	**D**	95.	**C**	120.	**D**	145.	**C**
21.	**D**	46.	**B**	71.	**B**	96.	**A**	121.	**E**	146.	**D**
22.	**A**	47.	**C**	72.	**C**	97.	**C**	122.	**C**	147.	**D**
23.	**B**	48.	**C**	73.	**E**	98.	**A**	123.	**B**	148.	**C**
24.	**B**	49.	**D**	74.	**B**	99.	**A**	124.	**A**	149.	**C**
25.	**E**	50.	**A**	75.	**D**	100.	**B**	125.	**B**	150.	**E**

FOUR

Explanations – **Test Number Four**

Question 1. C. Freud described a series of stages through which children pass as a part of normal development. These stages correspond to shifts of sexual energy from one erotic body part to the next.

The first phase is the oral phase from birth to 1 year. In the oral phase the infant's needs and expression are centered in the mouth, lips, and tongue. Tension is relieved through oral gratification. Those who do not complete the oral phase successfully can be very dependent in adulthood. Successful resolution of the oral stage allows the adult to both give and receive without excessive dependency or envy.

The next is the anal stage from ages 1 to 3 years. In the anal stage the child develops control of his anal sphincter. This phase is marked by increase in aggressive and libidinal drives. Control of feces gives the child independence, and the child struggles with the parent over separation. Successful completion of this stage leads to a sense of independence from the parent. Failure to complete this stage leads to obsessive–compulsive neuroses.

The phallic stage is from ages 3 to 5 years. In the phallic stage there is a focus on sexual interests and excitement in the genital area. The goal of this stage is to focus erotic interests in the genital area and lay the groundwork for gender identity. Poor resolution of this stage leads to the neuroses often associated with poor resolution of the oedipal complex. Successful resolution leads to a clear sense of sexual identity, curiosity without embarrassment, initiative without guilt, and mastery over things both internal and external.

The phallic stage is followed by latency, during which there is a decrease in sexual interest and energy. Latency lasts from age 5 years until puberty. It is a period of consolidating and integrating previous development in psychosexual functioning and developing adaptive patterns of functioning.

At puberty there is an increase in sexual energy. This time is described as the genital stage. It lasts from about ages 11–13 years until adulthood. In this stage, libidinal drives are intensified. There is a regression in personality organization, allowing for resolution of prior conflicts and the solidification of the adult personality. The goal is the ultimate separation from the parents and the development of non-incestuous object relations. Failure to complete this stage can lead to multiple complex outcomes. Freud felt that one must pass successfully through all of these stages to develop normal functioning as an adult.

Human Development

K&S Ch. 2

Question 2. A. Amaurosis fugax is a symptom of carotid artery territory ischemia. It presents as a sudden onset of transient loss of vision that manifests as a curtain or shade or veil usually over the central visual field. The duration of visual loss is generally brief, lasting about one to five minutes, and only infrequently exceeds thirty minutes in duration. When the episode concludes, vision is generally returned to normal. The event is then truly termed a transient ischemic attack (TIA), because of a duration less than twenty-four hours. In some cases, there is permanent visual loss due to retinal infarction. Amaurosis fugax is the only feature that can distinguish a middle cerebral artery syndrome from a carotid artery syndrome.

Vertebrobasilar territory ischemia would be expected to affect the cerebellum and/or brainstem. Classic posterior circulation ischemic symptoms include ataxia, nystagmus, vertigo, dysarthria, and dysphagia.

An ipsilateral Horner's syndrome can occur if the descending oculosympathetic fibers are disrupted. Crossed weakness (ipsilateral facial paresis, contralateral limb paresis) is indicative of brainstem involvement above the level of the area of decussation of the pyramids in the medulla.

Lenticulostriate territory ischemia affects the small penetrating branching arteries off of the middle cerebral artery that feed the striatum. Ischemia to this territory can produce lacunar infarcts of the internal capsule that result in a pure contralateral motor hemiparesis.

Anterior cerebral artery ischemia would be expected to produce a contralateral hemiparesis of the leg preferentially, because the cortical homuncular representation of the leg is situated parasagittally in the postcentral motor cortex.

Middle cerebral artery territory ischemia can take many different forms. If the lesion is in the dominant hemisphere, aphasia may result. Nondominant ischemia can result in hemineglect, anosognosia, visual and tactile extinction, aprosody of speech and contralateral limb apraxia.

Neurology

B&D Ch. 51

Question 3. A.   Norepinephrine (NE) is made in the locus caeruleus. Serotonin is made in the dorsal raphe nuclei. Dopamine is made in the substantia nigra. Acetylcholine is made in the nucleus basalis of Meynert.

Basic Neuroscience

K&S Ch. 3

Question 4. D.   The onset of back pain, followed by leg weakness and urinary incontinence is a classic manifestation of bilateral spinal cord pathology. In this case, the correct syndrome is a transverse myelitis because the deficits are closely preceded by an influenza vaccination. Transverse myelitis is a segmental inflammatory syndrome of the bilateral spinal cord. It is believed to be immunologic in origin and often follows an infection or vaccination, or is the direct result of demyelination due to multiple sclerosis (MS). Up to 40% of cases have no identifiable origin. The classic presentation is the rapid onset of bilateral leg weakness that presents with a clear-cut sensory level below the level of the lesion. Pain and temperature sensation are usually affected, but often proprioception and vibration sensation are spared. Urinary and/ or bowel incontinence are common findings. MRI of the spine is the imaging modality of choice. If both the spine and the brain show demyelination on MRI imaging the likelihood of the myelitis being the first manifestation of MS is greater than 50%. If the condition is proven to be a result of inflammation or demyelination, then high dose intravenous steroids are the initial acute treatment of choice.

Spinal cord metastases causing an acute cord compression would be expected to cause a similar presentation to myelitis as noted above, but one would expect the history to reveal some sort of primary cancer, such as that of the lung or prostate, that would precede the onset of spinal cord symptoms. Only about 15% of primary CNS tumors originate in the spinal cord. Emergent MRI must be performed to characterize the lesion. Treatment of acute cord compression due to metastatic lesions involves intravenous steroids, radiation therapy, and possible surgical decompression.

Vacuolar myelopathy is found almost uniquely in AIDS patients, and is similar to the condition noted in vitamin B12 deficiency. AIDS myelopathy is noted in about one-quarter of AIDS patients. The clinical picture is similar to that of myelitis or cord compression, but the timeline is usually much slower and more progressive, evolving over many months. The pathophysiology of AIDS-related vacuolar myelopathy may be due to viral release of cytokines that are neurotoxic in nature, or abnormalities in vitamin B12 utilization. Vitamin B12 levels are often normal in these cases. Antiretroviral therapy may not reverse the symptoms.

Acute disseminated encephalomyelitis (ADEM) is a monophasic demyelinating syndrome that follows a systemic infection or vaccination. It differs from transverse myelitis, because ADEM involves the whole CNS and is not simply localized to a segment of the spinal cord. ADEM usually results in multifocal signs and symptoms that include an encephalopathy. Brainstem and cerebral involvement are noted, as well as symptoms localizing to the spinal cord.

Neurology

B&D Chs 55&56

Question 5. B.   If different doctors can look at the same case and make the same diagnosis, the diagnosis is said to be reliable. In other words, it is consistent. Accuracy of the diagnosis is called validity. Descriptive validity means that the disorder has features that are characteristic enough to separate it from other disorders. Predictive validity means that the diagnosis allows the doctor to predict clinical course and treatment response. Construct validity means the diagnosis is based on underlying pathophysiology and the use of biologic markers to confirm the disease.

Statistics

K&S Ch. 4

Question 6. C. Horner's syndrome results from an interruption to the sympathetic fibers supplying the pupil, upper eyelid, facial sweat glands and facial blood vessels. The classic symptom triad is that of ptosis, miosis, and anhydrosis. Horner's syndrome can be seen as part of the lateral medullary stroke syndrome (Wallenberg's syndrome), carotid occlusion or dissection, high spinal cord lesions, neoplasms like Pancoast's tumor that affect the cervical ganglia, or intracranial hemorrhage. If the condition affects only the eye and not the sweat glands, the lesion usually localizes to the territory of the internal carotid artery. The other answers to this question need no explanation as they are simply nonsense distracters.

Neurology

B&D Ch. 77

Question 7. A. This question lists side effects that may be found with amphetamines. All of the answer choices except choice A, are central nervous system depressants and would be predicted to have effects opposite to many of those listed in the question, although there may be some similarities with certain symptoms. Amphetamine is a sympathomimetic.

Substance Abuse and Addictive Disorders

K&S Ch. 12

Question 8. D. Prosopagnosia is the inability to recognize familiar faces. It is associated classically with bilateral occipital–temporal lesions. It is often associated with agraphia and achromatopsia (inability to recognize colors and hues). It is almost always associated with visual field deficits. Anosognosia, the denial of disease or hemiparesis, is seen with lesions of the non-dominant hemisphere. Simultanagnosia is the inability to perceive a scene with multiple parts to it. The patient is only able to see and recognize individual elements of a multi-part scene, and cannot interpret the overall picture. Astereognosis refers to the inability to recognize and identify items by weight, texture and form alone, when the items are held in the hand. It is a form of tactile agnosia. Aprosodia is a deficit in the emotional aspect of expressive or receptive speech.

Neurology

B&D Chs 11,12&51

Question 9. E. With PCP use hypertension is often seen, not hypotension. Other symptoms include paranoia, nystagmus, catatonia, convulsions, hallucinations, mood lability, loosening of associations, violence, mydriasis, ataxia, and tachycardia. Treatment consists of haloperidol every 2–4 hours until the patient is calm. PCP can be detected in the urine up to eight days after ingestion.

Substance Abuse and Addictive Disorders

K&S Ch. 12

Question 10. B. Bell's palsy (VII nerve palsy) is a severe, acute, unilateral, complete facial paresis that evolves over 24–48 hours. The condition is often accompanied by pain behind the ear. Taste impairment and hyperacusis are frequent associated symptoms. The incidence is about 20 in 100 000. The syndrome is believed to be of viral etiology, and herpes simplex virus is thought to be the most frequent viral pathogen responsible for the condition. About 80–85% of patients improve completely within three months. Incomplete paralysis at onset is a better prognostic sign than complete paralysis. Treatment with acyclovir and prednisone is often administered, but remains controversial due to the etiological uncertainty of the disorder. The paralysis of Bell's palsy involves the entire face, whereas the facial paresis of a hemispheric stroke spares the upper third of the face (the brow and upper eyelid).

Neurology

B&D Ch. 70

Question 11. A.   This question focuses on Piaget's stages of cognitive development. Object permanence develops during the sensorimotor stage. There are several other questions on Piaget in this book. If you did not get this question correct, go back and review those questions and answer explanations. Know Piaget well!

Human Development

K&S Ch. 2

Question 12. A.   Syringomyelia refers to the constellation of signs and symptoms produced by a syrinx, a cavitation of the central spinal cord. The cavitation may be contiguous with a dilated central spinal canal, or it may be separate from a central canal. Most syringes occur in the cervical spinal cord. Most of those that develop from a central spinal canal are associated with an Arnold–Chiari type I or type II malformation. The classic presentation is that of a dissociated suspended sensory deficit usually in a cape or shawl pattern over the arms and upper trunk. There is impairment of pain and temperature sensation and preserved light touch, vibration and proprioception. These sensory deficits are combined with lower motor neuron signs (flaccidity, muscular atrophy, fasciculations) at or about the level of the lesion, as well as spinal long tract signs below the level of the lesion. Pain often accompanies a syrinx and can manifest as headache, neck pain, radicular pain, and segmental dysesthesia. MRI of the spine is the imaging modality of choice to best evaluate a syrinx.

Neurology

B&D Ch. 73

Question 13. E.   Urinary retention is a side effect of the belladonna alkaloids, but not of glue and benzene products. All of the other answer choices are possibilities for a patient sniffing glue daily for over 6 months. In addition to those contained in the question, side effects include slurred speech, ataxia, hallucinations, and tachycardia with ventricular fibrillation. This grouping of substances includes glue, benzene, gasoline, paint thinner, lighter fluid, and aerosols.

Substance Abuse and Addictive Disorders

K&S Ch. 12

Question 14. D.   Opsoclonus–myoclonus is a paraneoplastic movement disorder that is also called "dancing eyes–dancing feet" syndrome. It is seen most often in infants ages 6 to 18 months and in 50% or more of cases is associated with an infantile neuroblastoma. In adults, lung cancer is a common cause of this disorder. It can also be noted as a result of postviral encephalitis, multiple sclerosis, thalamic hemorrhage, and hyperosmolar coma. The condition presents as multifocal myoclonus and rapid dancing movements of the eyes. It is caused by lesions to the pause cells in the pons. Steroids or adrenocorticotropic hormone are effective treatment for this particular type of myoclonus. The other conditions noted in this question are distracters that are not related to opsoclonus–myoclonus.

Neurology

B&D Ch. 52G

Question 15. D.   Social phobia is characterized by a fear of one or more social or performance situations in which the person is exposed to unfamiliar people or possible scrutiny by others. The individual is afraid of acting in a way that would be embarrassing. Exposure to the situation almost always causes anxiety, and the person is aware that the fear is excessive. In this question, fear of scrutiny is the most definitive symptom of social phobia. The other choices could provoke anxiety in someone with some type of anxiety disorder but are neither necessarily limited to nor considered major diagnostic criteria for social phobia.

Anxiety Disorders

K&S Ch. 16

Question 16. E.   The Ramsay Hunt syndrome is a herpetic cranial neuritis that affects the facial (VII) and acoustic (VIII) nerves. The pathogen is of course the varicella-zoster virus (herpes zoster; chicken pox virus). The clinical presentation is that of a painful facial palsy, vertigo, ipsilateral hearing loss and vesicles in the external auditory canal and sometimes on the pinna. The infection is presumed to localize to the geniculate ganglion. Treatment is symptomatic. Recovery is often worse than in idiopathic Bell's palsy. The other answer choices are distracters.

Neurology

B&D Chs 53&69

Question 17. D. All of the answer choices given are true except for D. In cases of body dysmorphic disorder, medical, dental, or surgical treatment fails to solve the patient's preoccupation. The disorder consists of a preoccupation with an imagined defect in appearance. If a slight physical anomaly is present the concern is markedly excessive. The cause of this disorder is unknown, onset is usually slow, and marked impairment in functioning occurs. There is an association with mood disorders and in some studies as many as 50% of patients benefited from treatment with a serotonin-selective reuptake inhibitor. The body part of concern may change over the course of the disorder. Differential diagnosis should include anorexia, gender identity disorder, and conditions that can result in brain damage such as neglect syndromes.

Somatic Symptom Disorders

K&S Ch. 17

Question 18. B. Glioblastoma multiforme is the most common primary brain tumor in about 50% or more of patients over 60 years of age. Average survival is about one year after diagnosis with radiation therapy. Anaplastic astrocytoma has a bimodal peak in incidence in the first and third decades. Ependymomas make up about 5% of all brain tumors. They are the third most common CNS tumors in children. Meningiomas make up about 20–25% of all brain tumors. They are more likely to occur after 50 years of age, and occur about twice as frequently in females as in males. About 80% of meningiomas turn out to be benign. Acoustic neuromas are considered to be schwannomas (nerve sheath tumors). The peak incidence of acoustic neuromas is in the fourth and fifth decades.

Neurology

B&D Ch. 52

Question 19. D. Neuroimaging studies in obsessive–compulsive disorder (OCD) patients have demonstrated abnormalities in the caudate, thalamus, and orbitofrontal cortex. Functional neuroimaging by positron emission tomography (PET) scanning has demonstrated increased metabolism in the basal ganglia (predominantly in the caudate), the frontal lobes and the cingulate gyrus. CT and MRI of the brains of patients with OCD have demonstrated bilaterally smaller caudate nuclei than those seen in normal controls.

Laboratory Tests in Psychiatry

K&S Ch. 16

Question 20. D. Anton's syndrome is considered to be an agnosia characterized by cortical blindness. The lesion localizes to the bilateral occipital lobes, usually due to strokes, particularly in the calcarine cortex (Brodmann's area 17) and visual association cortex. The hallmark of the syndrome is that patients deny that they are blind and they confabulate. Patients may also suffer from visual hallucinations.

Neurology

B&D Ch. 14

Question 21. D. Signs of impending violence, or predictive factors for violence include alcohol and drug intoxication, recent acts of violence, command auditory hallucinations, paranoia, menacing behavior, psychomotor agitation, carrying weapons, frontal lobe disease, catatonic excitement, certain manic or agitated depressive episodes, violent ideation, male gender, ages 15–24 years, low socioeconomic status, and few social supports.

Management in Psychiatry

K&S Ch. 34

Question 22. A. Riluzole (Rilutek) is a glutamate antagonist and is FDA-approved in the treatment of amyotrophic lateral sclerosis (ALS). It has demonstrated mild to moderate improvement in the survival rate of ALS. It may also help patients remain in a milder disease state for a longer period of time. The medication comes in 50 mg tablets which are started at one per day at night and increased to twice daily after 1–2 weeks, if tolerated. Side effects include gastrointestinal upset, dizziness, fatigue, and liver enzyme elevation. The other answer choices are distracters.

Neurology

B&D Ch. 74

Question 23. B. Conversion disorder consists of one or more neurological symptoms that can not be explained by a medical condition. The symptoms are thought to be unconsciously produced in response to psychological conflict. Pseudoseizures can be common symptoms of conversion disorder. Conversion disorder can be associated with passive–aggressive, antisocial, histrionic, and dependent personality disorders. In obsessive–compulsive disorder a patient has intrusive unwanted thoughts that cause them to repeat a ritual or action to remove the anxiety associated with that thought. Nothing like that is described in this question. Somatization disorder presents as a patient who has a number of medical complaints involving several organ systems that can not be otherwise explained by a known medical condition. That is not the case in this question. Social phobia presents as a patient who has a fear of being in social situations or meeting new people. That has nothing to do with this question. Panic disorder presents as a patient who has recurrent and unexpected panic attacks. This patient is having pseudoseizures, not panic attacks.

Somatic Symptom Disorders

K&S Chs 16&17

Question 24. B. Primary central nervous system lymphoma occurs in AIDS patients in about 5% of cases. These lymphomas are most often of B-cell origin. Patients can present with a gradual onset of any of the following symptoms: headache, aphasia, hemiparesis, altered mental status, behavioral changes, and ataxia. Constitutional symptoms like fever and weight loss are generally absent. Diagnosis is established by MRI brain imaging. PCR testing on CSF revealing Epstein–Barr virus DNA helps to corroborate the diagnosis. Treatment with antiretroviral polypharmacy can help slow progression. None of the other tumor types mentioned in the answer choices are particularly associated with AIDS.

Neurology

B&D Ch. 53

Question 25. E. The development of the central nervous system is a very important area of study, as abnormal development is implicated in several clinical conditions, including schizophrenia. The central and peripheral nervous systems arise from the neural tube. The neural tube gives rise to the ectoderm, which becomes the peripheral nervous system, whereas the neural tube itself becomes the central nervous system. The second trimester of gestation is the peak of neuronal proliferation, with 250 000 neurons born each minute. Migration of neurons, guided by glial cells, peaks during the first 6 months of gestation. Synapse formation occurs at a high rate from the second trimester through age 10, but peaks around 2 years (toddler period) with as many as 30 million synapses forming per second. The nervous system is also actively myelinating its axons starting prenatally, and continuing through childhood, finishing in the third decade of life.

Basic Neuroscience

K&S Ch. 3

Question 26. E. AIDS dementia complex is a late complication of AIDS, particularly when the HIV infection is untreated and CD4 cell counts are low. Symptoms include poor attention and concentration, bradyphrenia, forgetfulness, poor balance, uncoordination, personality changes, apathy, and depression. Focal neurologic deficits are usually absent, such as hemiparesis or aphasia. Treatment involves administration of antiretroviral therapy.

Neurology

B&D Ch. 53

Question 27. E. All of the answer choices given are correct, with the exception of increased bone density. Anorexic patients tend to suffer from osteoporosis. They also have cachexia, loss of muscle mass, reduced thyroid metabolism, loss of cardiac muscle, arrhythmias, delayed gastric emptying, bloating, abdominal pain, amenorrhea, lanugo (fine baby-like hair), and abnormal taste sensation.

Feeding and Eating Disorders

K&S Ch. 23

Question 28. A. Central nervous system toxoplasmosis is the most frequent CNS opportunistic infection in the AIDS patient. It is noted in 10% or more of AIDS patients. The infection is caused by the parasite *Toxoplasma gondii*. Cerebral toxoplasmosis in the AIDS patient results most often from a resurgence of a previously acquired infection. The infection usually occurs in late-stage AIDS, when CD4 cell counts are less than 200/μL. CNS toxoplasmosis presents clinically with headache and focal neurological deficits with or without fever. Other possible manifestations include aphasia, seizures, and hemiparesis. In cases with significant progression, patients can develop confusion and lethargy that lead to coma. The diagnosis is made on the basis of CT or MRI brain imaging revealing a single lesion or multiple ring-enhancing lesions. Therapy is undertaken with pyrimethamine and sulfadiazine, or with clindamycin in sulfa-allergic patients. The other answer choices occur less frequently in AIDS patients. Cryptococcal meningitis, another important opportunistic infection in AIDS, as well as the other three answer choices, are explained elsewhere in this volume.

Neurology

B&D Ch. 53

Question 29. D. All choices given are correct, except for hyperkalemia. In purging, it is common to see a hypokalemic, hyperchloremic alkalosis. In addition, one may also see hypomagnesemia, pancreatic inflammation, increased serum amylase, esophageal erosion, and bowel dysfunction.

Feeding and Eating Disorders

K&S Ch. 23

Question 30. C. HIV-associated vacuolar myelopathy is the most common cause of spinal cord pathology in AIDS patients, and is seen in one-quarter to one-half of patients on autopsy. The disorder usually occurs in late-stage AIDS. The clinical picture is that of spasticity, gait instability, lower extremity weakness, loss of proprioception and vibration sensation, and sphincter dysfunction. Neurologic examination reveals a spastic paraparesis, hyper-reflexia and Babinski's signs. It is unusual to note a clear-cut sensory level on the trunk. Vitamin B12 levels are usually normal. Viral neurotoxic cytokines may contribute to the pathophysiology of the disease.

Distal sensory polyneuropathy is the most common peripheral nerve syndrome that complicates AIDS. It is seen in about one-third of AIDS patients. The clinical presentation is that of diminished ankle jerk reflexes, decreased pain, temperature, and vibration sensation, and possible paresthesia or numbness of the feet. The disorder is usually symmetrical. The condition frequently presents with lower extremity neuropathic pain. Treatment involves antiretroviral therapy and management of the pain with tricyclic antidepressants, anticonvulsants, or even narcotic analgesics if needed.

Neurosyphilis, progressive multifocal leukoencephalopathy, and HTLV-1 myelopathy are all explained elsewhere in this volume.

Neurology

B&D Ch. 53

Question 31. E. Central serous chorioretinopathy is a disease leading to detachment of the retina and has nothing to do with anxiety. Carcinoid syndrome can mimic anxiety disorders and is accompanied by hypertension, and elevated urinary 5-HIAA. Hyperthyroidism presents with anxiety in the context of elevated T3, T4 and exophthalmos. Hypoglycemia presents with anxiety and fasting blood sugar under 50 mg/dL. Signs and symptoms of diabetes may also be present with hypoglycemia (polyuria, polydipsia, and polyphagia). Hyperventilation syndrome presents with a history of rapid deep respirations, circumoral pallor, and anxiety. It responds well to breathing into a paper bag.

Anxiety Disorders

K&S Ch. 16

Question 32. E. Progressive multifocal leukoencephalopathy (PML) is a demyelinating disorder affecting AIDS patients with low CD4 counts. It results from an opportunistic infection by the JC virus, a form of human papilloma virus. It occurs in about 5% of patients with AIDS. Demyelination occurs preferentially in the subcortical white matter of the parietal and/or occipital lobes. Clinical presentation can involve hemiparesis, aphasia, sensory deficits, ataxia, and visual field deficits. Mental status may deteriorate progressively over time. MRI often reveals multiple or coalesced nonenhancing white matter lesions in the parietal or occipital lobes. CSF assay for the JC virus DNA by PCR can help confirm the diagnosis. There is no specific treatment for PML and mean survival is about two to four months after diagnosis. Antiretroviral therapy can reconstitute immune function, but often proves to be too

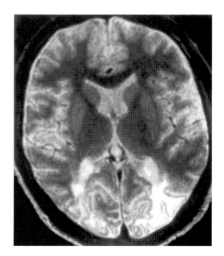

little too late. The other answer choices in this question are distracters and are explained elsewhere in this volume.

Neurology

B&D Ch. 53

Question 33. D. The distinction between social phobia and avoidant personality disorder can sometimes be confused. In a situation where the patient is afraid of almost all social situations, then avoidant personality disorder should be considered. Social phobia presents with a fear of one or more social situations. Avoidant personality disorder is defined by a pervasive pattern of social inhibition, feelings of inadequacy, and hypersensitivity to negative evaluation. This can be shown by avoiding activities involving interpersonal contact, unwillingness to get involved with people unless certain of being liked, showing fear in intimate relationships for fear of ridicule, preoccupation with criticism or rejection in social situations, viewing self as socially inept and being inhibited in new social situations or afraid to take risks for fear of embarrassment.

Anxiety Disorders

Personality Disorders

K&S Ch. 27

Question 34. D. Prion diseases are also known as transmissible spongiform encephalopathies. Prions are proteinaceous and infectious particles that are unlike bacteria or viruses. Prions are unique in that they can be passed on through heredity (chromosome 20), acquired by infection, or acquired spontaneously. Kuru is the prion disease endemic to the cannibalistic Fore people. The clinical presentation is that of progressive cerebellar ataxia. The progressive disease course generally leads to death in about twelve months from initial onset.

Gerstmann–Sträussler–Scheinker syndrome is an inherited form of prion disease. Symptoms begin to manifest in about the third or fourth decade. The disease is the slowest of the spongiform encephalopathies and can progress over several years. The clinical presentation depends on which mutation in the PRNP gene is acquired by the patient. The syndrome varies in nature and presents with any combination of ataxia, Parkinson's plus-like symptoms, or a progressive dementia.

Fatal familial insomnia occurs between ages 35 and 60 years. It presents with progressive insomnia and sympathetic autonomic hyperactivity, such as hyperhidrosis, tachycardia, hyperthermia, or hypertension. Mild cognitive impairment is usually noted. Other symptoms can include ataxia, tremor, myoclonus, confusion, or hallucinations.

Creutzfeldt–Jakob disease can be sporadic, iatrogenic or familial. CSF evaluation of 14-3-3 and Tau proteins is the diagnostic test of choice to confirm the disease. The classic sporadic disease usually affects those between ages 50 and 75 years. The downward clinical course is rapid and progresses towards death over 6 months to 2 years. The disease has three stages. Stage one presents with neuropsychiatric symptoms that can include fatigue, sleep disturbance, memory and concentration deficits, and personality changes. Stage two presents with generalized cognitive deficits, as well as significant psychiatric symptoms such as psychosis and hallucinosis. The third and final stage that precedes death is characterized by profound and severe dementia, with myoclonus and choreoathetosis. Treatment of the spongiform encephalopathies is palliative and symptomatic. There is no known cure for these diseases.

Devic's disease, also known as neuromyelitis optica, is believed to be a variant of multiple sclerosis (MS). The presentation is that of cervical myelopathy and bilateral optic neuropathy. In certain patients, the two conditions occur simultaneously, but in others, they occur at separate intervals, pointing more directly to a diagnosis of MS. Devic's disease is a disease of demyelination and has nothing to do with prions.

Neurology

B&D Chs 53&54

Question 35. E. Bipolar II disorder is characterized by at least one major depressive episode and at least one hypomanic episode during the patient's lifetime. There are no full manic episodes in bipolar II disorder. If criteria for a manic episode are met then the correct diagnosis is bipolar I disorder. Psychotic features can be found in bipolar I disorder during mania or depression but in bipolar II will occur only associated with depression as full mania is not present in bipolar II.

Bipolar Disorders

K&S Ch. 15

Question 36. A. Carotid artery occlusion presents with the triad of headache, ipsilateral Horner's syndrome, and contralateral hemiparesis. A resultant cerebral infarct can increase intracranial pressure and thereby cause headache. The Horner's syndrome itself can result in headache because of interruption of ascending sympathetic tracts from the superior cervical ganglion to the intracranial vessels and dura which are pain-sensitive structures.

Pontine hemorrhage is a neurologic emergency as it can lead to rapid death if the bleed is large. This hemorrhage type accounts for about 5% of all intracranial hemorrhages. Large bleeds in the basal tegmentum of the pons result in a clinical presentation characterized by quadriplegia, coma, decerebrate posturing, respiratory rhythm anomalies (apneustic breathing), pinpoint reactive pupils, hyperthermia, horizontal ophthalmoplegia, and ocular bobbing. The likely etiology of these bleeds is the rupture of small tegmental pontine penetrating arteries that originate from the trunk of the basilar artery.

Cerebral aneurysmal rupture results in a sudden explosive headache ("the worst headache of my life"), obtundation, nausea, vomiting, meningeal signs, neck pain, and photophobia. Aneurysms are discussed in further detail elsewhere in this volume, as are giant cell arteritis and Wallenberg's syndrome.

Neurology

B&D Chs 51&69

Question 37. C. Analysis of variance is a set of statistical procedures which compares two groups and determines if the differences are due to experimental influence or chance. Other answer choices were covered in Test Three.

Statistics

K&S Ch. 4

Question 38. B. The condition described in this question is of course that of a Bell's palsy (VII nerve palsy). Bell's palsy is characterized by a sudden, severe, unilateral infranuclear (i.e., involving both the upper and lower parts of the face) facial paresis. In serious cases, the brow droops, with widening of the palpebral fissure, and the eyelid cannot close completely. When the patient tries to close the affected eye with effort, the lid remains partially opened and the globe turns up and out. This sign is known as Bell's phenomenon. The incidence is about 20 per 100 000, with a peak in the third decade. The disorder is believed to be viral in origin and is thought to be most often due to occult herpes simplex infection. The facial paresis is often preceded by pain behind the ipsilateral ear, which may resolve. The facial paresis results soon thereafter and may evolve over one to two days, with maximal deficit within the first 72 hours. Eighty to eighty-five per cent of patients recover fully within 3 months. A 7 to 10-day course of oral acyclovir with an oral prednisone taper may shorten the course of the disorder, but studies have not demonstrated a clear-cut benefit to this approach.

Borrelia burgdorferi, the spirochete responsible for Lyme disease can result in a unilateral, or even bilateral Bell's palsy. This is often accompanied by an aseptic meningitis, which when combined with facial diplegia is termed Bannwarth's syndrome. Facial diplegia from Lyme disease is much less common than idiopathic Bell's palsy and the history should point to deer tick exposure in the outdoor setting at some time directly preceding the onset of symptoms.

Epstein–Barr virus, West Nile virus, and varicella zoster virus infections do not usually result in a Bell's palsy. Other conditions that can cause a VII nerve palsy include Guillain–Barré syndrome, sarcoidosis, and facial nerve tumors or metastases.

Neurology

B&D Ch. 70

Question 39. E. This question gives a clear description of autism. In autism the child displays a lack of ability to use and read nonverbal gestures, failure to develop appropriate peer relationships, lack of sharing enjoyment with other people, and lack of emotional reciprocity. They also show communication deficits such as delays in language development (not seen in Asperger's), inability to sustain conversation, repetitive or idiosyncratic use of language, and lack of make-believe play. They exhibit repetitive or stereotyped patterns of behavior such as preoccupation with areas of interest that are abnormal either in intensity or focus, adherence to inflexible ineffective routines, repetitive motor mannerisms, or persistent preoccupation with parts of objects. Some of the above mentioned symptoms appear before three years of age.

Neurodevelopmental and Pervasive Developmental Disorders

K&S Ch. 41

Question 40. D. This question points to a diagnosis of rabies virus infection. Rabies virus is transmitted to humans most often by wild animals such as bats, foxes, and raccoons, or by nonimmunized dogs. The incubation period is about one to two months. There is a prodromal period characterized by paresthesias, headache, and fever, which can then progress to generalized neurologic compromise, coma, and death. During the progressive phase of the illness, 80% or more of patients exhibit hydrophobia, which manifests as pharyngeal and nuchal spasms that are triggered by swallowing, smells, tastes, or sounds. These spasms can last up to several minutes in duration. The condition usually progresses to an encephalitis that is often accompanied by high fever that can rise up to 107°F, as well as autonomic hyperactivity, seizures, agitation and psychosis. Treatment begins with postexposure prophylaxis with rabies vaccine and antirabies immunoglobulin in patients who have never received immunization.

West Nile virus infection is an arbovirus infection that is endemic to many parts of the world. Mosquito bites from the genus *Culex* are frequent vectors of transmission of the virus to humans. Most infections in humans are asymptomatic. In about 20% of affected patients, the infection presents as a febrile condition after an incubation period of a few days to up to two weeks. Only 1 in 150 patients goes on to develop a meningitis or encephalitis picture. The infection may progress to the development of a demyelinating or axonal neuropathy. Diagnosis is made by detection of IgM antibodies in cerebrospinal fluid, or IgM and IgG antibodies in serum. Treatment is generally supportive. Patients with serious symptoms may respond to intravenous administration of anti-West Nile virus immunoglobulin.

Acute tetanus results from infection with the bacterium *Clostridium tetani*. This bacterium releases tetanospasmin, also known as tetanus toxin, which blocks GABA and glycine in the inhibitory interneurons in the spinal cord, and causes the characteristic muscle contractions that are seen in tetanus. The bacterial spores can live for years in dust and soil and when an open wound is inoculated with dirt that contains the spores, they can release the toxin that causes the disease. The toxin is taken up into the anterior horn cells by retrograde axonal transport. Trismus, or lockjaw, is a primary symptom of the disorder in over 75% of cases. Risus sardonicus, a sustained involuntary grimace resulting from uncontrollable facial muscle spasm, is another characteristic of tetanus. Laryngospasm can lead to respiratory compromise and death if the disorder is untreated. Cardiac arrest can also result from dysautonomia. Treatment begins with airway protection and intubation if there is respiratory compromise. Tetanus immune globulin given in a single intramuscular dose of 500 units neutralizes blood-borne toxin. Prevention of the disease by vaccination with anti-tetanus antibody vaccine following a dirty open wound is the cornerstone of disease management.

Clostridium botulinum is a bacteria that secretes a potent neurotoxin that blocks acetylcholine release at the neuromuscular junction and thus prevents neuromuscular transmission. The bacterium infects humans by its presence in tainted food or by wound contamination from dirt or soil containing the organism. Classic symptoms of botulism include dysphagia, dysarthria, ptosis, and diplopia. These symptoms rapidly progress to limb paralysis and eventually to paralysis of respiratory muscles that can lead to death if the condition is untreated. Gastrointestinal symptoms of nausea, vomiting, and diarrhea, often present with neurologic compromise after a 12–36-hour incubation period following ingestion of the toxin. Infants who consume unpasteurized honey may ingest spores and can present with weak cry, lethargy, floppiness, poor suck, and constipation. Diagnosis can be established by wound or stool culture. Electromyography and nerve conduction studies can reveal characteristic anomalies compatible with presynaptic neuromuscular blockade. Treatment is supportive, particularly with respect to airway protection, and trivalent equine antitoxin administration can reverse the effects of circulating toxin.

Epstein–Barr virus (EBV) infection can be asymptomatic, or it can present as infectious mononucleosis, with splenomegaly, pharyngitis, and cervical lymphadenopathy. Less than 1% of EBV infections present with neurologic manifestations, which can include meningitis, transverse myelitis, sensory polyneuropathy, or Guillain–Barré syndrome. EBV can be detected in the CSF of patients with AIDS-related primary CNS lymphoma.

Neurology
B&D Ch. 53

Question 41. D. The three receptor types associated with glutamate are AMPA, kainate, and *N*-methyl-D-aspartate (NMDA). Acetylcholine is associated with the nicotinic and muscarinic receptors. Norepinephrine is associated with the alpha 1, alpha 2, and beta receptors. Serotonin is associated with the various 5-HT receptors. GABA is associated with the GABA receptor. Opioids are associated with the mu and delta receptors. Dopamine is associated with the D1, D2, D3, D4 receptors.

Basic Neuroscience
K&S Ch. 3

Question 42. B.   This vignette depicts a patient with classic manifestations of Pick's disease. Pick's disease is one of the so-called frontotemporal dementias (FTDs). The frontal and temporal lobes are preferentially affected and pathological studies reveal localized "knife-edge" atrophy of these lobes, together with ballooned cells and intraneuronal inclusions, termed "Pick's inclusion bodies". These inclusions plus the finding of swollen neurons and gliosis have come to be termed Pick-type histology.

The clinical presentation can manifest either with predominant behavioral disturbance or with progressive language disturbance. In the first type, behavioral changes occur with poor judgment, inability to reason or plan, and impulsivity. Patients can display hyperorality and hypersexuality (similar to that in Klüver–Bucy syndrome) with both behavioral disinhibition and a lack of motivation.

Treatment is aimed at management of depression and behavioral problems. Antidepressant therapy with SSRI medication can be useful. Atypical antipsychotic agents may help with impulsivity and behavioral anomalies. The condition is invariably irreversible.

Hirano bodies are eosinophilic neuronal inclusions that can be seen in certain neurodegenerative diseases such as Creutzfeldt–Jakob disease and Alzheimer's dementia. Lewy bodies are cytoplasmic inclusions found in the substantia nigra and cortex of many patients with idiopathic Parkinson's disease and in the cerebral cortex of patient's with Alzheimer's dementia and diffuse Lewy body disease. Neurofibrillary plaques and tangles are the neuropathologic hallmark of Alzheimer's dementia. Severe white-matter demyelination can occur in several distinct diseases, particularly in multiple sclerosis, Binswanger's disease, acute disseminated encephalomyelitis, and progressive multifocal leukoencephalopathy.

Neurology

B&D Ch. 66

Question 43. A.   It is thought that a child's temperament at an age as young as 8 months is a function of his genes. At such a young age environmental factors play a small role in the child's temperament. As the child gets older, environmental factors will play a larger and larger role. Temperament has been examined by researchers and divided into several components. These include activity level, rhythmicity (of hunger, feeding, elimination, etc.), approach or withdrawal, adaptability, intensity of reaction, responsiveness, mood, distractibility, and attention span. There is a genetic component to why these vary among individuals, as well as the influence of parents, consequences of the child's behavior, and other environmental influences.

Psychological Theory and Psychometric Testing

K&S Ch. 2

Question 44. A.   The neuropathological hallmark of idiopathic Parkinson's disease is the finding of characteristic Lewy bodies in surviving neurons in the pars reticulata of the substantia nigra in the midbrain. The substantia nigra itself is depigmented, pale and demonstrates gliosis and neuronal loss. Lewy bodies have a pale halo and an eosinophilic center.

Hirano bodies are eosinophilic neuronal inclusions that can be seen in certain neurodegenerative diseases such as Creutzfeldt–Jakob disease and Alzheimer's dementia.

Amyloid and neuritic plaques are noted in Alzheimer's dementia. Amyloid may also be found in the cerebrovascular wall. Mesial temporal sclerosis is the pathological hallmark of brain tissue in those with temporal lobe epilepsy. The entorhinal cortex and hippocampi are characterized by neuronal loss and gliosis. Atrophy of the head of the caudate nucleus is found in Huntington's disease, but it does not correlate with the severity of the disease.

Neurology

B&D Chs 66,67&71

Question 45. C.   This question gives a description of someone who has schizotypal personality disorder. Schizotypal personality disorder is composed of a pervasive pattern of personal and social deficits characterized by ideas of reference, odd beliefs or magical thinking, unusual perceptual experiences, paranoid ideation, inappropriate affect, eccentric appearance, lack of close friends, and excessive social anxiety that has a paranoid flair.

Personality Disorders

K&S Ch. 27

Question 46. B. Fibromyalgia does not present with psychosis. Fibromyalgia is a controversial syndrome characterized by diffuse muscular and soft-tissue pain with multiple tender "trigger" points. The patient must have tenderness to palpation at eleven or more of eighteen specific tender points. Other clinical manifestations can include weakness, paresthesias, sleep disturbance, mood disturbance, headache, fatigue, muscle or joint stiffness, and dizziness. Neurological examination and all laboratory and clinical investigations are usually within normal limits. The cause of the disorder is not known. Treatment involves a good physician–patient relationship, exercise, avoiding a sedentary lifestyle and possibly the use of tricyclic antidepressants.

Neurology

B&D Ch. 73

Question 47. C. Pancreatic cancer has been associated with a high rate of depression. Patients present with apathy, decreased energy, and anhedonia. It should be a consideration in the clinician's mind whenever seeing middle-aged depressed patients. Cancer in general brings about many psychological reactions in patients. Fear of death, fear of abandonment and disfigurement, loss of independence, denial, anxiety, guilt, financial worries, and disruption in relationships all play a role. Of patients with cancer, 50% often have comorbid psychiatric diagnoses with adjustment disorder, major depressive disorder, and delirium being the most common.

Depressive Disorders

K&S Ch. 28

Question 48. C. This vignette depicts a classic neurologic emergency: acute epidural spinal cord compression (ESCC). In this case, the causative agent is likely to be a spinal metastasis from the patient's prostate cancer. Metastases from primary carcinoma of the breast, lung and prostate each make up 20% of the cause of ESCC. Back pain is the most frequent presenting feature in over 80% of cases. The back pain is usually progressive and increases with tumor growth over a period of up to 2 months before the onset of neurological deficits. Motor weakness is noted in about 80% of cases, and it predicts the post-treatment outcome much of the time. Sensory deficits are noted in about 75% of cases. Metastatic ESCC causes a spastic paraparesis or paraplegia with a sensory level that is usually several levels below the actual lesion. Bowel and bladder incontinence, urinary retention, or constipation, are observed in a majority of patients. Sagittal screening MRI imaging of the entire spine is the initial test of choice, if available, because only MRI and myelography can immediately identify and characterize the nature of the lesion and guide treatment. Treatment is undertaken acutely with parenteral corticosteroids and subacutely with radiation therapy. Decompressive laminectomy can be performed, but radiotherapy has of late produced results as good as a surgical approach. Chemotherapy is generally ineffective, because metastases causative of ESCC are usually not chemosensitive.

Neurology

B&D Ch. 52

Question 49. D. It is important to be able to distinguish conduct disorder from other childhood psychiatric diagnoses. In conduct disorder the patient shows a pattern whereby the rights of others and societal rules are violated. This presents as bullying other children, using weapons, physical fighting, cruelty to animals, stealing, fire setting, destroying property, truancy, or running away from home. Patients with ADHD can have many behavioral problems, but those problems are a result of inattention, hyperactivity, and impulsivity. ADHD does not show a pattern where the child is intentionally or malevolently being violent or destructive. Any such acts happen as a result of hyperactivity and poor impulse control. In depression children can become very irritable, withdrawn, and not wish to socialize. They may even act out as a result of how badly they are feeling. However this is different than a long-standing pattern of actively trying to carry out violence or do property damage regardless of mood state. In bipolar disorder children may break rules and have behavioral difficulties during manic and depressive episodes. However there will be a clear cycling pattern to their moods (and other symptoms), which corresponds to the times when their behaviors become problematic. One of the other important distinctions to make is between conduct disorder and oppositional defiant disorder (ODD). In ODD there is a pattern of negativistic, hostile, or defiant behavior directed at adults or authority figures. In conduct disorder the negative behavior is directed at all others regardless of whether they are authority figures or not. ODD behaviors are therefore more targeted and have less of a wide-ranging destructive nature than those of conduct disorder.

Disruptive, Impulse Control, Conduct Disorders, and ADHD

K&S Ch. 44

Question 50. A. Subacute combined degeneration is the result of a deficiency in vitamin B12 (cobalamin). Cobalamin deficiency manifests as macrocytic anemia, atrophic glossitis, and neurologic deficits. Neurologic symptoms include lesions to the lateral and posterior columns of the spinal cord (subacute combined degeneration), peripheral neuropathy, optic atrophy, and brain lesions. Spinal cord symptoms present as posterior column deficits, which can manifest as upper motor neuron limb weakness, spasticity, and Babinski's signs. Peripheral neuropathy can present as paresthesias and large fiber sensory impairment (loss of proprioception and vibration sensation). Cerebral symptoms present as behavioral changes, forgetfulness, and in severe cases, dementia and stupor. Sensory ataxia is demonstrated by a positive Romberg sign. There can also be a diffuse hyper-reflexia with absent ankle jerk reflexes. Deficiencies of vitamins B6, niacin, and folic acid are explained elsewhere in this volume.

Neurology

B&D Chs 57&76

Question 51. D. Victims of childhood incest often develop depressive feelings mixed with guilt, shame, and a feeling of permanent damage. Teens that undergo sexual abuse often show poor impulse control, self-destructive behavior, and suicidal behavior. Adults abused as children often have post-traumatic stress disorder and dissociative disorders. Incest is most often perpetrated by fathers, stepfathers or older siblings. It is defined as sexual relations between two people who are related or who society has deemed inappropriate to be sexually involved. Most reported cases involve father–daughter incest. In addition to depression, children involved in incest may present to the doctor with complaints of abdominal pain, genital irritation, separation-anxiety disorder, phobias, or school problems.

Trauma and Stress Related Disorders

K&S Ch. 32

Question 52. B. This question presents the classic lacunar stroke syndrome called pure motor hemiparesis. This lacunar syndrome classically localizes to the contralateral internal capsule. Two other possible locations of such a lacunar stroke are the contralateral basis pontis or corona radiata. The pure motor stroke presents without cortical deficits. There are no sensory or visual deficits. Aphasia, agnosia and apraxia, are all absent in a pure motor stroke. If both the thalamus and internal capsule are involved, one would expect to see a combined sensory-motor stroke, which manifests not only as a contralateral motor hemiparesis, but also as a contralateral hemisensory loss. The lesion localizes to ischemia in the territory of the small penetrating lenticulostriate arteries that originate off the proximal middle cerebral artery.

Neurology

B&D Ch. 51

Question 53. D. The amino acid neurotransmitters include GABA, glutamate, and aspartate. GABA is the main inhibitory neurotransmitter of the brain. Glutamate is the main excitatory neurotransmitter of the brain. The benzodiazepines, barbiturates and several anticonvulsants work through the action of GABA-A and not GABA-B. Lioresal, a muscle relaxant, works through GABA-B. The street drug PCP works primarily through the glutamate receptor. Cocaine works by blocking reuptake of serotonin, norepinephrine, and dopamine. It is also believed to increase glutamate in the nucleus accumbens, accounting for its habit-forming effects. Histamine is a biogenic amine neurotransmitter.

Basic Neuroscience

K&S Ch. 3

Question 54. D. Choreoathetosis is not a feature of Parkinson's disease (PD). The classic cardinal clinical features of idiopathic Parkinson's disease are akinesia (or bradykinesia), rigidity, resting tremor, and loss of postural reflexes. Tremor is an oscillating 3 to 5 Hz, seen more in the hands where it resembles pill-rolling, but also in the face, chin and the lower extremities. Bradykinesia refers to slowness of voluntary movements that make it difficult for the patient to dress, eat and maintain personal hygiene. Bradykinesia becomes most evident when a patient attempts to perform rapid alternating movements. Rigidity is often manifested as a cogwheeling when the extremities are passively mobilized. Loss of postural reflexes is also a hallmark of idiopathic PD, and is responsible for the many falls sustained by patients with the disease. Other associated clinical features include masked facies, decreased blink, micrographia, seborrhea, weight loss, constipation, and dysphagia. Gait is classically altered and patients walk with "petits pas" (small steps) and a shuffling gait. When they turn around, they turn "en bloc" (without swinging the hips and shoulders, much like a robot). Other autonomic features include orthostatic hypotension, sweating disorder, and urinary frequency. Other symptoms include sleep disturbance, restless legs, fatigue, anxiety, depression, cognitive and behavioral disturbances. These associated features are not present in every case, and are seen less frequently than the cardinal symptoms.

Neurology

B&D Ch. 71

Question 55. E.   Reading disorder is characterized by reading achievement being substantially below what is expected for the child's age, intelligence, and education. It interferes with academic achievement and activities of daily living that require reading skills. In the question given, the child's difficulties are all in situations where she may be asked to read. When children refuse to go to school, separation-anxiety disorder should also be considered. In this case however, the child likes to stay with friends and grandparents, so separation from her parents is not the issue. Children with reading disorder become depressed and demoralized. The diagnosis must be made with a standardized reading test, and pervasive developmental disorders, attention–deficit/hyperactivity disorder, and mental retardation must be ruled out. Treatment consists of understanding the child's deficits and developing an educational program to remedy them. The child must be given coping strategies such that they are not overwhelmed and discouraged. Coexisting emotional and behavioral problems should also receive treatment.

Neurodevelopmental and Pervasive Developmental Disorders

K&S Ch. 39

Question 56. A.   Myoclonus is not typically a symptom of botulism toxin poisoning. Botulism results from the ingestion of *Clostridium botulinum*, a bacterium that extrudes an exotoxin into the circulation and that blocks acetylcholine release at the neuromuscular junction. The bacterium infects humans by its presence in tainted food or by wound contamination from dirt or soil containing the organism. Classic symptoms of botulism include dysphagia, dysarthria, ptosis, diplopia, and urinary retention. Other systemic symptoms include dry mouth and lethargy. Pupillary reflexes are usually impaired. These symptoms rapidly progress to limb paralysis and eventually to paralysis of respiratory muscles that can lead to death if the condition is untreated. Gastrointestinal symptoms of nausea, vomiting, and diarrhea, often present with neurologic compromise after a 12 to 36-hour incubation period following ingestion of the toxin. Infants who consume unpasteurized honey may ingest spores and can present with weak cry, lethargy, floppiness, poor suck, and constipation. Diagnosis can be established by wound or stool culture. Electromyography and nerve conduction studies can reveal characteristic anomalies compatible with presynaptic neuromuscular blockade. Treatment is supportive, particularly with respect to airway protection, and trivalent equine antitoxin administration can help reverse the effects of circulating toxin.

Neurology

B&D Ch. 78

Question 57. D.   This question gives a clear case of oppositional defiant disorder (ODD). In ODD a child shows a pattern of negativistic, hostile, and defiant behavior directed at adults or authority figures. This behavior may include temper tantrums, arguing with adults, actively defying adults' requests or rules, deliberately annoying people, blaming others for their mistakes or misbehavior, being easily annoyed by others, being angry and resentful, or being spiteful or vindictive. The child in question should not meet criteria for conduct disorder to be diagnosed with ODD. The primary treatment for ODD is therapy for the child, and parental training to give parents management skills. Often behavioral therapy will be used to reinforce good behavior while ignoring or not reinforcing bad behavior.

Disruptive, Impulse Control, Conduct Disorders, and ADHD

K&S Ch. 44

Question 58. E. Balint's syndrome is a rare stroke syndrome resulting from ischemic lesions to the bilateral parietal-occipital lobes, or the occipital lobes alone. The condition is often a complication of vascular dementia and can occur after a series of strokes to the area involved. It can sometimes be the result of a "top of the basilar syndrome". The "top of the basilar syndrome" results from rostral basilary artery occlusion that is often embolic in origin. This results in infarction to the midbrain, thalamus and parts of the temporal and occipital lobes. "Top of the basilar syndrome" presents with delirium, peduncular hallucinosis (brainstem-induced visual hallucinations), obtundation, and memory deficits. There may be a gaze palsy, skew deviation of the eyes, ocular bobbing, impaired convergence, or convergence–retraction nystagmus.

Balint's syndrome presents with ocular apraxia (the inability to scan extrapersonal space appropriately with the eyes), optic ataxia (dysmetric or saccadic jerks that can impede vision and ocular focus), and deficits in visual attention. Simultanagnosia may also be noted, which is an inability to perceive a scene with multiple parts to it. The patient is only able to see and recognize individual elements of a multi-part scene, and cannot interpret the overall picture. The optic tracts and radiations are usually spared so visual fields are generally normal. Balint's syndrome can be accompanied by a complete or partial Gerstmann's syndrome if the dominant parietal lobe is affected in the area of the angular gyrus (Gerstmann's syndrome is explained elsewhere in this volume). Balint's syndrome may also result in visuoconstructional apraxia (the inability to put things in their proper place or order). The other answer choices are explained in other questions in this volume, and examination candidates are strongly recommended to review these lobar syndromes as they appear frequently on standardized tests.

Neurology

B&D Chs 51&66

Question 59. D. Although there are no specific behaviors that prove that sexual abuse has taken place, children that have been abused often behave in certain patterns. If very young children have detailed knowledge of sexual acts, they have usually witnessed or participated in sexual behavior. They express their sexual knowledge through play and may initiate sexual behavior with other children. Abused children can also be very aggressive. Other signs of sexual abuse include bruising, pain or itching of the genitals, genital or rectal bleeding, recurrent urinary tract infections, or the presence of sexually transmitted disease.

Trauma and Stress Related Disorders

K&S Ch. 32

Question 60. D. Anton's syndrome is considered to be an agnosia characterized by cortical blindness. The lesion localizes to the bilateral occipital lobes, usually due to strokes, particularly in the calcarine cortex (Brodmann's area 17) and visual association cortex. The arterial territory involved is that of the bilateral posterior cerebral arteries (PCAs). The hallmark of the syndrome is that patients are unaware or deny that they are blind and they confabulate. Patients may also suffer from visual hallucinations.

Prosopagnosia is the inability to recognize familiar faces. It is associated classically with bilateral occipital-temporal lesions. It is often associated with agraphia and achromatopsia (inability to recognize colors and hues). It is almost always associated with visual field deficits. Aphasia is a disorder of speech and language that can be expressive, receptive, or both. Aphasia occurs following lesions to the dominant hemisphere. Prosopagnosia often occurs following lesions of the occipitotemporal region. The lesion is usually either bilateral or on the right side. Apraxia is the inability to perform simple motor tasks that have been previously learned. Motor apraxia can result from lacunar infarcts to the internal capsule or pons, or from nondominant hemispheric strokes. Hiccups are often the result of phrenic nerve irritation. This is frequently caused by medication side effects such as dopa repletion therapy in Parkinson's disease.

Neurology

B&D Chs 14&66

Question 61. D. Dependent personality disorder (DPD) is the least likely of the answer choices given to present with violence. Patients with dependent personality disorder subordinate their needs to those of others, get others to assume responsibility for major areas of their life, lack self-confidence, and are uncomfortable when alone. They have an intense need to be taken care of that leads them to be clingy, submissive, and fear separation. They can not make decisions without an excessive amount of advice from others. Because of their submissiveness patients with DPD are less likely to become violent than patients with other disorders. People with the other personality disorders listed can be aggressive, outrageous, and at odds with others. Some patients with these disorders may have a clear history of violence. Treatment of dependent personality disorder consists of therapy to modify the patient's interpersonal interactions, and medication to deal with comorbid anxiety and depression.

Personality Disorders

K&S Ch. 27

Question 62. B. Chronic abuse of *n*-hexane or other hydrocarbon inhalants (glue, paint thinner) can lead to distal sensorimotor polyneuropathy. The first manifestation is usually numbness and distal paresthesia, which is subsequently followed by distal motor weakness. If inhalants continue to be abused, the motor weakness can worsen and can spread to involve the proximal muscles of both the arms and the legs. At low to moderate doses, the inhalants cause dysarthria, uncoordination, euphoria, and relaxation. Higher doses and more chronic exposure can lead to hallucinosis, psychosis, and seizures, as well as more systemic end-organ damage such as renal failure, bone marrow suppression, and hepatic failure.

Substance Abuse and Addictive Disorders

B&D Ch. 58

Question 63. D. Delusional disorder is characterized by a fixed false belief that is nonbizarre (i.e., may be possible…such as being poisoned, infected, followed, or having a disease). It is differentiated from schizophrenia by the lack of positive symptoms (no auditory or visual hallucinations, no thought disorganization). Tactile or olfactory hallucinations may be present. Apart from the direct impact of the delusion, the patient does not have a marked impairment in functioning. In the case of somatic delusions, the person believes he has some physical defect or medical condition. Treatment consists of antipsychotics in addition to psychotherapy.

The other answer choices do not fit the question stem. The patient does not have a neurological deficit, so conversion disorder is incorrect. He does not have auditory or visual hallucinations, and does not have significant negative symptoms and functional impairment, so schizophrenia is unlikely. There is no mention of depressive symptoms. This would not be considered hypochondriasis because hypochondriasis presents with an unreasonable obsession with a perceived medical problem that could be real. This case clearly presents a delusion that has no possible basis in reality, which would push it out of the realm of hypochondriasis.

Psychotic Disorders

K&S Ch. 14

Question 64. C. Stimulants such as cocaine typically lower the seizure threshold when abused to intoxication. In moderate doses, cocaine and the stimulants can produce wakefulness, alertness, mood elevation, diminished appetite, and increased performance in certain tasks. The stimulants can also result in psychosis and paranoia. There is also an increased risk of myocardial infarction with cocaine use. Systemic problems such as dehydration, rhabdomyolysis, and hyperthermia can also be noted. The most common neurologic adverse effect of cocaine and the stimulants is headache. In certain cases, the stimulants can produce myoclonus, encephalopathy, and seizures. Cocaine is the stimulant that is most likely to induce seizures. Smoking and intravenous administration of cocaine are more likely to induce seizures than intranasal use. Ischemic and hemorrhagic strokes can also result from cocaine use. Cocaine is the most significant cause of drug-induced stroke and accounts for about 50% of all cases. The mechanism of cocaine-induced stroke is believed to involve vasoconstriction, acute hypertension, and vasospasm.

Opioid ingestion and intoxication can produce a state of euphoria or dysphoria. Other possible adverse effects include hallucinations, dry mouth, nausea, vomiting, constipation, and urinary retention. Examination usually reveals pupillary constriction during acute intoxication. Autonomic disturbance such as hypotension and hypothermia can also be noted. Seizures are rare with opioid intoxication. Overdose can result in coma and respiratory compromise. Opioids do not usually cause seizures or lower the seizure threshold.

Phencyclidine (PCP) intoxication produces hallucinosis, dysphoria, and paranoia. Agitation, catatonia, and bizarre behavior are also common. At higher doses, PCP use can lead to stupor and coma. In overdose, rhabdomyolysis may result from agitation and dysautonomia such as fever, hypertension, and sweating. PCP can lower the seizure threshold, but less frequently than cocaine.

Tetrahydrocannabinol (THC), the primary active ingredient in marijuana, causes euphoria, depersonalization, and relaxation. Other effects of the drug include sleepiness, paranoia, and anxiety. High doses of THC can result in hallucinosis, panic, and even paranoia. Seizures are not generally noted with THC intoxication.

Alcohol has intoxicating effects that can cause sedation, memory impairment, uncoordination, dysarthria, euphoria, dysphoria, sleepiness, and acute confusion. Alcohol intoxication does not lower the seizure threshold, it in fact is protective against seizures, because of its agonistic effects at the GABA-A receptor. Alcohol withdrawal can lower the seizure threshold because of rapid desaturation of the GABA-A receptor, in much the same way as the benzodiazepines.

Substance Abuse and Addictive Disorders

B&D Ch. 58

Question 65. E. Mark, who has major depressive disorder, has the highest likelihood of completing suicide. About 95% of those who attempt or commit suicide have some form of psychiatric disorder. Major depressive disorder accounts for 80% of suicides, schizophrenia accounts for 10%, and dementia or delirium for 5%. Of those who have problems with alcohol, 15% attempt suicide, but the numbers are less than for those with depression. Personality disorders may contribute to suicide attempts, but numbers do not surpass those for depression, and often the two overlap. Mental retardation is not a significant risk factor for suicide. Always keep in mind that the best predictor of future suicidal behavior is past suicidal behavior.

Management in Psychiatry

K&S Ch. 34

Question 66. D. Meige's syndrome denotes the combination of blepharospasm (involuntary eyelid blinking) and oromandibular dystonia. Patients have involuntary contraction of the eyelids as well as the lower facial muscles in the area of the jaw, tongue, or neck. The treatment of choice is chemodenervation of the hyperactive muscles by Botulinum toxin type A injection. The tongue requires careful injection in these cases as it can fall back and occlude the airway if it is weakened too severely. The other answers are simply distracters.

Neurology

B&D Ch. 16

Question 67. D. The Tarasoff rule came as a result of the Tarasoff court case. In this case it was decided that a physician or therapist who has reason to believe that a patient might injure or kill someone must notify the potential victim, their family or friends, and the authorities.

The Durham rule is no longer used, but said that an accused is not responsible if his or her unlawful actions were the result of mental disease or defect.

The M'Naghten rule comes from British law, stating that a patient is guilty by reason of insanity if they have a mental disease such that they were unaware of the nature, quality, and consequences of their actions, and were incapable of realizing that their actions were wrong.

Ford vs Wainwright was a case that sustained the need for a patient to be competent in order to be executed. Also worthy of note is that psychiatrists are ethically bound not to participate in state mandated executions in any way.

Respondeat superior is a legal concept stating that a person at the top of a hierarchy is responsible for the actions of those at the bottom of the hierarchy.

Forensic Psychiatry

K&S Ch. 57

Question 68. A. Scanning speech is essentially a form of dysphasia that causes a cerebellar "dysmetria" of the speech pattern. It is also known as ataxic dysarthria. Lesions of the cerebellum such as strokes, degeneration, or tumor can cause this condition. Speech rhythm is usually irregular and choppy. This can also be accompanied by slow, labored speech pattern.

Neurology

B&D Ch. 12

Question 69. B.   As many as 40% of mothers may experience mood or cognitive symptoms during the postpartum period. Postpartum blues (or maternity blues) is a normal state of sadness, dysphoria, tearfulness, and dependence which may last for several days and is the result of hormonal changes and the stress of being a new mother.

Postpartum depression is more severe and involves neurovegetative signs and symptoms of depression and potential suicidality.

Postpartum psychosis can involve hallucinations and delusions, as well as thoughts of infanticide.

There is no DSM-recognized specific phobia regarding being a parent. The fear of the responsibility associated with parenthood may play a part in postpartum blues or postpartum depression, but is not a distinct entity.

Depressive Disorders

K&S Ch. 30

Question 70. D.   Aphemia is a motor speech disorder characterized by near muteness with normal reading, writing, and comprehension. Some experts consider aphemia to be the equivalent of pure speech apraxia; however, this remains a controversy. Aphemia is likely to result from lesions to the primary motor cortex or Broca's area. Patients are first mute, then they become able to speak with hesitancy and phonemic substitutions.

Aphasia is simply any acquired disorder of language. Aphasias can take multiple forms, including expressive, receptive, conduction, global, or transcortical varieties.

Agnosia is the inability to recognize and identify objects. Agnosias imply that the patient is able to see, hear, or touch the object to be identified and that the patient does not have a sensory or perceptual deficit that could impair perception of the object.

Apraxia is the inability to perform a skilled, learned, purposeful motor behavior, in the absence of other deficits that may impair motor functioning. Abulia resembles akinetic mutism. Patients display severe apathy, with affective blunting, amotivation, and immobility. There is an absence of spontaneous speech and movement. Patients retain awareness of their environment.

Neurology

B&D Chs 5&12

Question 71. B.   The N-methyl-D-aspartate (NMDA) receptor is one of the best known glutamate receptors. It has been found to play a role in learning and memory, as well as in psychopathology. The other glutamate receptors are known as the non-NMDA glutamate receptors. The NMDA receptor allows sodium, potassium, and calcium to pass through. It opens when bound by two glutamate molecules and one glycine molecule at the same time. The receptor can be blocked by physiological concentrations of magnesium, and bound by PCP and PCP-like substances.

Basic Neuroscience

K&S Ch. 3

Question 72. C.   Stupor refers to a state of unresponsiveness from which arousal only occurs with vigorous and repeated stimulation. It is on the continuum between alertness and coma. Alert patients are awake and in a normal state of arousal. Lethargic patients are sleepy but awake and arousable to alertness with stimulation. Coma implies a state of unarousable unresponsiveness. The persistent vegetative state follows coma. Patients lose cognitive functioning, but retain vegetative, or autonomic functioning (such as cardiac function, respiration, and blood pressure maintenance).

Neurology

B&D Ch. 5

Question 73. E.   Of the various somatoform disorders, the one with the best prognosis is conversion disorder. The somatoform disorders are characterized by physical symptoms suggestive of a medical condition but are not fully explained by a medical condition or substance abuse. The symptoms are not intentionally produced as in factitious disorders or malingering. Somatization disorder consists of complaints from various organ systems and has a poor prognosis. In hypochondriasis the patient is falsely convinced that he has a serious disease, often based on the misinterpretation of bodily symptoms or functions.

Hypochondriasis has a fair to good prognosis. Conversion disorder is the development of one or more neurological deficits that can not be explained by a known medical disorder. Psychological factors are often associated with the onset of the deficit. The prognosis is excellent. Somewhere from 90–100% of patients with conversion disorder are in remission within less than a month. Body dysmorphic disorder is characterized by the false belief or exaggerated perception that a body part is defective. The prognosis is usually poor and the disease is chronic. Pain disorder is marked by pain in one or more sites that is not fully accounted for by a medical condition. The prognosis is guarded and variable.

Somatic Symptom Disorders

K&S Ch. 17

Question 74. B. All of these answer choices are at least partly untrue, except for answer choice B. Comatose patients require a head CT scan prior to lumbar puncture (LP), in order to assess if there is a presence of a mass lesion or acute hemorrhage that could result in transtentorial or cerebellar herniation if a LP were to be performed.

Not every patient with Guillain–Barré syndrome (GBS) should be hospitalized in an intensive care unit. Mild forms of the disease can be monitored in a regular inpatient setting and bedside respiratory peak-flow monitoring can be assessed frequently to screen for acute respiratory compromise that could lead to death. Patients with GBS who deteriorate rapidly, or show signs of poor oxygenation, can be transferred to an intensive care or pulmonary unit for close monitoring, and intubation can be undertaken if deemed clinically necessary. The rule of "20-30-40" is a guide for determining if intensive care unit admission is needed. A vital capacity of less than 20 mL/kg, or a decline by 30% from baseline, or a maximal inspiratory pressure less than 30 cmH$_2$O, or expiratory pressure less than 40 cmH$_2$O, all indicate the need for ICU admission and close monitoring of respiratory status.

A positive grasp reflex is usually a pathological sign in an adult. It is a normal infantile reflex that is present at birth and usually disappears by 6 months of age. Persistence or redevelopment of the reflex in adulthood would be indicative of frontal lobe pathology and the grasp reflex is considered one of the frontal-release signs.

Cerebellar hemispheric lesions produce movement deficits that affect the ipsilateral side of the body to the lesion. This is due to the double-crossing of pathways. Ascending cerebellocortical tracts decussate in the midbrain and proceed to the contralateral cortex. Descending corticospinal tracts (the pyramidal tracts) decussate in the medulla to project to the contralateral body.

Bell's palsy is believed to be the result of a herpes simplex infection that affects the Gasserian ganglion. *Borrelia burgdorferi*, the spirochete responsible for Lyme infection, can indeed cause facial diplegia, but is a much rarer infection than that caused by the herpes simplex virus.

Neurology

B&D Ch. 76

Question 75. D. The American Psychiatric Association considers it unethical for a psychiatrist to accept a patient's estate after death. It is considered an exploitation of the therapeutic relationship. It is acceptable to accept a token bequest that you were unaware was in the will when the patient was alive. All of the other acts listed are ethical. Psychiatrists can not participate in executions (often asked on exams). Abandoning patients without arranging for follow-up care is unethical. It is unethical to release information about a patient to another party without the patient's permission. It is unethical to pay another doctor for sending you referrals. You can rent other doctors space in your office. And it is ethical to charge a fee for supervision.

Ethics

K&S Ch. 58

Question 76. A. The amygdala is necessary for the recall of emotional contexts of specific events and the experience of fear, pleasure, or other emotions associated with these events. Declarative or episodic memory (also known as short-term memory) requires the intact functioning of the hippocampus and parahippocampal areas (nucleus basalis of Meynert) of the medial temporal lobe for storage and retrieval of information. The other answers are distracters.

Basic Neuroscience

B&D Ch. 6

Question 77. C. Desipramine is the least anticholinergic of the tricyclic antidepressants (TCAs). Anticholinergic side effects are common with patients on TCAs, but tolerance develops over time. Amitriptyline, imipramine, trimipramine, and doxepin are the most anticholinergic. Amoxapine, nortriptyline and maprotiline are less so. Anticholinergic side effects include dry mouth, blurred vision, constipation, and urinary retention. Because of this last side effect desipramine would be the best choice for someone with prostatic hypertrophy. One should always keep in mind the potential for severe anticholinergic effects to lead to a delirium.

Psychopharmacology

K&S Ch. 36

Question 78. D. Children are expected to reach developmental milestones at the appropriate age. Standardized examination candidates should memorize these milestones, as questions concerning this material come up on many different examinations. Here are the milestones that need to be remembered:

- 2 months of age: cooing, smiling with social contact, holding head up 45°
- 4 months of age: laughing/squealing, sustaining social contact, grasping objects, weight bearing on legs
- 6 months of age: imitating speech sounds, single syllables, prefers mother, enjoys mirror, transferring objects hand to hand, raking grasp, sitting up with support
- 8 months of age: jabbering, playing peek-a-boo, patty-cake, waving bye-bye, sitting without support, creeping or crawling
- 12 months of age: speech specific to "dada/mama," playing simple ball games, able to adjust body to dressing, standing alone, able to use thumb-finger pincer grasp
- 14 months of age: one to two-word vocabulary, indicating desires by pointing, hugging parents, walking alone, stooping and recovering
- 18 months of age: six-word vocabulary, able to feed self, walking up stairs while hand is held, imitating scribbling
- 24 months of age: combining words, 250-word vocabulary, helping to undress, listening to picture stories, running well, making circular scribbles, copying a horizontal line
- 30 months of age: knows full name, refers to self as "I", pretending in play, helping put things away, climbing stairs alternating feet, copying a vertical line
- 36 months of age: counting three objects correctly, knowing age and sex, helping in dressing, riding a tricycle, standing briefly on one foot, copying a circle
- 48 months of age: telling a story, counting four objects, playing with other children, using toilet alone, hopping on one foot, using scissors to cut out pictures, copying a square and a cross
- 60 months of age: naming four colors, counting ten objects, asking about word meanings, domestic role playing, skipping, copying a triangle

Human Development

B&D Ch. 7

Question 79. A. This question is a case of exhibitionism. Exhibitionism is a paraphilia in which the patient has a recurrent urge to expose their genitals to strangers. Sexual arousal is brought about by the event. Cases are almost always men exposing themselves to women. Medroxyprogesterone acetate has been shown to be helpful in some cases, and is useful in any sexual disorder in which the patients are extremely hypersexual to the point of being out of control or dangerous. Other drugs such as antipsychotics and antidepressants have not been shown to be particularly useful in such cases. Some patients may improve with the sexual side effects of a serotonin-selective reuptake inhibitor, but it would not be the first choice for treatment.

Sexual Dysfunctions

K&S Ch. 21

Question 80. B. The clinical vignette described in this question involves a classic presentation of Hoover's sign. Hoover's sign is positive when a patient suspected of a hysterical or psychogenic hemiparesis does not give effort in the contralateral (unaffected) lower extremity when asked to push down on the bed with the paretic (affected) lower extremity. The examiner places a hand under the patient's heel on the unaffected side to feel if the patient is pushing down towards the bed in an attempt to give a full effort at raising the affected leg. In a real hemiparesis, the patient would be expected to make every effort to brace himself with the unaffected leg while trying to raise the paretic leg.

Hoffman's sign is the equivalent to a Babinski's sign, but it is noted in the upper extremity. The sign is positive when a flick of the distal phalange of the index or middle finger results in an adduction of the ipsilateral thumb. The sign, when present, indicates contralateral corticospinal tract damage that affects the upper extremity.

Lasègue's sign is present when straight-leg raising in a recumbent position results in reproduction of pain or paresthesia in the sciatic distribution. The sign can either be ipsilateral or crossed. The positive sign points to sciatic nerve compression due to mechanical interruption of the nerve trajectory, most often due to an intervertebral disk bulge or herniation at the lumbar or sacral level.

Romberg's sign is positive when a patient is asked to stand up straight with eyes closed and subsequently loses his balance. The presence of Romberg's sign usually signals a deficit localizing either to the posterior columns of the spinal cord (i.e., loss of proprioception and/or vibration sensation in the legs), or to cerebellar pathology, or both.

Gegenhalten refers to "clasp-knife" type rigidity that can be observed in the extremities in several types of disorders that can include stroke, multiple sclerosis, and catatonia.

Neurology

B&D Ch. 22

Question 81. E. Clomipramine is one of the tricyclic antidepressants. It has been useful in the treatment of patients with premature ejaculation, depression, panic, obsessive–compulsive disorder, phobias, and pain disorder. It has no use in treating psychosis. It carries with it the cardiac, autonomic, neurologic, sedative, and anticholinergic effects found with many of the tricyclic antidepressants. All tricyclic antidepressants should be avoided during pregnancy.

Psychopharmacology

K&S Ch. 35

Question 82. C. The only true emergency in neurology that requires immediate MRI imaging is acute epidural spinal cord compression (ESCC). If MRI is unavailable, the alternate imaging modality of choice is a spinal myelogram. The cause of spinal cord compression can be an intervertebral disk, metastatic carcinoma, or epidural hematoma. Metastases from primary carcinoma of the breast, lung and prostate each make up 20% of the cause of ESCC. Back pain is the most frequent presenting feature in over 80% of cases. The back pain is usually progressive and increases with tumor growth over a period of up to two months before the onset of neurological deficits. Motor weakness is noted in about 80% of cases, and it predicts the post-treatment outcome much of the time. Sensory deficits are noted in about 75% of cases. Metastatic ESCC causes a spastic paraparesis or paraplegia with a sensory level that is usually several levels below the actual lesion. Bowel and bladder incontinence, urinary retention, or constipation, are observed in a majority of patients. Sagittal screening MRI imaging of the entire spine is the initial test of choice, if available, because only MRI and myelography can immediately identify and characterize the nature of the lesion and guide treatment. Treatment is undertaken acutely with parenteral corticosteroids and subacutely with radiation therapy. Decompressive laminectomy can be performed, but radiotherapy has of late produced results as good as a surgical approach. Chemotherapy is generally ineffective, because metastases causative of ESCC are usually not chemosensitive. The other answers are clearly distracters and are discussed individually elsewhere in this volume.

Neurology

B&D Ch. 52

Question 83. C. The legal concept of parens patriae allows the state to intervene and act as a surrogate parent for those who are unable to care for themselves or who may harm themselves.

Actus reus means voluntary conduct. Mens rea means evil intent. Durable power refers to durable power of attorney, where a patient selects who they want to make decisions for them should they become incompetent to make those decisions for themselves. Respondeat superior is the concept that a person at the top of a hierarchy is responsible for the actions of those at the bottom of the hierarchy.

Forensic Psychiatry

K&S Ch. 57

Question 84. B.   Tiagabine (Gabitril) is the only agent that is a selective GABA reuptake inhibitor. It is FDA-approved as adjunctive treatment of partial complex seizures. Recent warnings have suggested that it can actually worsen or cause seizures. Gabapentin (Neurontin) is a GABA modulating agent that does not directly affect GABA receptors. It is FDA-approved for adjunctive therapy of partial complex seizures and postherpetic neuralgia. Pregabalin (Lyrica) is FDA-approved for adjunctive therapy in partial complex seizures and in neuropathic pain. Its mechanism of action is similar to that of gabapentin: it binds to the alpha-2-delta subunit of the voltage-gated calcium channel. Vigabatrin is not available on the US market. It is an irreversible inhibitor of GABA transaminase (the enzyme that metabolizes GABA) that is approved abroad in the adjunctive therapy of partial complex seizures. Lioresal (Baclofen) is a GABA-B agonist that is approved for spasticity in disorders such as stroke and multiple sclerosis.

Neurology

B&D Ch. 67

Question 85. E.   The trail-making test is a measure of executive function. The second part of the test consists of drawing lines between a series of letters and numbers in the correct order. For example, the patient would connect A-1-B-2-C-3, etc. The trail-making test is given as part of the Halstead–Reitan Test Battery.

Psychological Theory and Psychometric Testing

K&S Ch. 5

Question 86. C.   Memantine (Namenda) is an NMDA antagonist that is FDA-approved for the treatment of moderate to severe Alzheimer's dementia. It has a completely different mechanism of action to donepezil (Aricept), rivastigmine (Exelon), and galantamine (Reminyl), which are inhibitors of acetylcholinesterase that are FDA-approved for treatment of mild to moderate Alzheimer's dementia. There is now evidence to suggest that concomitant therapy with memantine and one of the cholinesterase inhibitors has measurable clinical advantages over therapy with either class of agent on its own. Neither of these two classes of agent attacks the true pathophysiology of Alzheimer's dementia, which is the formation of neurofibrillary plaques and tangles in the brain that lead to neuronal cell death. Memantine may reverse the process of apoptosis (preprogrammed cell death) that is believed to be intrinsic to the pathological basis of cell death in Alzheimer's dementia. Glutamate and NMDA hyperstimulation may lead to premature cell death by promoting calcium influx into neurons and this in turn leads to progression of Alzheimer's dementia. Memantine may slow disease progress by modulating and lessening the adverse effects of glutamate on the brain. The other answer choices are distracters and need no particular explanation.

Neurology

Psychopharmacology

B&D Ch. 66; also see www.namenda.com

Question 87. A.   It is the GABA-A receptor that has binding sites for the benzodiazepines. There are three types of GABA receptors, GABA-A, B, and C. There are no GABA-D or GABA-E receptors. The benzodiazepines increase affinity of the GABA-A receptor for GABA. The GABA-A receptor is a chloride ion channel.

Psychopharmacology

K&S Ch. 3

Question 88. A.   Vagal nerve stimulation has been FDA-approved since 1997 for adjunctive treatment of refractory partial complex epilepsy in patients over 12 years of age. It recently obtained FDA-approval in intractable major depressive disorder. The modality involves the invasive implantation of an electric stimulating device inside the chest cavity. The stimulator is connected to a wire that wraps around the left vagal nerve (the right vagal nerve is not clinically important in the management of epilepsy). The stimulator is programmed to cycle on for 30 seconds and off for 5 minutes throughout the day. Seizure frequency is typically reduced by about 50%. Side effects can include hoarseness from irritation of the adjacent recurrent laryngeal nerve, and throat tingling and/or coughing during actual stimulation. Vagal nerve stimulation is not as of yet approved for use in any other psychiatric disorder apart from depression.

Neurology

B&D Ch. 67

Question 89. D.   It is true that some studies have shown the efficacy of using carbamazepine in the treatment of alcohol withdrawal to be equal to that of the benzodiazepines. Carbamazepine is approved in the US for temporal lobe and generalized epilepsy as well as trigeminal neuralgia. It is metabolized by the liver and excreted by the kidneys. It causes its own autoinduction by hepatic enzymes that makes it necessary over time to give more medication to achieve the same blood levels. It also affects the metabolism of several other drugs. Carbamazepine has been associated with a transient decrease in white blood cell count and has been associated with an inhibition of colony-stimulating factor in the bone marrow. It has also been associated with severe blood dyscrasias such as aplastic anemia and agranulocytosis. A benign rash has been found in 10–15% of patients on carbamazepine, and a small percentage of these patients go on to develop serious rashes such as Stevens–Johnson syndrome, exfoliative dermatitis, erythema multiforme, or toxic epidermal necrolysis.

Psychopharmacology

K&S Ch. 35

Question 90. E.   Auscultation of the head that reveals a bruit is a classic hallmark of an arteriovenous malformation (AVM). Seizures are the presenting symptom of AVMs in about one-quarter to two-thirds of cases. Headaches occur in anywhere from 5 to 35% of cases. Hemorrhage from ruptured AVM tends to be intracerebral in location, rather than subarachnoid as in the case of a ruptured aneurysm. The other distracters are discussed elsewhere in this volume.

Neurology

B&D Ch. 51

Question 91. D.   The Draw-A-Person test is a projective test. It is administered by telling the patient to draw a person. Then the patient is asked to draw a person of the sex opposite that of the first drawing. The assumption is that the drawing of the patient's gender is representative of the self in the environment. The level of detail is also correlated with intelligence in children. The Halstead–Reitan battery is used to find the location and effects of certain brain lesions. It is not projective. The Stanford–Binet test is an intelligence test. The Wechsler–Bellvue test is a memory test. The Minnesota Multiphasic Personality Inventory (MMPI) is a self report inventory used to assess personality traits.

Psychological Theory and Psychometric Testing

K&S Ch. 5

Question 92. B.   The image depicts a classic colloid cyst of the third ventricle. This is a rare condition that presents in middle-aged adults. The cyst is a round, well-circumscribed lesion that is situated in the anterior aspect of the third ventricle. It appears as a "button nose" right in the middle of the ventricular system and this MRI image is a typical example of its appearance. Clinical presentation is that of intermittent headaches that result from increased intracranial pressure because of the ball-valve blockage of the passage of cerebrospinal fluid in the ventricular system. The blockage can even lead to brief intermittent drop attacks in certain patients. These cysts are composed of high concentrations of cholesterol and protein that give them their characteristic hyperintense appearance particularly on T2-weighted MRI brain imaging.

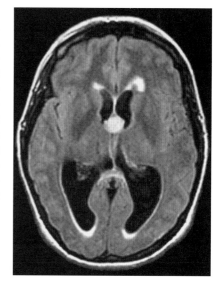

Neurology

B&D Ch. 52

Question 93. C.   Buprenorphine is a mixed opioid agonist/antagonist. It is used for the treatment of heroin addiction as an alternative to methadone. Aripiprazole is a mixed dopamine agonist/antagonist. Naltrexone is an opioid antagonist. Methadone is an opioid agonist. Gabapentin is an anticonvulsant, and is thus unrelated to the opioid receptors.

Basic Neuroscience

K&S Ch. 12

Question 94. D.   Hallevorden–Spatz syndrome is a rare autosomal recessive disease of childhood onset that presents with the combination of dementia and parkinsonism. The classic neuropathologic hallmark of the disorder is a rusty-brown discoloration of the medial globus pallidus and pars reticulata of the substantia nigra on autopsy. The discoloration is due to the accumulation of iron in the basal ganglia. The disorder is caused by an enzymatic deficiency in cysteine dioxygenase. This leads to increased levels of cysteine in the brain, which chelates iron. Free iron deposits in the basal ganglia and leads to free radical formation, neuronal demise, and ultimately death. Other features of the syndrome include optic atrophy, pigmentary retinopathy, psychomotor retardation and clinical signs of corticospinal tract damage.

Neurology

B&D Ch. 66

Question 95. C.   Anterograde amnesia is most often associated with alcohol abuse. Keep the Wernicke–Korsakoff syndrome in mind. Wernicke's encephalopathy is an acute disorder characterized by ataxia, vestibular dysfunction, confusion, and eye movement abnormalities. Korsakoff's syndrome is a chronic amnestic syndrome that can follow Wernicke's. It presents with impaired recent memory and anterograde amnesia. The patient may or may not confabulate as well. Long term memory is usually not affected. Treatment for both of these conditions is thiamine administration. If not treated early, permanent damage can take place and Korsakoff's syndrome can become permanent.

Substance Abuse and Addictive Disorders

K&S Ch. 12

Question 96. A.   Subacute combined degeneration is the result of a deficiency in vitamin B12 (cobalamin). Cobalamin deficiency manifests as macrocytic anemia, atrophic glossitis, and neurologic deficits. Neurologic symptoms include lesions to the lateral and posterior columns of the spinal cord (subacute combined degeneration), peripheral neuropathy, optic atrophy, and brain lesions. Spinal cord symptoms present as posterior column deficits, which can manifest as upper motor neuron limb weakness, spasticity, and Babinski's signs. Peripheral neuropathy can present as paresthesias and large fiber sensory impairment (loss of proprioception and vibration sensation). Cerebral symptoms present as behavioral changes, forgetfulness, and in severe cases, dementia and stupor. Sensory ataxia is demonstrated by a positive Romberg sign. There can also be a diffuse hyper-reflexia with absent ankle jerk reflexes. Treatment is undertaken with parenteral B12 injections intramuscularly.

Neurology

B&D Ch. 76

Question 97. C.   The appropriate action to take in the case presented is to increase the carbamazepine dose and take follow-up levels. This is because carbamazepine has an auto-induction phenomenon whereby it causes the induction of the hepatic enzymes which break it down. Thus, after starting at one dose, the enzymes are induced and break down more carbamazepine, thereby decreasing the serum level. The answer? Give more carbamazepine to bring serum levels back up. The informed clinician knows that this phenomenon will happen, and as such knows the patient is being honest. There is no need to switch to another medication if the carbamazepine was keeping the patient stable. Adding a serotonin-selective reuptake inhibitor would be a good way to flip the patient into overt mania, but not a good way to solve this problem. The patient in question has yet to meet criteria for hospitalization, so that would just be overly aggressive and unwarranted.

Psychopharmacology

K&S Ch. 36

Question 98. A.   Isoniazid (INH) exposure can cause a vitamin B6 (pyridoxine) deficiency. Most normal adults consume adequate amounts of vitamin B6 in their diets (1.5–2 mg daily). Hydralazine and penicillamine can also cause drug-induced vitamin B6 deficiency. These drugs interfere with vitamin B6 coenzyme activity. Vitamin B6 deficiency results in a distal sensorimotor peripheral neuropathy. Patients can develop distal paresthesias, sensory loss and motor weakness after six months of INH therapy if not on vitamin B6 supplementation. Pyridoxine supplementation of 100 mg daily needs to accompany INH therapy to avoid this untimely deficiency.

Vitamin A deficiency is rare and can occur with malabsorption syndromes like sprue and biliary atresia. The earliest manifestation is night blindness. Hypervitaminosis A is associated with pseudotumor cerebri which manifests as headache and papilledema. The other answer choices are distracters that are explained elsewhere in this volume.

Neurology

B&D Chs 57&76

Question 99. A. The answer to this question is undoubtedly choice A. Although borderline patients make frequent suicidal gestures, they are extremely impulsive. As such it is the psychiatrist's job to assume that any gesture could be potentially life-threatening and to take the threat seriously. Steps must be taken to protect these patients. Choices B and C are ridiculous and dangerous. Talking about suicide does not increase the risk that patients will try to harm themselves. Isolating them will offer them less support and increase their chances of harming themselves. Choice D is inappropriate because these patients can not be relied on to keep promises when they are in an impulsive, emotionally labile state. Giving these patients a benzodiazepine could potentially disinhibit them further and make it more likely that they would try to harm themselves.

Management in Psychiatry

K&S Ch. 33

Question 100. B. West Nile virus infection is an arbovirus (a form of flavivirus) infection that is endemic to many parts of the world. Mosquito bites from the genus *Culex* are frequent vectors of transmission of the virus to humans. Most infections in humans are asymptomatic. In about 20% of affected patients, the infection presents as a febrile condition after an incubation period of a few days to up to 2 weeks. Only one in 150 patients goes on to develop a meningitis or encephalitis picture. The infection may progress to the development of a demyelinating or axonal neuropathy. Diagnosis is made by detection of IgM antibodies in cerebrospinal fluid, or IgM and IgG antibodies in serum. Treatment is generally supportive. Patients with serious symptoms may respond to intravenous administration of anti-West Nile virus immunoglobulin.

Arenaviruses are rodent-borne and infect humans when a person comes into contact with infected rodent fecal matter. Lymphocytic choriomeningitis virus and Lassa fever virus are two examples of arenaviruses.

Filoviruses are represented by the Ebola and Marburg viruses. The reservoir of these viruses is not known. Infection can cause a severe hemorrhagic encephalitis with myositis and muscle pain. Treatment is supportive. Body fluids of these patients are highly contagious.

Retroviruses are represented by the well-known HIV, HTLV-1 and HTLV-2. The JC virus is a papovavirus and is the causative pathogen of progressive multifocal leukoencephalopathy that can develop in patients with advanced AIDS with low CD4 cell counts. JC virus can be detected in CSF by PCR amplification of its DNA.

Neurology

B&D Ch. 53

Question 101. B. You, being the skillful physician that you are, would order a lithium level on this patient! Why? Because the side effects of lithium intoxication include gastrointestinal upset such as nausea, vomiting, and diarrhea. Lithium can cause tremor, nephrogenic diabetes insipidus, acne, muscular weakness, hypothyroidism, weight gain, edema, leukocytosis, psoriasis, hair loss and cardiac dysrhythmias. When toxic it can also cause ataxia, slowed thinking, impaired memory, impaired consciousness, seizures, and death.

Psychopharmacology

K&S Ch. 36

Question 102. E. This question asks the exam taker to correlate the neuroanatomical location of a certain type of neurons with the function of the neurotransmitter particular to those neurons. The best answer to this question is choice E, acetylcholine. The basal forebrain is the location of the nucleus basalis of Meynert, which is the structure containing a high density of cholinergic neurons. These neurons project to the limbic system and the cerebral cortex. Alzheimer's disease is a result of cholinergic neuronal demise predominantly in the nucleus basalis of Meynert.

Acetylcholine is synthesized from acetylcoenzyme A and choline by the enzyme choline acetyltransferase in the synaptic nerve terminal. Acetylcholine is then stored in vesicles in the synaptic bouton. Once released into the synapse, it is inactivated and metabolized by acetylcholinesterase and the resultant choline is taken back up into the presynaptic terminal for reutilization.

Acetylcholine is responsible for maintaining short-term memory, attention, executive functioning, and novelty-seeking, which are mediated through the nucleus basalis of Meynert. In Alzheimer's dementia, acetylcholine is depleted and memory and executive functioning are compromised as a result. The Alzheimer's agents donepezil, rivastigmine, and galantamine are all acetylcholinesterase inhibitors and can increase levels of circulating acetylcholine in the nucleus basalis and throughout the brain, thereby improving symptoms of dementia to a limited extent. The other neurotransmitters offered in this question are distracters. Each one is explained in other questions in this volume.

Basic Neuroscience

K&S Ch. 3

Question 103. E.   The tricyclic antidepressants, venlafaxine, bupropion, and nefazodone block the reuptake of norepinephrine (and serotonin in some cases) into the presynaptic neuron. This leads to more norepinephrine in the synaptic cleft. Mirtazapine works by blocking presynaptic alpha-2 receptors, which stops feedback inhibition on the release of norepinephrine into the synaptic cleft. This results in more norepinephrine released into the synapse.

Psychopharmacology

K&S Ch. 3

Question 104. D.   PCP exerts its hallucinogenic effects by antagonism of N-methyl-D-aspartate (NMDA) receptors, which in turn prevents the influx of calcium ions into neurons. PCP also activates ventral tegmental dopamine which results in the reinforcing qualities of the drug. Tolerance to the physiologic effects of PCP can occur in humans, but dependence and physiologic withdrawal do not usually occur. PCP intoxication produces hallucinosis, dysphoria, and paranoia. Agitation, catatonia, and bizarre behavior are also common. At higher doses, PCP use can lead to stupor and coma. In overdose, rhabdomyolysis may result from agitation and dysautonomia such as fever, hypertension, and sweating. The other answer choices are simply distracters that need no explanation.

Substance Abuse and Addictive Disorders

K&S Ch. 12

Question 105. B.   The three best benzodiazepines for patients with liver dysfunction are temazepam, oxazepam, and lorazepam. This is an important little fact for the well-prepared test taker to know. They have short half lives, and do not have active metabolites. Other benzodiazepines are less desirable in patients with hepatic dysfunction.

Psychopharmacology

K&S Ch. 36

Question 106. C.   *Aspergillus* is a fungus that colonizes in the paranasal sinuses and can cause a hypersensitivity pneumonitis. Infection can originate from the lungs in immunocompromised patients. The fungus has a predilection for invading the posterior circulation and can cause vertebrobasilar strokes. The fungus causes a cerebral vasculitis by invasion of vessel walls. Sinus infection can extend to the brain by contiguous infiltration. Spinal cord compression can result from pulmonary Aspergillosis that extends to the thoracic vertebrae through the epidural space.

Histoplasma is a fungus that can cause an influenza-like infection with erythematous skin lesions and liver function abnormalities. In fewer than 20% of cases, there is a development of neurologic manifestations in the form of cerebritis, basilar meningitis, or CNS granuloma. Cerebral abscess is also a possible neurologic complication of histoplasmosis infection in about 40% of cases. Meningeal symptoms and signs of headache, fever and neck stiffness can also be noted in the neurologic form of the infection.

Candida albicans is one of the most common fungal organisms found in the human body. Neurologic infection is rare in immunocompetent hosts. In patients with immune compromise, candidal infection can manifest in the form of intracranial abscesses, vasculitis, and small vessel thrombosis. Candida can form mycotic intracerebral aneurysms that can rupture and cause parenchymal hemorrhage.

Pseudallecheria boydii is an uncommon fungal pathogen that can infect immunosuppressed patients. Clinical presentation is typically that of a meningitis or multiple brain abscesses.

Cryptococcus neoformans infection is discussed in detail elsewhere in this volume.

Neurology

B&D Ch. 53

Question 107. C. Adverse effects of fluoxetine that set it apart from other serotonin-selective reuptake inhibitors include headache, anxiety, and respiratory complaints. Other side effects include nausea, diarrhea, and insomnia. High blood pressure is found with patients on venlafaxine. Blurred vision can occur from anticholinergic medications. Shuffling gait can occur as a result of parkinsonian side effects of antipsychotics. Loss of consciousness occurs with sedatives.

Psychopharmacology

K&S Ch. 36

Question 108. B. The GABA-A receptor (the most predominant GABA receptor) is a chloride channel. Such a useful little fact for the prudent student to know!

Basic Neuroscience

K&S Ch. 3

Question 109. D. After making an error in psychodynamic psychotherapy, the best way to proceed is to briefly acknowledge that a mistake was made, and move on, focusing on the patient and their problems. Interpreting the patient's reaction can be seen as dismissive. It does not address the fact that the therapist made a mistake, not the patient. Ignoring the mistake will contaminate the patient's transference toward the therapist, potentially making him angry. Giving a long but clear explanation puts too much emphasis on the mistake. The emphasis should be on the patient and his behavior, not the therapist and hers. To profusely apologize is the wrong approach, as it is an over-reaction to a minor mistake. The goal is to acknowledge the mistake and move on, spending as little time focusing on the therapist and her actions and more time on the patient and his actions. Mistakes are a normal part of therapy, as the therapist is human. Dealing with them in a way that maintains boundaries and therapeutic neutrality will be in the best interest of the patient and the therapy.

Psychotherapy

K&S Ch. 35

Question 110. C. Identity diffusion is the failure to develop a cohesive self or self-awareness. Do not bother looking the other answer choices up. They are unrelated distracters, some of which are ludicrously unrelated to the question.

Psychological Theory and Psychometric Testing

K&S Ch. 2

Question 111. C. Treatment of children with separation-anxiety disorder should be multimodal. It should involve individual therapy for the child, medication to reduce anxiety, family therapy and education, and return to school which is graded if necessary (i.e., start with 1 hour per day, then increase to 2 hours, then 3 hours, etc.). The parental education should focus on giving the child consistent support but maintaining clear boundaries about the child's avoidant behaviors towards anxiety provoking situations.

Anxiety Disorders

K&S Ch. 48

Question 112. D. Naltrexone is an opioid antagonist that is often used as an adjunctive agent for alcohol abuse because it decreases craving and alcohol consumption. It is nowhere near 100% effective and its success is very much dependent on the patient's desire to stop drinking and the success of concurrent behavioral modification. It is not better than behavioral modification. Naltrexone has nothing to do with dopamine or the GABA receptor.

Psychopharmacology

K&S Ch. 36

Question 113. D. The anticholinergic activity of many psychiatric drugs (including tricyclic antidepressants like imipramine) can cause urinary hesitancy, dribbling, and urinary retention. These side effects occur especially with older men who have enlarged prostates. Treatment usually consists of bethanechol 10–30 mg three to four times daily.

Psychopharmacology

K&S Ch. 36

Question 114. B. The most important take home point from this question is that bipolar I disorder has equal prevalence for men and women. Major depression is more common in women than in men. There is no correlation between socioeconomic status and frequency of depression. There is a correlation between hypersecretion (not hyposecretion) of cortisol and increased depression. Only about 50% of those with major depressive disorder receive specific treatment.

Bipolar Disorders

K&S Ch. 15

Question 115. B. A child who is not speaking should first have her hearing checked. Phonological disorders are characterized by a child's inability to make age appropriate speech sounds. The child can not be diagnosed if the deficits are being caused by a structural or neurological problem, therefore these things must first be ruled out. Phonological disorder may present as substitutions of one sound for another, or omissions such as leaving the final consonant off of words. The treatment of choice is speech therapy, and recovery can be spontaneous in some children. Speech therapy is indicated if the child can not be understood, is over 8 years old, when self-image and peer relationships are being affected, when many consonants are misarticulated, and when the child is frequently omitting parts of words.

Diagnostic and Treatment Procedures in Psychiatry

K&S Ch. 41

Question 116. E. State-dependent learning is the facilitated recall of information in the same internal state or environment in which the information was originally obtained. An example of this is when someone learns a behavior when intoxicated with a drug. Without the drug they can not recall the behavior. When the drug is given to them again they remember the behavior. The other answer choices relate to learning and conditioning. The most important of them have been covered in their own separate questions. Others are just distracters.

Psychological Theory and Psychometric Testing

K&S Ch. 4

Question 117. C. This is a case of Wernicke's encephalopathy. Wernicke's, and its partner, Korsakoff's amnesia, are the result of thiamine deficiency often found in alcoholics. Wernicke's is an acute neurological disorder characterized by ataxia, confusion, vestibular dysfunction, and eye movement impairment. Wernicke's encephalopathy is reversible with treatment, but if it progresses into Korsakoff's amnesia, damage may be irreversible. Korsakoff's presents as impaired recent memory and anterograde amnesia. The treatment for these syndromes is thiamine, first intravenously in the case of an acute Wernicke's, then orally for as long as 3 to 12 months in the case of Korsakoff's amnesia. While other answer choices are good ideas, the primary goal is to prevent further brain damage by getting thiamine into the patient immediately.

Substance Abuse and Addictive Disorders

K&S Ch. 12

Question 118. B. Niacin is an essential nutrient also called nicotinic acid. Niacin deficiency, termed pellagra, occurs in individuals who consume corn as their main carbohydrate staple. Corn lacks niacin and tryptophan (which can be converted in the body to niacin). Bread is now niacin fortified, which has diminished the widespread problem of pellagra in most countries.

Pellagra causes the classic triad of the three Ds: dementia, dermatitis and diarrhea. Gastrointestinal problems present as diarrhea, anorexia, and abdominal discomfort. Skin manifestations present as a hyperkeratotic corporal rash over much of the body. The neurological manifestations can include depression, memory impairment, apathy, and irritability. A confusional state may result and may lead to stupor or coma. Oral doses of 50 mg three times daily of nicotinic acid can reverse the symptoms of pellagra.

The triad of neuropathy, retinopathy, and areflexia can result from a deficiency in vitamin E (α-tocopherol). Other manifestations can include ataxia, loss of proprioception and vibration sensation, nystagmus and external ophthalmoplegia.

The triad of neuropathy, ataxia, and dementia can result from vitamin B12 (cobalamin) deficiency. Symptoms present as paresthesias of the hands and feet, weakness, gait disturbance, depression, confusion, psychosis, peripheral neuropathy, and loss of position and vibration sensation. Myelopathic symptoms such as spastic paraparesis can occur, as well as visual disturbances as manifested by optic atrophy and visual loss. Treatment is undertaken with parenteral administration of vitamin B12 100 μg daily or 1000 μg twice weekly for 2 weeks.

Folate deficiency can result in a clinical picture that is similar in presentation to that of B12 deficiency. Elevated serum homocysteine is a surrogate marker for low folate levels. The deficiency can lead to neuropathy and/or spasticity due to spinal cord involvement. Treatment is initially undertaken with 1 mg of folate orally three times daily, followed by a maintenance dose of 1 mg daily. Answer choice A is a nonsense distracter and needs no explanation.

Neurology

B&D Ch. 57

Question 119. C. The best way to address a missed therapy session is to use neutral questioning to help explore why it happened. Ignoring the missed appointment is a mistake that can be misunderstood by the patient as the therapist not caring if she shows or not. Getting angry at the patient or punishing the patient is the wrong approach. It will only make the patient angry and less likely to reveal the emotional reasons for why the session was missed, and what meaning that has for the therapeutic relationship. In therapy, the patient's treatment of the therapist is a reflection of how he or she treats others in life as well. As such, aspects of the patient's behavior such as missed appointments should be noted and explored.

Psychotherapy

K&S Ch. 1

Question 120. D. Tachycardia, not bradycardia, is a symptom of cannabis intoxication. All other answer choices are also symptoms. Orthostatic hypotension is usually only seen with high doses of cannabis.

Substance Abuse and Addictive Disorders

K&S Ch. 12

Question 121. E. Akathisia is a subjective feeling of muscular tension caused by antipsychotic medication, which can cause restlessness, pacing, or an inability to stand still. Treatment consists of a beta adrenergic receptor antagonist such as propranolol. Other choices include anticholinergic medications such as benztropine. Benzodiazepines can be useful in some cases.

Psychopharmacology

K&S Ch. 36

Question 122. C. Clonidine works by agonist activity at presynaptic alpha-2 receptors. This leads to a decrease in the amount of neurotransmitter released into the synaptic cleft leading to decreased sympathetic tone and decreased arousal. In the case of opioid withdrawal the action of clonidine on the locus ceruleus is thought to be particularly important to the decrease in autonomic symptoms associated with withdrawal. Other answer choices are unrelated distracters.

Psychopharmacology

K&S Ch. 36

Question 123. B. Blockade of muscarinic cholinergic receptors is a common side effect of many drugs. Blockade leads to blurred vision, dry mouth, constipation, and difficulty urinating. When there is excessive blockade of this receptor, a patient can develop confusion and delirium. Alzheimer's disease has been postulated to be in part, the result of too little cholinergic activity. As such, drugs like donepezil block the enzyme acetylcholinesterase (which breaks down acetylcholine) and thereby increase cholinergic activity. This has been shown to be useful in the treatment of dementia. This is the opposite of blockade of muscarinic cholinergic receptors which one would postulate, would worsen the symptoms of Alzheimer's.

Psychopharmacology

K&S Ch. 3

Question 124. A.   While all of the lab tests involved in this question can be elevated in alcohol abuse, the most likely test to pick up alcohol abuse is the gamma-glutamyl transferase (GGT). It is elevated in 80% of those with alcohol-related disorders. The other tests are elevated at lower rates than 80% and as such will not pick up as many alcohol disorders as the GGT.

Laboratory Tests in Psychiatry

K&S Ch. 12

Question 125. B.   Pimozide (Orap) is a dopamine receptor antagonist which has been approved in the US for the treatment of Tourette's disorder. Haloperidol is also widely used for this indication. In Europe, pimozide is used as an antipsychotic medication for treatment of schizophrenia.

Psychopharmacology

K&S Ch. 36

Question 126. C.   The gene for amyloid precursor protein is found on chromosome 21. Amyloid precursor protein is broken down to form beta amyloid protein, which is a major component of senile plaques in Alzheimer's disease.

Neurocognitive Disorders

K&S Ch. 10

Question 127. D.   Heinz Kohut developed the school of self-psychology. Central to his theories of personality development is the idea that when parents mirror a child's behavior this functions as a form of empathy, which is necessary for personality development and the formation of healthy self-esteem. When this parental empathy is lacking, the sense of self does not develop properly and personality disorders develop. Patients then need others to fulfill functions that the self would normally handle. Oedipal conflict is a classic part of Freud's theories in which, greatly simplified, a child competes with the parent of the same sex for the attention of the parent of the opposite sex. The concept of the good enough mother came from Winnicott. He describes a holding environment that develops, where the good enough mother allows the child's true self to develop. He also gave us the concept of the transitional object. The paranoid–schizoid position and the depressive position are found in the work of Melanie Klein. The paranoid–schizoid position is a view of the world from the perspective of the infant, in which the whole world is split into good and bad elements. The depressive position occurs when the infant is able to view the mother ambivalently as having both positive and negative aspects.

Human Development

K&S Ch. 6

Question 128. D.   When erythromycin and carbamazepine are given together the carbamazepine levels are increased.

Psychopharmacology

K&S Ch. 36

Question 129. D.   Valproic acid should be avoided during pregnancy because of its propensity to cause neural tube defects in the developing fetus. It should not be used by nursing mothers, as it is excreted in breast milk. Should the continuation of valproic acid in pregnancy be an absolute necessity, risk of neural tube defects can be reduced by giving the patient 1–4 mg of folic acid per day. However switching to another medication is the best choice.

Psychopharmacology

K&S Ch. 36

Question 130. D.   Increased appetite, weight gain, and increased sleep make this question a case of atypical depression. The treatment of choice for atypical depression is the monoamine oxidase inhibitors (MAOIs). As such phenelzine is the answer, as it is the only MAOI listed.

Psychopharmacology

K&S Ch. 15

Question 131. C.   Venlafaxine carries the potential side effect of increasing blood pressure. For this reason a baseline blood pressure should be taken for anyone starting venlafaxine, and regular monitoring of blood pressure is a good idea. Increased blood pressure has been found particularly with doses over 300 mg per day, and lower doses have shown less hypertension. As such, caution must be used when giving this drug to anyone with preexisting hypertension.

Psychopharmacology

K&S Ch. 36

Question 132. D.   Interpersonal therapy (IPT) was developed to treat depression. It focuses on interpersonal behavior and social interaction. Patients are taught to rate their interactions with others and become aware of their own behavior. The therapist may give direct advice, help make decisions, and clarify conflicts.

Psychotherapy

K&S Ch. 35

Question 133. E.   Imprinting is the work of Konrad Lorenz. Imprinting implies that an animal has a critical period when it is sensitive to certain stimuli that elicit a specific behavioral response. For example, the baby goose has a period where it "imprints" on its mother and learns to follow her wherever she goes. If a person was the first moving object the goose saw it would imprint on that person and follow that person as if she were the mother. Nikolas Tinbergen conducted experiments both on animal behavior and on humans. He worked on measuring the power of certain stimuli to elicit specific behaviors from animals. He studied displacement activities, where in times when the urge to fight or flee would be equal, the animal would do some other activity to diffuse the tension. Humans also do this in times of stress. He described innate release mechanisms whereby animals have a specific response that is triggered by a releaser. A releaser is an environmental stimulus that prompts the specific response. Tinbergen also worked with human autistic children. He observed both the behavior of autistic children and normal children and postulated that in autistic children certain stimuli that are comforting to a normal child arouse fear in the autistic child. He postulates that this is part of what leads to the behavioral pattern found in autistic children.

Psychological Theory and Psychometric Testing

K&S Ch. 4

Question 134. E.   The hippocampus is one of the most important structures in the formation of memory. Other areas important to memory include some of the diencephalic nuclei and the basal forebrain. The amygdala also plays a role by rating the emotional content of memories thereby leading to stronger recall of more emotionally charged memories.

Basic Neuroscience

K&S Ch. 3

Question 135. E.   This is a difficult question unless you know all of the involved scales. It is easier if you know that the brief psychiatric rating scale (BPRS) is a scale used for schizophrenia and psychosis. This is the take-home point. The other scales listed all are mood disorder scales. Will the Montgomery Åsberg scale end up on a standardized test near you? Probably not. But the BPRS probably will, so remember it. It is a good idea to be familiar with the most common psychiatric rating scales such as the BPRS, Hamilton, and GAF (global assessment of functioning – axis V). We will not print the full scales in this text, but it is worth your time to be familiar with them.

Psychological Theory and Psychometric Testing

K&S Ch. 9

Question 136. C.   Sleep terror disorder is characterized by recurrent episodes of awakening and screaming during the first third of the night. The patient has intense fear, autonomic arousal, sweating, tachycardia, and rapid breathing. The patient is unresponsive to efforts of others to comfort him. There are no dreams recalled and there is amnesia for the event. Small doses of diazepam are often useful to stop the episodes.

Sleep Wake Disorders

K&S Ch. 24

Question 137. C.   Thioridazine (Mellaril) is one of the older typical antipsychotics that is not used as frequently since the advent of the atypicals. It is very sedating, causes orthostatic hypotension, has anticholinergic side effects, and has low rates of extrapyramidal symptoms. One of its more notable side effects is retrograde ejaculation, in addition to impotence. Patients on thioridazine can be told that retrograde ejaculation is not dangerous, but they will produce milky-white urine following orgasm.

Psychopharmacology

K&S Ch. 36

Question 138. C. Donepezil is an acetylcholinesterase inhibitor. All other answer choices are distracters. Donepezil is used to treat mild to moderate Alzheimer's disease. By blocking acetylcholinesterase, the drug leads to increased acetylcholine in the synaptic cleft which has been proven to slow decline in Alzheimer's disease.

Psychopharmacology

K&S Ch. 36

Question 139. B. Different cultures may present with culture-bound psychiatric syndromes, or different aspects of a certain disorder may be more prevalent in one culture than in another. With regard to depression, Chinese culture often presents with more somatic complaints and less focus on mood symptoms. Very often Chinese patients will come to the primary care physician or emergency room with somatic symptoms that are somewhat non-specific and are found to be driven by an underlying depressive disorder. Cultures have differences in how they view many things, including definitions of what constitutes health and sickness.

Cultural Issues in Psychiatry

K&S Ch. 4

Question 140. A. The amphetamines in general exert their effects through the dopaminergic system. However, ecstasy is a "designer amphetamine" which acts through both the dopaminergic and serotonergic systems. Had dopamine been given as an answer choice it would also have been acceptable. The other neurotransmitters listed are unrelated to ecstasy.

Substance Abuse and Addictive Disorders

K&S Ch. 12

Question 141. C. The field of child psychiatry developed out of the growth of child guidance centers in the early 1900s. Other answer choices are just distracters. Choice A happened after the early 1900s. Choice B happened before the early 1900s. Choice E took place in 1996 and is a bill relating to HIV testing. Choice D is unrelated to the US, as Freud lived in Vienna.

History of Psychiatry

K&S Ch. 36

Question 142. A. Sarcoidosis is a granulomatous disease that affects multiple organ systems. Neurological manifestations occur in about 5% of sarcoidosis patients. Up to 20% of neurologic manifestations present as a peripheral neuropathy. Cranial neuropathies, and in particular facial nerve palsy, are the most common manifestation of neurosarcoidosis, occurring in up to 75% of cases. The treatment of choice is systemic corticosteroid or immunosuppressive therapy. The diagnosis is established clinically, but can often be confirmed by muscle biopsy or an elevated level of angiotensin-converting enzyme (ACE) in the CSF. Other possible neurologic manifestations include cauda equina syndrome, mononeuropathy multiplex, peripheral sensorimotor polyneuropathy, diffuse meningo-encephalitis, uveitis, and polyradiculoneuropathy resembling Guillain–Barré syndrome.

Neurology

B&D Chs 49&76

Question 143. D. Trazodone is an antidepressant that is frequently used for insomnia. It is associated with priapism, which is a prolonged erection in the absence of sexual stimulation. Priapism is a potential medical emergency which can be treated by intracavernosal injection of epinephrine. Untreated priapism can also lead to impotence. Patients who start to develop priapism on trazodone should be switched to another medication.

Psychopharmacology

K&S Ch. 36

Question 144. C.   Low levels of cerebrospinal fluid serotonin are associated with increased aggression. Increased levels of dopamine are associated with increased aggression.

Basic Neuroscience

K&S Ch. 4

Question 145. C.   Mirtazapine is an antidepressant medication which works by antagonism of presynaptic alpha-2 adrenergic receptors leading to potentiation of serotonergic and noradrenergic neurotransmission. Mirtazapine is sedating, particularly at low doses, which is good for depressed patients with insomnia. It lacks the anticholinergic side effects of the tricyclics, and lacks the anxiogenic side effects of the serotonin-selective reuptake inhibitors. Mirtazapine is also notable for its lack of sexual side effects.

Psychopharmacology

K&S Ch. 36

Question 146. D.   Sleep changes characteristic of the elderly include both decrease in REM sleep and decrease in slow wave sleep. This is a useful little fact for the test-taker to remember.

Sleep Wake Disorders

K&S Ch. 24

Question 147. D.   A score of 70 on the global assessment of functioning (GAF) corresponds with "some difficulty in social, occupational, or school functioning, but generally functioning well, has some meaningful interpersonal relationships". A persistent failure to maintain personal hygiene is a GAF of 10. Major impairment in several areas is a GAF of 40. Superior functioning in all areas is a 100. No friends, unable to keep a job is a GAF of 30. It is a good idea to be familiar with the most common psychiatric rating scales such as the BPRS, Hamilton, and GAF (global assessment of functioning-axis V). We will not print the full scales in this text, but it is worth your time to be familiar with them.

Diagnostic and Treatment Procedures in Psychiatry

K&S Ch. 9

Question 148. C.   Kleine–Levin syndrome is a rare condition. (But not so rare on standardized tests!) It is marked by periods of hypersomnia with periods of normal sleep in between. During the periods of excessive sleep the patients wake up and experience apathy, irritability, confusion, voracious eating, loss of sexual inhibitions, disorientation, delusions, hallucinations, memory impairment, incoherent speech, excitation, and depression. The onset of the illness usually hits between 10 and 20 years of age, and it goes away by the time the patient is in his forties.

Disruptive, Impulse Control, Conduct Disorders, and ADHD

K&S Ch. 24

Question 149. C.   David has obsessive–compulsive personality disorder (OCPD). OCPD presents as a pervasive pattern of preoccupation with orderliness, perfectionism, and control. This preoccupation comes at the expense of openness, efficiency, and flexibility. The OCPD patient's perfectionism interferes with task completion. These patients are inflexible regarding moral and ethical issues. They devote time to work at the expense of leisure activities. They are reluctant to delegate tasks to others. They are characteristically rigid and stubborn. OCPD patients often can not discard old or worn-out objects even when they have no value. They will not give tasks to others without reassurance that the tasks will be done their way. They are miserly in spending and view money as something to be hoarded for catastrophes. David is not presenting with prominent anxiety symptoms, so generalized anxiety disorder is incorrect. He does not have obsessive thoughts, and compulsions to stop those thoughts, so obsessive–compulsive disorder is incorrect. If David had schizoid personality disorder we would see that he had no friends or close contacts and that this does not bother him. In this question David has few friends because he spends all of his time working. If David had avoidant personality disorder he would have a pattern of social inhibition, feelings of inadequacy, and hypersensitivity to negative evaluation. That pattern is not described in this question.

Personality Disorders

K&S Ch. 27

Question 150. E.   Cognitive behavioral therapy is founded on the principle that people make assumptions that affect their thoughts. Their thoughts then affect their mood. The goal of the therapy is therefore to uncover assumptions and thoughts that may be both faulty and automatic and determine how they contribute to changes in mood. Then the therapy aims to correct these faulty thoughts and stop them from being automatic.

The other answer choices are all appropriate pieces of psychodynamic therapy and psychoanalysis. They are not however part of cognitive behavioral therapy.

Psychotherapy

K&S Ch. 35

FIVE

Test Number Five

1. Blocking the H1 receptor will lead to which of the following?

   A. *Weight gain*

   B. *Dry mouth*

   C. *Orthostatic hypotension*

   D. *Elevated prolactin*

   E. *Urinary retention*

2. Needle electromyographic studies of muscles of patients with myasthenia gravis would be expected to reveal:

   A. *Delayed F-responses*

   B. *Slow nerve conduction velocities*

   C. *Decrementing response to repetitive stimulation*

   D. *Incrementing response to repetitive stimulation*

   E. *Increased motor latencies*

3. While working in the ER you evaluate a patient with confusion, myoclonus, diarrhea, hypotension, tachycardia and a normal CPK. The patient is not speaking. His family tells you that he was recently started on a new medication by his psychiatrist for treatment of bipolar disorder. They don't know the name of the medication or what kind of medication it was. Using your astute clinical skills and significant psychiatric knowledge you narrow the diagnosis down to either NMS or serotonin syndrome. But alas, you must pick one diagnosis for the medical record. Which one will it be and why?

   A. *NMS because the patient is confused*

   B. *NMS because rigidity is more commonly part of serotonin syndrome*

   C. *Serotonin syndrome because it commonly presents with hypotension*

   D. *NMS because it usually presents with normal CPKs*

   E. *Serotonin syndrome because it more commonly presents with myoclonus and GI symptoms*

 Full test available online - see inside front cover for details.

4. Which of the following MRI imaging anomalies is most closely associated with patients diagnosed with Huntington's disease?

    A. *Caudate head atrophy*

    B. *Cerebellar atrophy*

    C. *Generalized cortical atrophy*

    D. *Putamen atrophy*

    E. *Communicating hydrocephalus*

5. Which of the following must be present to meet DSM criteria for somatization disorder?

    A. *Three pain symptoms*

    B. *Two sexual symptoms*

    C. *Three pseudoneurological symptoms*

    D. *Two GI symptoms*

    E. *The illness must begin after age 30*

6. A 65-year-old woman is brought to the emergency room from a nursing home. She is noted to have cognitive impairment, delusions, masked facies, shuffling gait, cogwheel rigidity of the extremities, visual hallucinations, and agitation. She is medicated by the emergency room physician with 5 mg of intramuscular haloperidol with acute worsening of her muscular rigidity. The most likely diagnosis is:

    A. *Frontotemporal dementia*

    B. *Dementia with Lewy bodies*

    C. *Alzheimer's dementia*

    D. *Normal pressure hydrocephalus*

    E. *Vascular dementia*

7. Which one of the following is not an inhibitor of CYP450 1A2?

    A. *Amiodarone*

    B. *Tobacco*

    C. *Cimetidine*

    D. *Fluvoxamine*

    E. *Grapefruit juice*

8. Brain metastasis is most commonly due to which of the following:

    A. *Lung carcinoma*

    B. *Breast carcinoma*

    C. *Melanoma*

    D. *Prostate carcinoma*

    E. *Colorectal carcinoma*

9. The obligation to act in the patients best interests is known as:

   A. *Beneficence*

   B. *Fiduciary duty*

   C. *Nonmalfeasance*

   D. *Altruism*

   E. *Parens patriae*

10. The CT of the brain shown to the right depicts which one of the following pathologies:

   A. *Epidural hematoma*

   B. *Left middle cerebral artery infarction*

   C. *Subdural hematoma*

   D. *Sagittal sinus thrombosis*

   E. *Uncal herniation*

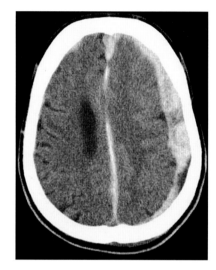

11. When considering schizophreniform disorder and brief psychotic disorder which one of the following statements is false?

   A. *A clear stressor is not needed for the diagnosis of brief psychotic disorder*

   B. *In schizophreniform disorder the patient returns to baseline functioning after the episode resolves*

   C. *Both conditions can present with hallucinations*

   D. *Schizophreniform disorder is ruled out when there is a medical condition present which could be causing psychotic symptoms*

   E. *The duration for brief psychotic disorder is at least 1 month but less than 6 months*

12. Which one of the following does not pertain to Parkinson's disease?

   A. *Resting 4 to 6 Hz tremor*

   B. *Considered a synucleinopathy*

   C. *Loss of pigment in the pars compacta of the substantia nigra*

   D. *Absence of eosinophilic, intraneuronal inclusions in the substantia nigra*

   E. *Impaired dopamine synthesis in the nigrostriatal tract*

13. You meet a new patient who describes episodes of distractibility, racing thoughts, increased goal directed activity, and elevated mood. These episodes last for 4 days and she is having one currently. She also describes past episodes lasting 3–4 weeks in which her mood is depressed and she experiences loss of appetite, fatigue, poor concentration and suicidal thoughts. Which of the following is the most accurate diagnosis?

    A. *Bipolar I disorder*

    B. *Bipolar II disorder*

    C. *Major depressive disorder*

    D. *Schizoaffective disorder bipolar type*

    E. *Cyclothymic disorder*

14. Which one of the following does not pertain to Wilson's disease?

    A. *Dementia*

    B. *Intention tremor, 4 to 6 Hz*

    C. *Kayser–Fleischer corneal rings*

    D. *Chronic hepatic dysfunction, cirrhosis*

    E. *Early onset, ages 15 to 45 years*

15. Which one of the following statements is false concerning development during the school-age years (ages 5–12)?

    A. *Children develop the ability to empathize with others during these years*

    B. *Children have a basic grasp of grammar and syntax and can understand word play*

    C. *Children learn social cues, rules and expectations*

    D. *Children become motivated by desire for approval and positive feedback*

    E. *Children have developed the capacity for abstract thinking*

16. Which one of the following movement disorders is not associated with dementia?

    A. *Parkinson's disease*

    B. *Wilson's disease*

    C. *Diffuse Lewy body disease*

    D. *Huntington's disease*

    E. *Primary torsion dystonia (dystonia musculorum deformans)*

17. What percentage of the general population has a diagnosable personality disorder?

    A. *5%*

    B. *10%*

    C. *25%*

    D. *50%*

    E. *70%*

18. Which one of the following CNS infections is most likely to produce ring-enhancing lesions on brain neuroimaging studies?

    A. *Tuberculosis*

    B. *CNS HIV-related lymphoma*

    C. *Cryptococcal meningitis*

    D. *Progressive multifocal leukoencephalopathy*

    E. *AIDS-related dementia complex (ARDC)*

19. Which one of the following would not correlate with the brain imaging finding of thin gyri, wide sulci and enlarged ventricles, (especially the third ventricle)?

    A. *Alzheimer's disease*

    B. *Chronic alcoholism or drug abuse*

    C. *A lacunar infarct of subcortical white matter*

    D. *Schizophrenia*

    E. *Trisomy 21 (Down's syndrome)*

20. A left-sided middle cerebral artery territory stroke is most likely to produce which of the following?

    A. *Impaired naming and repetition*

    B. *Preserved language functioning*

    C. *Right hemiparesis with leg weakness worse than the face and arm*

    D. *Receptive, fluent aphasia*

    E. *Speech paraphasias*

21. Dr. Smith, a psychiatrist, has been having sexual fantasies about one of his psychotherapy patients. He tells you this and gives you several reasons why the prohibition of sex with patients does not apply to this situation. Which of the following would be the most ethical advice you could give him?

    A. *He should continue to discuss the situation with colleagues to better define his sexual boundaries*

    B. *He should see the patient more frequently to use the strong feelings between them as a motivational tool for positive change in therapy*

    C. *He should share his fantasies with the patient*

    D. *He should transfer the patient's care to another psychiatrist*

    E. *He should stock his desk with condoms so that if they have sex in his office she does not become pregnant*

22. Alexia without agraphia is attributable to a stroke in which of the following arterial territories?

    A. *Middle cerebral*

    B. *Posterior cerebral*

    C. *Posterior communicating*

    D. *Vertebral*

    E. *Basilar*

23. You are studying two variables, a binary predictor variable and a continuous outcome variable. You want to know if the relationship between those two variables is due to chance alone. Which of the following tests would you use?

    A. *Analysis of variance*

    B. *Chi-square test*

    C. *T-test*

    D. *Negative predictive power*

    E. *Predictive validity*

24. Which of the following childhood disorders is accompanied by pectus excavatum, ocular lens dislocation, Marfan's habitus, mental retardation and scoliosis?

    A. *Homocystinuria*

    B. *Phenylketonuria*

    C. *Tay–Sachs disease*

    D. *Niemann–Pick disease*

    E. *Metachromatic leukodystrophy*

25. At what age can a child run well without falling, build a tower of six cubes, and engage in parallel play?

    A. *18 months*

    B. *2 years*

    C. *3 years*

    D. *4 years*

    E. *5 years*

26. Niemann–Pick disease is due to a deficiency in which one of the following?

    A. *Arylsulfatase-A*

    B. *Sphingomyelinase*

    C. *Hexosaminidase-A*

    D. *Hypoxanthine guanine phosphoribosyl transferase (HPRT)*

    E. *Phenylalanine hydroxylase*

27. A patient in treatment for bipolar disorder reports severe mid-upper abdominal pain radiating to the back, nausea, anorexia, fever and evidence of an acute abdomen. Pain is worse after eating and upon lying down. She is taking citalopram and valproic acid. Which of the following tests would be most useful in making a diagnosis?

    A. *Complete blood count*

    B. *Basic metabolic panel*

    C. *Liver function tests*

    D. *Amylase*

    E. *Prolactin level*

28. The most common inherited cause of infantile mental retardation is due to:

    A. *Arylsulfatase-A deficiency*

    B. *Hexosaminidase-A deficiency*

    C. *Trisomy 21*

    D. *Sphingomyelinase deficiency*

    E. *Trinucleotide repeat disorder causing long face, long ears and macro-orchidism*

29. Which one of the following is not a feature of trisomy 21?

    A. *Single palmar crease*

    B. *Short stature*

    C. *Brushfield spots on the iris*

    D. *Normal penis with small, firm testes and sterility*

    E. *Increased risk of dementia*

30. A child is brought to clinic with the following characteristics: elfin facies, short stature, hypoplastic teeth, mild mental retardation, friendly personality and gifted musically. This disorder is due to:

    A. Trisomy 21

    B. Autosomal microdeletion in chromosome 7q

    C. Deletion in chromosome 15q

    D. Deletion 45X0

    E. 47 XXY

31. Where should electrodes be placed in ECT to minimize cognitive impairment?

    A. Anterior bilateral placement

    B. Right unilateral placement

    C. Left unilateral placement

    D. Posterior bilateral placement

    E. Midline placement

32. Which one of the following is not a neurologic cause of autistic symptoms?

    A. Rett syndrome

    B. Fragile X syndrome

    C. Marfan syndrome

    D. Angelman syndrome

    E. Tuberous sclerosis

33. A patient suffering from depression is referred for ECT. Prior to ECT which of the following medications should be discontinued?

    A. Lithium

    B. Olanzapine

    C. Imipramine

    D. Thioridazine

    E. Selegiline

34. Which one of the following is not a feature of tuberous sclerosis?

    A. Cutaneous and conjunctival telangiectasias

    B. Mental retardation

    C. Seizures

    D. Shagreen patches

    E. Ash leaf spots

35. Which one of the following is considered a mature defense mechanism?

    A. Sublimation

    B. Displacement

    C. Repression

    D. Hypochondriasis

    E. Introjection

36. Hemianesthesia following a stroke with gradual return of sensory function and pain is due to a lesion of:

    A. *The corona radiata*
    B. *The spinothalamic tract*
    C. *The spinoreticular tract*
    D. *The thalamus*
    E. *The internal capsule*

37. Robert is arrested for assault and held in prison. Because of disorganized behavior a psychiatric evaluation is conducted by a forensic psychiatrist to determine Robert's fitness to stand trial for the charges. Robert reports that 1 month earlier he was evaluated for hearing voices in a local emergency room. What is the difference between the evaluation done by the forensic psychiatrist and the evaluation done by the emergency room psychiatrist?

    A. *Only the ER evaluation requires a full medication history*
    B. *Only the forensic evaluation contains details on Robert's memory*
    C. *The forensic psychiatrist does not have a doctor–patient relationship with Robert*
    D. *The ER evaluation will be the only one to contain recommendations*
    E. *Only the ER evaluation contains details on Robert's memory*

38. Burst-suppression wave pattern and periodic complexes seen on EEG are characteristic of which of the following?

    A. *Alzheimer's disease*
    B. *Parkinson's disease*
    C. *AIDS-related dementia complex*
    D. *Creutzfeldt–Jakob disease*
    E. *Delirium*

39. The symptoms of this disorder include dementia, incontinence and gait apraxia;

    A. *Normal pressure hydrocephalus*
    B. *Diffuse Lewy body disease*
    C. *Alzheimer's disease*
    D. *Progressive supranuclear palsy*
    E. *Wernicke–Korsakoff syndrome*

40. An intracranial bleed that causes brief loss of consciousness, followed by an initial lucid period then further deterioration thereafter, is a result of damage to:

    A. *Bridging veins*
    B. *Middle meningeal artery*
    C. *Aneurysm of the posterior communicating artery*
    D. *Reticular activating system*
    E. *Frontal lobes*

41. At which age will the majority of children be able to play pat-a-cake?

    A. *10 months*
    B. *2 months*
    C. *17 months*
    D. *2 years*
    E. *10 weeks*

42. An HIV-positive patient develops incoordination, lack of attention and motivation and memory loss that are gradual in onset. CSF is normal on lumbar puncture. MRI of the brain reveals confluent white matter changes on T2 sequencing, no mass effect and no gadolinium enhancement. The most likely diagnosis is:

    A. *Progressive multifocal leukoencephalopathy*

    B. *CNS lymphoma*

    C. *CNS toxoplasmosis*

    D. *Cryptococcal meningitis*

    E. *HIV-related dementia*

43. Which one of the following is not a substrate for CYP 2D6?

    A. *Aripiprazole*

    B. *Bupropion*

    C. *Codeine*

    D. *Duloxetine*

    E. *Haloperidol*

44. Which of the following disorders characteristically presents with festinating gait, postural instability and truncal rigidity?

    A. *Alcoholic cerebellar atrophy*

    B. *Alzheimer-type dementia*

    C. *Normal pressure hydrocephalus*

    D. *Parkinson's disease*

    E. *Tropical HTLV-1 paraparesis*

45. Billy and Susan are out at a bar. They spend the evening drinking heavily. They each drink 10 beers. As the evening comes to an end they both vomit and pass out on the floor. An ambulance is called and they are brought into the ER. Susan is found to have a higher blood alcohol level than Billy. Why is this so?

    A. *Susan drank more*

    B. *Susan has a higher body water content than Billy*

    C. *Billy metabolizes more alcohol in his gastric mucosa*

    D. *Susan urinates less frequently than Billy*

    E. *Susan is morbidly obese*

46. A 70-year-old patient presents with severe left hemicranial headache of acute onset with left eye visual loss. He also presents with aches, pains and stiffness in the extremities for several weeks. MRI of the brain reveals T2 periventricular white matter hyperintensities. Serum sedimentation rate is 110 mm/h. Which of the following is the next most important step in management?

    A. *Obtain a temporal artery biopsy.*

    B. *Begin treatment with high dose prednisone.*

    C. *Begin treatment with broad-spectrum intravenous antibiotics*

    D. *Obtain a magnetic resonance arteriogram*

    E. *Begin treatment with intravenous acyclovir*

47. Which of the following conditions is not a potential effect of low folate levels?

    A. *Fatigue*

    B. *Panic attacks*

    C. *Agitation*

    D. *Delirium*

    E. *Dementia*

48. Which of the following agents is most appropriate for acute abortive therapy of migraine headache?

    A. *Naratriptan*

    B. *Divalproex sodium*

    C. *Topiramate*

    D. *Desipramine*

    E. *Gabapentin*

49. A depressed patient comes to you with brittle hair, weight gain, muscle weakness, dry skin, constipation, and cold intolerance. Which is the most appropriate next step in management?

    A. *Start sertraline*

    B. *Refer the patient for a head CT*

    C. *Check TSH level*

    D. *Check serum glucose*

    E. *Prescribe sertraline plus Colace*

50. A patient reports a history of sudden onset of severe headache, vomiting, collapse, and preservation of consciousness. On examination there are no lateralizing neurologic signs but there is some neck stiffness noted. This clinical picture is most characteristic of:

    A. *Epidural hemorrhage*

    B. *Subdural hemorrhage*

    C. *Acute venous sinus thrombosis*

    D. *Intracerebral hemorrhage*

    E. *Subarachnoid hemorrhage*

51. Internuclear ophthalmoplegia is a characteristic finding in patients with which of the following:

    A. *Amyotrophic lateral sclerosis*

    B. *Myasthenia gravis*

    C. *Multiple sclerosis*

    D. *Huntington's chorea*

    E. *Progressive supranuclear palsy*

52. Demyelinating neuropathy is most often accompanied by which of these findings on electrodiagnostic studies?

    A. *Fibrillations and positive sharp waves*

    B. *Delayed sensory latency*

    C. *Decreased motor amplitude*

    D. *Conduction block*

    E. *Decremental response to repetitive stimulation*

53. Which of the following is not one of the DSM signs of cannabis intoxication?

   A. *Conjunctival injection*

   B. *Diuresis*

   C. *Increased appetite*

   D. *Dry mouth*

   E. *Tachycardia*

54. A 30-year-old patient presents with depression and personality changes over several years. His family reports ongoing irritability, impulsivity, and odd social behaviors. On exam you note mild hyper-reflexia, mild bradykinesia, increased eye blinking and tongue impersistence. You note he is very fidgety. His father died of dementia in his 50 s. The most likely diagnosis in this case is:

   A. *Early-onset Alzheimer's disease*

   B. *Wilson's disease*

   C. *Huntington's disease*

   D. *Corticobasal degeneration*

   E. *Frontotemporal dementia*

55. Caution should be exercised when prescribing which one of the following to a patient on carbamazepine because the combination will increase carbamazepine levels?

   A. *Cyclosporine*

   B. *Doxycycline*

   C. *Erythromycin*

   D. *Phenobarbital*

   E. *Theophylline*

56. Which of the following disorders is known to be precipitated by chiropractic adjustments?

   A. *Lumbosacral subluxation*

   B. *Brachial plexitis*

   C. *Vertebral artery dissection*

   D. *Sacroiliac dislocation*

   E. *Anterior spinal artery occlusion*

57. A patient presents with acute onset of right facial paresis involving the forehead and lower face equally. The paresis was preceded by right ear and mastoid pain and loud noises and low pitch sounds ipsilaterally. This presentation is most likely to be:

   A. *Bell's palsy*

   B. *Trigeminal neuralgia*

   C. *Facial dystonia*

   D. *Acute lateral medullary infarct*

   E. *Left-sided Horner syndrome*

58. The pharmacologic treatment of choice for postherpetic neuralgia is:

    A. *Topiramate*

    B. *Duloxetine*

    C. *Carbamazepine*

    D. *Desipramine*

    E. *Gabapentin*

59. In which brain area can characteristic lesions be seen that are associated with coma due to carbon monoxide poisoning?

    A. *Cingulate gyrus*

    B. *Globus pallidus*

    C. *Corona radiata*

    D. *Corpus callosum*

    E. *Thalamus*

60. Persistent limb rigidity and spasms, also known as stiff-person syndrome is often related to:

    A. *High titers of JC virus antigen*

    B. *High titers of HTLV-1 virus antigen*

    C. *Circulating lupus anticoagulant*

    D. *Autoantibodies against glutamic acid decarboxylase*

    E. *Autoantibodies against nicotinic receptors*

61. Why does mirtazapine decrease nausea?

    A. *5-HT2 antagonism*

    B. *5-HT3 antagonism*

    C. *5-HT2 agonism*

    D. *Alpha-2 antagonism*

    E. *Alpha-2 agonism*

62. A 6-year old girl presents with 6 months of headache, vomiting, diplopia, gait unsteadiness and falls. T1-weighted sagittal MRI brain imaging reveals the scan. The most likely diagnosis is:

    A. *Glioblastoma*

    B. *Neuroblastoma*

    C. *Arachnoid cyst*

    D. *Medulloblastoma*

    E. *Hemangioblastoma*

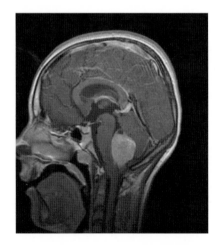

63. Which one of the following happens in 50% of families following the death of a child?

    A. *One of the remaining children commits suicide*

    B. *One parent dies*

    C. *Neglect of the remaining children*

    D. *Parental divorce*

    E. *Physical abuse of surviving children*

64. Which area of the brain, when damaged minimally, can induce unconsciousness?

    A. *Limbic system*

    B. *Reticular formation*

    C. *Internal capsule*

    D. *Thalamus*

    E. *Cerebral cortex*

65. Which of the following is most likely to be found on neuroimaging of schizophrenics?

    A. *Decreased metabolic activity in the frontal lobes*

    B. *Increased size of the lateral ventricles*

    C. *Increased cerebral asymmetry*

    D. *Increased size of the fourth ventricle*

    E. *Decreased size of the thalamus*

66. A patient suffers an injurious fall down a flight of stairs. Neurologic examination reveals right biceps weakness, absent right biceps reflex, right shoulder and arm pain with pain radiating to the right thumb. The likely diagnosis is:

    A. *C-6 radiculopathy*

    B. *Biceps tendon tear*

    C. *Radial neuropathy*

    D. *Ulnar neuropathy*

    E. *Cervical myelopathy*

67. Which of the following is not a common symptom of narcolepsy?

    A. *Sleep attacks*

    B. *Sleep-onset REM period*

    C. *Catalepsy*

    D. *Sleep paralysis*

    E. *Cataplexy*

68. A deficiency of which vitamin is associated with subacute combined degeneration of the posterior columns of the spinal cord?

    A. *Vitamin E*

    B. *Vitamin D*

    C. *Vitamin B12*

    D. *Vitamin B6*

    E. *Vitamin A*

69. Which of the following neurologic signs would be more indicative of vascular dementia rather than a dementia of the Alzheimer type?

    A. *Anomic aphasia*

    B. *Constructional apraxia*

    C. *Anosognosia*

    D. *Extensor plantar responses*

    E. *Short-term memory loss*

70. A 75-year-old man displays paranoid ideation and suspiciousness. He is unable to dress himself or manage his activities of daily living, such as cooking or cleaning. He does not have memory loss, difficulty identifying people or objects, driving a car or using a telephone or a pen. Head CT scan reveals the image. The likely diagnosis is:

    A. *Pick's disease*

    B. *Late-onset schizophrenia*

    C. *Lewy-body dementia*

    D. *Alzheimer's dementia*

    E. *Medication-induced psychosis with parkinsonism*

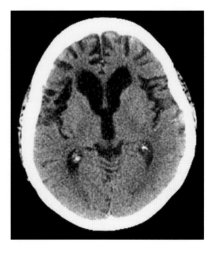

71. Which of the following deficits is associated with the condition known as hyperkalemic periodic paralysis?

    A. *Sodium channel inactivation*

    B. *Calcium channel inactivation*

    C. *Potassium channel inactivation*

    D. *Chloride channel inactivation*

    E. *Nicotinic cholinergic transmission blockade*

72. Which is the most reliable cerebrospinal fluid (CSF) finding in patients in the chronic progressive phase of multiple sclerosis?

    A. *Myelin basic protein concentration*

    B. *Total protein concentration*

    C. *Presence of oligoclonal bands*

    D. *Acellularity of the CSF*

    E. *Immunoglobulin G concentration*

73. Mirtazapine works via action on which of the following receptors?

    A. *Dopamine type 2*

    B. *Alpha 2*

    C. *Glutamate*

    D. *Alpha 1*

    E. *GABA*

74. The most useful treatment for acute cluster headaches in men is:

    A. *Indomethacin*

    B. *Oxygen therapy with a triptan medication*

    C. *Immediate-release oxycodone with acetaminophen (Percocet)*

    D. *Butalbital and acetaminophen (Fioricet)*

    E. *Methysergide*

75. The chronic headache syndrome known as hemicrania continua is most responsive to:

    A. *Indomethacin*

    B. *Oxygen therapy with a triptan medication*

    C. *Immediate-release oxycodone with acetaminophen (Percocet)*

    D. *Butalbital and acetaminophen (Fioricet)*

    E. *Methysergide*

76. Which of the following combination of risk factors is most important to control when considering the prevention of lacunar strokes?

    A. *Hypertension and hyperlipidemia*

    B. *Hypertension and obesity*

    C. *Hyperlipidemia and obesity*

    D. *Hypertension and tobacco smoking behavior*

    E. *Hyperlipidemia and diabetes*

77. A 1-day-old neonate is found to have this MRI image of the brain. The most likely diagnosis is:

    A. *Arnold–Chiari Type I malformation*

    B. *Arnold–Chiari Type II malformation*

    C. *Dandy–Walker malformation*

    D. *Arachnoid cyst*

    E. *Anencephaly*

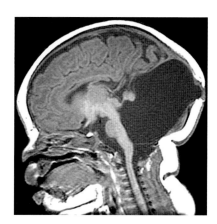

78. A 5-year-old boy is evaluated and found to have developmental delay, aggressivity, temper tantrums and overeating behavior. The boy had hypotonia as an infant. The most likely diagnosis is:

    A. Prader–Willi syndrome

    B. Fragile X syndrome

    C. Trisomy 21

    D. Williams syndrome

    E. Angelman syndrome

79. Which of the following syndromes is characterized by a rapidly progressing dementia with exaggerated startle response and violent unprovoked myoclonus?

    A. Progressive multifocal leukoencephalopathy

    B. Subacute sclerosing panencephalitis

    C. Spongiform encephalopathy

    D. Cytomegalovirus encephalitis

    E. Herpes encephalitis

80. Which one of the following complications of HIV disease is caused by a central nervous system (CNS) infection by JC virus?

    A. CNS lymphoma

    B. CNS toxoplasmosis

    C. Cryptococcal meningitis

    D. Progressive multifocal leukoencephalopathy

    E. Neurocystercircosis

81. Which of the following is the most common complication of idiopathic intracranial hypertension (pseudotumor cerebri)?

    A. Exopthalmos

    B. Visual impairment

    C. Gait disorder

    D. Uncal herniation

    E. Hypovitaminosis A

82. Which of the following is achieved during Piaget's developmental stage of concrete operations?

    A. Conservation

    B. Animistic thinking

    C. Deductive reasoning

    D. Object permanence

    E. Egocentricity

83. Male sexual behavior in the seventh decade is characterized by which of the following?

    A. Decreased time to ejaculation

    B. Decreased time to erection

    C. No change in sex drive

    D. No change in penile turgidity

    E. Absence of ejaculation upon orgasm

84. Infantile secure attachment is associated with which of the following outcomes?

    A. *Higher intellectual ability in adolescence and adulthood*

    B. *Educational success throughout childhood and adolescence*

    C. *Physical coordination and later athletic ability*

    D. *Emotional and social competence*

    E. *Easy temperament in childhood*

85. A young girl performs in a school play and revels in the praise and pride displayed to her by her mother. In Kohut's theory of self-psychology, this child is experiencing:

    A. *Idealization*

    B. *Good-enough mothering*

    C. *Mastery*

    D. *Primary narcissism*

    E. *Mirroring*

86. According to Margaret Mahler's stages of separation–individuation the period from 10 to 18 months of age during which the infants' ability to move autonomously increases their exploration of the outer world is known as:

    A. *Object constancy*

    B. *Rapprochement*

    C. *Practicing*

    D. *Differentiation*

    E. *Symbiosis*

87. Which of the following is an example of declarative memory?

    A. *Priming*

    B. *Retention and recall of facts*

    C. *Skills and habits*

    D. *Simple classical conditioning*

    E. *Non-associative learning*

88. The "addictive" nature of gambling behavior and the disorder of pathological gambling can best be explained by theories of:

    A. *Operant conditioning*

    B. *Classical conditioning*

    C. *Drive and neurotic impulses*

    D. *Self-psychology and pathological narcissism*

    E. *Habituation and sensitization*

89. A patient with depression tells the therapist about a variety of unpleasant personal circumstances that have occurred in the past week, worries about friends being sad and withdrawn, and a reluctance to watch the news on television because "the only news on television is bad news." In the theory of cognitive psychology, this type of behavior is best formulated as:

    A. *Learned helplessness*

    B. *Selective attention bias*

    C. *Catastrophizing*

    D. *Automatic negative thoughts*

    E. *Information overload*

90. A clinical test that detects 96% of patients with a certain disease, but also produces many false positives in patients without the disease, is deemed to have:

    A. *High sensitivity and high specificity*

    B. *Low sensitivity and high specificity*

    C. *Low sensitivity and low specificity*

    D. *High sensitivity and low specificity*

    E. *Low overall clinical utility*

91. Which of the following classes of psychotropic medications has the best documented treatment effects for agitation in the demented patient?

    A. *Antipsychotics*

    B. *Mood stabilizers*

    C. *Benzodiazepines*

    D. *Selective serotonin reuptake inhibitor antidepressants*

    E. *Tricyclic antidepressants*

92. A television news program reports that a famous actress has been seen in public exhibiting verbal outbursts and unexplained violent behavior directed at people and property. A well-known psychiatrist appears on the program and when asked about the actress, states she is likely suffering from bipolar disorder and possibly substance abuse. Which of the following best qualifies the ethics of the psychiatrist's on-air affirmations?

    A. *It is ethical because the actress is a public figure*

    B. *It is ethical unless there is conflict of interest involved*

    C. *It is unethical because the psychiatrist has never examined the actress*

    D. *It is unethical because the psychiatrist was paid to appear on-air and make such statements*

    E. *It is ethical because the psychiatrist is acting under the constitutional rights of freedom of speech and freedom of the press*

93. Transcranial magnetic stimulation (Neurostar TMS®) was cleared by the FDA in 2008 for in-office treatment of major depressive disorder. The area of the brain that is treated with electromagnetic stimulus application is first mapped by finding the motor threshold at the area on the motor strip corresponding to the thumb and fingers. Following the discovery of the best area of motor threshold by this mapping, the ongoing treatment is applied to approximately which of the following brain areas?

    A. *Left cingulate gyrus*

    B. *Left parietal lobe*

    C. *Left dorsolateral prefrontal cortex*

    D. *Right parietal lobe*

    E. *Right dorsolateral prefrontal cortex*

94. Transcranial magnetic stimulation (Neurostar TMS®) was cleared by the FDA in 2008 for in-office treatment of major depressive disorder. Which one of the following correctly classifies the type of patient history for which this treatment is indicated?

  A. *For patients who failed to achieve satisfactory benefit from one antidepressant medication at an adequate dose and duration in the current episode*

  B. *For patients who failed to achieve satisfactory benefit from two antidepressant medications at an adequate dose and duration in the current episode*

  C. *For patients who failed to achieve satisfactory benefit from three antidepressant medications at an adequate dose and duration in the current episode*

  D. *For patients who failed to achieve satisfactory benefit from at least one antidepressant medication with at least one augmenting agent (second antidepressant or antipsychotic agent) at adequate doses and duration in the current episode*

  E. *For patients who failed to achieve satisfactory benefit from at least one antidepressant agent at an adequate dose and duration in the current episode, or who could not tolerate the side effects of antidepressant agents or who did not wish to take antidepressant agents*

95. A patient comes to you 3 weeks after witnessing a child hit by a car. Since then she has been having feelings of detachment and feels "in a daze." She has recurrent thoughts and dreams about the event. She describes depersonalization. She has avoided discussing the event with friends and family and her sleep has been poor. What is the most appropriate diagnosis?

  A. *Post-traumatic stress disorder*

  B. *Major depressive disorder*

  C. *Acute stress disorder*

  D. *Panic disorder*

  E. *Primary insomnia*

96. Which one of the following properties of atypical antipsychotics is hypothesized to be responsible for these medications to be less likely to produce extrapyramidal side effects?

  A. *Decreased binding to D2 receptors*

  B. *Rapid dissociation from D2 receptors*

  C. *Affinity for muscarinic cholinergic receptors*

  D. *Binding to multiple other dopamine receptors besides D2 receptors*

  E. *Higher affinity for D1 receptors*

97. Which of the following choices is a risk factor for developing conversion disorder?

  A. *High socioeconomic status*

  B. *Little education*

  C. *High intelligence*

  D. *Urban setting*

  E. *Lack of military service*

98. Neurotoxicity due to methylenedioxymethamphetamine (MDMA) is associated with deficits in neurons that produce which of the following neurotransmitters?

  A. *Dopamine*

  B. *Norepinephrine*

  C. *Acetylcholine*

  D. *Serotonin*

  E. *Glutamate*

99. A high score on the MMPI infrequency scale (scale F) is most consistent with which one of the following diagnoses?

    A. *Major depressive disorder*

    B. *Histrionic personality disorder*

    C. *Malingering*

    D. *Obsessive–compulsive disorder*

    E. *Hypochondriasis*

100. When triiodothyronine is added to a tricyclic antidepressant for augmentation, the clinician needs to be cautious if:

    A. *The patient is an older woman over 50 years of age*

    B. *The patient has subclinical hypothyroidism*

    C. *The patient has a history of hypertension*

    D. *The patient has a history of cognitive deficits with depression*

    E. *The patient relapsed while on a previously effective tricyclic antidepressant*

101. One of your patients has been taking zolpidem for sleep recently and started having sleep walking episodes on the medication. She finds these episodes to be disturbing. She asks you about taking eszopiclone instead. Which of the following possible responses to her question is most accurate?

    A. *Eszopiclone is a bad choice because she will develop tolerance over time*

    B. *Eszopiclone can also cause sleep walking*

    C. *Eszopiclone works as a melatonin receptor agonist*

    D. *Eszopiclone is used to treat both sleep and depression*

    E. *Unlike with zolpidem, hallucinations do not occur with eszopiclone*

102. As part of doing blood-work for an alcoholic patient you decide to order a GGT (gamma-glutamyl transpeptidase). How long after the patient stopped drinking would you expect the GGT to return to normal?

    A. *2 days*

    B. *3 weeks*

    C. *10 days*

    D. *8 weeks*

    E. *5 days*

103. A schizophrenic patient asks his doctor to bill his insurance company as if he had an adjustment disorder instead of schizophrenia because he is concerned about the stigma that schizophrenics face. What should the doctor do?

    A. *Agree to bill for an adjustment disorder because the stigma is real*

    B. *Kick the patient out of her practice and refuse to see him again*

    C. *Explore the reasons behind the request and explain why this is something she is not comfortable doing*

    D. *Suggest she bill the visit as psychotic disorder NOS because, though it is not accurate, it is closer to the truth than adjustment disorder*

    E. *Agree to bill as an adjustment disorder as long as the patient spends time exploring their feelings surrounding the request and their feelings about the diagnosis*

104. Which of the following is not one of the psychiatric symptoms that can result from adrenal insufficiency?

    A. *Delirium*

    B. *Psychosis*

    C. *Mania*

    D. *Depression*

    E. *Irritability*

105. Which of the following is true about administering different mood stabilizers together?

    A. *Valproic acid will increase lamotrigine levels*

    B. *Lamotrigine will increase valproic acid levels*

    C. *Valproic acid will decrease lamotrigine levels*

    D. *Valproic acid will decrease carbamazepine levels*

    E. *Carbamazepine will increase lithium levels*

106. Which of the following neurochemical changes would you expect to see in a patient with increased aggression?

    A. *Increased serotonin*

    B. *Decreased dopamine*

    C. *Decreased testosterone*

    D. *Decreased GABA*

    E. *Decreased acetylcholine*

107. Which one of the following statements is false concerning motor development during infancy?

    A. *The cerebellum is not fully formed until 1 year of age*

    B. *Myelination of peripheral nerves is not complete until 2 years of age*

    C. *The grasp and tonic neck reflexes begin to develop between 2 and 6 months*

    D. *Fine pincer grasp develops around 9 to 12 months*

    E. *The ability to sit without support occurs at 6 months*

108. Which of the following is a risk factor for neuroleptic-induced tardive dyskinesia?

    A. *Anxiety disorder*

    B. *Migraine headaches*

    C. *Lower socioeconomic class*

    D. *Advanced age*

    E. *Male gender*

109. Which of the following statements about benzodiazepines is correct?

    A. *Clonazepam has a rapid rate of absorption*

    B. *Alprazolam has a half life of 2.5 hours*

    C. *Diazepam has a half life of 200 hours*

    D. *Lorazepam is considered a short acting benzodiazepine*

    E. *Clonazepam is considered a short acting benzodiazepine*

110. Which of the following anxiety disorders has equal rates in both males and females?

    A. *Panic disorder*

    B. *Generalized anxiety disorder*

    C. *Social phobia*

    D. *Obsessive–compulsive disorder*

    E. *Specific phobia*

111. Which of the following is part of the correct schedule for monitoring WBC count when using clozapine?

    A. *Weekly WBC for the first 6 weeks then every other week thereafter*

    B. *Daily WBC for the first week, then weekly for the next 6 months*

    C. *Weekly WBC for the first 6 months then monthly thereafter*

    D. *Daily WBC for the first week after discontinuation of clozapine*

    E. *Weekly for the first 6 months then biweekly for 6 months then monthly thereafter*

112. The following choices are potential side effects of lithium except:

    A. *Hair loss*

    B. *Tremor*

    C. *Confusion*

    D. *Neural tube defects*

    E. *Seizures*

113. Which of the following is most correct regarding management of alcohol withdrawal symptoms?

    A. *IV thiamine and dextrose should be given for the first 9 days*

    B. *If alprazolam is used it should be given BID*

    C. *Disulfiram should be given during withdrawal*

    D. *One should choose clonazepam over lorazepam in a hepatically impaired patient*

    E. *If lorazepam is used it should be given QID*

114. Which of the following terms refers to spastic contractions of discrete muscle groups such as the neck, tongue, eyes or back?

    A. *Akathisia*

    B. *Tardive dyskinesia*

    C. *Acute dystonia*

    D. *Blepharospasm*

    E. *Tardive dystonia*

115. Which one of the following is not an inducer of CYP3A4?

    A. *Carbamazepine*

    B. *Oxcarbazepine*

    C. *Phenytoin*

    D. *Fluoxetine*

    E. *Rifampin*

116. Suzie goes to the emergency room with a pain in her right leg. Prior to initiating treatment the physician obtains informed consent. This is an example of which of the following ethical principles?

    A. *Competence*

    B. *Justice*

    C. *Autonomy*

    D. *Parens patriae*

    E. *Nonmaleficence*

117. The average number of ECT treatments needed to treat depression is:

    A. *1–3*

    B. *6–12*

    C. *15–20*

    D. *25–30*

    E. *35–45*

118. Which of the following is not included in the SCID (Structured Clinical Interview for DSM IV Axis I Diagnosis)?

    A. *Mood episodes*

    B. *Anxiety disorders*

    C. *Functional Impairment*

    D. *Eating disorders*

    E. *Mood disorders differential*

119. Which of the following is true regarding self-disclosure in psychotherapy?

    A. *It is always prohibited*

    B. *It is acceptable if it helps the therapist feel more comfortable*

    C. *It is acceptable for the therapist to share their real feelings as long as they don't lie*

    D. *It is acceptable if it is done solely for the benefit of the patient*

    E. *It is never prohibited*

120. A 67-year-old male carries a diagnosis of bipolar disorder and is being treated with carbamazepine. His family brings him to the emergency room because he has become confused and disoriented over the past 2 days. He is afebrile and has no neurological deficits. Although you could reasonably order any of the following tests to evaluate his condition, which of the following is most important that you check given the patient's history?

    A. *Head CT*

    B. *Chest X-ray*

    C. *Urinalysis*

    D. *Basic metabolic panel*

    E. *TSH*

121. Which of the following medications would be the best choice for a patient with psychosis and impaired hepatic function?

    A. *Olanzapine*

    B. *Quetiapine*

    C. *Paliperidone*

    D. *Ziprasidone*

    E. *Risperidone*

122. A general consensus among experienced clinicians and researchers is known as:

    A. *Face validity*

    B. *Descriptive validity*

    C. *Predictive validity*

    D. *Construct validity*

    E. *Positive predictive power*

123. Which one of the following statements is false concerning desvenlafaxine extended release tablets (Pristiq)?

    A. *Desvenlafaxine may cause orthostasis and hyponatremia in the elderly*

    B. *Dosage should be adjusted in patients with renal disease*

    C. *Monitoring must be conducted for increase in suicidality during treatment, especially in children and teens*

    D. *Taking desvenlafaxine in combination with an MAOI may precipitate a serotonin syndrome*

    E. *Desvenlafaxine has no impact on blood pressure, unlike venlafaxine*

124. Which of the following GAF scores would be most appropriate for a patient who has impaired reality testing and has major impairment in work functioning and family interactions?

    A. *5*

    B. *15*

    C. *75*

    D. *35*

    E. *65*

125. Which of the following changes can be seen in the sleep of elderly human subjects?

    A. *Gradual phase retardation*

    B. *Increased REM sleep*

    C. *Decreased Stage I sleep*

    D. *Increased sleep efficiency*

    E. *Decreased Stage III and Stage IV sleep*

126. Which one of the following statements is false concerning atomoxetine (Strattera)?

    A. *Atomoxetine works as a norepinephrine reuptake inhibitor*

    B. *Full results are seen within 2 weeks of initiating treatment with atomoxetine*

    C. *Once daily dosing of atomoxetine works well for most patients*

    D. *Most common side effects include dizziness and reduced appetite*

    E. *Atomoxetine carries a black box warning for suicidality*

127. Which of the following famous therapists suggested that empathic failures in the mother lead to developmental arrest in the child at a stage when the child needs others to help perform self-object functions?

    A. *Melanie Klein*

    B. *Heinz Kohut*

    C. *Jacques Lacan*

    D. *Adolph Meyer*

    E. *B. F. Skinner*

128. Naltrexone extended release injectable suspension (Vivitrol) is indicated for treatment of which of the following disorders?

    A. *Major depressive disorder*

    B. *Generalized anxiety disorder*

    C. *Psychosis*

    D. *Alcohol dependence*

    E. *Cocaine withdrawal*

129. Which of the following rating scales is used to evaluate severity of depression?

    A. *GAF*

    B. *HAM-D*

    C. *PANSS*

    D. *BPRS*

    E. *CAGE*

130. Which of the following medications is a serotonin and norepinephrine reuptake inhibitor, lacks significant antihistaminic effects, can cause withdrawal symptoms if stopped abruptly, and has an indication for neuropathic pain?

    A. *Mirtazapine*

    B. *Quetiapine*

    C. *Nefazodone*

    D. *Paroxetine*

    E. *Duloxetine*

131. Which one of the following foods can be consumed when taking an MAOI?

    A. *Aged cheese*

    B. *Cured meats*

    C. *Smoked fish*

    D. *Vodka*

    E. *Caviar*

132. A 19-year-old male is brought into the emergency room after his family noticed an acute change in his behavior. He is aggressive, assaultive, and belligerent. On exam it is noted that he has nystagmus, slurred speech, a perioral rash, and a tremor. His family reports that he became out of control while in the garage and kicked a hole through the garage door. He has no prior psychiatric history. What is his most likely diagnosis?

    A. *Bipolar disorder*

    B. *Psychotic disorder NOS*

    C. *Panic disorder*

    D. *Inhalant intoxication*

    E. *Antisocial personality disorder*

133. Which one of the following is not a clinical feature of narcolepsy?

    A. *Cataplexy*

    B. *Increased REM latency*

    C. *Hypnagogic hallucinations*

    D. *Associated with human leukocyte antigen HLA-DR2 in most cases*

    E. *Sleep paralysis*

134. Jimmy has IQ testing as part of an evaluation for behavioral disturbances. His IQ score is 45. Based on this information Jimmy is:

    A. *Not mentally retarded*

    B. *Mildly mentally retarded*

    C. *Moderately mentally retarded*

    D. *Severely mentally retarded*

    E. *Profoundly mentally retarded*

135. Which of the following statements is correct concerning clozapine?

    A. *Smoking will not affect clozapine levels*

    B. *Risk of agranulocytosis is dose related*

    C. *Clozapine carries high risk of prolactin elevation*

    D. *Doses of clozapine greater than 600 mg/day carry a much higher risk of seizures than lower doses*

    E. *Adding lithium to clozapine lowers the chances of NMS*

136. Which one of the following is false concerning delusional disorder?

    A. *Non-bizarre delusions are present*

    B. *The patient meets criteria A for schizophrenia*

    C. *There is a preservation of functioning*

    D. *"Erotomanic" is a subtype*

    E. *"Somatic" is a subtype*

137. Which of the following is the most significant risk factor for post-traumatic stress disorder and the best predictor of symptom development following exposure to trauma?

    A. *A family history of anxiety or depression*

    B. *The availability of psychiatric care immediately following the trauma*

    C. *Low socioeconomic status*

    D. *Being single, divorced or widowed*

    E. *The nature, severity and duration of exposure to the trauma*

138. Which of the following correctly describes the likelihood of patients with schizophrenia committing homicide as compared with the general population at large?

    A. *Half as likely*

    B. *Equally likely*

    C. *Twice as likely*

    D. *Five times as likely*

    E. *Ten times as likely*

139. A new patient comes to you asking for help with depression. She states that she has had a very low mood recently and has been feeling overwhelmed. She has a 2-month-old daughter at home and keeping up with a new baby has been hard for her. She reports constant fatigue, listlessness, and weight loss. She states that her libido is down and she is very upset because she could not breast feed her baby due to lack of milk production. Her concentration is normal. She bursts into tears and states that she doesn't think she can be a good mother. Which of the following would be the most appropriate next step in the management of this case?

    A. *Start psychotherapy only*

    B. *Start an antidepressant*

    C. *Start a benzodiazepine*

    D. *Send patient for endocrine bloodwork*

    E. *Report the case to child protective services*

140. Which of the following choices about avoidant personality disorder is most accurate?

    A. *It is often misdiagnosed as paranoid personality disorder*

    B. *These patients tend to be indifferent to praise or criticism*

    C. *Affective instability is a key component of the disorder*

    D. *These patients avoid social interaction out of fear of shame or ridicule*

    E. *These patients are unable to discard worthless objects*

141. Which one of the following is not a possible psychiatric manifestation of Acute Intermittent Porphyria?

    A. *Anxiety*

    B. *Dementia*

    C. *Depression*

    D. *Psychosis*

    E. *Delirium*

142. The prevalence of Alzheimer's disease in those patients over age 85 years is:

    A. *Less than 5%*

    B. *5 to 10%*

    C. *11 to 20%*

    D. *21 to 40%*

    E. *41 to 50%*

143. Which of the following statements concerning psychiatrists and suicide is most accurate?

    A. *The law imposes liability on the psychiatrist whenever a patient commits suicide*

    B. *A psychiatrist is expected to foresee all possible harm that may come to a patient*

    C. *The law views suicide as predictable in all cases*

    D. *No-Harm contracts are dependable legal protection for the psychiatrist*

    E. *Psychiatrists must document risk assessment and appropriate interventions to meet the standard of care when treating a suicidal patient*

144. Which of the following is the correct criterion for a covered disability according to the Americans with Disabilities Act (ADA)?

    A. *It is due to a substance-related disorder*

    B. *It is due to a general medical condition*

    C. *It seriously affects social functioning at work*

    D. *It substantially limits one or more major life activities*

    E. *It causes significant impairment in the workplace*

145. Which one of the following is false concerning the homeless mentally ill?

    A. *The numbers of homeless mentally ill continue to grow*

    B. *A significant number of homeless mentally ill are also dependent on alcohol or other substances of abuse*

    C. *Street dwellers usually have schizophrenia, substance abuse or both*

    D. *Episodically homeless have personality disorders, substance abuse or mood disorders*

    E. *Traditional mental health systems are often very effective at treating the homeless once they are enrolled in treatment*

146. Which one of the following situations is considered ethical behavior for a psychiatrist?

    A. *Having sex with a current patient*

    B. *Noting romantic feelings between therapist and patient then discontinuing therapy, then beginning a sexual relationship*

    C. *Transferring the case to another doctor, then waiting for one year, then beginning a sexual relationship with the former patient*

    D. *Taking on a new patient with whom you had been sexually involved several years ago, but are not currently*

    E. *Never having sex with a patient or ex-patient, ever, under any circumstances*

147. Which of the following medications is a partial nicotine agonist which decreases craving and withdrawal in patients trying to stop smoking?

    A. *Bupropion*

    B. *Buspirone*

    C. *Nicotine gum*

    D. *Nicotine nasal spray*

    E. *Varenicline*

148. The treatment of choice for organophosphate insecticide exposure and poisoning is:

    A. *Pralidoxime and atropine*

    B. *Flumazenil*

    C. *Intravenous fluids and ventilation*

    D. *Naloxone*

    E. *Dimercaprol or penicillamine*

149. Which one of the following is false regarding HIPAA?

    A. *Authorization must be obtained for release of health information except for routine uses such as provider payment or healthcare operations*

    B. *Patients must have access to written notice of their privacy rights*

    C. *Patients have a right to know how their protected information is kept and disclosed*

    D. *Patients have a right to copies of their medical record*

    E. *Patients may control who receives their information but not how the information is communicated*

150. One of your patients asks you to give them information about Mirtazapine. If you made all of the following statements to the patient, which one would be considered factually inaccurate?

    A. *Mirtazapine blocks serotonin reuptake*

    B. *Mirtazapine causes minimal sexual dysfunction*

    C. *Mirtazapine can be very sedating*

    D. *Mirtazapine is a potent H1 receptor antagonist*

    E. *Mirtazapine can cause weight gain*

FIVE

Answer Key – **Test Number Five**

1. **A**	26. **B**	51. **C**	76. **D**	101. **B**	126. **B**
2. **C**	27. **D**	52. **D**	77. **C**	102. **D**	127. **B**
3. **E**	28. **E**	53. **B**	78. **A**	103. **C**	128. **D**
4. **A**	29. **D**	54. **C**	79. **C**	104. **C**	129. **B**
5. **D**	30. **B**	55. **C**	80. **D**	105. **A**	130. **E**
6. **B**	31. **B**	56. **C**	81. **B**	106. **D**	131. **D**
7. **B**	32. **C**	57. **A**	82. **A**	107. **C**	132. **D**
8. **A**	33. **A**	58. **E**	83. **C**	108. **D**	133. **B**
9. **B**	34. **A**	59. **B**	84. **D**	109. **A**	134. **C**
10. **C**	35. **A**	60. **D**	85. **E**	110. **D**	135. **D**
11. **E**	36. **D**	61. **B**	86. **C**	111. **E**	136. **B**
12. **D**	37. **C**	62. **D**	87. **B**	112. **D**	137. **E**
13. **B**	38. **D**	63. **D**	88. **A**	113. **E**	138. **B**
14. **B**	39. **A**	64. **B**	89. **B**	114. **C**	139. **D**
15. **E**	40. **B**	65. **B**	90. **D**	115. **D**	140. **D**
16. **E**	41. **A**	66. **A**	91. **A**	116. **C**	141. **B**
17. **B**	42. **E**	67. **C**	92. **C**	117. **B**	142. **D**
18. **A**	43. **B**	68. **C**	93. **C**	118. **C**	143. **E**
19. **C**	44. **D**	69. **D**	94. **A**	119. **D**	144. **D**
20. **A**	45. **C**	70. **A**	95. **C**	120. **D**	145. **E**
21. **D**	46. **B**	71. **A**	96. **B**	121. **C**	146. **E**
22. **B**	47. **B**	72. **C**	97. **B**	122. **A**	147. **E**
23. **C**	48. **A**	73. **B**	98. **D**	123. **E**	148. **A**
24. **A**	49. **C**	74. **B**	99. **C**	124. **D**	149. **E**
25. **A**	50. **E**	75. **A**	100. **C**	125. **E**	150. **A**

FIVE

Explanations **– Test Number Five**

Question 1. A.

Blocking the H1 receptor leads to weight gain and sedation. You should also be familiar with the effects of blocking some other receptors. Blocking acetylcholine receptors leads to dry mouth, constipation, blurry vision, urinary retention, and cognitive dysfunction. Blocking alpha 1 adrenergic receptors leads to orthostatic hypotension and drowsiness. Blocking dopamine receptors can lead to EPS and elevated prolactin.

Basic Neuroscience

K&S Ch. 3

Question 2. C.

The diagnostic evaluation of myasthenia gravis (MG) is multifaceted. Timed endurance tasks such as prolonged upgaze, holding outstretched arms in abduction, or vital capacities are useful office-based physical examination evidence of fatigability. Weakness improvement upon edrophonium chloride (Tensilon) injection is a useful sign, though false-negative and false-positive results are known to occur. The detection of acetylcholine receptor antibodies (AChR-ab) in serum is another useful corroborative test that has 70% sensitivity in ocular myasthenia and 80% sensitivity in generalized disease.

Repetitive nerve stimulation by needle EMG may demonstrate a decrementing response: a reduction of the compound muscle action potential, potentiated after one minute of exercise, consistent with a poly-synaptic transmission defect. The sensitivity of repetitive stimulation is about 75%. The demonstration of increased "jitter" by single-fiber EMG is the most sensitive test for MG. The sensitivity ranges from 80% in ocular myasthenia to close to 100% in moderate generalized MG. Using AChR-ab, repetitive stimulation and single-fiber EMG identifies all MG cases.

Neurology

B&D Ch. 78

Question 3. E.

This question may be a bit odd, but it covers an important point nonetheless. It is asking you to compare NMS and serotonin syndrome. This can be a very tricky task as they both present with many of the same symptoms. Both present with mental status changes, autonomic instability, diaphoresis, and mutism. Both can have elevated CPKs but high CPKs are more common in NMS because of the muscular rigidity. To make the decision between the two the key point is that serotonin syndrome presents with myoclonus, hyper-reflexia and GI symptoms, whereas NMS presents with muscle rigidity. Now some may argue that serotonin syndrome can present with rigidity also...and they're right. But when we take the whole clini-cal picture into account the myoclonus, GI symptoms and normal CPK would push the decision in the direction of the serotonin syndrome over NMS. In the real world hopefully the patient's family members or doctor could tell you what the new medication was, which would greatly influence your diagnosis.

Psychopharmacology

K&S Ch. 36

Question 4. A.

Classically, MRI studies of the brains of patients with Huntington's disease (HD) reveal caudate and cerebral atrophy. Besides taking a fastidious family history, blood should be drawn and DNA testing conducted for the Huntington's genetic anomalies. HD is caused by a mutation on chromosome 4 caus-ing an unstable expansion of CAG repeats.

The atrophy of the caudate alters the appearance and configuration of the frontal horns of the lateral ventricles, because the inferolateral borders do not reveal the typical bulge formed by the head of the caudate nucleus. Also, in general, the ventricles are diffusely enlarged. Further discussion of HD can be found in other questions in this volume.

Neurology

B&D Ch. 71

Question 5. D. This question tests how well you know your DSM criteria for somatization disorder. For somatization disorder you need four pain symptoms, two GI symptoms, one sexual symptom and one pseudoneurological symptom. These symptoms may present over a period of several years. The illness must begin before age 30. The symptoms either cannot be explained by a medical condition or are out of proportion to the symptoms/impairment one would expect given the medical condition. The symptoms are not intentionally produced or feigned. More women get the illness than men, and it often presents as a dramatic patient who is very vague about details of their symptoms.

Somatic Symptom Disorders

K&S Ch. 17

Question 6. B. The core features of dementia with Lewy bodies (DLB) include visual hallucinations, fluctuating cognition and parkinsonism. Two features are required to diagnose clinically probable DLB and one is required to diagnose clinically possible DLB. Rapid eye movement (REM) sleep behavior disorder, and neuroleptic sensitivity, as well as low uptake in basal ganglia on fluorodopa PET and SPECT scans are now considered "suggestive" clinical criteria. In general, the clinical picture of mild parkinsonism with more severe dementia and marked visual hallucinations and paranoid delusions should trigger consideration of the diagnosis of DLB.

Parkinsonian features of DLB may respond well to L-dopa therapy, but usually only temporarily and sometimes with the undesirable side effect of causing agitated delirium or hallucinations. Some patients also suffer from orthostatic hypotension. There is no definitive diagnostic test for DLB, although PET scans sometimes reveal reduced activity in the posterior parietal cortical regions.

Neurocognitive disorders

B&D Ch. 66

Question 7. B. All of the choices listed are inhibitors of CYP450 1A2 except tobacco, which is an inducer. Other inducers of 1A2 include charbroiled meats, and cruciferous vegetables.

Psychopharmacology

K&S Ch. 3

Question 8. A. Intracranial metastatic carcinoma is more frequently seen than primary brain tumors. Most carcinomas metastasize to the brain via hematogenous spread. About one-third of brain metastases originate in the lung and about half that number originate in the breast. The third most frequent source is melanoma, followed by the gastrointestinal tract, in particular the colon and the rectum. This is followed in frequency by cancers of the kidney. The remainder are accounted for by cancers of the thyroid, liver, gallbladder, testicle, pancreas, uterus, and ovaries.

Neurology

B&D Ch. 52F

Question 9. B. Fiduciary duty is the obligation to work in the patient's best interests. Beneficence is an obligation to help patients and relieve suffering. Nonmaleficence is the duty to do no harm. Altruism is putting the needs of others before your own needs. Parens patriae is a doctrine that allows the state to intervene and act as a surrogate parent for those who cannot take care of themselves.

Ethics

K&S Ch. 58

Question 10. C. Most subdural hematomas occur over the convexity of the cerebral hemispheres. Bleeding into the subdural space is usually a result of tearing of one or more of the bridging veins that cross the space to reach the venous sinuses. In 50–80% of patients there is a history of head trauma. Headache due to subdural hematoma can occur due to chronic expansion of the lesion. Other symptoms that can be caused by chronic subdural hematoma include cognitive deficits, personality changes, subacute dementia, dizziness and excessive sleepiness. Headache is the single most common symptom and is more common in younger patients, who have less atrophy than the elderly. In the presence of atrophy a larger collection of blood can accumulate before it expands and deforms pain-sensitive structures.

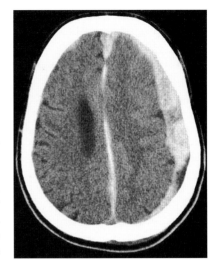

The photo attached to this question most likely represents a subacute subdural hematoma. An acute bleed would initially be hyperdense, but gradually becomes more isodense after a period of one or more weeks. The fluid then becomes more hypodense (with respect to the cortex) over a period of two to six weeks.

Neurology

B&D Ch. 69

Question 11. E.   This question compares schizophreniform disorder with brief psychotic disorder to see if you know some of the key differences. Both disorders present with schizophrenia-like symptoms (i.e., criteria A symptoms). In both disorders the patient returns to baseline functioning after the disturbance resolves. In brief psychotic disorder there is often a stressor which precedes the episode, but there does not need to be one. In making the diagnosis the DSM allows us to describe the episode as "with marked stressor", "without marked stressor", or "with postpartum onset." The key point to keep in mind is the time difference. Brief psychotic disorder lasts from 1 day to 1 month. Schizophreniform disorder lasts from 1 month to 6 months. After 6 months the psychosis can be called schizophrenia (assuming schizophrenia criteria are met). Either diagnosis is ruled out if there is a medical condition present that could be causing the symptoms. In that case one would diagnose psychotic disorder secondary to a medical condition.

Psychotic Disorders

K&S Ch. 14

Question 12. D.   The core features of Parkinson's disease are resting tremor, rigidity, postural instability and hypokinesia/bradykinesia. The classic parkinsonian tremor is seen in the initial presentation of about seventy percent of patients with the disuase. The 4 to 6-per-second characteristic "pill-rolling" tremor of thumb and fingers is seen in about half of the patients with Parkinson's disease. The tremor is typically seen when the hands are still (hence the term *resting tremor*).

The most replicable finding in idiopathic Parkinson's disease is loss of pigmented cells in the substantia nigra and other pigmented dopaminergic tracts. Recall that there must be a loss of at least 80% of dopaminergic cell bodies before the clinical symptoms and signs of Parkinson's disease begin to manifest. PD traditionally has been considered a non-genetic disorder; however, around 15% of individuals with PD have a first-degree relative who has the disease. At least 5% of people are now known to have forms of the disease that occur because of a mutation of one of several specific genes.

Mutations in specific genes have been conclusively shown to cause PD. These genes code for alpha-synuclein (SNCA), parkin (PRKN), leucine-rich repeat kinase 2 (LRRK2 or dardarin), PTEN-induced putative kinase 1 (PINK1), DJ-1 and ATP13A2. In most cases, people with these mutations will develop PD. In terms of pathophysiology, PD is considered a synucleinopathy due to an abnormal accumulation of alpha-synuclein protein in the brain in the form of Lewy bodies, as opposed to other diseases such as Alzheimer's disease where the brain accumulates tau protein in the form of neurofibrillary tangles. Nevertheless, there is clinical and pathological overlap between tauopathies and synucleinopathies. A classical Lewy body is an eosinophilic cytoplasmic inclusion that consists of a dense core surrounded by a halo of 10-nm wide radiating fibrils, the primary structural component of which is alpha-synuclein. These are found pervasively in the substantia nigra of patients with Parkinson's disease.

Neurology

B&D Ch. 71

Question 13. B. The answer to this question is bipolar II disorder because the patient meets criteria for hypomania as well as major depressive episodes. The important learning point here is to distinguish mania from hypomania. To qualify for mania one needs symptoms for at least a week. If the core symptom is euphoria, three additional symptoms are needed. If the core symptom is irritability, four additional symptoms are needed. Additional symptoms can include grandiosity, decreased need for sleep, pressured speech, flight of ideas, distractibility, increased goal directed activity, or excessive involvement in pleasurable activities. One must demonstrate impairment in social or occupational functioning, need for hospitalization, or presence of psychosis as part of the picture of mania.

Hypomania lasts for at least 4 days. The same criteria for symptoms apply, but the patient does not experience disturbance in social or occupational functioning, require hospitalization, or become psychotic as part of the symptom picture.

To qualify for cyclothymic disorder a patient must have 2 years with periods of hypomania and depressive symptoms that don't meet criteria for MDD.

Major depressive disorder is not the correct answer choice because the patient meets criteria for a bipolar diagnosis based on her hypomanic episodes. Schizoaffective disorder is ruled out by the absence of any psychotic symptoms in the patient's description. Bipolar I disorder is incorrect because the patient does not meet criteria for manic episodes.

Bipolar Disorders

K&S Ch. 15

Question 14. B. Wilson's disease (hepatolenticular degeneration) is a rare heredodegenerative disorder affecting 1–2/100 000 individuals. It is an autosomal recessive disorder of copper metabolism localizing to mutations on chromosome 13, in the *ATP7B* gene. Many patients present in childhood with signs and symptoms of liver dysfunction that span the spectrum from cirrhosis to fulminant liver failure. Some patients present with hemolytic anemia, hypersplenism and kidney failure. Neurological signs and symptoms can be seen in up to half of patients with Wilson's disease. These CNS manifestations can include parkinsonism, postural and kinetic tremor, ataxia, titubation, chorea, seizures, dysarthria, and dystonia. Dementia may be present and is most often mild. Psychiatric manifestations can also be seen and include mood and personality disorders, behavioral changes and psychosis. When neurologic manifestations are seen, ophthalmological exam almost inevitably demonstrates the presence of Kayser–Fleischer rings due to copper deposition in Descemet's membrane. Treatment is classically accomplished by copper chelation with D-penicillamine. Note that answer B is correct because the classic 4–6 Hz intention tremor is generally associated with idiopathic Parkinson's disease and not Wilson's disease.

Neurology

B&D Ch. 71

Question 15. E. The school-age years (ages 5–12) include many important milestones. All of those listed are correct with the exception of choice E. The ability to think abstractly usually develops during adolescence and coincides with the stage that Piaget coined "formal operations." In this stage the person can manipulate data and emotions in the environment in a constructive manner using their own experience and a hypothetical or "what if" framework. It is not a skill that usually develops during the school-age years.

Human Development

K&S Ch. 2

Question 16. E. This answer refers to what is currently termed childhood-onset generalized primary dystonia. This disease entity was formerly known as Oppenheim's dystonia or *dystonia musculorum deformans*. The disease prevalence is about 1.4 in 100 000. Most cases that start early in childhood are DYT1 dystonia, resulting from a mutation in the torsin A gene (*TOR1A*) on chromosome 9q32-34. The prevalence of DYT1 is as high as 20 to 30 per 100 000 and is commonly seen in individuals of Ashkenazi Jewish decent. Early symptoms are characterized by an action-induced dystonia of the leg or the arm. In about

70% of affected individuals, dystonic movements spread to the trunk and other limbs and the condition generalizes over about 5 years. Laryngeal and pharyngeal dystonia remain rare in this disorder. Cognition is generally intact. The other four movement disorders in answers A through D are all associated with a dementing process. These disorders are described in other questions in this volume.

Neurology

B&D Ch. 71

Question 17. B.   Ten to fifteen percent of the general population has a diagnosable personality disorder.

Personality disorders

K&S Ch. 27

Question 18. A.   Approximately 1% of tuberculosis infections are complicated by neurologic disease, such as intracerebral tuberculoma, tuberculous meningitis, or tuberculous spine involvement with myelopathy (Pott's disease). TB meningitis usually follows a subacute course with low-grade fever, headache and intermittent nausea and vomiting. This is followed by more severe headache, neck stiffness, altered mentation, and cranial nerve palsies. The diagnosis is made by identifying tubercle bacilli on CSF acid-fast bacilli (AFB) smear or culture. CSF examination reveals normal or elevated opening pressure, elevated protein (80–400 mg/dL), low glucose (<40 mg/dL), and pleocytosis (averaging 200 to 400 WBC/μL with lymphocytic predominance). Tuberculomas, the parenchymal form of TB, are single or multiple brain or spinal cord lesions. CT or MRI may show low- or high-intensity lesions with ring enhancement. The other answer choices, B through E, are among the most common CNS manifestations of HIV disease. These diseases do not classically present with ring-enhancing lesions on neuroimaging. Be sure to read up on these other AIDS-related disorders, as they do appear frequently on standardized examinations.

Neurology

B&D Ch. 53C

Question 19. C.   The finding of thin gyri, wide sulci and enlarged ventricles on neuroimaging studies is typically indicative of cortical atrophy. With normal aging, there is mild to moderate progressive enlargement of the ventricles, sulci and cisternal spaces. In neurodegenerative disorders, such as Alzheimer's disease, atrophy is excessive and premature. Chronic alcoholism and drug abuse can cause early cerebral atrophy. More typically though, chronic alcohol use causes cerebellar atrophy which can result in truncal ataxia due to the preferential involvement of the vermis over the cerebellar hemispheres. The classic symptoms of cerebellar atrophy due to alcohol use are gait unsteadiness and a wide-based gait. Brain imaging of patients with schizophrenia can also reveal generalized cortical atrophy with enlargement of the ventricular spaces. Trisomy 21 (Down's syndrome) leads to an early onset of Alzheimer-like changes in the brain. Trisomy 21 leads to increased levels of amyloid precursor protein (APP), because it is expressed on chromosome 21. Increase in amyloid deposition occurs as a result of the increase in APP. A single lacunar infarct of the subcortical white matter would not be expected to be accompanied by generalized cortical atrophy.

Neurology

B&D Ch. 66

Question 20. A.   Middle cerebral artery (MCA) infarction is one of the most common types of strokes. The clinical picture varies depending on whether the site of occlusion is in the stem, superior division, inferior division, or lenticulostriate branches.

A stem occlusion typically produces a large hemispheric infarction with contralateral hemiplegia, conjugate eye deviation towards the side of the infarct, hemianesthesia and homonymous hemianopia. Associated global aphasia occurs if the dominant hemisphere is involved. Hemineglect occurs in cases of nondominant hemispheric involvement.

A Broca-type aphasia is more common in upper division MCA infarcts because of the preferential involvement of the anterior branches of the upper division when occluded. Answer choice A is the best response to this question because a perisylvian infarct would almost certainly impair naming and repetition, producing a perisylvian aphasia. Answer B is incorrect because a dominant hemisphere infarct in the MCA territory would almost certainly involve some kind of language functioning impairment. Answer choice C is incorrect because the left MCA territory stroke would cause a right hemiparesis with face and arm weakness that is worse than the leg. This is so, because the anterior cerebral artery irrigates the part of the motor strip responsible for lower extremity movement. Answers D and E are features of a Wernicke-type aphasia. Wernicke's area is indeed within the MCA territory, particularly the inferior branch, but is less likely to be affected than Broca's area.

Neurology

B&D Chs 12A&51A

Question 21. D.
There is only one ethical answer here, and that is to transfer the patient's care to another psychiatrist. There are no exceptions to the rule prohibiting sex between psychiatrist and patient. Regardless of circumstances, his processing of the matter or what he tells the patient, having a sexual relationship is prohibited. He can no longer serve a neutral therapeutic role in this case. It must be transferred to another psychiatrist.

Ethics

K&S Ch. 58

Question 22. B.
Pure alexia without agraphia is classically caused by a stroke in the left posterior cerebral artery (PCA) territory, particularly in the splenium of the corpus callosum. This syndrome was initially described by Dejerine in 1892. Patients can write, but they cannot read their own writing. Speech, auditory comprehension and repetition are intact. Naming, particularly for colors, may be deficient. Dejerine postulated that this syndrome was due to a disconnection between the intact right visual cortex and left hemisphere language centers. Associated signs may include: right hemianopia or superior quadrantanopia, short-term memory loss and the absence of motor and sensory signs.

Neurology

B&D Ch. 12A

Question 23. C.
A binary variable has two possible values ...such as yes or no, positive or negative, male or female. A continuous variable will fall somewhere on a range, such as age, height, or weight. Independent Variables (predictor variables) are contributing factors to a result or predictors of a certain outcome within an experimental study. They are the variables that are manipulated by the experimenter. Dependent variables (outcome variables) are the outcomes that the independent variables contributed to or predicted. A dependent variable is the variable that is not manipulated by the experimenter.

To answer this type of question, first ask yourself two more questions. How many variables are there? Are they binary or continuous? Then consider the following:

The Chi-Square test is used for 1 binary predictor variable and 1 binary outcome variable. The T-test is used for 1 binary predictor variable and 1 continuous outcome variable. The ANOVA test is used for 2 or more binary predictor variables and 1 continuous outcome variable. Correlation is used for 1 continuous predictor variable and 1 continuous outcome variable. Regression Analysis is used with two or more continuous or binary variables and 1 continuous outcome variable.

Statistics

K&S Ch. 4

Question 24. A.
Homocystinuria is an inborn error of amino acid metabolism. Three types of enzymatic deficiencies are possible: homocysteine methyltransferase, methylene tetrahydrofolate reductase and cystathione-β-synthetase. The accumulation of homocysteine in the blood leads to endothelial injury and premature atherosclerosis. Patients can present with marfanoid habitus, livedo reticularis, malar flush, ectopia lentis, glaucoma, myopia, optic atrophy, mental retardation, spasticity, seizures, psychiatric problems, osteoporosis, and a high likelihood of intracranial arterial or venous thrombosis. Death can result from myocardial infarction, stroke or pulmonary embolism. Raised plasma homocysteine levels may be an independent risk factor for coronary artery disease, cerebrovascular disease, or peripheral artery occlusive disease. Elevated homocysteine levels can effectively be lowered by administration of folic acid, sometimes needing the addition of pyridoxine (vitamin B6) and vitamin B12.

Phenylketonuria is an amino acidopathy resulting from an enzyme deficiency, specifically phenylalanine hydroxylase. The pattern of inheritance is autosomal recessive. Other symptoms may include: delayed mental and social skills, head size significantly below normal, hyperactivity, jerking movements of the arms or legs, mental retardation, seizures, skin rashes, tremors, and unusual positioning of hands. If the condition is untreated or foods containing phenylalanine are not avoided, a "mousy" or "musty" odor may be detected on the breath and skin and in urine. The unusual odor is due to a buildup of phenylalanine substances in the body.

Tay–Sachs disease is the infantile form of hexosaminidase-A deficiency. The pattern of inheritance is autosomal recessive. It is caused by a mutation in the *HEXA* gene on chromosome 15. Infants with the disorder appear to develop normally for the first 6 months after birth. Then, as nerve cells become distended with gangliosides, a relentless deterioration of mental and physical abilities occurs and progresses inexorably. The child becomes blind, deaf, unable to swallow, and develops atrophy and paralysis. Death usually occurs before age four. The disease has no known treatment or cure.

Metachromatic leukodystrophy (MLD) is yet another lysosomal storage disease of infancy. This disorder results from a deficiency in arylsulfatase A. Again, its pattern of inheritance is autosomal recessive. In the late infantile form, which is the most common form of MLD (50–60%), affected children begin having difficulty walking after the first year of life, usually at 15–24 months. Symptoms include muscle wasting and weakness, muscle rigidity, developmental delays, progressive loss of vision leading to blindness, convulsions, impaired swallowing, paralysis, and dementia. Children may become comatose. Untreated, most children with this form of MLD die by age 5, often much sooner. There is no cure for MLD, and no standard treatment. It is a terminal illness. Treatment options for the future are currently being investigated. These include gene therapy, enzyme replacement therapy (ERT), substrate reduction therapy (SRT), and potentially enzyme enhancement therapy (EET).

Neurology

B&D Chs 51A&62

Question 25. A.   Knowing childhood developmental stages is important for standardized psychiatry exams. A child is capable of running well without falling, building a tower of six cubes, and engaging in parallel play by 18 months of age.

Human development

K&S Ch. 2

Question 26. B.   Niemann–Pick disease is a sphingomyelinase deficiency that is categorized as a lysosomal storage disease of infancy. The pattern of inheritance is autosomal recessive. There are essentially 2 types of Niemann–Pick disease that are further categorized in subtypes A, B, C and D, depending on specific genetic loci of mutation. Symptoms are related to the organs in which they accumulate. Enlargement of the liver and spleen (hepatosplenomegaly) may cause reduced appetite, abdominal distension and pain as well as thrombocytopenia secondary to splenomegaly. Sphingomyelin accumulation in the central nervous system (including the cerebellum) results in unsteady gait (ataxia), slurring of speech (dysarthria) and discoordinated swallowing (dysphagia). Basal ganglia dysfunction causes abnormal posturing of the limbs, trunk and face (dystonia) and upper brainstem disease results in impaired voluntary rapid eye movements (supranuclear gaze palsy). The type A disease has a very poor prognosis, with most cases resulting in death by age 18 months. Patients with types B and C disease often live into their adolescent years with a better prognosis. Current and future treatment research focuses on enzyme replacement therapy and gene therapy.

Hexosaminidase-A deficiency is Tay–Sachs disease. Arylsulfatase-A deficiency is metachromatic leukodystrophy. Phenylalanine deficiency is phenylketonuria. Hypoxanthine guanine phosphoribosyltransferase (HGPRT) deficiency results in hyperuricemia and Lesch–Nyhan syndrome. Lesch–Nyhan syndrome, unlike the other diseases noted in this question, is an X-linked recessive disease. It is a disorder of purine and pyrimidine metabolism. These diseases of inborn errors in metabolism are all explained further in other questions in this volume.

Neurology

B&D Ch. 62

Question 27. D.   Depakote has the potential to cause pancreatitis which will lead to an increased serum amylase and the symptoms described in this question. Another concern with valproic acid would be hepatitis, for which one would want to look at liver function tests but hepatitis would most likely present with right upper quadrant pain, nausea, vomiting, diarrhea, fever, coca-cola urine and jaundice.

Psychopharmacology/Lab Tests in Psychiatry

K&S Ch. 36

Question 28. E. The disease described in answer choice E is that of fragile X syndrome. Fragile X syndrome is the most common inherited cause of infantile mental retardation and the most common single-gene cause of autism. Of course, this question is constructed to try to trick you by not giving you the disease name, but forcing you to extrapolate the disease name from its presenting symptoms. Fragile X results in a spectrum of intellectual disability ranging from mild to severe as well as physical characteristics such as an elongated face, large or protruding ears, and larger testes (macro-orchidism), behavioral characteristics such as stereotypical movements (e.g. hand-flapping), and social anxiety.

Fragile X syndrome is associated with the expansion of the CGG trinucleotide repeat affecting the Fragile X mental retardation 1 (*FMR1*) gene on the X chromosome, resulting in a failure to express the fragile X mental retardation protein (FMRP), which is required for normal neural development. Depending on the length of the CGG repeat, an allele may be classified as normal (unaffected by the syndrome), a premutation (at risk of fragile X associated disorders), or full mutation (usually affected by the syndrome). A definitive diagnosis of fragile X syndrome is made through genetic testing to determine the number of CGG repeats. The mode of transmission is X-linked dominant.

There is currently no drug treatment that has shown benefit specifically for fragile X syndrome. However, medications are commonly used to treat symptoms of attention deficit and hyperactivity, anxiety, and aggression. Supportive management is important in optimizing functioning in individuals with fragile X syndrome, and may involve speech therapy, occupational therapy, and individualized educational and behavioral programs.

Neurology

B&D Ch. 40

Question 29. D. The signs and symptoms of Down's syndrome (trisomy 21) are characterized by the neotenization of the brain and body to the fetal state. Down's syndrome (DS) is characterized by decelerated maturation (neoteny), incomplete morphogenesis (vestigia) and atavisms. Individuals with Down's syndrome may have some or all of the following physical characteristics: microgenia (abnormally small chin), oblique eye fissures with epicanthic skin folds on the inner corner of the eyes (formerly known as a mongoloid fold), muscle hypotonia (poor muscle tone), a flat nasal bridge, a single palmar fold, a protruding tongue (due to small oral cavity, and an enlarged tongue near the tonsils) or macroglossia, "face is flat and broad", a short neck, white spots on the iris known as Brushfield spots, excessive joint laxity including atlantoaxial instability, excessive space between large toe and second toe, a single flexion furrow of the fifth finger, a higher number of ulnar loop dermatoglyphs and short fingers. They also tend to have a single palmar crease (also called a "simian crease" for its resemblance to that in apes and monkeys). Growth parameters such as height, weight, and head circumference are smaller in children with DS than with typical individuals of the same age. Adults with DS tend to have short stature and bowed legs – the average height for men is 5 feet 1 inch (154 cm) and for women is 4 feet 9 inches (144 cm). Individuals with DS are also at increased risk for obesity as they age and tend to be "round in shape". Individuals with trisomy 21 often develop early-onset Alzheimer's type dementia and die young from its complications. This occurs because the amyloid precursor protein gene is expressed on chromosome 21 which these patients possess in triplicate. Stunted growth and mental retardation are seen in virtually 100% of trisomy 21 patients. Small genitalia are seen in at least 75% of cases and in most cases these individuals are sterile.

Neurology

B&D Chs 40&66

Question 30. B. Answer choice B refers to Williams' syndrome. The syndrome is a result of an autosomal microdeletion on chromosome 7q11. Features of the disorder include cardiac valvular stenosis, hypotonia, hyperacusis, short stature and "elfin" facies, low nasal bridge, unusual ease with strangers and pleasant demeanor, developmental delay and strong language skills. Prevalence is 1 in 7500 to 20 000 births. The disorder has no known cure and is strongly associated with attention deficit–hyperactivity disorder.

The distracters in this question are described in greater detail in other questions in this volume. Trisomy 21 is of course, Down's syndrome. Deletion in chromosome 15q is Angelman syndrome. Deletion of 45 XO refers to Turner's syndrome. Klinefelter's syndrome is a result of an extra sex chromosome 47 XXY.

Neurology

B&D Ch. 7

Question 31. B.   Right unilateral placement of the electrodes in ECT has been shown to minimize cognitive impairment and memory deficits. If unilateral electrode placement fails to improve the patient's symptoms after four to six treatments the placement may be switched to bilateral, which can be more effective but carries a higher risk of side effects.

Diagnostic and Treatment Procedures in Psychiatry

K&S Ch. 36

Question 32. C.   Marfan's syndrome is an inherited autosomal dominant connective tissue disease associated with defects in fibrillin. Features include arachnodactyly, joint laxity, extreme limb length, pectus carinatum or excavatum, aortic valvular insufficiency and subluxation of the lens. Marfan's syndrome is also associated with dilatation of the aortic root and coarctation of the aorta, mitral valve prolapse and mitral annulus calcification with regurgitation. Dissection of the ascending aorta is also a possible occurrence, following from dilatation of the aortic root. Saccular intracranial aneurysms or carotid artery dissection are also possible. Patients with Marfan's syndrome are recommended to undergo annual echocardiogram screening and to avoid contact sports.

The other answer choices are all inherited disorders that present with either mental retardation, autistic features, or both, and they are explained in the answer material of other questions in this volume. Marfan's syndrome is not associated with either mental retardation or autism.

Neurology

B&D Ch. 51A

Question 33. A.   Lithium can prolong seizure activity during ECT and should be discontinued. Antipsychotics are fine during ECT, with the exception of clozapine which causes late appearing seizures during ECT. TCAs and MAOIs are fine to continue during ECT.

Diagnostic and Treatment Procedures in Psychiatry

K&S Ch. 36

Question 34. A.   The major features of tuberous sclerosis (TS) include facial angiofibromas or forehead plaque, nontraumatic ungual or periungual fibroma, hypomelanotic macules (ash leaf spots), shagreen patch, multiple retinal hamartomas, cortical tuber, subependymal nodule, subependymal giant astrocytoma, cardiac rhabdomyoma, lymphangiomyomatosis and renal angiomyolipoma. The predominant neurologic manifestations of TS are seizures, mental retardation and behavioral abnormalities. Seizures of various types occur in eighty to ninety percent of patients with TS. Tuberous sclerosis comes up quite a bit on standardized examinations and you should know the major features, imaging appearance and genetic facts of this disorder. These are reviewed in other questions in more detail.

Cutaneous and conjunctival telangiectasias are seen in the disorder known as ataxia–telangiectasia (AT). This is a neurodegenerative disorder that begins in childhood as slowly progressing ataxia. Later, other features develop, in particular, telangiectasias (small dilated blood vessels), immunodeficiency and sensitivity to ionizing radiation. The telangiectasias typically involve the earlobes, sclera, bridge of the nose and less commonly, the eyelids, necks, antecubital and popliteal fossae. AT is an autosomal recessive neurocutaneous disorder, affecting both sexes equally with a prevalence of 1 in 40 000 to 100 000. Nearly all patients with AT have elevated alphafetoprotein levels and about 80% have reduced serum IgA, IgE or IgG. The gene associated with AT is the large gene at chromosome 11q22-23. Approximately 10 to 15% of AT patients develop a lymphoid malignancy by early adulthood.

Neurology

B&D Ch. 65

Question 35. A.   Sublimation is a mature defense mechanism. Displacement and repression are neurotic defense mechanisms. Hypochondriasis and introjection are immature defense mechanisms. For your exam you must not only know what each defense mechanism is but also be able to say which are mature and which are immature.

Psychological Theory and Psychometric Testing

K&S Ch. 4

Question 36. D. Thalamic lesions are usually responsible for sensory deficits of cerebral origin. The thalamus receives its blood supply from the thalamoperforate branches of the posterior cerebral arteries. In some individuals, both thalami are supplied by one posterior cerebral artery, thus unilateral arterial occlusion may result in bilateral thalamic infarction. Thalamic pain syndrome sometimes results following thalamic sensory stroke. The pain is typically spontaneous and localized to the distal arm and leg and is exacerbated by contact and stress.

Neurology

B&D Ch. 28

Question 37. C. When a forensic psychiatrist is evaluating a case they are doing so for a third party, such as the court. As such there is no assumption of confidentiality the way there normally would be with a psychiatrist. The forensic psychiatrist should tell the patient this at the beginning of the interview. The information collected is expected to be shared with a third party and is not expected to remain confidential. If there is no confidentiality and no therapeutic alliance there is no doctor–patient relationship. Both evaluations should include a medication history and basic elements of the mental status exam and mini mental status exam such as memory, as would any complete psychiatric examination regardless of setting. Both evaluations will contain recommendations. ER recommendations will focus on the next step in treatment whereas forensic recommendations will focus on the particular legal issues being decided and the impact of the patient's illness upon those issues.

Forensics

K&S Ch. 58

Question 38. D. The typical EEG findings in Creutzfeldt–Jakob disease (CJD) are periodic sharp wave complexes (PSWCs) which may be preceded by less specific frontal intermittent rhythmical delta activity. These characteristic EEG abnormalities can be seen in about 70% of patients with CJD.

EEG findings in Alzheimer's dementia are dependent on timing. Early in disease course, the EEG may be normal, or show an alpha rhythm at or just below normal. As the disease progresses, generalized slowing ensues. Delirium is most often characterized by generalized slow wave activity on EEG. If triphasic waves are seen, these are indicative of a metabolic cause in an unresponsive patient. Previously, it was thought that these triphasic waves were diagnostic of hepatic encephalopathy, but other metabolic causes such as uremia, hypoxia, hyponatremia and hyperosmolarity can also produce this EEG abnormality. There are no particular classic EEG abnormalities associated directly with either Parkinson's disease or HIV-related dementia.

Neurology

B&D Chs 32A&66

Question 39. A. The classic triad of dementia, urinary incontinence and gait apraxia is the clinical picture of normal pressure hydrocephalus (NPH). The gait problems resemble those in Parkinson's disease, though they abate after gait is initiated. Cognitively, patients can present with deficits in speed of mental processing, decreased memory functioning, poor abstraction and difficulty with set-shifting tasks. Other common features include depression, hypersomnia, abulia and apathy. The gait disturbance and incontinence are believed to be a result of pressure on and distortion of descending white matter pathways. The cognitive symptoms are thought to be due to pressure on anterior cortical structures. Neuroimaging studies usually show ventricular enlargement of the lateral, third and fourth ventricles. Treatment of NPH is placement of a ventricular peritoneal shunt. Successful response to shunting ranges from 25 to 80% of cases. The other distracters in answers B through E are explained in detail in other questions in this volume.

Neurology

B&D Ch. 66

Question 40. B. The clinical picture here is that of the epidural hematoma. Notice that nowhere in this question is the phrase "epidural hematoma" mentioned. You are asked to extrapolate this from the data given. Epidural hematomas are located between the inner table of the skull and the dura. They typically occur when a skull fracture tears the middle meningeal artery or one of its branches. Epidural hematomas have a lens-shaped appearance and smooth inner border, because as they enlarge, they strip the dura away from the inner table of the skull. The classic clinical presentation is as described in this question: a brief loss of consciousness, followed by an intercurrent period of lucidity and then a later deterioration. Recall that damage to the bridging veins usually causes a subdural hematoma, which is often seen in alcoholics who have head injury that goes undetected. An intracranial aneurysmal rupture would present as a subarachnoid hemorrhage and "the worst headache of my life" scenario. Damage to the reticular activating system (in the brainstem) would likely cause unconsciousness and, if protracted, coma. Frontal lobe damage from traumatic brain injury, for example, can result in loss of executive functioning and planning ability, impulsivity, inappropriate behavior and mood swings.

Neurology

B&D Ch. 50B

Question 41. A. Because it is an often asked developmental milestone, it is good to know that pat-a-cake occurs for most children around 10 months.

Human Development

K&S Ch. 2

Question 42. E. This is a great question, because it takes you through the commonest CNS manifestations of AIDS. The best answer here is HIV-related dementia (AIDS-related dementia complex or ARDC). ARDC is the commonest complication of late untreated HIV disease. Early symptoms usually consist of problems with attention and concentration. Many patients have a slowness of thought (bradyphrenia). Complex tasks may become difficult to accomplish and may take longer due to these problems. Social withdrawal, apathy, depression and fatigue are all commonly seen in ARDC. There are generally psychomotor deficits noted as well. These can include gait incoordination and rigidity and slowness of gait. Fine and skilled hand and finger movements are affected early in the course of ARDC.

Diffuse cerebral atrophy is almost always seen on brain MRI and CT imaging in ARDC patients. In some patients, MRI may show nonspecific white matter abnormalities in the hemispheres and less commonly in the thalamus and basal ganglia. CSF examination in ARDC reveals mild mononuclear pleocytosis and mildly elevated protein in about 60% of cases. Specialized CSF studies may also reveal intrathecal IgG synthesis and a presence of oligoclonal bands. These findings are seen in other conditions such as multiple sclerosis and so their diagnostic value in ARDC is uncertain. Please note that the other four answer choices, A through D, are explained in other questions in this volume. Do study them, because they can and do appear on standardized examinations.

Neurology

B&D Ch. 53A

Question 43. B. The CYP450 2D6 enzyme has a long list of substrates. All of the choices listed in the question are substrates except bupropion, which is an inhibitor. Other inhibitors include citalopram, duloxetine (this is both a substrate and an inhibitor), escitalopram, fluoxetine, methadone, paroxetine, sertraline, and TCAs. Bupropion is a substrate of 2B6.

Psychopharmacology

K&S Ch. 3

Question 44. D. This is a simple question really, but some will find it tricky because it asks about the less common symptoms and signs of Parkinson's disease (PD). You can never study Parkinson's disease enough for standardized examinations in psychiatry. This topic comes up time and time again on neurology questions, because there is a strong overlap with behavioral and psychiatric presentation in this disorder. We've discussed the disorder in many questions in this book BUT we want to give you some of the essential bullet points now:

- Pathology = depigmentation and neuronal loss in the substantia nigra and presence of Lewy bodies and pale bodies
- Pathologic hallmark is dopaminergic underactivity in the striatum
- 60 to 85% of striatal dopamine and nigral neurons must be lost before symptoms of PD arise
- Prevalence is 100 to 200 per 100 000 population
- Cardinal features = resting tremor (4 to 7 Hz), rigidity, postural instability and bradykinesia

- Tremor is called "pill-rolling" as it resembles the rolling of the finger tips over a pill surface

- Festination, or a festinating gait, refers to the tendency of the patient to propulse involuntarily while standing or walking, or to retropulse and fall.

- Manifestations are usually asymmetrical early in the disease and become bilateral later on in the course

- Levodopa–carbidopa is the mainstay of therapy. Other important antiparkinsonian agents include dopamine agonists, monoamine oxidase inhibitors, anticholinergics.

Remember that alcoholic cerebellar atrophy presents with truncal ataxia for the most part, because the cerebellar vermis is preferentially affected. The vermis is responsible for truncal balance and smooth movement around the midline.

Neurology

B&D Ch. 71

Question 45. C. When compared to men, women have less alcohol dehydrogenase in their gut. As such men metabolize more alcohol in their gut leading to lower blood alcohol levels. Women have a lower body water content compared to men so that the alcohol is distributed in less water and is therefore more concentrated. The question said they both drank the same amount, so choice A is wrong. There is no evidence that Susan urinates more than Billy or that it can be assumed that a woman would urinate more than a man. The question stem says nothing about either of their weight so we can't make any assumptions. If you chose answer choices A, D, or E, you made assumptions about data that was not provided in the question stem. This is a common way that people get questions wrong. Never insert data into the question that the test writer didn't give you.

Substance Abuse

K&S Ch. 12

Question 46. B. Here we have another question that asks you to jump directly to appropriate management from symptom presentation only. The question bypasses asking you what the disease entity is, because that would clearly be too simple: temporal arteritis. Temporal arteritis (TA) is a vasculitis found in the elderly patient. If left undiagnosed and untreated it can frequently lead to permanent blindness. Headache is the most common symptom, experienced by about 72% of patients at some point during this condition and seen in one-third of patients on initial presentation. More than half of the patients with TA present concomitantly with polymyalgia rheumatica, which consists of aching in proximal and axial joints, proximal myalgias and often significant morning stiffness. Jaw claudication is a common associated symptom and presents initially in about 4% of patients with TA. Amaurosis fugax is one the most ominous symptoms as it evolves to partial or total blindness in 50% of cases, if left untreated. The most often recognized lab abnormality in TA is the erythrocyte sedimentation rate (ESR) which is elevated in most cases (85 ± 32 mm). Diagnosis is then confirmed by temporal artery biopsy. Nevertheless, it is essential to treat early, even before biopsy is done or results are known, with high-dose oral prednisone, to avoid the onset of irreversible visual loss. Prednisone should be initiated at 40 to 60 mg daily and maintained for at least 1 month before beginning a cautious taper.

Neurology

B&D Ch. 69

Question 47. B. Low levels of folate can lead to fatigue, agitation, delirium, dementia, psychosis, and paranoia. It is seen commonly in alcoholics. Low folate does not cause panic attacks.

Lab Tests in Psychiatry

K&S Ch. 10

Question 48. A. This is a simple question. Answer choices B through E are all preventative (prophylactic) treatments of migraines. Divalproex sodium and topiramate are both in fact FDA-approved for preventative therapy of migraine headache. Desipramine is of course a tricyclic antidepressant that is used off-label for neuropathic pain. It is also effective in the prevention of migraine and this is an off-label use, as well. Gabapentin is an anticonvulsant agent, FDA-approved for seizure and post-herpetic neuralgia. It too is used off-label for the prevention of migraine. The triptans, including sumatriptan, naratriptan, eletriptan, rizatriptan, are abortive agents for migraines. Their mechanism of action is as agonists at 5-HT1B and 5-HT1D receptors. These agents modulate the excitability of cells in the trigeminal nucleus caudalis (TNC), which receives input from the trigeminal nerve.

Neurology

B&D Ch. 69

Question 49. C.   This patient is clearly hypothyroid. If you miss that fact and treat the depression and not the thyroid you will get the question wrong and mistreat the patient. Symptoms of hypothyroidism include depression, weakness, stiffness, poor appetite, constipation, menstrual irregularities, slowed speech, apathy, impaired memory, hallucinations, or delusions. This is a very common test question. Make sure you get it right when it shows up on an exam near you!

Somatic Symptom Disorders

K&S Ch. 10

Question 50. E.   Rupture of an intracranial aneurysm or AVM results in a subarachnoid hemorrhage, which may extend into the brain parenchyma. The headache associated with this bleed is usually sudden in onset and explosive. It's often described by patients as "the worst headache of my life." The headache is often accompanied by vomiting. Hydrocephalus may develop, resulting from intraventricular blood that distorts the midline structures. Noncontrast head CT confirms the diagnosis by revealing blood in the subarachnoid cisterns or in the parenchyma. If CT confirms the presence of blood in the subarachnoid spaces, lumbar puncture should be avoided to prevent a possible herniation or further bleeding. Subarachnoid hemorrhage generally indicates the need for cerebral angiography. Note that 80 to 85% of aneurysms arise from the arteries of the anterior circulation: the anterior communicating artery, posterior communicating artery or middle cerebral artery. In contrast, 15 to 20% of aneurysms arise from the posterior circulation. The majority of these aneurysms are found at the bifurcation of the basilar artery or at the origin of the posterior inferior cerebellar artery on the vertebral artery.

Neurology

B&D Chs 49,51C&69

Question 51. C.   Damage to the medial longitudinal fasciculus (MLF) between the third and sixth cranial nerve nuclei interrupts transmission of neural impulses to the ipsilateral medial rectus muscle. Adducting saccades of the ipsilateral eye are impaired. The nystagmus-like movement of the typical abduction is in fact overshoot dysmetria. Upward-beating and torsional nystagmus are often present. The classic cause of this lesion is a demyelinating lesion of the brainstem in multiple sclerosis. There are many other possible causes of internuclear ophthalmoplegia (INO). These include pontine stroke, intrinsic tumor, drug intoxication, and chemotherapy with radiation therapy. INO can be caused by myasthenia gravis and progressive supranuclear palsy, but certainly less often than in multiple sclerosis.

Neurology

B&D Ch. 36

Question 52. D.   When focal injury to myelin arises, conduction along the affected nerve fibers may alter. This can result in conduction slowing or conduction block along the nerve fibers. This conduction defect can be seen on nerve conduction studies. More than 50% decrement of both the compound muscle action potential (CMAP) amplitude and area across the lesion usually is the criterion for definite conduction block.

Fibrillation potentials are the electrophysiological markers of muscle denervation. These are elicited on needle electromyographic (EMG) studies and are usually seen with positive sharp waves. Based on their distribution, they are useful in localizing lesions to the anterior horn cells of the spinal cord, ventral root, plexus, or peripheral nerve. Positive sharp waves may appear within 2 weeks of acute denervation; however, fibrillation potentials do not become full until about 3 weeks after axonal loss.

After acute focal axonal damage, the distal nerve segment undergoes Wallerian degeneration. Nerve conduction studies classically demonstrate unelicitable or low CMAP amplitudes. Decremental response to slow repetitive stimulation is a hallmark of postsynaptic neuromuscular junction disorders like myasthenia gravis.

Neurology

B&D Ch. 32B

Question 53. B.   Signs of cannabis intoxication include conjunctival injection, increased appetite, dry mouth, and tachycardia. Impaired motor coordination, euphoria, anxiety, sensation of slowed time, impaired judgment, and social withdrawal may also be found. Diuresis is not one of the side effects.

Substance Abuse and Addictive Disorders

K&S Ch. 12

Question 54. C.   Huntington's disease (HD) is an autosomal dominant neurodegenerative disorder characterized by progressive movement disorder associated with psychiatric and cognitive decline, culminating in a terminal state of dementia and immobility. Prevalence is about 10 per 100 000. HD usually begins between ages 30 and 55 years. About 60% of patients present initially with motor signs, about 15% with behavioral signs and about 25% with both motor and behavioral signs. A change in the ability to generate saccadic eye movements and their speed is often the earliest sign. Eventually, a blink or head thrust may be required to initiate saccadic eye movements. The motor disorder usually begins with clumsiness and fidgetiness that evolves into chorea. In addition to chorea, HD patients have bradykinesia and motor impersistence, with difficulty sustaining ongoing movement. The gait often resembles a marionette, lurching, swaying, dipping and bobbing. Dysarthria and dysphagia progressively impair communication and nutrition. Mean survival is 17 years. Most patients wind up wheelchair or bedbound and perish from complications that include pneumonia and head injury. HD is dominantly inherited and caused by an unstable expanded CAG trinucleotide repeat in exon 1 of the HD gene on the tip of the short arm of chromosome 4. Essentially all patients with 40 or more CAG repeats in the HD gene will develop the clinical illness. The direct DNA test for the CAG repeat expansion in the *huntingtin* (*HD*) gene, formerly called *IT15*, is highly sensitive and specific. The pathology of HD includes prominent neuronal loss and gliosis in the caudate nucleus and putamen, along with regional and more diffuse atrophy. No treatment has yet been proven to improve disease progression. The use of tetrabenazine has been found to be effective in reducing chorea in HD patients and is now FDA-approved and available in the USA for this labeled use.

Neurology

B&D Ch. 71

Question 55. C.   Carbamazepine will interact with all of the drugs listed in this question. Erythromycin will increase carbamazepine levels. Phenobarbital and theophylline will decrease carbamazepine levels. Carbamazepine will decrease doxycycline and cyclosporine levels.

Psychopharmacology

K&S Ch. 36

Question 56. C.   Extracranial vertebral artery dissection presents with high cervical pain sometimes radiating to the occipital region, as well as posterior circulation transient ischemic attacks (TIAs) or stroke. Vertebral artery dissection can occur spontaneously, but most commonly, it is due to trauma, which can be dramatic (cervical fractures and dislocation) or subtle (abrupt turning of the neck, chiropractic manipulation, or simple hyperextension of the neck such as sometimes used for shaving under the chin). Anticoagulation is the mainstay of treatment for extracranial vertebral dissection, when there is ischemic symptomatology. The results are usually favorable, unless the patient already has a fixed deficit.

Pain in the arm can result from damage to the brachial plexus. Infiltrative or inflammatory lesions of the brachial plexus produce severe brachialgia, with pain radiating down the arm and spreading into the shoulder region. Radiation to the ulnar two fingers suggests origin in the lower brachial plexus, and radiation to the upper arm, forearm, and thumb suggests an upper brachial plexopathy. Causes of brachial plexopathy include traction and heavy impact. Sporting injuries in bicycling, football, snowmobiling, skiing, and horseback riding can all cause plexus injury. Rucksack paralysis is another form of brachial plexus injury from the traction and pressure on the brachial plexus exerted by heavy backpack straps to the shoulders. Other plexus injuries can be caused by metastatic disease or radiation-induced injury in the cancer patient.

Sacroiliac joint syndrome is a major source of low back pain. Pain can present on one side of the lower back and radiate down to the hip or thigh. Pain often worsens upon walking up stairs. Patrick's test or single leg standing test often exacerbates the pain. NSAIDs are first-line therapy in patients with joint inflammation. Sacroiliac joint corticosteroid injection can provide temporary pain relief.

Anterior spinal artery syndrome results in spinal cord infarction and has been seen more frequently because of increased numbers of invasive surgical procedures, such as vascular and thoracoabdominal surgeries. The anterior horns and anterolateral tracts are affected (corticospinal tract involvement below the level of the lesion), resulting in loss of bowel and bladder control and sexual dysfunction. A sensory deficit develops, sparing the posterior columns, involving only the spinothalamic tracts. Spinal shock with areflexia is expected initially, followed by later onset of spasticity.

Neurology

B&D Chs 24,29,44&46

Question 57. A.   Bell's palsy is a self-limited, monophasic facial nerve palsy of acute or subacute onset. In 60% of patients, pain accompanies the facial weakness, impaired lacrimation in 60%, taste changes in 30 to 50% and hyperacusis in 15 to 30%. MRI of the internal auditory canal often demonstrates enhancement of the facial nerve, most often at the geniculate ganglion. Eighty five percent of patients recover normal facial function within 3 weeks. Bell's palsy occurs with increased frequency during pregnancy and is associated with a poorer recovery rate. Residual abnormalities after Bell's palsy occur in 12% of patients, persistent severe facial weakness in 4%, and synkinetic contraction and twitching of the upper and lower facial muscles in 17%. Aberrant regeneration involving the lacrimal gland may lead to tearing with facial muscle contraction (syndrome of "crocodile tears"), particularly during eating. The finding of spontaneous fibrillation in facial muscles on EMG 10 to 14 days after onset of facial weakness is a predictor of poor outcome. Bell's palsy can be recurrent, but in these cases other causes such as Lyme disease or sarcoidosis must be considered. Bilateral facial palsy is also common with acute inflammatory demyelinating polyneuropathy. Bell's palsy is considered to be idiopathic, but herpes simplex virus and varicella zoster virus reactivation in the geniculate ganglion have been implicated in its pathogenesis. Early administration of corticosteroids and acyclovir is common practice and may enhance recovery.

The classic triad of Horner's syndrome from sympathetic dysfunction is that of ipsilateral ptosis, miosis and facial anhidrosis. Later medullary syndrome (Wallenberg's syndrome) typically results from occlusion of the posterior inferior cerebellar artery and produces sensory loss on the ipsilateral face, from trigeminal involvement, plus loss of pain and temperature sensation from the contralateral body, from damage to the ascending spinothalamic tract. Motor findings include ipsilateral cerebellar ataxia, bulbar weakness resulting in dysarthria and dysphagia, and Horner's syndrome.

Neurology

B&D Chs 16,28&70

Question 58. E.   The pain of postherpetic neuralgia (PHN), described as continuous deep aching, burning sharp, stabbing, and shooting, and triggered by light touch over the affected dermatomes, is often debilitating and difficult to treat. Tricyclics (amitriptyline or desipramine), selective serotonin reuptake inhibitors (sertraline or nefazodone hydrochloride), anticonvulsants (carbamazepine and gabapentin), oral opioids (oxycodone), and topical capsaicin cream or lidocaine patches are helpful in about 50% of patients. Note that gabapentin is the best answer to this question because it is specifically FDA-approved for PHN and carbamazepine and desipramine are used off-label.

PHN occurs in anywhere from 8 to 70% of patients following herpes zoster (the shingles, which is varicella-zoster virus reactivation of the dorsal root ganglion). Herpes zoster is characterized by sharp or burning radicular pain sometimes associated with fever, malaise and rash. The cutaneous eruption begins as an erythematous maculopapular rash and progresses to grouped clear vesicles that continue to form for 3 to 5 days. These become pustules by 3 to 4 days and form crusts by 10 days. Pain usually disappears as the vesicles fade.

Neurology

B&D Ch. 75

Question 59. B.   Carbon monoxide exposure occurs mainly in miners, gas workers, and garage employees. Other exposures occur with poorly ventilated home heating systems, stoves and suicide attempts. The neurotoxic effects of carbon monoxide relate to intracellular hypoxia. Carbon monoxide binds to hemoglobin with high affinity to form carboxyhemoglobin. Acute toxicity leads to headache, disturbances of consciousness and other behavioral changes. Motor abnormalities can occur with pyramidal and extrapyramidal deficits. Seizures may occur and focal cortical deficits sometimes develop. Pathological examination shows hypoxic and ischemic damage in the cerebral cortex as well as in the hippocampus, cerebellar cortex, and basal ganglia. Lesions are also present diffusely in the cerebral white matter.

Neurology

B&D Ch. 58

Question 60. D. In approximately 80% of patients with stiff-person syndrome, the disorder develops as non-paraneoplastic phenomenon in association with diabetes and polyendocrinopathy and, often, antibodies to glutamic acid decarboxylase. Characteristic of stiff-person syndrome is fluctuating rigidity of the axial musculature with superimposed spasms. Muscle stiffness primarily affects the lower trunk and legs, but it can extend to the arms, shoulders and neck. The usual precipitating factors of muscle spasms are emotional upset and auditory or somesthetic stimuli. The rigidity disappears during sleep and after local or general anesthesia. The paraneoplastic form of stiff-person syndrome is usually associated with breast and lung cancers and Hodgkin's disease. The main autoantigen of the paraneoplastic form of stiff-person syndrome is amphiphysin. Treatment of the tumor and the use of corticosteroids may improve paraneoplastic stiff-person syndrome. IVIg is useful in patients with non-paraneoplastic stiff-person syndrome. GABA-enhancing agents, such as benzodiazepines, gabapentin, and baclofen, provide symptomatic relief.

Neurology

B&D Ch. 52G

Question 61. B. Mirtazapine has 5-HT3 receptor antagonism which is thought to be responsible for its antinausea effect. This same receptor antagonism is responsible for the antinausea properties of ondansetron.

Psychopharmacology

K&S Ch. 36

Question 62. D. The clinical manifestations of a medulloblastoma, located in the fourth ventricle, are the result of increased intracranial pressure (ICP) and obstructive hydrocephalus. Headache is the most common initial symptom and usually precedes diagnosis by 4 to 8 weeks. Intractable nausea and vomiting occur frequently, characteristically in the morning. Personality changes, namely irritability, are an early feature. Lethargy, diplopia, head tilt and truncal ataxia are other features that can help lead to diagnosis. Common signs on physical examination are papilledema, ataxia, dysmetria, and cranial nerve involvement. Abducens nerve palsy, secondary to increased ICP, is a cause of diplopia and head tilt. Torticollis can be a sign of cerebellar tonsil herniation.

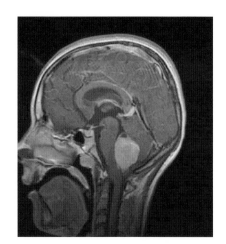

Neurology

B&D Ch. 52E

Question 63. D. In 50% of families where a child dies, parental divorce follows.

Depressive Disorders

K&S Ch. 28

Question 64. B. For the individual to be rendered unconscious by a traumatic brain lesion, either the reticular activating system must be involved or diffuse injury to both hemispheres. The functioning of the awake mind requires the ascending inputs referred to as the reticular activating system, with its way stations in the brainstem and thalamus, as well as an intact cerebral cortex. Bilateral lesions of the brainstem or the thalamus produce coma. Very diffuse lesions of the hemispheres produce an "awake" patient who shows no responsiveness to the environment, a state sometimes called *coma vigil* or *persistent vegetative state*, as in the recent Terry Schiavo case. Patients with very slight responses to environmental stimuli are said to be in a *minimally conscious state*.

Neurology

B&D Ch. 6

Question 65. B. Neuroimaging of schizophrenics demonstrates increased size of the lateral ventricles. PET scan and fMRI of schizophrenics will show decreased metabolic activity in the frontal lobes. Know these facts for your exam.

Laboratory Tests in Psychiatry

K&S Ch. 13

Question 66. A. Symptoms of cervical radiculopathy often appear suddenly. Acute trauma is often the cause of nerve root contusion or disk herniation that results in cervical radiculopathy. In patients younger than age 45, disk herniation is more likely to be the cause. With increasing age, degenerative changes resulting in neural foraminal stenosis are more likely to be the causative factors. Pain is usually in the neck with radiation to an arm. Headache may also be a symptom. The C5, C6, and C7 roots are the ones most commonly involved in cervical spondylosis, because they are at the level of greatest mobility. Lesions at the C4–C5 level affect the C5 root, causing pain, paresthesias and sometimes loss of sensation over the shoulder, with weakness of the deltoid, biceps, and brachioradialis muscles. The biceps and supinator reflexes may be lost. Lesions at the C5–C6 level affect the C6 root and cause paresthesias in the thumb or lateral distal forearm and weakness in the brachioradialis, biceps or triceps. The biceps and brachioradialis reflexes may be diminished or inverted. Lesions at the level of C6–C7 affect the C7 root and cause paresthesias, usually in the index, middle or ring fingers, and weakness in C7-innervated muscles, such as the triceps and pronators. The triceps tendon reflex may be diminished. Remember that myelopathy (compromise of the spinal cord) generally causes hyperreflexia and not diminished or absent reflexes, particularly early on in the course of the condition.

Typical findings in cervical myelopathy are a combination of leg spasticity, upper extremity weakness or clumsiness, and sensory changes in the arms, legs or trunk. Some patients experience leg or trunk paresthesia induced by neck flexion (Lhermitte's sign).

Neurology

B&D Ch. 73

Question 67. C. Narcolepsy consists of irresistible attacks of sleep that occur daily for at least 3 months. They involve cataplexy (loss of muscle tone during attacks often associated with strong emotion) and REM sleep during episodes often leading to hypnopompic or hypnagogic hallucinations and sleep paralysis. Catalepsy is also known as waxy flexibility and is seen in catatonic schizophrenia.

Sleep Wake Disorders

K&S Ch. 24

Question 68. C. Subacute combined degeneration (SCD) refers to the combination of spinal cord and peripheral nerve pathology associated with vitamin B12 (cobalamin) deficiency. Patients often complain of unsteady gait and distal paresthesias. The neurologic examination may demonstrate evidence of posterior column, pyramidal tract and peripheral nerve involvement. Cognitive, behavioral and psychiatric manifestations can also occur. Personality change, cognitive dysfunction, mania, depression and psychosis, have all been reported. Dementia is often comorbid with cobalamin deficiency; however the causative association is unclear. Cobalamin deficiency-associated cognitive impairment is more likely to improve when impairment is mild and of short duration.

Neurology

B&D Ch. 9

Question 69. D. Extensor plantar responses (Babinski signs) are indicative of a lesion of the corticospinal tracts i.e. upper motor neuron involvement. The other four answers are clearly cardinal features of a dementia of the Alzheimer type. Alzheimer's dementia does not typically involve lesions to the descending motor tracts, unless some other ischemic or hemorrhagic process is accompanying the dementia. That is not to say that vascular dementia does not present with aphasia, apraxia, agnosia or memory loss. Vascular dementia (or multi-infarct dementia as it was formerly called) typically includes a history of clinical strokes with focal neurological signs and symptoms and "stepwise" cognitive decline. Epidemiological studies find that the prevalence of vascular dementia ranges from 3 to 21%. In autopsy studies of late-life dementia, 15 to 20% of the patients are reported to have had vascular dementia.

Neurology

B&D Ch. 66

Question 70. A.   This scan and the question vignette are indicative of a frontotemporal dementia (FTD), one of which is Pick's disease. The scan demonstrates classic preferential atrophy of the frontal and temporal lobes with occipitoparietal sparing. This kind of imaging finding is known as "knife-edge" atrophy of the frontal and temporal lobes and was characterized histologically by ballooned cells and intraneuronal inclusions (Pick cells and Pick bodies). Criteria focus on loss of insight, easy distractibility, reduced concern or empathy for others, emotional lability or withdrawal, impulsiveness, poor self-care, perseveration, features of the Klüver–Bucy syndrome, and diminished verbal output. There is a second type of presentation of FTD, which is characterized by early and progressive change in language, with problems of expression of language or severe naming difficulty and problems with word meaning. Males and females are affected

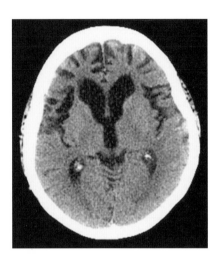

equally. Mean duration of illness is approximately 8 years, with a range from 2 to 15 years. FTD makes up 10–15% of the neurodegenerative dementias in clinical autopsy series.

Neurology

B&D Ch. 66

Question 71. A.   The potassium-sensitive periodic paralysis and myotonias are associated with mutations in the α-subunit of the sodium channel; the gene is located on chromosome 17q. Inheritance of potassium-sensitive periodic paralysis is autosomal dominant, with strong penetrance and involvement of both sexes. Symptom onset occurs in infancy or early childhood. An infant may cry in an altered or unusual manner, or may be found lying quietly in the crib. The first attack often occurs during the first few weeks of school because of the enforced sitting. The predominant symptom is weakness provoked by potassium exposure. Myotonia may be present, but the overwhelming difficulty is recurrent bouts of paralysis. Many patients have two kinds of attacks, light and heavy. A light attack is characterized by fatigue and mild weakness usually dissipates in under an hour. A heavy attack, in contrast, may be associated with more severe paralysis, during which the patient may not be able to rise from a chair or a bed. The frequency can vary from two or three mild attacks a day to episodes months apart.

Neurology

B&D Ch. 79

Question 72. C.   CSF findings on their own cannot make or exclude the diagnosis of MS. The CSF is grossly normal in MS, being clear, colorless and under normal pressure. Total leukocyte count is normal in two thirds of patients. CSF protein (or albumin) level is normal in the majority of patients with MS. Albumin levels are elevated in only 20–30% of patients. A common finding in MS is an elevation of CSF immunoglobulin levels. The increase is predominantly IgG, but the synthesis of IgA and IgM is also increased. Oligoclonal bands (OCBs) have been found in 85 to 95% of patients with clinically definite MS. The presence of OCBs in monosymptomatic patients predicts a significantly higher rate of progression to MS than the absence of bands: 25% versus 9% at 3 years' follow-up. The pattern of banding remains relatively consistent in individual patients during the disease course, though bands may be added over time.

Neurology

B&D Ch. 54

Question 73. B.   Mirtazapine works via alpha 2 antagonism on the presynaptic neuron. This blocks a feedback loop causing more serotonin and norepinephrine to be released into the synaptic cleft.

Psychopharmacology

K&S Ch. 36

Question 74. B.   Cluster headache is classified by at least five repeated attacks that are severe or very severe unilateral, orbital, supraorbital and/or temporal pain lasting 15 to 180 minutes if left untreated. The headache must be accompanied by one of the following: ipsilateral conjunctival injection or lacrimation; ipsilateral nasal congestion and/or rhinorrhea; ipsilateral eyelid edema; ipsilateral forehead and facial swelling; ipsilateral miosis and/or ptosis; a sense of restlessness or agitation. Attacks have a frequency from one every other day to eight per day. Cluster headache is predominantly a disease of men. Onset typically begins in the third decade of life. Periodicity is a cardinal feature of cluster headache. The first cluster of attacks tends to last, on average, for 6 to 12 weeks and is followed by a remission period that lasts from months to years.

The pain is strictly unilateral and almost always remains on the same side of the head from cluster to cluster. The pain is felt generally in the retro-orbital and temporal regions (upper syndrome) but may be maximal in the jaw or cheek (lower syndrome). It is often described as being boring or stabbing in nature, like a hot poker going through the eye or poking the eye. During the episode, patients tend to avoid the recumbent position because lying down tends to exacerbate the pain.

The pathogenesis of cluster headache is not entirely understood. The pain is likely mediated by the activation of trigeminal nerve pathways and the autonomic symptoms are due to parasympathetic outflow and sympathetic dysfunction. The periodicity suggests a defect in CNS cycling mechanisms that is likely related to hypothalamic dysfunction.

Acute symptomatic therapy is best accomplished by administering of oxygen, subcutaneous sumatriptan, and subcutaneous or intramuscular DHE. Oxygen delivered at a flow rate of 8 to 10 L/min via a nonrebreathing face mask can be dramatically effective for aborting a cluster attack. Methysergide is utilized as maintenance prevention of cluster attacks. It is dosed from 4 to 10 mg per day and prevents cluster headache in about 60% of patients. Typically, NSAIDs, butalbital combination preparations, and oral narcotics are not particularly effective in aborting cluster attacks.

Neurology

B&D Ch. 69

Question 75. A.   Hemicrania continua is characterized by a continuous unilateral headache of moderate intensity. The female to male ratio is about 2 to 1 and the average age of onset is 28 years. The disorder is usually continuous and unremitting; however, in certain cases it can resemble a prolonged unilateral migraine attack of several days to weeks in duration, with headache-free remissions. The continuous headache is typically punctuated by painful unilateral exacerbations lasting twenty minutes to several days. These periods of increased pain intensity are accompanied by one or more autonomic features. Primary stabbing headache ("ice-pick headache") is often a feature of this disorder, usually on the ipsilateral side, and usually during a period of exacerbation. Hemicrania continua patients respond completely to prophylactic indomethacin. Cases of hemicrania continua have been reported that have not recurred after stopping indomethacin. It is therefore reasonable to withdraw treatment periodically. Other agents that may produce a response include: methysergide, acetaminophen with caffeine, lamotrigine, gabapentin, topiramate, verapamil, melatonin, dihydroergotamine, corticosteroids, and lithium.

Neurology

B&D Ch. 69

Question 76. D.   Lacunar infarcts are small ischemic infarctions in the deep regions of the brain or brainstem that range in diameter from 0.5 to 15.0 mm. Lacunes usually occur in patients with longstanding arterial hypertension, current cigarette smoking and diabetes mellitus. The most frequent sites of involvement are the putamen, basis pontis, thalamus, posterior limb of the internal capsule and the caudate nucleus. Multiple lacunar infarcts are strongly associated with arterial hypertension and diabetes mellitus. Studies indicate that arterial hypertension leads to microvascular changes characterized by fibrinoid angiopathy, lipohyalinosis, and microaneurysm formation. Control of hypertension, prevention of microangiopathy, and use of platelet antiaggregants are essential in the management of patients with lacunar infarcts.

Neurology

B&D Ch. 51A

Question 77. C.   The Dandy–Walker malformation consists of a ballooning of the posterior half of the fourth ventricle, often but not always associated with nonopening of the foramen of Magendie. In addition, the posterior cerebellar vermis is aplastic, and there may be heterotopia of the inferior olivary nuclei, pachygyria of the cerebral cortex, and other cerebral and sometimes visceral anomalies. Obstructive hydrocephalus usually ensues, but if treated promptly, the prognosis may be good. Neurological handicaps, such as spastic diplegia and mental retardation, probably relate more to the associated malformations of the brain than to the hydrocephalus.

Chiari malformations involve a displacement of the tonsils and posterior vermis of the cerebellum through the foramen magnum, compressing the spinomedullary junction. The simple form is termed Chiari type I malformation. Type II involves an additional downward displacement of a distorted lower medulla and dysplasia of medullary nuclei and is a constant feature of lumbosacral meningomyelocele. Chiari type III malformation is actually a cervical spina bifida with cerebellar encephalocele.

Anencephaly is a failure of the closing of the anterior neuropore at 24 days' gestation. Death in utero occurs in approximately 7% of anencephalic pregnancies, 34% are born prematurely and 53% at term. Stillbirth occurs in 20% of these deliveries. The prenatal diagnosis of anencephaly is by examination of amniotic fluid for elevation of alpha-fetoprotein and confirmation is by sonographic imaging as early as 12 weeks' gestation.

Neurology

B&D Ch. 60

Question 78. A.   Prader–Willi syndrome (PWS) is a genetically defined mental retardation syndrome. It is caused by a deletion on chromosome 15q11–q13. If the individual inherits the deletion from a maternal chromosome 15, the result is Angelman's syndrome; if the mutation is on a paternal chromosome 15, the result is PWS. Mean IQ range in PWS is 70, with a spectrum ranging from profound mental retardation to average intelligence. Language function is impaired by oromotor dysfunction. PWS patients have a knack for doing jigsaw puzzles and demonstrate good visuospatial strength. Executive functioning is impaired and characterized by obsessive skin picking. There is a high likelihood of autism in PWS patients. Social functioning is often impaired by the internalizing and externalizing of problems, as well as by ADHD. With maternal uniparental disomy, psychosis and aggressive behaviors can be seen in young adults with PWS. Hypothalamic dysfunction in PWS results in overeating behavior leading to truncal obesity in many patients. The other four answer choices to this question are also genetically defined mental retardation syndromes. Explanations of these can be found in other questions in this volume.

Neurology

B&D Ch. 61

Question 79. C. Creutzfeldt–Jakob disease (CJD) is a rapidly progressive spongiform degeneration of the brain secondary to the accumulation of misfolded prion proteins. Three other human prion diseases have been described: kuru (in New Guinea), Gerstmann–Straussler–Scheinker syndrome , and fatal familial insomnia. Because these diseases are now believed to be caused by a "proteinaceous infectious particle", they are often referred to as prion diseases. Do read up on these other prion diseases; they do appear once in a while on board-style examinations. CJD affects men and women equally and typically manifests in late middle age. Peak incidence is in the 55–70-year age group. Symptoms can appear gradually over a period of weeks, or more suddenly. Approximately one-third of patients exhibit mental deterioration, one-third exhibit physical disabilities (especially incoordination), and another third exhibit mixed mental and physical abnormalities. Memory loss, accompanied by either cerebellar or visual–oculomotor signs are frequent at the disease onset. As the illness evolves, these symptoms are joined by pyramidal and extrapyramidal signs and a variety of involuntary movements, especially myoclonus. A small number of patients present with sleep and autonomic disorders that mimic familial fatal insomnia. Progressive mental deterioration terminates in mutism and global dementia. Death commonly occurs within 6 months of disease onset. Three laboratory tests are used to aid the diagnosis: EEG, CSF analysis, and brain MRI. In its most pathognomonic form, when the disease is fulminant, the EEG reveals a one- or two-cycle per second slow-wave triphasic spiking activity. The CSF is analyzed in two ways: for 14-3-3 protein kinase inhibitor and for tau protein. The presence of elevated levels of either one of these two markers has a sensitivity and specificity for CJD in the 90% range. Finally, in sporadic disease, the MRI may reveal a symmetrical or sometimes unilateral hyperintense signal in the basal ganglia. The other distractors are discussed elsewhere in other questions in this volume. Please do study them as well; they do pop up on standardized tests a great deal.

Neurology

B&D Ch. 66

Question 80. D. The JC virus is a polyomavirus and is ubiquitous; up to 85% of individuals have antibodies to the virus by age 9 years. The JC virus is the etiological agent of progressive multifocal leukoencephalopathy (PML). The kidneys are thought to be the site of latent JC viral persistence. Reactivation of the virus associated with immunosuppression results in hematogenous spread of the virus to the brain. Foci of PML are frequently located in proximity to blood vessels. PML occurs in patients with impaired cell-mediated immunity such as those with AIDS, chronic lymphocytic leukemia, Hodgkin's disease, other lymphomas, sarcoidosis, organ transplantation, and lupus. The JC virus preferentially infects myelin-producing oligodendrocytes, resulting in cell lysis and demyelination. Focal neurologic deficits, seizure activity and cognitive impairment characterized by memory impairment, psychomotor retardation, and inattentiveness characterize the clinical presentation of PML. There is no proven therapy for PML, but clinical trials are ongoing. The average length of survival from the onset of symptoms to death is 1 to 4 months, but a small percentage of patients reportedly have improved spontaneously and survived for several years.

The etiologic agent responsible for CNS lymphoma is Epstein–Barr virus (EBV). EBV is detectable from a majority of primary CNS lymphomas in AIDS patients and to a lesser degree from primary CNS lymphomas in immunocompetent individuals. The clinical presentation is that of progressive personality changes, seizures, and signs of increased intracranial pressure. The other answer choices to this question are discussed in greater detail elsewhere in this volume. Do study all of these CNS manifestations of HIV, because you are likely to come upon these questions on your board-style examination.

Neurology

B&D Ch. 53B

Question 81. B. The major morbidity associated with idiopathic intracranial hypertension (aka pseudotumor cerebri), is visual loss related to optic nerve dysfunction. Patients should satisfy the modified Dandy's criteria: (1) signs and symptoms due to increased intracranial pressure; (2) a normal result on neurological examination except for an abducens palsy; (3) neuroimaging excluding a mass lesion or other cause of elevated intracranial pressure; and (4) normal CSF parameters, except an elevated opening pressure (>250 mmH$_2$O). Patients are usually young, obese females who may complain of headache, transient visual obscurations (seconds), pulsatile intracranial noises, or double vision. Almost uniformly, patients have papilledema. Typically, visual acuity and color are preserved, but optic nerve-related visual field defects, which are best detected with computerized threshold perimetry, are present in more than 90% of patients and include enlarged blind spots, generalized constriction, and inferior nasal field loss. Hypervitaminosis A is one of many purported causes of idiopathic intracranial hypertension. Treatment involves reducing intracranial pressure. Acetazolamide is an inhibitor of carbonic anhydrase that lowers CSF production and pressure. It is given in a dose of 250 mg twice daily, which can be increased to 1 g/day. Some patients undergo repeated lumbar punctures with CSF removal to maintain lower CSF pressures. If vision is threatened, surgery is usually contemplated. Lumboperitoneal shunting and optic nerve sheath fenestration are the procedures of choice, although the latter has not been proven beneficial in follow-up studies.

Neurology

B&D Ch. 59

Question 82. A. Here is yet another look at Piaget's theory of development. This material comes up very frequently on standardized tests so it is imperative to study and memorize. The developmental stage of concrete operations refers to ages 7 to 11 years. During this period, children are able to act on real, concrete and perceivable objects and events that surround them. Egocentric thought (characteristic of the stage of preoperational thought), is replaced by operational thought. Children gain the ability to see things from other people's perspectives. *Conservation* and *reversibility* are the two abilities that children demonstrate in the stage of concrete operations. Conservation refers to the ability to recognize that although the shape of objects may change, the objects still maintain or conserve characteristics that enable them to be recognized as the same. Reversibility is the ability to understand the relation between things, that one thing can turn into another and then back again.

Human Development

K&S Ch. 4

Question 83. C. Men do not lose their sex drive as they age, unless there are specific physical and/or psychological factors underlying this problem. As is the case with women, lack of desire in men can be of either physical or psychological origin.

Physical causes:

- Alcoholism – quite common. Tobacco use: frequent and its role is underestimated in loss of sexual drive
- Abuse of drugs such as cocaine
- Obesity – quite common; slimming down will often help
- Anemia – unusual, unless the man has been bleeding for any reason
- Hyperprolactinemia – a rare disorder where the pituitary gland produces too much of the hormone prolactin
- Prescribed drugs – particularly Proscar, a tablet used for prostate problems
- Low testosterone level – contrary to what many people think, this is rare, except in cases where some injury or illness has affected the testicles
- Any major disease such as diabetes

Psychological causes:

- Depression – very common
- Stress and overwork
- Hang-ups from childhood
- Latent homosexuality
- Serious relationship problems with your partner

Sexual desire has been described as a "longing for sexual union", it associates with certain behaviors that are more linked to arousal and states of fear, concern and enhanced attention to others, and sexual cue displays such as lip biting and touching. In keeping with the correlation between sexual desire and arousal, sexual desire is mediated by gonadal estrogens and androgens.

Enhanced focus, concern and attention toward the desired other has not only been associated with increased arousal by means of testosterone, but also with elevated concentrations of central dopamine and norepinephrine, and decreased levels of central serotonin. Other forms of physiological arousal associated with enhanced levels of dopamine include increased energy, exhilaration, euphoria, sleeplessness, loss of appetite, trembling, pounding heartbeat, and accelerated breathing. This same increased arousal is also a feature of attraction, and is the suggested cause of feelings of exhilaration, ecstasy, intrusive thinking about the love object, regarding them as unique, and a craving for emotional union with this partner or potential partner.

Human development

K&S Ch. 21

Question 84. D.   Attachment theory was first set forth by John Bowlby, a British psychoanalyst. Attachment is defined as the emotional tone between children and caregivers, manifested by the infant's seeking and clinging to the caregiver closely, such as the mother. It is well-accepted that a person's psychological health and sense of well-being depend to a great extent on the quality of relationships and attachments to others, particularly those attachments that were laid down in childhood with caregivers. People with a secure attachment style are highly invested in relationships and tend to behave without much possessiveness or fear of rejection.

Human Development

K&S Ch. 4

Question 85. E.   Heinz Kohut, an Austrian-born American psychoanalyst was best known for his development of self psychology, an influential school of thought within psychodynamic/psychoanalytic theory which helped transform the modern practice of analytic and dynamic treatment approaches. Though he initially tried to remain true to the traditional analytic viewpoint with which he had become associated and viewed the self as separate but coexistent to the ego, Kohut later rejected Freud's structural theory of the id, ego, and superego. He then developed his ideas around what he called the tripartite (three-part) self. According to Kohut, this three-part self can only develop when the needs of one's "self states," including one's sense of worth and well-being, are met in relationships with others. In contrast to traditional psychoanalysis, which focuses on drives (instinctual motivations of sex and aggression), internal conflicts, and fantasies, self psychology thus placed a great deal of emphasis on the vicissitudes of relationships. Kohut demonstrated his interest in how we develop our "sense of self" using narcissism as a model. If a person is narcissistic, it will allow him to suppress feelings of low self-esteem. By talking highly of himself, the person can eliminate his sense of worthlessness.

Kohut initially proposed a bipolar self compromising two systems of narcissistic perfection: (1) a system of ambitions and, (2) a system of ideals. Kohut called the pole of ambitions the narcissistic self (later, the grandiose self), while the pole of ideals was designated the idealized parental imago. According to Kohut, these poles of the self represented natural progressions in the psychic life of infants and toddlers.

Kohut argued that when the child's ambitions and exhibitionistic strivings were chronically frustrated, arrests in the grandiose self led to the preservation of a false, expansive sense of self that could manifest outwardly in the visible grandiosity of the frank narcissist, or remain hidden from view, unless discovered in a narcissistic therapeutic transference (or self-object transference) that would expose these primitive grandiose fantasies and strivings. Kohut termed this form of transference a mirror transference. In this transference, the strivings of the grandiose self are mobilized and the patient attempts to use the therapist to gratify these strivings (this is essentially what is displayed between child and mother in this examination question).

Kohut proposed that arrests in the pole of ideals occurred when the child suffered chronic and excessive disappointment over the failings of early idealized figures. Deficits in the pole of ideals were associated with the development of an idealizing transference to the therapist who becomes associated with the patient's primitive fantasies of omnipotent parental perfection.

Kohut believed that narcissistic injuries were inevitable and, in any case, necessary to temper ambitions and ideals with realism through the experience of more manageable frustrations and disappointments.

It was the chronicity and lack of recovery from these injuries (arising from a number of possible causes) that he regarded as central to the preservation of primitive self systems untempered by realism.

Human Development

K&S Ch. 6

Question 86. C.　　Margaret Mahler, was a pioneer in object-relations psychoanalysis. Her six stages of separation–individuation come up on almost every standardized examination in psychiatry. Here is the list in correct order:

1. *Normal autism* (birth to 2 months): sleep periods predominate over arousal periods. This stage hearkens back to fetal and intrauterine life for the infant.

2. *Symbiosis* (2 to 5 months): Mother–infant is perceived as a single fused entity. Developing perceptual abilities gradually enable infants to distinguish the inner from the outer world.

3. *Differentiation* (5 to 10 months): Distinctness from mother is appreciated. Progressive neurological development and increased alertness draw the infant's attention away from self to the outer world.

4. *Practicing* (10 to 18 months): The ability to move autonomously increases the child's exploration of the outer world.

5. *Rapprochement* (18 to 24 months): Children move away from their mothers and come back for reassurance. As they slowly realize their helplessness and dependence, the need for independence alternates with the need for closeness.

6. *Object constancy* (2 to 5 years): Children gradually comprehend and are reassured by the permanence of mother and other important people, even when not in their presence.

Human Development

K&S Ch. 2

Question 87. B.　　Memory can be divided into three system categories: episodic, semantic and procedural. Episodic memory is mediated by the medial temporal lobes, anterior thalamic nuclei, mamillary bodies, fornix and prefrontal cortex. It involves explicit, declarative awareness. An example of episodic memory would be remembering what you ate for a meal a day earlier, or what you did on your last vacation. Semantic memory is mediated by the inferolateral temporal lobes. It too involves explicit, declarative awareness. Examples of semantic memory include knowing who the first President of the United States was, or knowing the difference between a bus and a train. Procedural memory is mediated by the basal ganglia, cerebellum and supplementary motor area. It involves either implicit or explicit, nondeclarative awareness. Examples of procedural memory include operating a motor vehicle (explicit) or learning how to type your telephone number without thinking about it (implicit).

Neurocognitive Disorders

K&S Ch. 3

Question 88. A.　　Burrhus Frederic "B. F." Skinner, was an American behaviorist, author, inventor, social philosopher and poet. Skinner invented the operant conditioning chamber, innovated his own philosophy of science called radical behaviorism, and founded his own school of experimental research psychology – the experimental analysis of behavior. Skinner's theory of learning and behavior is known as operant conditioning. In operant conditioning, an animal is active and behaves in a way that produces a reward. Thus, learning occurs as a consequence of action. Gambling behavior occurs due to the reinforcement schedule known as a *variable–interval schedule*. Reinforcement in this schedule, occurs after variable intervals (of time). As such, the response rate does not change between reinforcements. The animal responds at a steady rate to get the reward when it is available.

Human Development

K&S Ch. 4

Question 89. B.　　*Selective perception* (or attention) is a broad term to identify the behavior all people exhibit to tend to "see things" based on their particular frame of reference. Selective perception may refer to any number of cognitive biases in psychology related to the way expectations affect perception. For instance, several studies have shown that students who were told they were consuming alcoholic beverages (which in fact were non-alcoholic) perceived themselves as being "drunk", exhibited fewer physiological symptoms of social stress, and drove a simulated car similarly to other subjects who had actually consumed alcohol. The result is somewhat similar to the placebo effect. A cognitive bias is a pattern of deviation in judgment that occurs in particular situations, leading to perceptual distortion, inaccurate judgment, illogical interpretation, or what is broadly called irrationality.

Learned helplessness, as a technical term in animal psychology and related human psychology, means a condition of a human person or an animal in which it has learned to behave helplessly, even when the opportunity is restored for it to help itself by avoiding an unpleasant or harmful circumstance to which it has been subjected. Learned helplessness theory is the view that clinical depression and related mental illnesses may result from a perceived absence of control over the outcome of a situation. Organisms which have been ineffective and less sensitive in determining the consequences of their behavior are defined as having acquired learned helplessness. Martin Seligman's experiments and theory of learned helplessness began at the University of Pennsylvania in 1967, as an extension of his interest in depression. Quite by accident, Seligman and colleagues discovered that the conditioning of dogs led to outcomes that opposed the predictions of B.F. Skinner's behaviorism, then a leading psychological theory. In the learned helplessness experiment an animal is repeatedly hurt by an adverse stimulus which it cannot escape. Eventually the animal will stop trying to avoid the pain and behave as if it is utterly helpless to change the situation. Finally, when opportunities to escape are presented, this learned helplessness prevents any action. The only coping mechanism the animal uses is to be stoical and put up with the discomfort, not expending energy getting worked up about the adverse stimulus.

Cognitive distortions are exaggerated and irrational thoughts, identified in cognitive therapy and its variants, which in theory perpetuate some psychological disorders. The theory of cognitive distortions was presented by David Burns in *The Feeling Good Handbook* in 1989, after studying under Aaron T. Beck. Eliminating these distortions and negative thoughts is said to improve mood and discourage maladies such as depression and chronic anxiety. The process of learning to refute these distortions is called "cognitive restructuring". *Magnifying or minimizing* a memory or situation such that they no longer correspond to objective reality, is one of many types of cognitive distortion. This is common enough in the normal population to popularize idioms such as "make a mountain out of a molehill." In depressed clients, often the positive characteristics of *other people* are exaggerated and negative characteristics are understated. There is one subtype of magnification: *catastrophizing*, which is the inability to foresee anything other than the worst possible outcome, however unlikely, or experiencing a situation as unbearable or impossible when it is just uncomfortable.

Psychological Theory and Psychometric Testing

K&S Chs 15&35

Question 90. D.   *Sensitivity and specificity* are statistical measures of the performance of a binary classification test, also known in statistics as classification function. Sensitivity (also called recall rate in some fields) measures the proportion of actual positives which are correctly identified as such (e.g., the percentage of sick people who are correctly identified as having the condition). Specificity measures the proportion of negatives which are correctly identified (e.g., the percentage of healthy people who are correctly identified as not having the condition). These two measures are closely related to the concepts of type I and type II errors. A perfect predictor would be described as 100% sensitivity (i.e., predict all people from the sick group as sick) and 100% specificity (i.e., not predict anyone from the healthy group as sick), however theoretically any predictor will possess a minimum error bound known as the Bayes error rate. For any test, there is usually a trade-off between the measures. The sensitivity of a test is the proportion of people who have the disease who test positive for it. It is calculated by taking the number of true positives and dividing by the number of true positives plus the number of false negatives. It is the probability of a positive test given that the patient is ill. If a test has high sensitivity then a negative result would suggest the absence of disease.

Specificity relates to the ability of the test to identify negative results. Consider the example of the medical test used to identify a disease. The specificity of a test is defined as the proportion of patients who do not have the disease who will test negative for it. Specificity is calculated by taking the number of true negatives and dividing by the number of true negatives plus the number of false positives. It is the probability of a negative test given that the patient is well. If a test has high specificity, a positive result from the test means a high probability of the presence of disease.

Statistics

K&S Ch. 4

Question 91. A.   Atypical antipsychotics are the most thoroughly studied class of medications for patients with dementia who are agitated, and are the most common drugs used in clinical practice. They are better tolerated than typical neuroleptic agents, with less risk of causing extrapyramidal syndrome (EPS). In the absence of contraindications such as serious extrapyramidal dysfunction (e.g., EPS, parkinsonism), an atypical neuroleptic agent should be initiated at the lowest effective dosage and titrated weekly. Tremor, rigidity, dystonia, and dyskinesia are identified in a significant number of patients at baseline and may be exacerbated by the use of atypical antipsychotics, particularly when these agents are taken at higher dosages. Physicians must use caution when increasing dosages and observe the patient closely for the emergence of EPS. Although the use of the conventional antipsychotic agent haloperidol (Haldol) is discouraged in long-term care facilities, it is widely used in the management of delirium and acute agitation in other settings. Haloperidol has been used with acceptable side effects in the management of behavior disorders of dementia. If used, it should be prescribed at low dosages and for short periods (typically days), after which the patient should be switched to another agent such as an atypical antipsychotic. Benzodiazepines should not be considered first-line therapy for management of chronic behavior disorders of dementia, even in patients with prominent anxiety. Chronic benzodiazepine use may worsen the behavior abnormality because of the amnestic and disinhibitory effects of these drugs. In clinical practice, benzodiazepine use should be limited to management of acute symptoms that are unresponsive to redirection or other agents. Anticonvulsant agents typically are used when psychotic behaviors result in aggressive behavior. Increasing evidence supports the use of divalproex (Depakote) or carbamazepine (Tegretol). These drugs are recommended as second-line agents in patients with inadequate response to antipsychotic agents. Tricyclic antidepressants should be avoided in demented patients, and in particular those with agitation, because of their anticholinergic effects, which can worsen both the agitation and the underlying dementia.

Psychopharmacology

K&S Ch. 10

Question 92. C.   Psychiatrists are held to ethical principles and standards by the American Psychiatric Association that are higher than other physicians are held to by the American Medical Association. On occasion, psychiatrists are asked to render an opinion about individuals who are public figures, or individuals who have revealed information about themselves through the public media. Psychiatrists are permitted to share their expertise about psychiatric issues in general with the public. However, it is unethical for psychiatrists to offer a professional opinion about a specific individual unless they have examined the individual and been granted proper authorization for such a statement.

Ethics

K&S Ch. 59

Question 93. C.   Transcranial magnetic stimulation (TMS) is a noninvasive method to cause depolarization or hyperpolarization in the neurons of the brain. TMS uses electromagnetic induction to induce weak electric currents using a rapidly changing magnetic field; this can cause activity in specific or general parts of the brain with minimal discomfort, allowing the functioning and interconnections of the brain to be studied. A variant of TMS, repetitive transcranial magnetic stimulation (rTMS), has been tested as a treatment tool for various neurological and psychiatric disorders including migraines, strokes, Parkinson's disease, dystonia, tinnitus, depression and auditory hallucinations. In 2008 Neuronetics, Inc, a privately held company in the United States received FDA clearance for its NeuroStar TMS device for the in-office treatment of major depressive disorder. The treatment protocol involves the application of electromagnetic stimulation to the standardized treatment location which is over the left prefrontal cortex, determined by moving the TMS coil 5 cm anterior to the MT location along a left superior oblique plane with a rotation point about the tip of the patient's nose. Treatment for depression involves 20–30 sessions of about 40 minutes each over a 4–6 week period.

Diagnostic and Treatment Procedures in Psychiatry

www.neuronetics.com

Question 94. A.   NeuroStar TMS Therapy is indicated for the treatment of major depressive disorder in adult patients who have failed to achieve satisfactory improvement from one prior antidepressant medication at or above the minimal effective dose and duration in the current episode. NeuroStar TMS Therapy noninvasively stimulates the left prefrontal cortex of the brain to treat the symptoms of major depression. It requires 4 to 6 weeks of treatment. Transcranial magnetic stimulation (TMS) is a noninvasive method to cause depolarization or hyperpolarization in the neurons of the brain. TMS uses electromagnetic induction to induce weak electric currents using a rapidly changing magnetic field; this can cause activity in specific or general parts of the brain with minimal discomfort, allowing the functioning and interconnections of the brain to be studied. A variant of TMS, repetitive transcranial magnetic stimulation (rTMS), has been tested as a treatment tool for various neurological and psychiatric disorders including migraines, strokes, Parkinson's disease, dystonia, tinnitus, depression and auditory hallucinations. In 2008 Neuronetics, Inc, a privately held company in the United States received FDA clearance for its NeuroStar TMS device for the in-office treatment of major depressive disorder.

Diagnostic and Treatment Procedures in Psychiatry

www.neuronetics.com

Question 95. C.   This patient has acute stress disorder. Remember that depersonalization and derealization are part of the criteria for ASD, but not PTSD. ASD lasts for 2 days to 4 weeks, whereas PTSD must last for 4 weeks or more. Major symptom clusters for both disorders include re-experiencing, avoidance, and increased arousal.

Anxiety Disorders

K&S Ch. 16

Question 96. B.   The mechanisms behind atypical antipsychotic (AAP) action are not clear. All antipsychotics work on the dopamine system but all vary in regards to the affinity to the dopamine receptors. There are five types of dopamine receptors in humans. There are the "D1-like" group which are types 1 and 5 which are similar in structure and drug sensitivity. The "D2-like" group includes dopamine receptors 2, 3 and 4 and have a very similar structure but very different sensitivities to antipsychotic drugs.

The "D1-like" receptors have been found to not be clinically relevant in therapeutic action. If D1 receptors were a critical component of the mechanism of AAP blocking just the D1 receptor would improve the psychiatric symptoms that are exhibited. If D1 receptor binding was a critical component of the action of antipsychotics they would need to be present in maintenance dosages. This is not seen. They are not present or present in low or negligible levels which would not even maintain the elimination of the symptoms that are seen.

The "D2-like" group of dopamine receptors are classified together based on structure but not drug sensitivity. It has been shown that D2 receptor blockade is necessary for action. All antipsychotics block D2 receptors to some degree, but the affinity of the antipsychotics vary from drug to drug and it has been hypothesized that it is the varying in affinities that causes a change in effectiveness.

One theory for how atypicals work is the "fast-off" theory. This theory of antipsychotic action is that AAP have low affinities for the D2 receptor and only bind loosely to the receptor and are rapidly released. In fact, the AAP bind more loosely to the D2 receptor than dopamine itself. The AAP effectively interfere with the phasic release of endogenous dopamine. The AAP transiently bind and rapidly dissociate from the D2 receptor to allow normal dopamine transmission. It is this transient binding that keeps prolactin levels normal, spares cognition and obviates EPS.

From a historical point of view there has been interest in the role of serotonin and treatment with the use of antipsychotics. Experience with LSD suggests that 5-HT2A receptor blockade may be a promising method of treating schizophrenia. One problem with this is the fact that psychotic symptoms caused by 5-HT2 receptor agonists differs substantially from the symptoms of schizophrenic psychoses. One promising factor of this is where the 5-HT2A receptors are located in the brain. They are localized on hippocampal and cortical pyramidal cells and have a high density in the fifth neocortex layer where the inputs of various cortical and subcortical brain areas are integrated. This makes the blocking of this receptor an interesting area considering these areas in the brain are of interest in the development of schizophrenia. This is an area of research that could prove convincing but has not yielded any convincing results. Evidence points to the fact that serotonin is not sufficient to produce an antipsychotic effect but serotonergic activity in combination with D2 receptor blockade may be responsible.

Psychopharmacology

K&S Ch. 36

Question 97. B. Conversion disorder is highest among rural populations, those with little education, low intelligence, low socioeconomic status, and military personnel who have had combat exposure.

Somatic Symptom Disorders

K&S Ch. 17

Question 98. D. Serotonin is involved in the mechanism of action of two major substances of abuse: LSD (lysergic acid diethylamide) and MDMA (ecstasy; methylenedioxymethamphetamine). The serotonin system is the major site of action of LSD, but exactly how it exerts its hallucinogenic effects is not well-understood. MDMA has dual effects: blocking the reuptake of serotonin and inducing the massive release of the serotonin contents of serotonergic neurons. In animals, it is well understood that MDMA produces selective, long-lasting damage to serotonergic nerve terminals. Users of MDMA show differences in neuroendocrine responses to serotonergic probes, and studies of former MDMA users show global and regional decreases in serotonin transporter binding, as measured by positron emission tomography.

Substance Abuse and Addictive Disorders

K&S Chs 3&12

Question 99. C. The MMPI has several validity and clinical scales. There are three validity scales, the lie scale (L scale), the infrequency scale (F scale), and the suppressor scale (K scale). The infrequency scale is useful in identifying malingering, illiteracy, confusion, psychosis, and panic. The lie scale focuses on socially desirable behaviors that are rarely practiced to test if the patient is being honest in answering the questions. The suppressor scale is used to decrease false positives and false negatives. There are 10 clinical scales which focus on specific symptom clusters.

Psychological Theory and Psychometric Testing

K&S Ch. 5

Question 100. C. Thyroid hormone can be used in psychiatry on its own, or as an augmenting agent for depressive or bipolar disorder. Liothyronine (Cytomel) is the synthetic oral replacement of endogenous T3 (tri-iodo-thyronine). Several controlled trials have demonstrated that liothyronine can convert about 50% of antidepressant nonresponders into responders. The dosage of liothyronine is 25 to 50 µg a day added to patient's antidepressant regimen. Adverse events occur infrequently with liothyronine when given at the dosage noted above. The most common adverse effects are weight loss, palpitations, transient head-ache, abdominal cramps, diarrhea, sweating, tachycardia, and increased blood pressure. Thyroid hormones should not be taken by patients with cardiac disease, angina, or hypertension. The hormones are contraindicated in thyrotoxicosis and uncorrected adrenal insufficiency and in patients with acute myocardial infarctions. Thyroid hormones can potentiate the effects of warfarin. They can increase the insulin requirements of diabetic patients and the digitalis requirements of patients with cardiac disease. Coadministration of thyroid hormones with SSRIs, tricyclics, lithium or carbamazepine can mildly lower serum thyroxine and raise serum thyrotropin levels. Thus, close serum monitoring is warranted in these patients that may require an increase in dosage of or initiation of thyroid hormone supplementation.

Psychopharmacology

K&S Ch. 36

Question 101. B. Eszopiclone is probably best known to most of us as Lunesta. It is a non-benzodiazepine hypnotic medication. It is only indicated for sleep (not depression or anything else for that matter). It does not lead to tolerance over time. Both zolpidem (Ambien) an eszopiclone can lead to hallucinations, sleep walking or other abnormal behaviors. So given this patients sleep walking, eszopiclone may not be the best alternative. As for choice C... the sleep medication famous for being a melatonin agonist is ramelt-eon (Rozerem). I'm sure you will come across it again elsewhere in this book!

Psychopharmacology

K&S Ch. 36

Question 102. D. GGT (gamma-glutamyl transpeptidase) is the most sensitive marker for alcohol abuse. In can be elevated in as many as ¾ of patients with alcohol dependence. It can also be increased by obesity, fatty liver, medications, as well as other types of liver disease. It usually takes up to 8 weeks for the GGT to return to normal following cessation of alcohol consumption.

Laboratory Tests in Psychiatry

K&S Ch. 12

Question 103. C.   You cannot lie to the insurance company. That would be simply unethical. The important therapeutic work to do is to understand the request and why the patient is making it, and help him explore his feelings about it. Giving a different false diagnosis is no more ethical than calling it an adjustment disorder, and kicking the patient out of your office is abdication of your responsibility as a therapist to help the patient cope with their illness.

Ethics

K&S Ch. 58

Question 104. C.   Adrenal insufficiency (a.k.a. Addison's disease) is a condition in which there is decreased production of mineralocorticoids, glucocorticoids, and sex hormones by the adrenal gland. There are primary, secondary and tertiary causes. Primary comes from direct damage to the adrenal gland. Secondary comes from pituitary disease. Tertiary comes from malfunction of the hypothalamus. This condition is fair game for a psychiatry exam because it can present with psychiatric symptoms. Most commonly these include depression, apathy, and irritability, but psychosis and delirium are also possible. Mania is not a common presentation. Patients may also experience fatigue, weight loss, hyperpigmentation, hypotension, nausea, vomiting, salt craving, dizziness, joint and muscle pain. Treatment consists of IV hydrocortisone in acute cases and treatment with prednisone or oral hydrocortisone in chronic cases.

Somatic Symptom Disorders

K&S Ch. 28

Question 105. A.   When giving lamotrigine and valproic acid together lamotrigine levels are elevated and valproic acid levels are decreased. When giving lamotrigine and carbamazepine together lamotrigine levels are decreased. Valproic acid will increase carbamazepine levels. Because lithium is cleared renally it will not affect the levels of lamotrigine, valproic acid, or carbamazepine.

Psychopharmacology

K&S Ch. 36

Question 106. D.   This question touches on the neurochemical changes that we associate with aggression. In aggressive patients we would expect to find increased dopamine, decreased serotonin, decreased GABA, increased testosterone, and increased acetylcholine.

Basic Neuroscience

K&S Ch. 3

Question 107. C.   This question tests your knowledge of motor development during infancy. Choice C is incorrect because the grasp and tonic neck reflexes begin to recede between 2 to 6 months. All other choices are correct and are good markers to keep in mind to measure normal development. Motor development should be looked at in conjunction with cognitive and social development when evaluating a young child for psychiatric reasons.

Human Development

K&S Ch. 2

Question 108. D.   Tardive dyskinesia (TD) is a delayed effect of antipsychotics. It is rarely seen until after 6 months of treatment. The disorder manifests as abnormal, involuntary, irregular choreoathetoid movements of the muscles of the trunk, limbs and head. Perioral movements are the most common and manifest as darting, twisting and protruding movements of the tongue, as well as chewing, lateral jaw movements, lip puckering and facial grimacing. In severe cases, torticollis, retrocollis, pelvic thrusting and trunk twisting can be seen. Dyskinesia disappears during sleep and is exacerbated by stress and anxiety. TD develops in about 10 to 20% of patients treated for more than a year. About 20 to 40% of patients with long-term psychiatric hospitalization have TD. Women are more likely to develop TD than men. Children, patients over 50 years of age and those with brain damage or mood disorders, are also at greater risk. Between 5 and 40% of all cases of TD remit and between 50 and 90% of all mild cases of TD remit. TD is less likely to remit in elderly patients than in young patients, however.

Management in Psychiatry

K&S Ch. 36

Question 109. A.
This question tests some important facts about commonly used benzodiazepines. Let's review the data. Clonazepam has a rapid rate of absorption, a half-life of 34 hours, and is considered long acting. Alprazolam has a medium rate of absorption, a half-life of 12 hours, and is considered short acting. Diazepam has a rapid rate of absorption, a half-life of 100 hours, and is considered long acting. Lorazepam has a medium rate of absorption, a half-life of 15 hours, and is considered short acting.

Psychopharmacology

K&S Ch. 36

Question 110. D.
For most anxiety disorders the rates are higher for women than for men.

The only anxiety disorder with equal rates between men and women is obsessive–compulsive disorder.

Anxiety Disorders

K&S Ch. 16

Question 111. E.
Appropriate monitoring of WBC count for patients on clozapine is as follows. First get a baseline WBC before the drug is started. Then monitor WBC weekly for the first 6 months…then biweekly for the next 6 months…then monthly thereafter. Following discontinuation of clozapine monitor weekly WBC for 4 consecutive weeks.

Laboratory Tests in Psychiatry

K&S Ch. 36

Question 112. D.
Common side effects of lithium include sedation, confusion, tremor, hair loss, nephrogenic diabetes insipidus, polyuria, polydipsia, acne, weight gain, nausea, diarrhea, and hypothyroidism. Lithium toxicity can lead to coma, seizures and death. Neural tube defects are caused in fetuses when the mother takes Depakote. When pregnant women take lithium it causes Ebstein's anomaly, which is a cardiac malformation of the tricuspid valve. Risk of Ebstein's anomaly are greatest when lithium is taken during the first trimester.

Psychopharmacology

K&S Ch. 36

Question 113. E.
This question looks at management of alcohol withdrawal. During alcohol withdrawal it is preferable to use long acting benzodiazepines such as chlordiazepoxide. As such alprazolam, which is short acting, is not a good choice. It would also have to be dosed more frequently than BID to actually cover the patient for 24 hours. IV thiamine and dextrose should be given for the first 3 days then switch to PO thiamine. Some argue that after the first IV dose, that the doses for the remainder of the 3 days can be given IM then switched to PO. Regardless of which method you advocate, giving the meds IV for 9 days is clearly wrong. Disulfiram is an aversive treatment used to stop a patient from drinking again who is currently detoxed and sober. It will make the patient sick if they have a drink while on the medication. It is not used to manage withdrawal. In a hepatically impaired patient one would choose lorazepam over clonazepam. This can be remembered by the phrase "Tolerated by Our Liver" or TOL – which stands for Temazepam, Oxazepam, Lorazepam – the three benzos safe to use in hepatic impairment. When using lorazepam for alcohol withdrawal it should be dosed QID for even coverage, then tapered off over three days.

Substance Abuse and Addictive Disorders

K&S Ch. 12

Question 114. C.   Acute dystonia is a rapid onset spastic contraction of discrete muscle groups such as the neck, eyes, back or tongue. Akathisia is a sensation of restlessness and an irresistible urge to move parts of the body. Tardive dyskinesia is a choreoathetoid movement of the tongue, mouth, face, extremities or trunk that is involuntary and irregular. Blepharospasm is an involuntary spasm of the muscles surrounding the eye. Tardive dystonia is a slow sustained twisting movement of the limbs, trunk and neck. It usually occurs late in onset following treatment with antipsychotics.

Psychopharmacology

K&S Ch. 12

Question 115. D.   All choices listed are inducers of CYP450 3A4 except fluoxetine, which is an inhibitor. Other inhibitors include calcium channel blockers, cimetidine, grapefruit juice, and antifungals.

Psychopharmacology

K&S Ch. 3

Question 116. C.   Asking the patient to consent to treatment is an example of respecting a patient's autonomy. Autonomy is the belief that a patient has a right to control what happens to their own bodies and make decisions freely and without coercion. All of the other choices are legal or ethical terms which will be the subject of their own questions throughout this text. Pay attention to them the next time you see them.

Ethics

K&S Ch. 58

Question 117. B.   On average depressed patients require 6–12 ECT treatments to treat depression. Some cases may require as many as 30 treatments, but these are the exception rather than the rule. Treatments are often given three times per week with one seizure per treatment. The use of more than one seizure per episode has no proven advantages. The preference is for unilateral electrode placement because it lessens memory impairment from the procedure. If a patient fails to improve after six unilateral treatments then bilateral electrode placement should be considered.

Diagnostic and Treatment Procedures in Psychiatry

K&S Ch. 36

Question 118. C.   The SCID does not include functional impairment. However functional impairment is covered in the SCAN (Schedule for Clinical Assessment in Neuropsychiatry) and the SCAN is thought to give a broader assessment of psychosocial function than the SCID. The SCID covers the following topics: General overview (demographics, medical, psych services and med use histories), mood episodes, psychotic symptoms, psychotic disorders differential, mood disorders differential, substance use, anxiety disorders, somatoform disorders, eating disorders, and adjustment disorders.

Diagnostic and Treatment Procedures in Psychiatry

K&S Ch. 5

Question 119. D.   Self-disclosure by the therapist is only acceptable when it is done solely for the benefit of the patient. It must be the patient's needs that drive the disclosure. The therapist must be very careful not to disclose things for their own benefit. Whether the disclosures are true is irrelevant. The focus of therapy should always be on the patient. That's what matters.

Psychotherapy

K&S Ch. 1

Question 120. D.   To boil this question down to its most basic facts, you have an elderly patient who is looking delirious and is on carbamazepine. Though there are a myriad of possible explanations for why an elderly patient can be delirious, the astute psychiatrist knows that carbamazepine has a vasopressin-like effect which can lead to hyponatremia. Therefore one of the first things you would want to look for in a confused patient on carbamazepine is the basic metabolic panel, more specifically the sodium level.

Psychopharmacology

K&S Ch. 36

Question 121. C.   Of all the medications listed all are metabolized by the liver except paliperidone (Invega). Paliperidone is 80% excreted through the kidney so you must be careful in using it in patients with renal impairment. It is a good choice for patients with hepatic impairment however. Paliperidone is the active metabolite of risperidone. Risperidone is metabolized through the liver.

Psychopharmacology

K&S Ch. 36

Question 122. A.   Validity is the degree to which an instrument measures what it is intended to measure. There are different types of validity. Face validity means a diagnosis is based on a general consensus among experienced clinicians and researchers. Descriptive validity means that a diagnosis is based on characteristic features that distinguish it from other disorders. Predictive validity means that a diagnosis will allow clinicians to accurately predict treatment response and clinical course. Construct validity means that a diagnosis is based on an understanding of the underlying pathophysiology. Positive Predictive Power is the ability of a positive test result to predict disease. It is calculated as true positives divided by true positives plus false positives.

Statistics

K&S Ch. 4

Question 123. E.   Desvenlafaxine extended release tablets are approved for treatment of MDD in adults. Desvenlafaxine is an SNRI. The usual dosage is 50 mg PO QD. Care must be taken with the dose in renally compromised patients and in the elderly. Side effects include orthostasis, hyponatremia (especially in the elderly) and hypertension, much like venlafaxine. There is a black box warning to monitor for suicidality especially for children and teens, as there is with all of the SSRIs and SNRIs.

Psychopharmacology

Physicians Desk Reference, 64th edition 2010, PDR Network LLC, Montvale NJ USA, p 3564

Question 124. D.   This patient would qualify for a GAF of 35, which represents impaired reality testing or communication and major impairment in functioning in several areas. The GAF scale is fair game for standardized exams. We will not reproduce the whole scale here but you should spend some time familiarizing yourself with the details before your exam. Some rough guidelines are that anyone above 60 has minor symptoms and is mostly functioning well. Anyone below 20 is either persistently dangerous to self or others or has severely impaired functioning. A score of 30 to 50 fit in between these extremes. Just knowing these rough landmarks you could have answered this question without memorizing every detail of the whole scale. Make sure you have some landmarks of your own in mind before your exam!

Diagnostic and Treatment Procedures in Psychiatry

K&S Ch. 7

Question 125. E.   A large proportion of the elderly population complains of difficulty in initiating and maintaining sleep, early-morning awakening, unrefreshing sleep, and daytime sleepiness. Many resort to napping. Polysomnographic investigations have supported these findings, and have revealed a gradual decrease in stages 3 and 4 sleep (delta sleep; aka slow-wave sleep) and an increase in stage 1 sleep. There may also be a decreased amount of REM sleep in the elderly. Additionally, sleep efficiency progressively decreases and the propensity for daytime napping increases, although it is still a matter of investigation as to whether the elderly are truly sleepier during the day. There also appears to be a progressive advance in the sleep/wake times with aging, related to a gradual phase advance in the internal biological clock; this may explain the common complaint of seniors that they fall asleep early in the evening, yet awaken much earlier than desired in the morning and cannot fall back to sleep easily. Because aging is also associated with an increased risk for medical and psychiatric disorders, which can also disrupt sleep, it may be difficult to ascertain, in any individual case, whether the sleep-related alterations are a "normal" consequence of the aging process itself or secondary to other disorders.

Sleep Wake Disorders

K&S Ch. 24

Question 126. B. Atomoxetine is a norepinephrine reuptake inhibitor approved for the treatment of ADHD in both children and adults (ages 6 years and above). It may take up to 10 weeks after starting treatment to reach optimal effect. Once daily dosing works well for most patients. Most common side effects include dizziness, reduced appetite, and dyspepsia. Similar to the SSRIs, atomoxetine carries a black box warning for suicidality. It is metabolized primarily by the liver and reports suggest that combination of atomoxetine with stimulants is well tolerated and effective.

Psychopharmacology

K&S Ch. 36

Question 127. B. The theory that empathic failures in the mother lead to developmental arrest in the child at a stage when the child needs others to help perform self-object functions is the work of Heinz Kohut. He specifically applied this theory to narcissism and later expanded it to other pathology as well. He viewed the development of self-esteem and self-cohesion as more important than sexuality or aggression. Object relations theory is best represented by the work of Melanie Klein. Object relations theory is known for the schizoid, paranoid and depressive positions as well as tension between the true and false self. Other famous therapists listed in this question are the subject of their own questions elsewhere in this text.

Psychological Theory and Psychometric Testing

K&S Ch. 4

Question 128. D. Vivitrol (naltrexone extended release injectable suspension) is a long acting injection of naltrexone used to control cravings in alcohol dependence. Naltrexone pills are often used to control alcohol craving in those trying to maintain sobriety and this injectable form of naltrexone aims to increase compliance and lower rates of relapse. It is given as a 380 mg IM injection every 4 weeks. Vivitrol was FDA-approved for opioid relapse prevention in 2010.

Psychopharmacology

http://www.vivitrol.com/

Question 129. B. The HAM-D (Hamilton depression rating scale) is used to evaluate depression. The GAF (Global Assessment of Functioning) rates overall level of functioning and is not linked to any one illness. The PANSS (Positive and Negative Symptom Scale) rates severity of psychosis. The BPRS (Brief Psychiatric Rating Scale) rates severity of psychosis. The CAGE is a questionnaire used to evaluate alcohol abuse.

Diagnostic and Treatment Procedures in Psychiatry

K&S Ch. 5

Question 130. E. The medication described in the question stem is Duloxetine (Cymbalta). It inhibits reuptake of both serotonin and norepinephrine. It has an indication for neuropathic pain. It lacks significant cholinergic, antihistaminic and alpha adrenergic effects. The side effect profile is similar to the SSRIs, however it is worth noting that abrupt discontinuation will give clear withdrawal symptoms (yes, paroxetine is known for this as well) and unlike the other SNRI venlafaxine, hypertension is not common with duloxetine. Of note, duloxetine is also FDA-approved for treatment of fibromyalgia.

Psychopharmacology

K&S Ch. 36

Question 131. D. Patients taking an MAOI have dietary restrictions to avoid hypertensive crisis. All of the foods listed in the question are restricted except for vodka. Small amounts of clear alcohol may be used, but patients should avoid tap beer, red wines, some white wines, and aged sherry.

Psychopharmacology

K&S Ch. 36

Question 132. D. This is a case of inhalant intoxication. This patient has been sniffing something out in the garage. The perioral rash should be a big clue. When inhalants contact the skin it dries out leading to small cracks which allow bacteria to enter. A dermatitis can develop which looks like a nonspecific contact hyperactivity reaction or perioral eczema. It is known as a "huffer's rash." Criteria for inhalant intoxication include recent exposure to volatile inhalants followed by change in behavior. The patient often becomes agitated, belligerent, assaultive, or apathetic. If bad enough this state can progress into a delirium, coma, or be fatal. The patient also must have 2 of a possible 13 neurologic signs. These signs include dizziness, nystagmus, incoordination, slurred speech, unsteady gait, lethargy, depressed reflexes, psychomotor retardation, tremor, muscle weakness, blurry vision, stupor, and euphoria.

Substance Abuse and Addictive Disorders

K&S Ch. 12

Question 133. B. Narcolepsy is a sleep disorder characterized by excessive daytime sleepiness with sleep attacks, as well as other characteristics that are manifested by the intrusion of REM sleep into wakefulness. The onset of the disorder in most cases is in adolescents and young adults, with a peak incidence between ages 15 and 30. The classic sleep attack, which occurs in virtually 100% of narcoleptic patients, is an irresistible desire to fall asleep in inappropriate circumstances and at inappropriate places (e.g., while talking, driving, eating, playing, walking, running, working, sitting, listening to lectures, watching television or movies, during sexual intercourse, or when involved in boring or monotonous circumstances). These spells last for a few minutes to as long as 20 to 30 minutes. The patient generally feels refreshed on waking. There are wide variations in frequency of attacks, anywhere from daily, weekly, monthly, or every few weeks to months. Attacks generally persist throughout the patient's lifetime, although fluctuations and rare temporary remissions may occur. Patients often show a decline in performance at school and work and encounter psychosocial and socioeconomic difficulties as a result of sleep attacks and excessive daytime sleepiness (EDS). Sudden loss of tone in all voluntary muscles except the respiratory and ocular muscles characterizes cataplexy. The attacks are triggered by emotional factors such as laughter, rage, or anger more than 95% of the time. The attacks may be complete or partial and are rarely unilateral. Most commonly, the patient may momentarily have head nodding, sagging of the jaw, buckling of the knees, dropping of objects from the hands, dysarthria, or loss of voice, but sometimes they may slump or fall forward to the ground for a few seconds. The duration is usually a few seconds to a minute or two, and consciousness is retained completely during the attack. An EEG recording shows evidence of wakefulness during brief cataplectic spells, but if the attack lasts longer than 1 to 2 minutes, the EEG shows REM sleep. This is indicative of decreased REM latency during attacks. In approximately 25 to 50% of patients, sleep paralysis is noted, generally months to years after the onset of narcoleptic sleep attacks. The sudden apparent paralysis of one or both sides of the body or one limb occurs either during sleep onset (hypnagogic) or on awakening (hypnopompic) in the morning. The patient is unable to move or speak and is frightened, although he or she retains consciousness. The attacks last from a few minutes to 15 to 20 minutes. In 20 to 40% of narcoleptic patients, hypnagogic hallucinations occur either at sleep onset or on awakening in the morning and generally appear months to years after the onset of sleep attacks. Hallucinations are most commonly vivid and visual (and often fear-inducing), but are sometimes auditory, vestibular, or somesthetic in nature. In 30% of patients, three of the four major manifestations of the narcoleptic tetrad (sleep attacks, cataplexy, sleep paralysis, and hypnagogic hallucinations) occur together, and in about 10% of cases all four major features occur together. Disturbed night sleep is commonly noted in 70 to 80% of patients. In approximately 20 to 40% of cases, automatic behavior, characterized by repeated performance of a single function such as speaking or writing in a meaningless manner or driving on the wrong side of the road or to a strange place without recalling the episode, is noted. These episodes of automatic behavior may result from partial sleep episodes, frequent lapses, or microsleeps. In patients with narcolepsy, HLA typing may be performed because most of the patients with narcolepsy show positivity for HLA DR2DQ1, and DQB1*0602 antigens.

Sleep Wake Disorders

K&S Ch. 24 and B&D Ch. 72

Question 134. C. Jimmy is moderately mentally retarded. The ranges you should memorize for the exam are as follows. Above 70 is not mentally retarded; 50–70 is mild mental retardation; 35–50 is moderate mental retardation; 20–35 is severe mental retardation. Less than 20 is profound mental retardation.

Neurodevelopmental and Pervasive Developmental Disorders

K&S Ch. 5

Question 135. D. This question covers some important facts about clozapine. Doses greater than 600 mg/day substantially increase the chance of developing seizures than lower doses. Clozapine is very anticholinergic and antihistaminic and has high likelihood of leading to weight gain and metabolic syndrome. NMS occurs rarely but adding lithium to clozapine increases the chances of developing NMS. Agranulocytosis can occur at any dose and is not dose related. Because of its impact on the CYP450 system, smoking can decrease clozapine levels.

Psychopharmacology

K&S Ch. 36

Question 136. B. In delusional disorder the patient usually has a non-bizarre delusion of at least 1 month duration. They do not have any other psychotic symptoms that would classify them as schizophrenic. As such, criteria A are not met and there is a relative preservation of function. In some cases the patient may have olfactory or tactile hallucinations but these are directly linked in some way to the delusional theme. The DSM specifies several subtypes. These subtypes are erotomanic, grandiose, jealous, persecutory, somatic, mixed and unspecified.

Psychotic Disorders

K&S Ch. 14

Question 137. E. Most people do not experience PTSD symptoms, even when faced with severe trauma. The lifetime prevalence of PTSD is about 6.7%, as per the National Comorbidity Study. As per that same study about 60% of males and 50% of females had experienced some significant trauma. Evidence points to a "dose–response" relationship between the degree of trauma and the likelihood of symptoms. The subjective meaning of the trauma to the individual is also extremely important. The predisposing vulnerability factors in PTSD are as follows:

1. Presence of childhood trauma.

2. Borderline, paranoid, dependent, or antisocial personality disorder traits.

3. Inadequate family or peer supports.

4. Female gender.

5. Genetic predisposition to mental illness.

6. Recent life stressors.

7. Perception of an external locus of control to the trauma (natural cause) as opposed to an internal one (human cause).

8. Recent alcohol abuse.

Anxiety Disorders

K&S Ch. 16

Question 138. B. Schizophrenic patients are no more likely to commit homicide than anyone in the general population at large. When a schizophrenic patient does commit murder, it may be for unpredictable or bizarre reasons due to delusions and/or hallucinations. Predictors of future homicidal behavior include a prior history of violence, dangerous behavior while hospitalized, and delusions or hallucinations involving this kind of violence. By contrast, schizophrenic patients are more prone to suicide attempts and completed suicide than the general population at large. Suicide attempts are made by 20 to 50% of schizophrenic patients. Long-term rates of suicide among schizophrenic patients are estimated at 10 to 13%. This reflects about a 20-fold increase in the suicide rate over the general population. The most important predictor of suicide in schizophrenic patients is the presence of a major depressive episode.

Psychotic Disorders/Public Policy

K&S Ch. 13

Question 139. D. This is a tricky question that can easily fool you if you are not familiar with the symptoms of Sheehan's syndrome. Sheehan's syndrome is a postpartum pituitary necrosis that can lead to chronic symptoms which can easily be mistaken for depression and misdiagnosed. Symptoms of Sheehan's syndrome include failure to lactate, hypotension, weight loss, loss of secondary sex characteristics, scant menses, constant fatigue, and diminished libido. These symptoms can develop months or even years after the birth. Diagnosis of Sheehan's syndrome is made by first looking for history of failure to make breast milk or failure to resume menstruation after birth. If suspected, pituitary hormone levels are checked followed by MRI to examine the pituitary. Important to keep in mind is that DSM criteria for postpartum depression states that it must onset within 4 weeks of the birth. When we consider this patient in light of our knowledge of Sheehan's it is clear that an endocrine workup to rule out the disease must be our first step, especially considering her failure to produce breast milk. To immediately treat the situation as if she has a major depressive disorder or anxiety disorder from the stress of the new baby would be missing a very important diagnostic rule out. There is no evidence of child abuse given here and as such child protective services should not be called.

Somatic Symptom Disorders

K&S Ch. 3

Question 140. D.   This question focuses on avoidant personality disorder. Patients with this disorder tend to avoid interpersonal interaction out of fear of shame and ridicule. They are hypersensitive to negative evaluation by others. They are unwilling to get involved with others without certainty of being liked. They are inhibited interpersonally because of fears of inadequacy. They see themselves as inferior to others. They are often misdiagnosed as dependent personality disorder and in some cases are very hard to distinguish from generalized social phobia.

Other answer choices reflect characteristics of other personality disorders:

"These patients tend to be indifferent to praise or criticism" – schizoid.

"Affective instability is a key component of the disorder" – borderline.

"These patients are unable to discard worthless objects" – OCPD.

Personality Disorders

K&S Ch. 27

Question 141. B.   Acute intermittent porphyria is one of the medical illnesses that is fair game for a psych exam because of the prominence of psychiatric symptoms in its presentation. It is a disorder of heme synthesis which leads to a buildup of porphyria. This leads to the classic triad of abdominal pain, peripheral neuropathy, and psychiatric disturbance. Psychiatric symptoms may come in the form of delirium, psychosis, depression, or anxiety (sorry, no dementia). The diagnosis is confirmed by looking for metabolites of porphyrins in the urine. This is the illness thought responsible for the "madness" of King George III.

Somatic Symptom Disorders

K&S Ch. 10

Question 142. D.   Most studies point to a prevalence of Alzheimer's disease of about 20–40% in the 85 years and over age range. Other statistics of note include the fact that 50 to 60% of patients that are demented have Alzheimer's disease. The second most common type of dementia is vascular dementia which accounts for approximately 15 to 30% percent of all dementia cases. Alzheimer's disease is slightly more prevalent in women than in men throughout the life cycle, about 1.3 to 1. Vascular dementia is more prevalent in men than women and is most common in the 60 to 70 age range. About 10 to 15% of patients have comorbid Alzheimer's disease and vascular dementia.

Neurocognitive Disorders/Public Policy

K&S Ch. 10

Question 143. E.   It is important to understand legal issues surrounding the suicidal patient. The law does not impose liability on the psychiatrist whenever a patient commits suicide. It asks whether the suicide was foreseeable and how a reasonable psychiatrist would have addressed the likelihood of harm. All potential harm is not viewed as foreseeable or predictable. The standard of care calls for documentation of risk assessment and implementation of appropriate precautions to protect the patient. No-harm contracts between therapist and patient do not protect the therapist from liability in the event of a suicide.

Forensic Psychiatry

K&S Ch. 57

Question 144. D. The definition of "disability" under the Americans with Disabilities Act (ADA) reflects the intent of Congress to prohibit the specific forms of discrimination that persons with disabilities face. While individuals with disabilities may experience the types of discrimination that confront other groups, they also may encounter unique forms of discrimination because of the nature of their disabilities and the effect that their present, past, or perceived conditions have on other persons. The purpose of the ADA is to eliminate discrimination that confronts individuals with disabilities. Since the definition of the term "disability" under the ADA is tailored to the purpose of eliminating discrimination prohibited by the ADA, it may differ from the definition of "disability" in other laws drafted for other purposes. For example, the definition of a "disabled veteran" is not the same as the definition of an individual with a disability under the ADA. Similarly, an individual might be eligible for disability retirement but not be an individual with a disability under the ADA. Conversely, a person who meets the ADA definition of "disability" might not meet the requirements for disability retirement.

The statutory definition – with respect to an individual, the term "disability" means

(A) a physical or mental impairment that substantially limits one or more of the major life activities of such individuals;

(B) a record of such an impairment; or

(C) being regarded as having such an impairment.

A person must meet the requirements of at least one of these three criteria to be an individual with a disability under the Act.

Public Policy
K&S Chs 2&8

Question 145. E. The homeless mentally ill are a significant public policy concern. Their population continues to grow with large numbers of homeless people carrying a psychiatric diagnosis. Many of them are also dependent on substances. Street dwellers tend to be schizophrenic with substance abuse. Episodically homeless tend to have personality disorders, substance abuse, and mood disorders. These of course are generalizations and exceptions can be found. Traditional mental health delivery systems often fail to successfully treat the homeless due to a variety of factors. Successful treatment for this population is often very non-conventional including street outreach programs.

Public Policy
K&S Ch. 4

Question 146. E. This is an easy one. No sex with patients or former patients…ever, under any circumstances. No former sexual partners as current patients either.

Ethics
K&S Ch. 58

Question 147. E. Varenicline (Chantix) is a partial nicotine agonist that decreases withdrawal and cravings as well as blocks the reinforcing effects of nicotine. Whereas nicotine replacement and bupropion have been shown to double quit rates, varenicline triples quit rates. Take note of its warning for behavioral changes such as hostility, agitation, depression, suicidal thoughts either during treatment of after stopping treatment. The most common side effect is nausea.

Psychopharmacology
K&S Ch. 12

Question 148. A. Treatment of organophosphate poisoning involves intravenous administration of pralidoxime (1 g) together with atropine (1 mg) given subcutaneously every 30 minutes until sweating and salivation are controlled. Pralidoxime accelerates reactivation of the inhibited acetylcholinesterase, and atropine is effective in counteracting muscarinic effects, although it has no effect on the nicotinic effects such as neuromuscular cholinergic blockade with weakness or respiratory depression. It is important to ensure adequate ventilatory support before atropine is given. The dose of pralidoxime can be repeated if no obvious benefit occurs, but in refractory cases it may need to be given by intravenous infusion, the dose being titrated against clinical response. Functional recovery may take approximately 1 week, although acetylcholinesterase levels take longer to reach normal levels. Measurement of paraoxonase status may be worthwhile as a biomarker of susceptibility to acute organophosphate toxicity; this liver and serum enzyme hydrolyzes a number of organophosphate compounds and may have a role in modulating their toxicity.

Chelation therapy with either water-soluble derivatives of dimercaprol (DMSA or DMPS) or penicillamine is effective in controlling the systemic effects of acute arsenic poisoning and may prevent the development of neuropathy if it is started within hours of ingestion. Lead encephalopathy is managed supportively, but corticosteroids are given to treat cerebral edema, and chelating agents (dimercaprol or 2,3-dimercaptopropane sulfonate) are prescribed also.

Poisoning

B&D Ch. 58

Question 149. E. HIPAA stands for Health Insurance Portability and Accountability Act. It contains rules to protect the transmission and confidentiality of patient information. The privacy rule is one that is very relevant to psychiatric practice. It applies to all protected health information whether on paper, electronic, or spoken. Some of the important points to keep in mind are as follows: Patients have a right to a written copy of their privacy rights. They also have a right to know how their protected information will be stored and disclosed. Patients have a right to a copy of their medical record. This does not include psychotherapy notes. Authorization must be obtained from the patient for release of their health information. Exclusions to this rule involve routine uses such as treatment, obtaining payment from the insurance company, or health care operations. Patients do have the right to dictate how their information is communicated. For example they can tell a doctor not to call their home phone number and only call their cell phone in order to protect their privacy, or dictate a specific address to which all confidential information must be sent.

Forensic Psychiatry

K&S Ch. 57

Question 150. A. To answer this question correctly you needed to know the mechanism of action of Mirtazapine. Mirtazapine works through antagonism at presynaptic alpha-2 receptors thereby potentiating the actions of serotonin and norepinephrine. It does NOT block reuptake of serotonin or norepinephrine. It is a potent H1 antagonist which explains why it is sedating and causes increased appetite and weight gain. It has minimal sexual side effects.

Psychopharmacology

K&S Ch. 36

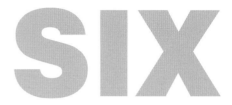

Test Number Six

1. Which of the following enzymes is responsible for the metabolism of trazodone?

   A. *CYP 2D6*

   B. *CYP 1A2*

   C. *CYP 2C19*

   D. *CYP 3A4*

   E. *CYP 2C9*

2. A young man presents to the emergency room with a complaint of several days of progressive lower extremity weakness and numbness bilaterally. History reveals he had a flu-like illness for about ten days prior to coming to the hospital. Examination confirms the lower extremity weakness, as well as loss of sensation to all sensory modalities below the middle of the thorax. Deep tendon reflexes are brisker below the waist than above and plantar reflexes are extensor bilaterally. The patient complains of recent episodes of urinary incontinence. The rest of the neurological and physical examinations are unremarkable. A lumbar puncture reveals 23 mononuclear cells, a protein level of 37 mg/dL and normal glucose. The most likely diagnosis is:

   A. *Spinal epidural abscess*

   B. *Anterior spinal artery infarction*

   C. *Acute transverse myelitis*

   D. *Acute inflammatory demyelinating polyneuropathy*

   E. *Spinal metastasis*

3. Which of the following medications has FDA approval for treatment of bipolar maintenance, thereby treating both mania and depression?

   A. *Topiramate*

   B. *Carbamazepine*

   C. *Lamotrigine*

   D. *Valproic acid*

   E. *Gabapentin*

 Full test available online - see inside front cover for details.

4. Which one of the follow sleep stages correlates with childhood somnambulism as measured by an electroencephalogram (EEG)?

    A. *Rapid eye movement sleep (REM)*

    B. *Stage II*

    C. *Stage III*

    D. *Stage IV*

    E. *Stage I*

5. Which of the following pregnancy categories should be given to a drug where animal studies show adverse fetal effect and no human studies are available?

    A. *Category A*

    B. *Category B*

    C. *Category C*

    D. *Category D*

    E. *Category E*

6. A 60-year-old man with diabetes mellitus is seen by an outpatient psychiatrist because the family states he is not making any sense. When asked what is wrong, the man states: "Thot blegging at bremull fee gelking." This expression has normal intonation, but no one can understand it. The man is able to respond to other questions with similar expressions, but he cannot execute any instructions. The most likely diagnosis is:

    A. *Wernicke's aphasia*

    B. *Balint's syndrome*

    C. *Gerstmann's syndrome*

    D. *Schizophrenic word salad*

    E. *Conduction aphasia*

7. Which of the following would the American Psychiatric Association consider unethical?

    A. *Accepting a cup of coffee from a patient*

    B. *Charging a patient for missed visits*

    C. *Selling your used car to a patient*

    D. *Releasing information about a patient to their insurance company*

    E. *Maintaining a separate set of psychotherapy notes in addition to the medical record*

8. A 75-year-old woman develops a sudden onset of right-foot and leg paralysis. Her right arm, hand and face are only very slightly affected. There is no visual field deficit or aphasia. Over the ensuing weeks she is found to have lack of spontaneity, abulia and loss of bladder control. Which of the following vascular territories would be implicated in this stroke?

    A. *Right anterior choroidal artery*

    B. *Left anterior cerebral artery*

    C. *Small subcortical vessels*

    D. *Deep penetrating vessels supplying the frontal lobes*

    E. *Superior frontal branch of the right middle cerebral artery*

9. Which of the following medications is excreted unchanged in the urine?

   A. *Sertraline*

   B. *Olanzapine*

   C. *Risperidone*

   D. *Lamotrigine*

   E. *Gabapentin*

10. A 55-year-old woman was found wandering the local bus terminal in a confused and disoriented state. She could recall her name, but not how she got to the bus terminal or why she was there. Her daughter went to pick her up at the local hospital thereafter and tried to reorient her mother many times. Nevertheless, her mother kept asking repetitive questions, even about information she had just been given about her location. Neurologic examination was normal, as were brain MRI and EEG. Within 12 hours the woman's symptoms subsided entirely. The most likely diagnosis of her problem was:

    A. *Attention-seeking behavior*

    B. *An acute dissociative state*

    C. *An epileptic fugue state*

    D. *Alcohol intoxication*

    E. *Transient global amnesia*

11. Giving a patient nefazodone and trazodone at the same time will lead to which of the following?

    A. *Decreased trazodone levels*

    B. *Decreased nefazodone levels*

    C. *Increased trazodone levels*

    D. *Increased nefazodone levels*

    E. *Induction of CYP 3A4*

12. Which of the following procedures would confirm the diagnosis of non-epileptic seizure?

    A. *Hypnotic suggestion*

    B. *Videotelemetry*

    C. *Magnetic resonance imaging brain scan (MRI)*

    D. *Observation for a 24-hour period*

    E. *Electroencephalogram (EEG) between episodes*

13. One of your patients on neuroleptic medication complains of symptoms of akathisia. Which of the following is the most appropriate treatment?

    A. *Benztropine*

    B. *Bromocriptine*

    C. *Nimodipine*

    D. *Propranolol*

    E. *Clonidine*

14. Lancinating facial pain that is sometimes triggered by minor sensory stimuli, is best treated initially with which of the following drugs?

    A. *Lioresal*

    B. *Transdermal lidocaine patch*

    C. *Eletriptan*

    D. *Carbamazepine*

    E. *Capsaicin*

15. In the management of patients with acute ischemic stroke, administration of which of the following agents within 48 hours of the onset of stroke has been shown to have a beneficial effect in reducing the risk of recurrent stroke, disability, and death?

    A. *Aspirin*

    B. *Heparin*

    C. *Recombinant tissue plasminogen activator (rTPA)*

    D. *Enoxaparin*

    E. *Clopidogrel*

16. A 35-year-old woman experiences numbness in both hands during her second trimester of pregnancy. The numbness involves the thumb, forefinger and middle finger of both hands. She reports that the dorsal part of the hand is not affected. She often awakens in the morning with aching of her arms, from the shoulder area to the hands. The most likely diagnosis is:

    A. *Ulnar entrapment neuropathies*

    B. *Brachial plexopathy*

    C. *Median neuropathies at the wrist*

    D. *Thoracic outlet syndrome*

    E. *C6 radiculopathies due to cervical spondylosis*

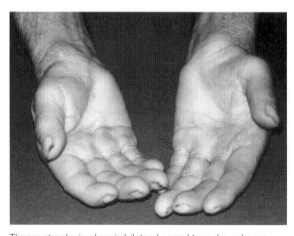

Thenar atrophy in chronic bilateral carpal tunnel syndrome

17. Which of the following anxiety disorders is most common?

    A. *Panic disorder*

    B. *Obsessive–compulsive disorder*

    C. *Post-traumatic stress disorder*

    D. *Specific phobia*

    E. *Generalized anxiety disorder*

18. The association of skin tumors, Lisch nodules of the iris, and abundant café au lait spots is diagnostic of a mutation in which of the following genes?

    A. *NACP (alpha-synuclein gene)*

    B. *NF-1 (neurofibromatosis 1 gene)*

    C. *ATM (ataxia telangiectasia gene)*

    D. *TSC-1 (tuberous sclerosis gene 1)*

    E. *NF-2 (neurofibromatosis 2 gene)*

19. Culture correlates most with which of the following factors?

    A. *Race*

    B. *Age*

    C. *Gender*

    D. *Nationality*

    E. *Ethnicity*

20. A 30-year-old patient presents to the emergency room 2 weeks after starting a crash fad diet to lose weight. The chief complaint is abdominal and extremity pain. The patient is anxious, tachycardic, disoriented and pale on examination, and seems to be responding to hallucinations. The family history from collaterals reveals that the patient's father suffers similar episodes at times. The most likely diagnosis is:

    A. *Acute intermittent porphyria*

    B. *Huntington's disease*

    C. *Hemophilia B*

    D. *Bipolar I disorder*

    E. *Anorexia nervosa with hallucinogen intoxication*

21. Which one of the following interactions might one expect when a thiazide diuretic is added on to a patient taking psychiatric medication?

    A. *Decreased clozapine level*

    B. *Decreased valproic acid level*

    C. *Increased lithium level*

    D. *Increased clozapine level*

    E. *Decreased lithium level*

22. Which of the following agents has been shown to reduce the accumulation of plaques and disability in patients with relapsing remitting multiple sclerosis?

    A. *Prednisone*

    B. *Interferon beta-1a*

    C. *Tizanidine*

    D. *Lioresal*

    E. *Intravenous gammaglobulin (IV IgG)*

23. A bulimic patient admits to you that she has been using large quantities of ipecac on a daily basis. Which of the following medical issues should you be most concerned with?

    A. *Cardiomyopathy*

    B. *Shortening of QTc interval*

    C. *Leukocytosis*

    D. *Increased serum amylase*

    E. *Infection*

24. The major clinical features of Binswanger's disease include a gait disorder, a pseudobulbar state and:

    A. *Urinary incontinence*

    B. *Aphasia*

    C. *Constructional apraxia*

    D. *Dementia*

    E. *Diplopia*

25. At which one of the following ages can children respond to simple directions and understand pronouns?

    A. *16 months*

    B. *23 months*

    C. *30 months*

    D. *40 months*

    E. *60 months*

26. A 32-year-old patient was referred for neurologic evaluation due to hand shaking. The history reveals that the shaking is present only when using the hands and is particularly bad when writing or bringing a cup to the mouth while drinking. Stress worsens the shaking. The shaking improves when the patient drinks a glass of wine. The patient's older sibling also suffers from a similar disorder. From this history, the most likely diagnosis is:

    A. *Alcohol-withdrawal tremor*

    B. *Wilson's disease*

    C. *Spinocerebellar ataxia*

    D. *Early onset Parkinson's disease*

    E. *Essential tremor*

27. At what age can children use language to tell a story, share ideas, and discuss alternatives?

    A. *10 months*

    B. *20 months*

    C. *30 months*

    D. *50 months*

    E. *60 months*

28. A palsy of the sixth cranial nerve is associated with which one of the following alcohol-related disorders?

    A. *Cerebellar degeneration*

    B. *Wernicke's encephalopathy*

    C. *Marchiafava–Bignami syndrome*

    D. *Alcohol-related delirium*

    E. *Korsakoff's syndrome*

29. Which of the following tests would be most helpful in trying to understand deficits in a patient with right hemisphere disease?

A. *Boston diagnostic aphasia examination*

B. *Sentence completion test*

C. *Word association technique*

D. *Judgment of line orientation test*

E. *Thematic apperception test*

30. A 68-year-old patient presents to an outpatient neurologist with marked gait abnormality, slow movements and asymmetric rigidity of the upper extremities. Eye examination reveals mild impairment in both upward and downward voluntary vertical gaze. Further history reveals that levodopa therapy only improved the slowness and rigidity modestly. Several years later, the patient is found to have impairment in voluntary horizontal as well as vertical gaze. Oculocephalic reflexes were normal. The patient's most likely diagnosis is:

A. *Pseudobulbar palsy*

B. *Olivopontocerebellar atrophy*

C. *Striatonigral degeneration*

D. *Progressive supranuclear palsy*

E. *Dentatorubral degeneration*

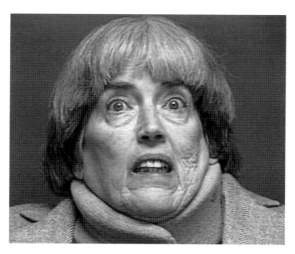

Typical facial expression of a patient with progressive supranuclear palsy, illustrating worried or surprised appearance, with furrowed brow and fixed expression of lower face.

31. All of the following are mature defenses except:

A. *Humor*

B. *Introjection*

C. *Altruism*

D. *Anticipation*

E. *Suppression*

32. A 50-year-old patient consults a neurologist for a gradually progressive and intermittent involuntary turning of the neck to the left. At times the patient complains of pain in the sternocleidomastoid muscle and head tremor. These symptoms are exacerbated by anxiety and stress. The most appropriate treatment for this condition is:

A. *Divalproex sodium*

B. *Olanzapine*

C. *Botulinum toxin*

D. *Levodopa/carbidopa*

E. *Benztropine*

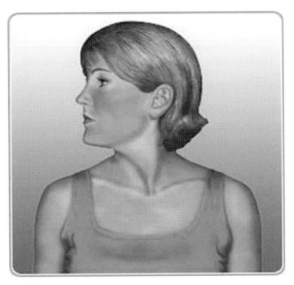

A patient with cervical dystonia (torticollis) with head rotation to the right demonstrating marked hypertrophy of the left sternocleidomastoid muscle.

33. All of the following are possible causes for anorgasmia except:

A. *Alcohol*

B. *TCAs*

C. *Diabetes*

D. *Spinal chord damage*

E. *Methylphenidate*

34. A 16-year-old patient is reported to have episodes of muscle jerks that involve the whole body and absence episodes during which the patient seems dazed for a few seconds. The EEG shows bursts of 4 to 6 Hz polyspike and wave activity. The most likely diagnosis in this case is:

A. *Juvenile myoclonic epilepsy*

B. *Nonepileptic seizures*

C. *Cataplexy*

D. *Petit-mal epilepsy*

E. *Rolandic epilepsy*

35. Upon graduation from residency you start a new practice in your home town. You go to a local internist and a local psychologist and tell them that for every patient they refer you, you will pay them $100. This arrangement is…

   A. *Ethical because people need doctors and you need patients*

   B. *Unethical because it puts the doctor's interests ahead of the patient's*

   C. *Ethical because all parties involved benefit in some way*

   D. *Ethical because the referring clinician is fairly compensated for his referral*

   E. *Unethical because the primary care physician should know how to treat depression and should not need to refer to you*

36. Multifocal myoclonus in a comatose patient is most likely indicative of a:

   A. *Brainstem infarct*

   B. *Metabolic encephalopathy*

   C. *Non-convulsive status epilepticus*

   D. *Subarachnoid hemorrhage*

   E. *Posterior fossa tumor*

37. Which of the following famous therapists developed the "epigenetic principle"?

   A. *Erik Erikson*

   B. *Melanie Klein*

   C. *B.F. Skinner*

   D. *Harry Stack Sullivan*

   E. *Heinz Kohut*

38. A 60-year-old patient with hypertension and diabetes consults a neurologist for left periorbital pain and diplopia. Examination reveals paralysis of abduction of the left eye. Which of the following is the most probable diagnosis?

   A. *Left pontine stroke*

   B. *Pseudotumor cerebri*

   C. *Diabetic sixth nerve palsy*

   D. *Myasthenia gravis*

   E. *Optic neuritis*

39. Which one of the following is not an appropriate DSM specifier used for substance-induced anxiety disorder?

   A. *With generalized anxiety*

   B. *With panic attacks*

   C. *With obsessive–compulsive symptoms*

   D. *With phobic symptoms*

   E. *With delayed onset*

40. A 35-year-old patient presents with headache, fever, seizures, confusion, stupor and coma that evolve over a period of a week. The EEG demonstrates periodic lateralized high-voltage sharp waves emanating from the left temporal region, as well as slow-wave complexes repeating at 2- to 3-second intervals. The brain CT scan shows a low-density lesion in the left temporal lobe. The most likely diagnosis in this case is:

   A. *Listeria meningitis*

   B. *HIV encephalitis*

   C. *St. Louis encephalitis*

   D. *Herpes simplex encephalitis*

   E. *Cryptococcal meningitis*

41. Which of the following is the most important factor in distinguishing pain disorder from chronic pain syndromes?

    A. *The pain is severe enough to warrant clinical attention*

    B. *The patient suffers disability from the pain*

    C. *No physical lesion is found on imaging studies*

    D. *Substance abuse and character pathology may complicate the picture*

    E. *The pain is attributed to psychological factors*

42. A 65-year-old man presents with 3 months of progressive limb weakness, worse on the right than the left. He has trouble swallowing liquids. Neurologic examination reveals normal cranial nerve function, but extensor neck muscle weakness. He has motor weakness in both distal and proximal muscles, which include the quadriceps, dorsal foot flexors, and especially the extensor pollicis longus. The upper extremity motor examination is significant for wrist and finger flexor weakness. Deep tendon reflexes are preserved and normal throughout. Muscle tone, coordination and gait are normal. The rest of the physical examination is normal. Laboratory values reveal mildly elevated serum creatine kinase. Which one of the following is the most likely diagnosis?

    A. *Myasthenia gravis*

    B. *Inclusion body myositis*

    C. *Polymyalgia rheumatica*

    D. *Dermatomyositis*

    E. *Polymyositis*

43. Which of the following brain pathways starts in the ventral tegmental area and projects to the frontal cortex?

    A. *Tuberoinfundibular pathway*

    B. *Nigrostriatal pathway*

    C. *Mesolimbic pathway*

    D. *Mesocortical pathway*

    E. *Ventral amygdalofugal pathway*

44. Which one of the following mitochondrial disorders is the most common?

    A. *Leber's hereditary optic neuropathy*

    B. *Myoclonus epilepsy with ragged-red fibers (MERRF)*

    C. *Mitochondrial encephalopathy, myopathy, lactic acidosis, and stroke-like episodes (MELAS)*

    D. *Kearns–Sayre syndrome (KSS)*

    E. *Maternally-inherited myopathy with cardiomyopathy*

45. Yves has a preoccupation with sexual fantasies involving being beaten, bound and humiliated. Which of the following terms best describes him?

    A. *Voyeurism*

    B. *Transvestic fetishism*

    C. *Fetishism*

    D. *Frotteurism*

    E. *Sexual masochism*

46. Botulinum toxin is FDA-approved for a number of movement disorders including cervical dystonia and blepharospasm. Its mechanism of action at the neuromuscular junction involves:

    A. *Inhibition of acetylcholine release from presynaptic terminals*

    B. *Blockade of voltage-dependent calcium channels*

    C. *Inhibition of acetylcholine synthesis at the neuromuscular junction*

    D. *Inhibition of acetylcholinesterase*

    E. *Blockade of the nicotinic acetylcholine receptors in muscle*

47. All of the following are symptoms of nicotine withdrawal except:

    A. *Depressed mood*

    B. *Bradycardia*

    C. *Somnolence*

    D. *Increased appetite*

    E. *Irritability*

48. A 58 year old patient with chronic atrial fibrillation develops aphasia and right hemiparesis acutely while watching television at home one evening at 8:00 pm. In the emergency room, the neurologic examination reveals moderate right hemiparesis and an expressive aphasia. A head CT scan done at 9:30 pm reveals no acute lesion. The most appropriate therapy in the emergency room is:

    A. *Aspirin*

    B. *Clopidogrel*

    C. *Intravenous heparin*

    D. *Low-molecular weight heparin*

    E. *Intravenous tissue plasminogen activator (rTPA)*

49. A man in his 30s is convinced that he has Lou Gehrig's disease. Despite negative evaluations by several physicians he is still convinced that he has it. He comes to you convinced that the proper diagnosis has been missed. Your workup is negative but he remains convinced that he has the disease despite your efforts at reassurance. What is the most appropriate diagnosis?

    A. *Somatization disorder*

    B. *Factitious disorder*

    C. *Malingering*

    D. *Hypochondriasis*

    E. *Lou Gehrig's disease*

50. A 70-year-old woman complains of leg stiffness while ambulating and lower extremity spasms while trying to sleep. Neurologic examination reveals a markedly stiff-legged gait, with leg adduction while walking. Lower extremity tone is increased with a spastic catch. Knee jerk reflexes are hyperactive and ankle jerk reflexes elicit clonus. Romberg testing reveals sway when the patient closes her eyes. The most likely diagnosis in this case is:

    A. *Parkinson's disease*

    B. *Restless legs syndrome*

    C. *Cervical spondylosis*

    D. *Alcoholic cerebellar degeneration*

    E. *Senile gait disorder*

51. A patient comes to you reporting sexual difficulties. She wants to have sex but is unable to get sexually excited. She fails to develop appropriate genital swelling and lubrication for intercourse. She denies any pain during intercourse. What is the most appropriate diagnosis?

    A. *Sexual aversion disorder*

    B. *Female sexual arousal disorder*

    C. *Female orgasmic disorder*

    D. *Vaginismus*

    E. *Dyspareunia*

52. A 60-year-old patient with hypertension complains of subacute painless visual loss of the right eye. Neurologic examination is normal apart from the blindness and a right afferent pupillary defect. A brain MRI scan reveals several periventricular white matter hyperintensities on T2 image sequencing. There are no lesions of the corpus callosum noted. The most likely diagnosis in this case is:

    A. *Optic neuritis*

    B. *Temporal arteritis*

    C. *Closed-angle glaucoma*

    D. *Retinal vein occlusion*

    E. *Ischemic optic neuropathy*

53. Intoxication with which one of the following can cause nystagmus?

    A. *Heroin*

    B. *LSD*

    C. *Methadone*

    D. *Nicotine*

    E. *Phencyclidine*

54. According to the American Academy of Neurology, an essential diagnostic criterion for the declaration of brain death prior to organ donation for transplantation requires:

    A. *A magnetic resonance imaging (MRI) scan with diffuse cortical damage*

    B. *A positive apnea test*

    C. *Neurologic consultation*

    D. *Two flat or isoelectric electroencephalographs (EEGs) in 24 hours*

    E. *Absence of deep tendon reflexes*

55. When considering the cytochrome P450 system which one of the following statements is false?

    A. *CYP2D6 and CYP3A4 are two important enzymes psychiatrists must understand*

    B. *Fluoxetine is a potent inhibitor of CYP2D6*

    C. *A CYP450 inhibitor will decrease the plasma levels of a drug over time*

    D. *Genetic polymorphisms in the CYP2D6 gene can make some patients rapid metabolizers*

    E. *Paroxetine is a potent inhibitor of CYP2D6*

56. A 47-year-old patient complains of gradual progressive weakness over the past 3–4 months, particularly in the right upper extremity. Neurologic examination demonstrates muscular atrophy of the right forearm and intrinsic muscles of the right hand. Deep tendon reflexes are brisk and plantar responses are extensor. Electrodiagnostic studies reveal widespread fasciculations, fibrillations, and positive sharp waves. This clinical picture most likely represents a diagnosis of:

   A. Multiple sclerosis

   B. Cervical spondylosis

   C. Chronic inflammatory demyelinating polyneuropathy

   D. Amyotrophic lateral sclerosis

   E. Myasthenia gravis

57. Which of the following is the most likely age for a patient on neuroleptics to develop tardive dyskinesia?

   A. 18 years

   B. 25 years

   C. 35 years

   D. 45 years

   E. 65 years

58. A 62-year-old patient presents with a first seizure with focal onset and secondary generalization. The most likely cause of this seizure is:

   A. Subarachnoid hemorrhage

   B. Glioblastoma multiforme

   C. Temporal lobe epilepsy

   D. Alcohol withdrawal

   E. Temporal arteritis

59. Interactions with which one of the following medications will increase lamotrigine levels?

   A. Oral contraceptives

   B. Valproic acid

   C. Carbamazepine

   D. Phenytoin

   E. Phenobarbital

60. Which of the following brain imaging techniques measures neuronal glucose metabolism?

   A. Electroencephalography (EEG)

   B. Magnetic resonance spectroscopy (MRS)

   C. Single photon emission computerized tomography (SPECT)

   D. Positron emission tomography (PET)

   E. Functional magnetic resonance imaging (fMRI)

61. Which one of the following inhibits the abnormal involuntary movements associated with Huntington's disease?

   A. Haloperidol

   B. Stereotactic thalamotomy

   C. Pramipexole

   D. Lioresal

   E. Benztropine

62. Which one of the following disorders presents with a gait disturbance characterized by involuntary acceleration?

    A. *Huntington's disease*

    B. *Alcohol intoxication*

    C. *Parkinson's disease*

    D. *Astasia–abasia*

    E. *Guillain–Barré syndrome*

63. The classic triad of symptoms present in meningitis includes fever, neck stiffness, and which of the following?

    A. *Tachycardia*

    B. *Alteration of sensorium*

    C. *Vomiting*

    D. *Syncope*

    E. *Headaches*

64. Which one of the following is not usually seen in Guillain–Barré syndrome?

    A. *CSF pleocytosis*

    B. *Elevated CSF protein*

    C. *Areflexia*

    D. *Motor loss with paresthesia*

    E. *Ascending paralysis*

65. Which type of intracranial hemorrhage frequently requires surgical intervention in order to improve the outcome?

    A. *Pontine hemorrhage*

    B. *Thalamic hemorrhage*

    C. *Putaminal hemorrhage*

    D. *Temporal lobe hemorrhage*

    E. *Cerebellar hemorrhage*

66. Stiff-person syndrome, causing persistent limb rigidity and spasms, is often correlated with the presence of:

    A. *High titers of JC virus antigen*

    B. *Circulating lupus anticoagulant*

    C. *Autoantibodies against glutamic acid decarboxylase*

    D. *Elevated methyl-malonic acid levels*

    E. *Elevated syphilis (Treponema pallidum) titers*

67. Gustatory special sensory auras localize to which area of the brain?

    A. *Cingulate gyrus*

    B. *Dorsolateral prefrontal cortex*

    C. *Occipital neocortex*

    D. *Insular cortex*

    E. *Parietal cortex*

68. A man presents with sudden onset left neck pain, left eyelid droop, left pupillary miosis, left facial anhydrosis, right hemiparesis and expressive aphasia. The most likely cause is:

    A. *Left internal carotid artery dissection*

    B. *Left vertebral artery dissection*

    C. *Middle cerebral artery CVA*

    D. *Posterior inferior cerebellar artery lesion.*

    E. *Demyelination*

69. A 40-year-old man presents to the ER complaining of subacute onset of daily headaches, blurred and double vision, fever, vertigo, joint pains and a feeling that his "eyeballs are popping out" of his head. On examination he has left-sided ptosis and inability to adduct and abduct the left eye fully. On primary gaze, his right eye looks straight and his left eye is slightly deviated to the left. Brain MRI reveals inflammatory changes in the cavernous sinus. The most likely diagnosis is:

    A. *Complicated migraine*

    B. *Tolosa–Hunt syndrome*

    C. *Cavernous sinus thrombosis*

    D. *CNS lyme disease (borreliosis)*

    E. *CNS sarcoidosis*

70. Which of the following benzodiazepines is metabolized by glucuronidation?

    A. *Lorazepam*

    B. *Diazepam*

    C. *Triazolam*

    D. *Clonazepam*

    E. *Alprazolam*

71. Which of the following is the most common side effect of selective serotonin reuptake inhibitors (SSRIs) early in treatment, leading to discontinuation by patients?

    A. *Sleeplessness*

    B. *Sexual dysfunction*

    C. *Gastrointestinal distress*

    D. *Headache*

    E. *Agitation/anxiety*

72. Anterior capsulotomy and/or cingulotomy have been demonstrated to be effective in cases of treatment failure with which of the following severe disorders?

    A. *Tourette's syndrome*

    B. *Schizophrenia*

    C. *Bipolar disorder*

    D. *Antisocial personality disorder*

    E. *Obsessive–compulsive disorder*

73. A patient on lithium for bipolar disorder reports feeling slow, dull and unable to concentrate, despite an excellent response in terms of mood stability. The most likely reason for this is that the patient is:

    A. Somatisizing

    B. Accurately reporting side effects

    C. Abusing other substances

    D. Rationalizing noncompliance

    E. Undervaluing normal mood

74. Which of the following choices accounts for about half of all completed suicides?

    A. Schizophrenia

    B. Personality disorders

    C. Alcohol abuse

    D. Major depression and bipolar disorder

    E. Organic brain syndromes

75. Which of the following is not one of the therapist's tasks in a group therapy setting?

    A. Formulate goals

    B. Decide on an open vs. closed group

    C. Maintenance of a therapeutic environment

    D. Choose frequency and length of group

    E. Suppression of catharsis

76. Which of the following blood tests is the most important to monitor in a patient taking carbamazepine?

    A. Creatinine

    B. Fasting glucose

    C. Complete blood count (CBC)

    D. Lipid profile

    E. Thyroid function tests (TSH and free T4)

77. At which of the following ages can children use a wide range of grammatical forms such as plurals, past tense, negatives and questions?

    A. 5 months

    B. 10 months

    C. 17 months

    D. 30 months

    E. 40 months

78. Which of the following agents is contraindicated in patients taking clozapine?

    A. Carbamazepine

    B. Fluoxetine

    C. Clonazepam

    D. Lithium

    E. Nortriptyline

79. Which one of the following cognitive enhancing agents is an NMDA receptor antagonist?

   A. *Galantamine*

   B. *Donepezil*

   C. *Rivastigmine*

   D. *Memantine*

   E. *Tacrine*

80. Which one of the following is not a symptom of organophosphate exposure or poisoning?

   A. *Lacrimation*

   B. *Salivation*

   C. *Diarrhea*

   D. *Vomiting*

   E. *Mydriasis*

81. *Clostridium tetani* causes trismus and dysphagia in those patients that acquire it by:

   A. *Activating glutamate receptors*

   B. *Inhibiting GABA and glycine release in the brain and spinal cord*

   C. *Blocking acetylcholine release at the neuromuscular junction*

   D. *Blocking acetylcholinesterase in cholinergic synapses*

   E. *Blocking calcium-mediated muscular contraction*

82. Low-voltage, mixed frequency background with sleep spindles and K complexes are typically seen on electroencephalograms (EEGs) during which phase of sleep?

   A. *Stage I*

   B. *Stage II*

   C. *Stage III*

   D. *Stage IV*

   E. *REM sleep*

83. In normal young adults, what percentage of total sleep time is spent in REM sleep?

   A. *5%*

   B. *0%*

   C. *20%*

   D. *25%*

   E. *35%*

84. Emergency room treatment of patients with MAOI-related hypertensive crisis, may involve administration of which of the following agents?

   A. *Diazepam*

   B. *Hydrochlorothiazide*

   C. *Phentolamine*

   D. *Bromocriptine*

   E. *Dantrolene*

85. The emergency room treatment of an acute serotonin syndrome involves stopping the offending agent(s) and then:

    A. *Administering dantrolene*

    B. *Hemodialysis*

    C. *Administering bromocriptine*

    D. *Supporting vital signs and functions*

    E. *Administering oral or intramuscular lorazepam*

86. Which of the following factors is most closely associated with child abuse and neglect?

    A. *Low socioeconomic status*

    B. *Child with behavioral problems*

    C. *Single-parent household*

    D. *Large family size*

    E. *Female child under 12 years of age*

87. A patient is doing individual therapy in an interpersonal psychotherapy (IPT) framework for depression. In the first five sessions, the patient and therapist come to identify the patient's unresolved grief due to the recent death of the patient's spouse as the area of greatest concern, and this is related to the patient's current feelings of depression. Which of the following will be the focus of the next phase in the patient's treatment?

    A. *Identifying and testing the validity of the patient's maladaptive assumptions*

    B. *Finding new activities and relationships to offset the patient's loss*

    C. *Providing the patient with a corrective emotional experience in the treatment*

    D. *Resolving guilt about conflicted feelings towards the patient's spouse*

    E. *Reframe the patient's catastrophizing and fortune-telling over the spouse's death*

88. When dialectical behavioral therapy is used to treat patients with borderline personality disorder, the word "dialectical" refers to therapeutic strategies focused on:

    A. *Alleviating psychic tension between the id and its fantasies and the superego and its responsibilities*

    B. *Going over traumatic events and analyzing their impact on the patient*

    C. *Reframing cognitive distortions and finding underlying mechanisms to negative thoughts*

    D. *Role-play that seeks to improve patient's interpersonal relationships*

    E. *Seeking for synthesis between seemingly contradictory ideas and emotions*

89. A 35-year-old patient presents with longstanding history of orderliness and alphabetizing and color-coding of all his belongings. This behavior can take him up to 2 hours every day to accomplish and he is often late for work in the mornings due to his inability to stop this behavior. The patient denies obsessive thoughts and cannot explain the ongoing need to alphabetize, color-code and order everything. The most probable diagnosis in this case is:

    A. *Impulse control disorder NOS*

    B. *Obsessive–compulsive personality disorder*

    C. *Body dysmorphic disorder*

    D. *Anxiety disorder NOS*

    E. *Obsessive–compulsive disorder*

90. Which one of the following would not be considered a case of pedophilia?

    A. *A 60-year-old elementary school teacher has clandestine sex with a 12-year-old neighbor*

    B. *A 20-year-old female camp counselor has clandestine sex with a 17-year-old male camper*

    C. *A 25-year old man has clandestine sex with his 13-year-old female cousin*

    D. *A grandfather has clandestine sex with his 9-year-old granddaughter*

    E. *A married couple, in their 30s, who are middle-school teachers at the same school, have a ménage-à-trois with an 11-year-old male student at their home*

91. An 11-year-old elementary school student is given a trial of methylphenidate for ADHD, inattentive type. The dose is titrated appropriately by the psychiatrist, but the student continues to complain of the core symptoms of ADHD. The next medication to be tried should be:

    A. *Guanfacine*

    B. *Clonidine*

    C. *Bupropion*

    D. *Dextroamphetamine*

    E. *Venlafaxine*

92. A 45-year-old woman is raped on an inner-city street late one night. She tells no one about the incident. The next day, her co-workers note that she is absent from work and a week later she is found 50 miles away in a nearby town mumbling incoherently to herself and wandering the streets. When taken to the local hospital emergency room she is initially unable to recall her name, her address, her birth date or her telephone number. This presentation is most compatible with a diagnosis of:

    A. *Dissociative amnesia*

    B. *Dissociative fugue*

    C. *Dissociative identity disorder*

    D. *Post-traumatic stress disorder*

    E. *Acute stress disorder*

93. Which of the following categories of disorders classically has a female to male ratio of about 10 to 1?

    A. *Substance-abuse disorders*

    B. *Sexual disorders*

    C. *Eating disorders*

    D. *Dissociative disorders*

    E. *Personality disorders*

94. The diagnosis of encopresis is seen to occur most frequently in children with which of the following in their history?

    A. *Sexual abuse*

    B. *Attention deficit–hyperactivity disorder*

    C. *Conduct disorder*

    D. *Oppositional defiant disorder*

    E. *Learning disorders*

95. Which subtype of schizophrenia tends to present at an older age at onset and is associated with less regression in mental faculties, emotional responses and behavior than the other subtypes?

    A. *Undifferentiated*

    B. *Residual*

    C. *Catatonic*

    D. *Disorganized*

    E. *Paranoid*

96. The impulse control disorder of chronic pathological gambling is believed to be associated with which of the following biological markers?

    A. *Decreased uptake in the brain on fluorodopa PET scans*

    B. *Decreased dopamine levels in the nucleus accumbens*

    C. *Increased serotonin and norepinephrine activity in the raphe and locus ceruleus*

    D. *Decreased plasma MHPG levels and decreased platelet MAO activity*

    E. *Decreased glutamate activity at NMDA receptors in the brain*

97. Which one of the following is not typically associated with juvenile conduct disorder?

    A. *Children with history of abuse or domestic violence victimization*

    B. *Children of underemployed parents*

    C. *Children with onset of serious violations of rules prior to 15 years of age*

    D. *Children with low plasma dopamine β-hydroxylase levels*

    E. *Children with greater right frontal EEG activity at rest*

98. A patient brings her daughter in for evaluation because she thinks the child may have autism. The child had normal development until 7 months of age. Since then she has decreased socializing, begun repetitive wringing hand movements, and appears psychomotor retarded. Her head circumference has not been keeping up with the growth curve according to her pediatrician. Which of the following is the most likely diagnosis?

    A. *Autism*

    B. *Asperger's disorder*

    C. *Pervasive developmental disorder NOS*

    D. *Childhood disintegrative disorder*

    E. *Rett's disorder*

99. Which of the following famous psychoanalysts is responsible for the concepts of the "collective unconscious" and "archetypes"?

    A. *Erich Fromm*

    B. *Kurt Goldstein*

    C. *Edith Jacobson*

    D. *Carl Jung*

    E. *Otto Kernberg*

100. A 5-year-old child presents with confusion, increased salivation, lacrimation, fasciculations, miosis, tachycardia and hypertension. Which of the following poisons can cause these manifestations?

    A. *Opium*

    B. *Strychnine*

    C. *Botulism*

    D. *Hexane*

    E. *Organophosphate insecticide*

101. Which of the following benzodiazepines is phase II metabolized but not phase I metabolized?

    A. *Diazepam*

    B. *Clonazepam*

    C. *Lorazepam*

    D. *Alprazolam*

    E. *Triazolam*

102. Which pregnancy category are benzodiazepines?

    A. *Category A*

    B. *Category B*

    C. *Category C*

    D. *Category D*

    E. *Category E*

103. Which of the following is the most common cause of malpractice claims against psychiatrists?

    A. *Sexual assault*

    B. *Improper termination*

    C. *Suicide or attempted suicide*

    D. *Boundary violations*

    E. *Medication error*

104. Which of the following is the most appropriate treatment for premature ejaculation?

    A. *SSRIs*

    B. *Yohimbine*

    C. *Testosterone*

    D. *Alprostadil*

    E. *Sildenafil*

105. Which of the following disorders is not more common in males?

    A. *Autism*

    B. *Obsessive–compulsive disorder*

    C. *Attention deficit–hyperactivity disorder*

    D. *Exhibitionism*

    E. *Pathological gambling*

106. For a socially harmful act to be considered a crime it must contain which of the following?

    A. *Parens patriae*

    B. *Mens rea*

    C. *Respondeat superior*

    D. *Substituted judgment*

    E. *Justice*

107. A patient with severe panic disorder comes to you for help. Which of the following is the most effective treatment you can offer her?

    A. *Psychodynamic psychotherapy*

    B. *An SSRI*

    C. *Cognitive behavioral therapy*

    D. *A tricyclic antidepressant*

    E. *Cognitive behavioral therapy plus an SSRI*

108. Which of the following is not a common comorbidity associated with social phobia?

    A. *Drug abuse*

    B. *Conversion disorder*

    C. *Alcohol abuse*

    D. *Other anxiety disorders*

    E. *Major depressive disorder*

109. You start a patient in your practice on an SSRI for treatment of panic disorder. Which of the following medications can you add that will be effective, FDA-approved for panic disorder, and lead to a more rapid response?

    A. *Buspirone*

    B. *Gabapentin*

    C. *Propranolol*

    D. *Topiramate*

    E. *Clonazepam*

110. An elderly bipolar patient is brought into the emergency room. He was found comatose at home by his son. His serum sodium is 115 mmol/L. Which of the following medications is the most likely cause of his sodium imbalance?

    A. *Lithium*

    B. *Olanzapine*

    C. *Carbamazepine*

    D. *Quetiapine*

    E. *Topiramate*

111. Which of the following is not part of the recommended monitoring for patients taking risperidone?

    A. *Weight*

    B. *Blood pressure*

    C. *Glucose*

    D. *Thyroid function tests*

    E. *Lipid profile*

112. A psychotherapist you work with recently lost his teenage daughter in a car accident. He proceeded to tell all of his patients about this recent loss. This revelation to his patients is problematic because;

    A. *He should not reveal personal information to a patient*

    B. *The only personal information he can reveal is his educational history*

    C. *Openly sharing his grief will help his patients to understand him*

    D. *It is driven by his personal needs rather than the needs of the patient*

    E. *He should only reveal this information to patients who have also lost children*

113. Which of the following statistical measures would be used to quantify the degree of agreement between two raters in a study?

    A. *Point prevalence*

    B. *Period prevalence*

    C. *Lifetime prevalence*

    D. *Kappa*

    E. *Correlation coefficient*

114. A female therapist is doing psychodynamic psychotherapy with a 29-year-old woman. She has been discussing issues surrounding her marriage and her relationship with her mother, who was distant emotionally when the patient was growing up. The patient becomes angry with the therapist when she requests therapy sessions three times per week and the therapist states that she cannot accommodate that with her schedule. She accuses the therapist of disliking her. This is an example of which of the following?

    A. *Rejection by the therapist*

    B. *Delusion of an erotomanic nature*

    C. *Transference on the part of the patient*

    D. *A precursor to stalking by the patient*

    E. *Displacement of anger onto the therapist*

115. Which of the following is not an indication for neurological imaging in a psychiatric patient?

    A. *New onset psychosis*

    B. *Acute mental status change with neurological abnormalities*

    C. *Delirium of unknown etiology*

    D. *Acute mental status change in a 65 year old patient*

    E. *Mania*

116. Which of the following types of therapy is considered the "gold standard" for treatment of obsessive–compulsive disorder?

    A. *Exposure with response prevention*

    B. *Motivational enhancement therapy*

    C. *Dialectical behavior therapy*

    D. *Dynamic psychotherapy*

    E. *Psychoanalysis*

117. A 35-year-old woman with bipolar disorder gives birth to a child with an abnormally formed tricuspid valve. Which of the following medications was she most likely taking?

    A. *Haloperidol*

    B. *Lithium*

    C. *Valproic acid*

    D. *Lamotrigine*

    E. *Carbamazepine*

118. Which of the following is not one of the psychological issues of pregnancy?

    A. *Pregnancy as a means of self-realization*

    B. *Fear of inadequate mothering*

    C. *Projection of hope onto the child to be*

    D. *Absence of desire for sexual activity*

    E. *Unconscious ambivalence about the effect on the dyadic relationship*

119. The son of a 95-year-old woman with severe dementia asks that his mother be deemed incompetent. This decision must be made by:

    A. *The son*

    B. *The psychiatrist*

    C. *The internist*

    D. *The hospital administrator*

    E. *The court*

120. In which of the following tests is a patient presented with geometric figures for about 10 seconds then asked to draw them from memory?

    A. *Benton Visual retention test*

    B. *Weschler memory scale*

    C. *Bender visual motor gestalt test*

    D. *Wisconsin card sorting test*

    E. *Mini mental status exam*

121. Which of the following defense mechanisms is considered immature?

    A. *Anticipation*

    B. *Schizoid fantasy*

    C. *Altruism*

    D. *Humor*

    E. *Suppression*

122. Lithium has been associated with which one of the following?

    A. *Neutropenia*

    B. *Hyperparathyroidism*

    C. *Pancreatitis*

    D. *Hepatic failure*

    E. *Eosinophilic colitis*

123. You are screening Thomas for brief psychodynamic psychotherapy. Which of the following is a sign that he is an appropriate candidate?

    A. *He sticks his hand down his pants and smears feces on your office chair*

    B. *He is fighting with both of his parents*

    C. *He takes sertraline every day*

    D. *He has one friend who he talks to twice per year*

    E. *He is able to identify and discuss his feelings*

124. Which of the following is most associated with object relations theory?

    A. *Melanie Klein*

    B. *Carl Jung*

    C. *Jean Baker Miller*

    D. *Anna Freud*

    E. *Sigmund Freud*

125. Joe Lehobo is a cachectic crack addict. Dr. Medpusher wants to convince Joe to stop using crack, but Joe is ambivalent and denies that crack use is a problem for him. How should Dr. Medpusher proceed?

    A. *Prescribe fluoxetine*

    B. *Dialectical behavior therapy*

    C. *Motivational enhancement therapy*

    D. *Electroconvulsive therapy*

    E. *Involuntary hospitalization*

126. Jim is a pediatrician in a local hospital. He is trying to raise money to build a new treatment center for children with developmental disabilities. He asks you to solicit your patients for contributions. You should agree to solicit funds from:

    A. *Only former patients*

    B. *No patients*

    C. *Only wealthy patients because this is a good cause and they have money to give*

    D. *Only patients with intact reality testing*

    E. *Elderly patients who can leave a donation to the hospital in their will*

127. An explanatory statement that links a feeling to its unconscious meaning is known as:

    A. *Confrontation*

    B. *Clarification*

    C. *Interpretation*

    D. *Empathic validation*

    E. *Affirmation*

128. A psychiatrist routinely receives free dinners, play tickets, and short trips from a pharmaceutical representative. Which of the following statements concerning this situation is correct?

    A. *There is no evidence that gifts influence physicians behavior*

    B. *This situation represents a conflict of interest for the psychiatrist*

    C. *This situation is ethical if no single gift is worth more than $500*

    D. *Self-regulation by physicians is the most effective way to deal with this issue*

    E. *Whereas doctors are not influenced by this behavior, support staff such as nurses, physicians assistants and secretaries are*

129. You have to interview a patient using an interpreter. Which of the following is the best way to proceed?

    A. *Speak in English but very loudly*

    B. *Look at the patient while speaking*

    C. *Look at the interpreter while speaking*

    D. *Address all questions to the interpreter and let her ask the patient.*

    E. *Make sure you not only have an interpreter but also the patient's family in the room so that they can all translate*

130. In which of the following theories does human development move through predetermined steps and stages wherein each stage has its own characteristics and needs that must be negotiated before moving forward?

    A. *Levinson's developmental theory*

    B. *The epigenetic view of development*

    C. *Vaillant theory of happy childhood*

    D. *Neurodevelopmental theory*

    E. *Normality as process*

131. Which of the following tests is not considered routine monitoring for patients taking lithium?

    A. *Complete blood count*

    B. *Serum electrolytes*

    C. *24-hour urine for creatinine and protein*

    D. *Blood urea nitrogen and creatinine*

    E. *Thyroid function tests*

132. A patient has a panic attack and then worries significantly about having more attacks. How long must he worry to meet DSM criteria for panic disorder?

    A. *1 week*

    B. *2 weeks*

    C. *1 month*

    D. *3 months*

    E. *6 months*

133. Your patient's mother dies. Shortly thereafter she begins to show signs of depression. How much time must pass following her mother's death before she can be diagnosed with major depressive disorder?

    A. *6 months*

    B. *3 months*

    C. *2 months*

    D. *1 month*

    E. *2 weeks*

134. Which of the following drugs is known for a severe hyperthermic syndrome that can progress to disseminated intravascular coagulation, rhabdomyolysis, liver and kidney failure, as well as death?

    A. *Heroin*

    B. *Gamma-hydroxybutyrate*

    C. *Flunitrazepam*

    D. *Methylenedioxymethamphetamine*

    E. *Ketamine*

135. Giving a patient CBT plus an SSRI for social anxiety disorder will most likely result in which of the following?

    A. *Better results than an SSRI alone*

    B. *Better results than CBT alone*

    C. *Poor results for refractory cases*

    D. *No initial benefit over monotherapy with either an SSRI or CBT in most cases*

    E. *Poorer response than psychodynamic psychotherapy alone*

136. Which of the following is least likely to cause weight gain?

    A. *Clozapine*

    B. *Olanzapine*

    C. *Valproic acid*

    D. *Lamotrigine*

    E. *Lithium*

137. Which of the following is not a component of skills training for patients with addictions?

    A. *Changing beliefs*

    B. *Stress management techniques*

    C. *Increasing assertiveness*

    D. *Examining unconscious symbolism behind fears*

    E. *Improving interpersonal communication*

138. Which of the following is considered incorrect concerning seclusion and restraint?

    A. *Seclusion and restraint are considered ethical when no less restrictive alternative is available*

    B. *A nurse observing a seclusion may extend the seclusion time if she feels the patient is still agitated*

    C. *A written order from an M.D. is needed to seclude a patient*

    D. *Seclusion orders are time limited*

    E. *The patient's condition while in seclusion should be regularly reviewed and documented*

139. Which of the following daily methadone doses is the best to block cravings and result in reduction of subsequent drug use for the average patient?

    A. *10 mg*

    B. *20 mg*

    C. *40 mg*

    D. *80 mg*

    E. *100 mg*

140. A homeless man comes to your emergency room with a long history of alcohol use. He has been living in a local park and prostituting himself to other men for money to buy alcohol. Because the weather has been warm he has been bathing in local ponds and streams. He has been drinking excessively lately and requests detoxification. You must decide whether to send him to inpatient or outpatient detoxification. Which of the following factors will affect your decision most?

    A. *Length of time living in the park*

    B. *Condom use*

    C. *Social supports*

    D. *Source of alcohol*

    E. *History of delirium tremens*

141. A 23-year-old male with severe obsessions, compulsions and tics comes to you for evaluation. Which of the following would be the best medication combination for this patient?

   A. *Citalopram plus lorazepam*

   B. *Paroxetine plus buspirone*

   C. *Sertraline plus naltrexone*

   D. *Fluoxetine plus alprazolam*

   E. *Fluvoxamine plus haloperidol*

142. Which of the following choices does not present with psychotic symptoms?

   A. *Major depressive disorder*

   B. *Hypomanic episodes*

   C. *Delirium*

   D. *Bipolar mixed episodes*

   E. *Manic episodes*

143. A patient comes to you and reports recurrent hypomanic episodes but denies any depressive symptoms. What is her diagnosis?

   A. *Bipolar I disorder*

   B. *Bipolar II disorder*

   C. *Cyclothymic disorder*

   D. *Substance induced mood disorder*

   E. *Bipolar disorder NOS*

144. Which of the following medical conditions can present with panic attacks, elevated blood pressure, flushing and tremulousness?

   A. *Crohn's disease*

   B. *Raynaud's phenomenon*

   C. *Hypothyroidism*

   D. *Hyperparathyroidism*

   E. *Pheochromocytoma*

145. Which of the following could be expected for a patient with social phobia as compared to the general population?

   A. *Increased number of friendships*

   B. *Higher level of education*

   C. *Lower rates of suicide*

   D. *Poorer marital function*

   E. *Increased success in career advancement*

146. Regularly scheduled primary care appointments are a crucial and standard part of treating which one of the following diagnoses?

   A. *Panic disorder*

   B. *Major depressive disorder*

   C. *Hypochondriasis*

   D. *Post-traumatic stress disorder*

   E. *Delusional disorder somatic type*

147. Which of the following factors does not increase the chances that an elderly patient will commit suicide?

    A. *Alcohol dependence*

    B. *Widowed*

    C. *Good physical health*

    D. *Unemployed*

    E. *Socially isolated*

148. You have a patient on clozapine who develops a WBC count between 2000 and 3000. What is your next step in management?

    A. *Continue clozapine and repeat WBC/ANC*

    B. *Stop clozapine. You may re-challenge if WBC count increases in future*

    C. *Continue clozapine. Draw twice-weekly WBC/ANC*

    D. *Continue clozapine. Draw weekly WBC/ANC for the next 4 weeks*

    E. *Stop clozapine. You may not re-challenge this patient in future*

149. Prolongation of the QTc interval above which of the following is an indication to stop a QTc-prolonging neuroleptic?

    A. *100 milliseconds*

    B. *200 milliseconds*

    C. *300 milliseconds*

    D. *400 milliseconds*

    E. *500 milliseconds*

150. You are doing a shift in the emergency room and a patient comes in complaining of depressed mood. On further questioning you discover that he is also suffering from fatigue and cognitive inefficiency. He provides you with a list of medications prescribed by his primary care physician. Of the following medications, which one could be responsible for exacerbating the patient's symptoms?

    A. *Interferon*

    B. *Ranitidine*

    C. *Verapamil*

    D. *Modafinil*

    E. *Amoxicillin*

SIX

Answer Key – **Test Number Six**

1.	D	26.	E	51.	B	76.	C	101.	C
2.	C	27.	E	52.	E	77.	E	102.	D
3.	C	28.	B	53.	E	78.	A	103.	C
4.	D	29.	D	54.	B	79.	D	104.	A
5.	C	30.	D	55.	C	80.	E	105.	B
6.	A	31.	B	56.	D	81.	B	106.	B
7.	C	32.	C	57.	E	82.	B	107.	E
8.	B	33.	E	58.	B	83.	D	108.	B
9.	E	34.	A	59.	B	84.	C	109.	E
10.	E	35.	B	60.	D	85.	D	110.	C
11.	C	36.	B	61.	A	86.	A	111.	D
12.	B	37.	A	62.	C	87.	B	112.	D
13.	D	38.	C	63.	E	88.	E	113.	D
14.	D	39.	E	64.	A	89.	E	114.	C
15.	A	40.	D	65.	E	90.	B	115.	E
16.	C	41.	E	66.	C	91.	D	116.	A
17.	D	42.	B	67.	D	92.	B	117.	B
18.	B	43.	D	68.	A	93.	C	118.	D
19.	E	44.	C	69.	B	94.	A	119.	E
20.	A	45.	E	70.	A	95.	E	120.	A
21.	C	46.	A	71.	C	96.	D	121.	B
22.	B	47.	C	72.	E	97.	C	122.	B
23.	A	48.	E	73.	B	98.	E	123.	E
24.	D	49.	D	74.	D	99.	D	124.	A
25.	B	50.	C	75.	E	100.	E	125.	C

126.	B
127.	C
128.	B
129.	B
130.	B
131.	C
132.	C
133.	C
134.	D
135.	D
136.	D
137.	D
138.	B
139.	D
140.	E
141.	E
142.	B
143.	E
144.	E
145.	D
146.	C
147.	C
148.	B
149.	E
150.	A

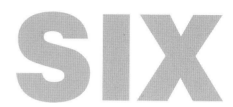

Explanations – **Test Number Six**

Question 1. D.   Trazodone is metabolized by the CYP 3A4 enzyme.

Psychopharmacology

K&S Ch. 36

Question 2. C.   Acute and subacute transverse myelitis (TM) is defined as the development of isolated spinal cord dysfunction over hours or days in patients in whom no evidence exists of a compressive lesion. Approximately 37% of patients reported a preceding febrile illness. TM is an acute myelopathic process that is presumed to be autoimmune in origin. Patients present with motor and sensory deficits below the lesion, usually in the form of a paraplegia. The abnormalities are typically bilateral but may be asymmetrical. MRI may show enhancement in the spinal cord, which has an appearance that differs subtly from that in involvement in multiple sclerosis. CSF analysis is nondiagnostic. TM is a clinical diagnosis. The primary differential diagnosis is between multiple sclerosis and neuromyelitis optica. Only about 7% of patients with TM go on to develop multiple sclerosis by clinical criteria.

Anterior spinal artery infarction usually causes paraparesis and spinothalamic sensory loss below the level of the lesion. Dorsal column function is preserved. Rarely, one segmental branch of the anterior spinal artery can be involved with unilateral spinal cord damage and monoparesis or hemiparesis. Spinal metastasis can cause a central cord deficit, but this is unusual in a young patient such as the one presented in this question!

Neurology

B&D Chs 23&54

Question 3. C.   Lamotrigine has FDA approval for bipolar maintenance and has demonstrated efficacy in both mania and depression. Topiramate is approved for seizures and migraines but is used off label for mania. Carbamazepine is approved for treatment of acute mania. Valproic acid has been demonstrated to be effective for acute mania. Gabapentin is approved for seizures, post-herpetic neuralgia, and neuropathic pain.

Psychopharmacology

K&S Ch. 36

Question 4. D.   Somnambulism (sleepwalking) is a parasomnia. It is common in children between ages 5 and 12. Sometimes it persists in adulthood or rarely begins in adults. Sleepwalking begins with the abrupt onset of motor activity arising out of slow-wave sleep (stage IV) during the first one-third of sleep. Episodes generally last less than 10 minutes. There is a high incidence of positive family history. Injuries and violent activity have been reported during sleepwalking episodes, but generally, individuals can negotiate their way around the room. Rarely, the occurrence of homicide has been reported and sometimes abnormal sexual behavior occurs. Sleep deprivation, fatigue, concurrent illness, and sedatives may act as precipitating factors. Treatment involves taking appropriate precautions to prevent wandering and troublesome behaviors. Medications that may improve the condition include imipramine and benzodiazepines. Remember also, that sleep terrors occur during the same stage of sleep as sleepwalking (stage IV, also called slow-wave sleep).

Neurology

B&D Ch. 68

Question 5. C.   The pregnancy categories are as follows:

Category A – Controlled studies show no risk. Generally considered safe.

Category B – Animal studies show no risk. No human studies available. Caution advised.

Category C – Animal studies show adverse fetal effect. No human studies available. Weigh risks and benefits.

Category D – Positive evidence of human fetal risk. Weigh risk and benefit.

Psychopharmacology

K&S Ch. 36

Question 6. A.   In Wernicke's aphasia, expressive speech is fluent but comprehension is impaired. The speech pattern is effortless and sometimes even excessively fluent (logorrhea). Speech is devoid of meaning, containing verbal paraphasias, neologisms, and jargon productions. This speech pattern is referred to as paragrammatism. Naming in Wernicke's aphasia is deficient, often with bizarre, paraphasic substitutions for the correct name. Auditory comprehension is impaired, sometimes even for simple nonsense questions. Deficient semantics is the major cause of the comprehension disturbance in Wernicke's aphasia, along with disturbed access to the internal lexicon. Repetition is impaired. Reading comprehension usually is affected in a fashion similar to that observed for auditory comprehension, but occasional patients show greater deficit in one modality than in the other. Writing also is impaired, but in a manner quite different from that of Broca's aphasia. The patient usually has no hemiparesis and can grasp the pen and write easily. The lesions of patients with Wernicke's aphasia usually involve the posterior portion of the superior temporal gyrus, sometimes extending into the inferior parietal lobule.

In 1909, Balint described a syndrome in which patients act blind, yet can describe small details of objects in central vision. The disorder is usually associated with bilateral hemisphere lesions, often involving the parietal and frontal lobes. Balint's syndrome involves a triad of deficits: (1) psychic paralysis of gaze, also called *ocular motor apraxia,* or difficulty directing the eyes away from central fixation; (2) *optic ataxia,* or incoordination of extremity movement under visual control (with normal coordination under proprioceptive control; and (3) impaired visual attention. These deficits result in the perception of only small details of a visual scene, with loss of the ability to scan and perceive the "big picture." Patients with Balint's syndrome literally cannot see the forest for the trees. Some but not all patients have bilateral visual field deficits.

A second partial Balint's syndrome deficit is *simultanagnosia,* or loss of ability to perceive more than one item at a time, first described by Wolpert in 1924. The patient sees details of pictures, but not the whole. Many such patients have left occipital lesions and associated pure alexia without agraphia; these patients can often read "letter-by-letter," or one letter at a time, but they cannot recognize a word at a glance.

Anomic aphasia refers to aphasic syndromes in which naming, or access to the internal lexicon, is the principal deficit. Spontaneous speech is normal except for the pauses and circumlocutions produced by the inability to name. Comprehension, repetition, reading, and writing are intact, except for the same word-finding difficulty in written productions. Isolated, severe anomia may indicate focal left hemisphere pathology. The angular gyrus is the purported site of lesions producing anomic aphasia, but lesions there usually produce other deficits as well, including alexia and the four elements of Gerstmann's syndrome: agraphia, right–left disorientation, acalculia, and finger agnosia, or inability to identify fingers.

Conduction aphasia is an uncommon but theoretically important syndrome that can be recognized by its striking deficit of repetition. Most patients have relatively normal spontaneous speech, although some make literal paraphasic errors and hesitate frequently for self-correction. Naming may be impaired, but auditory comprehension is preserved. Repetition may be disturbed to seemingly ridiculous extremes, such that a patient who is capable of self-expression at a sentence level, and can comprehend conversation, may be unable to repeat even single words. Associated deficits include hemianopia in some patients; right-sided sensory loss may be present, but right hemiparesis usually is mild or absent. The lesions of conduction aphasia usually involve either the superior temporal or inferior parietal region. Conduction aphasia has been advanced as a classical disconnection syndrome. Wernicke originally postulated that a lesion disconnecting Wernicke's and Broca's areas would produce this syndrome; Geschwind later pointed to the arcuate fasciculus, a white matter tract traveling from the deep temporal lobe, around the sylvian fissure, to the frontal lobe, as the site of disconnection.

Most psychotic patients speak in an easily understood, grammatically appropriate manner, but their behavior and speech content are abnormal. Only rarely do schizophrenics speak in "clang association" or "word salad" speech. Sudden onset of fluent, paraphasic speech in a middle-aged or elderly patient should always be suspected of representing a left hemisphere lesion with aphasia.

Neurology

B&D Ch. 12A

Question 7. C.   Accepting a small gift from a patient is acceptable under certain circumstances. The details of the case are important in determining whether or not to accept the gift. Exploitation involves using the therapeutic relationship for personal gain, such as hiring a patient, or going into business with a patient. You can not have any business interactions with a patient aside from their paying you for treatment. Charging for missed visits is considered ethical. Releasing information to the patient's insurance company is ethical. You should only release as much information as is necessary to process the claim or pre-approve the visit etc. It is ethical to keep a separate set of psychotherapy notes for your therapy patients that are not part of the medical record and to which the patient is not entitled access.

Ethics

K&S Ch. 58

Question 8. B.   Anterior cerebral artery (ACA) territory infarctions are uncommon. They occur in patients with vasospasm after subarachnoid hemorrhage caused by ACA or anterior communicating artery aneurysm. Excluding these causes, the percentage of acute cerebral infarcts that are in the ACA territory is less than 3%. The characteristics of ACA infarction vary according to the site of involvement and the extent of collateral blood flow. Contralateral weakness, involving primarily the lower extremity and, to a lesser extent, the arm, is characteristic of infarction in the territory of the hemispheric branches of the ACA. Other characteristics include abulia, akinetic mutism (with bilateral mesiofrontal damage), impaired memory or emotional disturbances, transcortical motor aphasia (with dominant hemispheric lesions), deviation of the head and eyes toward the lesion, paratonia (gegenhalten), discriminative and proprioceptive sensory loss (primarily in the lower extremity), and sphincter incontinence. An anterior disconnection syndrome with left arm apraxia caused by involvement of the anterior corpus callosum can be seen. Pericallosal branch involvement can cause apraxia, agraphia, and tactile anomia of the left hand. Infarction of the basal branches of the ACA can cause memory disorders, anxiety, and agitation. Infarction in the territory of the medial lenticulostriate artery (artery of Heubner) causes more pronounced weakness of the face and arm without sensory loss caused by this artery's supply of portions of the anterior limb of the internal capsule.

The anterior choroidal artery syndrome is often characterized by hemiparesis caused by involvement of the posterior limb of the internal capsule, hemisensory loss caused by involvement of the posterolateral nucleus of the thalamus or thalamocortical fibers, and hemianopia secondary to involvement of the lateral geniculate body or the geniculocalcarine tract. The visual field defect with anterior choroidal artery syndrome infarcts is characterized by a homonymous defect in the superior and inferior visual fields that spares the horizontal meridian. In a small number of patients, left spatial hemineglect with right hemispheric infarctions and a mild language disorder with left hemispheric infarctions may occur. With bilateral infarctions in the anterior choroidal artery syndrome territory, there can be pseudobulbar mutism and a variety of other features, including facial diplegia, hemisensory loss, lethargy, neglect, and affect changes.

Other answer choices are discussed in detail elsewhere in this volume.

Neurology

B&D Ch. 51A

Question 9. E.   Of the choices given only gabapentin is excreted unchanged in the urine. It has no interaction with the CYP 450 system and no liver metabolism. The other choices are first metabolized in the liver and their metabolites are subsequently excreted in the urine and/or feces.

Psychopharmacology

K&S Ch. 36

Question 10. E.   Transient amnesia is a temporary version of amnestic syndrome. The most striking example of transient amnesia is the syndrome of transient global amnesia, lasting from several to 24 hours. In this syndrome, an otherwise cognitively intact individual suddenly loses memory for recent events, asks repetitive questions about his or her environment, and sometimes confabulates. During the episode, the patient has both anterograde and retrograde amnesia, as in the permanent amnestic syndrome. As recovery occurs, however, the retrograde portion "shrinks" to a short period, leaving a permanent gap in memory of the brief retrograde amnesia before the episode and the period of no learning during the episode. The syndrome is of unknown cause but can be closely imitated by disorders of known etiology, such as partial complex seizures, migraine, and possibly transient ischemia of the hippocampus on one or both sides. Studies do not prove an ischemic etiology for transient global amnesia; rather, they indicate transient dysfunction in the hippocampus or its connections. Drug intoxication, alcoholic "blackouts," and minor head injuries can also produce transient amnesia.

Neurology

B&D Ch. 6

Question 11. C.   Nefazodone inhibits CYP3A4 thereby increasing trazodone levels.

Psychopharmacology

K&S Ch. 36

Question 12. B.   Psychogenic nonepileptic seizures are episodes of movement, sensation, or behaviors that resemble epileptic seizures, but do not have a neurologic origin; rather, they are somatic manifestations of psychologic distress. Inpatient video-electroencephalography monitoring is the gold standard for the diagnosis of nonepileptic seizures. Definitive diagnosis is made when a patient is observed having typical seizures without accompanying EEG abnormalities. From 5 to 10% of outpatient epilepsy patients and 20 to 40% of inpatient epilepsy patients have psychogenic nonepileptic seizures. Such patients inevitably have comorbid psychiatric illnesses, most commonly depression, post-traumatic stress disorder, other somatoform and dissociative disorders, and character pathology, especially borderline personality disorder or traits. Many patients have a history of sexual or physical abuse. Up to 40% of patients with nonepileptic seizures also have true epileptic seizures. Between 75 and 85 percent of patients with psychogenic nonepileptic seizures are women. Treatment involves discontinuation of antiepileptic drugs in patients without concurrent epilepsy and referral for appropriate psychiatric care. As an auxiliary investigation of suspected psychogenic seizures, plasma prolactin concentrations may provide additional supportive data. Plasma prolactin concentrations frequently are elevated after tonic–clonic seizures and less frequently after complex partial seizures. Serum prolactin levels almost invariably are normal after psychogenic seizures, although such a finding does not exclude the diagnosis of true epileptic seizures. Elevated prolactin levels, however, also may be present after syncope and with the use of drugs such as antidepressants, estrogens, bromocriptine, ergots, phenothiazines, and antiepileptic drugs. Although a number of procedures are employed to help distinguish epileptic from nonepileptic seizures, none of these procedures have both high sensitivity and high specificity. No procedure attains the reliability of EEG-video monitoring, which remains the standard diagnostic method for distinguishing between the two.

Neurology

B&D Ch. 2

Question 13. D.   Beta blockers are first line treatment for akathisia. Benzodiazepines may also help in some cases. Anticholinergics like benztropine are not helpful. Bromocriptine is a mixed dopamine agonist/antagonist useful in neuroleptic malignant syndrome, Parkinson's disease, elevated prolactin, and cocaine withdrawal. Nimodipine is a calcium channel blocker (useless for akathisia). Clonidine is an alpha 1 agonist which is useful in treating hypertension, aggression, attention deficit hyperactivity disorder, and opiate withdrawal.

Psychopharmacology

K&S Ch. 36

Question 14. D.   Characteristic of trigeminal neuralgia (TN), *tic douloureux*, is paroxysmal lancinating attacks of severe facial pain. TN has an incidence of approximately 4 per 100 000, with a large majority of cases occurring spontaneously. Both genders experience the disorder with a slight female predominance, and it is most common after the age of 50. Characteristics of classic TN include an abrupt onset and termination of unilateral brief electric shock-like pain. Pain often is limited to the distribution of one or two (commonly the second and third) divisions of the trigeminal nerve. Trivial stimuli, including washing, shaving, smoking, talking, and brushing the teeth (trigger factors), can evoke the pain. Some areas in the nasolabial fold or chin may be particularly susceptible to stimulation (trigger areas). In individual patients, stereotypical pain attacks recur with the same intensity and distribution. Most affected patients are symptom-free between attacks and clinical examination is usually normal. Attacks of TN occur in clusters and remissions can last for months. The cause of the pain attacks is unknown. Compression of the trigeminal nerve by benign tumors and vascular anomalies may play a role in the development of clinical symptoms.

Carbamazepine is the drug of first choice for treatment of TN. Both controlled and uncontrolled studies confirm its clinical efficacy. Carbamazepine monotherapy provides initial symptom control in as many as 80% of the patients. Of those initially responding to the drug, approximately 75% will continue to have long-term control of pain attacks. Controlled studies demonstrate that baclofen and lamotrigine are superior to placebo for treatment of TN. In the experience of many clinicians, baclofen is just as effective as carbamazepine and often better tolerated. Baclofen could be an alternate choice for initial drug therapy. Other medications that may be effective include oral gabapentin, clonazepam, oxcarbazepine, topiramate, and phenytoin. If a patient is not satisfied with single-medication therapy, adding another oral medication may offer additional benefit. Intravenous lidocaine or phenytoin may be effective for some severe refractory cases of TN. These treatments carry additional risks, however, and require close cardiovascular monitoring. Opioid analgesics are not effective for TN.

Neurology

B&D Ch. 44

Question 15. A.   Aspirin, the oldest and most commonly used nonprescription drug in the world, is the standard medical therapy for prevention of stroke in patients with transient cerebral ischemia, as well as for reducing the risk for recurrent stroke and postoperative strokes after carotid endarterectomy (CEA). Aspirin is effective, inexpensive, and safe if started within 48 hours of acute ischemic stroke. Meta-analyses have shown that aspirin reduces the combined risk for stroke, MI, and vascular death by approximately 25%. The optimal dose of aspirin remains a source of controversy among neurologists. The range of acceptable management includes daily doses ranging between 50 and 1300 mg of aspirin. There is a suggestion that aspirin is also effective in doses as low as 30 mg daily. The mechanism of action of aspirin is the irreversible inhibition of platelet function by inactivation of cyclo-oxygenase. The antiaggregant effect is seen within 1 hour after administration. Aspirin is also anti-inflammatory, antioxidant, and may increase fibrinolytic activity up to 4 hours after administration. The main side effect of aspirin is gastric discomfort. Gastrointestinal hemorrhage occurs in 1 to 5% of cases.

Evidence from several clinical studies favors the use of platelet antiaggregants as the first line of therapy in patients at high risk for stroke. These agents are indicated for secondary prevention of stroke. There appears to be no evidence to support the use of aspirin in primary prevention of stroke among low-risk middle-aged people. Results of primary prevention trials do not support the use of aspirin for primary stroke prevention. However, aspirin 81 mg every other day was effective in primary prevention of stroke in older women. Although aspirin did not offer a long-term protective effect among 372 asymptomatic patients with carotid bruits and greater than 50% carotid stenosis on duplex ultrasonography, many physicians continue its use in patients with carotid bruits or asymptomatic carotid stenosis under the assumption that it may be effective. Data regarding intraplaque hemorrhage caused by platelet antiaggregants are conflicting.

Oral anticoagulation with warfarin is indicated for primary and secondary prevention of stroke in patients with nonventricular atrial fibrillation. Ticlopidine and clopidogrel are structurally related thienopyridines that have antiplatelet effects. Ticlopidine reduces the relative risk for death or nonfatal stroke by 12% in comparison with aspirin. Ticlopidine acts primarily by irreversibly inhibiting the adenosine 5[1] diphosphate pathways of the platelet membrane. It also reduces plasma fibrinogen levels and increases erythrocyte deformability. The recommended dosage of ticlopidine, in most of the world, is

250 mg twice a day. Ticlopidine has more side effects than aspirin, including diarrhea, nausea, dyspepsia, and rash. The Clopidogrel versus Aspirin in Patients at Risk of Ischemic Events study (CAPRIE) assessed the relative efficacy of clopidogrel (75 mg daily) and aspirin (325 mg daily) in reducing the incidence of ischemic stroke, MI, or symptomatic atherosclerotic peripheral arterial disease. The results of this study showed that clopidogrel was modestly more effective (8.7% relative risk reduction) than aspirin in reducing the combined risk for ischemic stroke, MI, and vascular death in patients with atherosclerotic vascular disease. Clopidogrel is a platelet adenosine diphosphate receptor antagonist. Overall, the tolerability of clopidogrel was excellent, with no increased incidence of neutropenia, and a lower incidence of gastrointestinal hemorrhage and peptic, gastric, or duodenal ulcers when compared with aspirin. Despite this evidence, Aspirin is still the recommended treatment of choice 48 hours following an ischemic cerebrovascular event.

Neurology

B&D Ch. 51A

Question 16. C. Carpal tunnel syndrome is by far the most common entrapment neuropathy. This entrapment occurs in the tunnel through which the median nerve and flexor digitorum tendons pass. Because the transverse carpal ligament is an unyielding fibrous structure forming the roof of the tunnel, tenosynovitis or arthritis in this area often produces pressure on the median nerve. Symptoms consist of nocturnal pain and paresthesias, most often confined to the thumb, index, and middle fingers. Patients complain of tingling numbness and burning sensations, often awakening them from sleep. Referred pain may radiate to the forearm and even as high as the shoulder. Symptoms are often worse after excessive use of the hand or wrist. Objective sensory changes may be found in the distribution of the median nerve, most often impaired two-point discrimination, pinprick and light touch sensation, or occasionally hyperesthesia, in the thumb and index fingers, with sparing of the thenar eminence. Thenar (abductor pollicis brevis muscle) weakness and atrophy may be present with prolonged entrapment (see photo below).

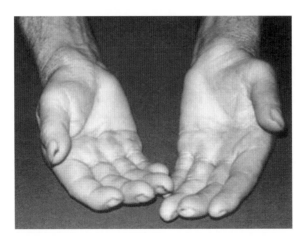

Thenar atrophy in chronic bilateral carpal tunnel syndrome

The syndrome is frequently bilateral and usually of greater intensity in the dominant hand. A positive Tinel's sign, in which percussion of the nerve at the carpal tunnel causes paresthesias in the distribution of the distal distribution of the median nerve, is present in approximately 60% of affected patients, but is not specific for carpal tunnel syndrome. Flexing the patient's hand at the wrist for 1 minute (Phalen's maneuver) or hyperextension of the wrist (reversed Phalen's maneuver) can reproduce the symptoms.

Approximately one in five pregnant women reports nocturnal hand paresthesias, primarily during the last trimester, often associated with peripheral edema. Excessive weight gain and fluid retention increase the occurrence of these complaints. This irritation can be expected to disappear spontaneously within weeks after parturition. During pregnancy, conservative therapy is indicated. Splitting of the wrist in the neutral position is helpful. Additionally, some physicians inject corticosteroids into the carpal tunnel. When hand muscles supplied by the median nerve weaken, surgical decompression using fiberoptic techniques is indicated.

Although it is frequently (mis)diagnosed, neurogenic thoracic outlet syndrome is a rare entity, seen only once or twice a year in busy EMG laboratories. Most patients are women. The mean age at onset is 32 years, but patients as young as 13 and as old as 73 years have been reported. Pain is usually the first symptom, with either aching noted on the inner side of the arm or soreness felt diffusely throughout the limb. Tingling sensations accompany pain and are felt along the inner side of the forearm and in the hand. In many cases, cervical spine roentgenograms disclose small bilateral cervical ribs or enlarged down-curving C7 transverse processes.

Arm pain and weakness are the cardinal manifestations of idiopathic brachial plexopathy. It occurs in all age groups, particularly between the third and seventh decades of life. Men are affected two to three times more often than women; there appears to be a higher incidence among men engaged in vigorous athletic activities, such as weight lifting, wrestling, and gymnastics. Although half of the cases seem unrelated to any precipitating event, in others the plexopathy follows an upper respiratory tract infection, a flu-like illness, an immunization, surgery, or psychological stress, or it occurs postpartum. The illness begins with the abrupt onset of intense pain, described as sharp, stabbing, throbbing, or aching, located in a variety of sites, including the shoulder, scapular area, trapezius ridge, upper arm, forearm, and hand. The pain may last from hours to many weeks, and then it gradually abates. Lessening of pain is associated with the appearance of weakness. This may have been present during the painful period but was not appreciated because the pain prevented the patient from moving the limb. Weakness may progress for 2 to 3 weeks after the onset of pain. Although pain subsides in most patients, it may continue for several weeks after weakness has reached its peak, and, rarely, it recurs episodically for a year or more. On examination, approximately one half of patients have weakness in muscles of the shoulder girdle, one third have weakness referable to both upper and lower parts of the plexus, and approximately 15% have evidence of lower plexus involvement alone. The natural history of brachial plexus neuropathy is benign; improvement occurs in the vast majority of patients, even in those with considerable muscle atrophy.

Neurology

B&D Chs 75,76&81

Question 17. D. Specific phobia is the most common anxiety disorder. It is the most common mental disorder among women and the second most common among men (after substance abuse). This fact takes many psychiatrists by surprise however, because most patients with specific phobia do not seek medical attention.

Statistics

K&S Ch. 16

Question 18. B. Neurofibromatosis (NF) is actually two separate diseases, each caused by a different gene. NF type 1 (NF1), or von Recklinghausen's disease, is the most common of the neurocutaneous syndromes, occurring in approximately 1 in 3000 people. NF type 2 (NF2) is characterized by bilateral vestibular schwannomas and often is associated with other brain or spinal cord tumors. NF2 occurs in only 1 in 35 000 to 50 000 people. Inheritance for both is an autosomal dominant pattern, but approximately half of NF1 cases result from a spontaneous mutation. The clinical features of both conditions are highly variable. A mutation of the 60-exon *NF1* gene on chromosome 17q causes NF1. The *NF1* gene product, neurofibromin, is a GTPase-activating protein, functioning to inhibit *ras*-mediated cell proliferation. Despite identification of approximately 100 mutations of *NF1* in various regions of the gene, none correlates to a specific clinical phenotype. Several patients have developed a somatic *NF1* mutation affecting only a limited region of the body. With this segmental NF, one extremity may have café-au-lait lesions, subcutaneous neurofibromas, and other signs of NF, but the rest of the body is unaffected. Similarly, some patients with only gonadal mosaicism have no outward manifestations of NF1 but have multiple affected offspring. A mutation of the *NF2* gene on chromosome 22 causes NF2. The NF2 protein product is *schwannomin* or *merlin*. The *NF2* gene suppresses tumor function. Dysfunction of the *NF2* gene accounts for the occurrence of multiple central nervous system (CNS) tumors in patients with NF2. The diagnostic criteria for NF1 and NF2 are as follows:

Neurofibromatosis Type 1 (any two or more)

- Six or more café-au-lait lesions more than 5 mm in diameter before puberty and more than 15 mm in diameter afterward
- Freckling in the axillary or inguinal areas
- Optic glioma
- Two or more neurofibromas or one plexiform neurofibroma
- A first-degree relative with neurofibromatosis type 1
- Two or more Lisch nodules
- A characteristic bony lesion (sphenoid dysplasia, thinning of the cortex of long bones, with or without pseudarthrosis)

Neurofibromatosis Type 2

- Bilateral VIII nerve tumor (shown by magnetic resonance imaging, computed tomography, or histological confirmation)
- A first-degree relative with neurofibromatosis type 2 and a unilateral eighth nerve tumor
- A first-degree relative with neurofibromatosis type 2 and any two of the following lesions: neurofibroma, meningioma, schwannoma, glioma, or juvenile posterior subcapsular lenticular opacity

Lisch nodules are pigmented iris hamartomas that are pathognomonic for NF1. Lisch nodules do not cause symptoms; their significance lies in their implications for the diagnosis of NF1. Lisch nodules are often not apparent during early childhood; therefore, their absence does not exclude the diagnosis of NF1. Rarely, children with NF1 have retinal hamartomas, but these usually remain asymptomatic. Optic nerve gliomas are the most common CNS tumors caused by NF1. About 15% of patients with NF1 have unilateral or bilateral optic glioma. Patients with NF2 have few cutaneous lesions. To meet criteria for NF2, patients must go on to develop bilateral schwannomas of the auditory nerve (acoustic neuromas), proven on neuroimaging or by postexcisional biopsy.

Neurology

B&D Ch. 65

Question 19. E.   Culture correlates most with ethnicity. People can be of the same race, age, gender, or nationality and have very different cultures.

Cultural Issues in Psychiatry

K&S Ch. 4

Question 20. A.   The porphyrias are caused by enzymatic defects in the heme biosynthetic pathway. Porphyrias with neuropsychiatric symptoms include acute intermittent porphyria (AIP), variegated porphyria (VP), hereditary mixed coproporphyria (HMP), and plumboporphyria (extremely rare and autosomal recessive), which may give rise to acute episodes of potentially fatal symptoms such as neurovisceral crisis, abdominal pain, delirium, psychosis, neuropathy, and autonomic instability. AIP, the most common type reported in the United States, follows an autosomal dominant pattern of inheritance and is due to a mutation in the gene for porphobilinogen deaminase. The disease is characterized by attacks that may last days to weeks, with relatively normal function between attacks. Infrequently, the clinical course may exhibit persisting clinical abnormalities with superimposed episodes of exacerbation. The episodic nature, clinical variability, and unusual features may cause symptoms to be attributed to somatization, conversion, or other psychiatric conditions. Attacks may be spontaneous, but are typically precipitated by a variety of factors such as infection, alcohol use, pregnancy, anesthesia, and numerous medications that include antidepressants, anticonvulsants, and oral contraceptives.

Porphyric attacks usually manifest with a triad consisting of abdominal pain, peripheral neuropathy, and neuropsychiatric symptoms. Seizures may also occur. Abdominal pain is the most common symptom, which can result in surgical exploration if the diagnosis is unknown. A variety of cognitive and behavioral changes can occur, including anxiety, restlessness, insomnia, depression, mania, hallucinations, delusions, confusion, catatonia, and psychosis. The diagnosis can be confirmed during an acute attack of AIP, HMP, or VP by measuring urine porphobilinogens. Acute attacks are treated with avoidance of precipitating factors (e.g., medications), intravenous hemin, intravenous glucose, and pain control.

Neurology

B&D Chs 9&62

Question 21. C. Lithium is cleared through the kidneys. It is reabsorbed in the proximal tubules with sodium. When a thiazide diuretic is added it leads to sodium depletion which in turn causes the reabsorbtion of sodium and lithium in the proximal tubules. This increased lithium reabsorbtion added to the lower fluid levels as a result of the diuretic can lead to an increased lithium level and lithium toxicity. Valproic acid and clozapine are metabolized through the liver and would not be effected by a thiazide diuretic.

Psychopharmacology

K&S Ch. 36

Question 22. B. The first medication approved by the FDA for use in MS was recombinant interferon beta-1b (Betaseron). Interferon beta-1b is administered subcutaneously every other day by self-injection. Side effects include influenza-like symptoms, which usually diminish over weeks to months, depression, and reactions at the injection site. The mechanism of action of interferon beta-1b is currently unknown, but may relate to anti-proliferative effects, cytokine changes, effects at the blood-brain barrier, and alterations of T-cell subsets.

Glatiramer acetate (formerly known as copolymer 1) (Copaxone) is a synthetic polypeptide administered by daily sub-cutaneous injection. Patients receiving glatiramer acetate have a 29% reduction in relapse rate over 2 years. The mechanism by which glatiramer acetate may work in humans is unknown, but may relate to interference with antigen presentation and induction of regulatory cells (Th2) that traffic to the CNS and induce bystander suppression of immune responses.

Tizanidine and Lioresal are muscle relaxing agents that are used to relieve some of the spasticity caused by multiple sclerosis. These are not disease-modifying agents. Prednisone, an oral corticosteroid, is given following an acute MS exacerbation to reduce the disease burden of an acute attack. Acute attacks are typically treated with intravenous corticosteroids. Indications for treatment of a relapse include functionally disabling symptoms with objective evidence of neurological impairment. Thus, mild sensory attacks are typically not treated. In the past, corticotropin and oral prednisone were primarily used. More recently, treatment with short courses of intravenous methylprednisolone, 500 to 1000 mg daily for 3 to 7 days, with or without a short prednisone taper, has commonly been used.

Neurology

B&D Ch. 54

Question 23. A. The most likely effects of ipecac abuse are cardiomyopathy, enlarged heart, increased QTc interval, increased CK-MB, decreased ejection fraction, tricuspid or mitral valve insufficiency, dysrythmia, low WBC, and increased LFTs. One would not expect pancreatitis (leading to an increase in amylase) or infection.

Feeding and Eating Disorders/Lab Tests in Psychiatry

K&S Ch. 23

Question 24. D. *Subcortical arteriosclerotic encephalopathy* (SAE), also known as Binswanger's disease, is a form of subcortical vascular dementia. Originally described in younger patients with hypertension (age 50 to 65), this disorder is characterized by a gradual (or stepwise) progressive dementia associated with frequent clinical strokes, motor and sensory deficits and seizures, multiple subcortical infarcts, and white matter lesions (WML; leukoaraiosis). Clinically, it may be difficult to differentiate from the *état lacunaire* described by Pierre Marie in patients with multiple subcortical ischemic lesions, including gray matter structures. SAE, however, is associated with more extensive WMLs, with ventricular enlargement. Both syndromes can have cortical infarcts and *état crible*, dilatation of the penetrating arteries' perivascular spaces. Although once believed to be rare, SAE is detected easily on CT or MRI, and the diagnosis is entertained more frequently when patients with cognitive decline have scans that show extensive subcortical WMLs. MRI can document that white matter abnormalities accompany the subcortical lacunes in a majority of cases. Therefore, the term used to describe this entity is *subcortical ischemic vascular dementia*, which incorporates subcortical WMLs and lacunar infarctions under the same subtype.

Gradual onset of cognitive difficulties is the first sign in more than half of the cases. Memory deficits, apathy, and slowed thinking are prominent. These memory deficits tend to be most prominent for delayed recall, with relative sparing of recognition memory, at least in comparison with this aspect of cognitive function in vascular dementia. Acute episodes of neurological dysfunction may occur at the onset or during the course; weakness, discoordination, and slurred speech are typical. Frequent falls often are reported. In some instances, these variable neurological signs and symptoms are absent, and the patient experiences only slowly progressing mental deterioration; such cases initially may be diagnosed as neurodegenerative disease such as Alzheimer's disease (AD).

Because the clinical picture is similar to that of MID (multi-infarct dementia with cortical strokes), cases with Binswanger's disease probably are included as MID in population studies. The population incidence and prevalence are unknown.

Neurology

B&D Ch. 66

Question 25. B.   At 23 months children can respond to simple directions and understand pronouns. They can also follow action commands and begin to understand complex sentences.

Human Development

K&S Ch. 2

Question 26. E.   Essential tremor (ET) is one of the most common movement disorders. In population-based studies, the prevalence increases steadily with age, occurring in up to 10% of patients older than age 60 years. The prevalence is higher in men than in women and in whites than in nonwhites. In its purest form, ET is a monosymptomatic illness characterized by gradually increasing amplitude postural and kinetic tremor of the forearms and hands (with or without involvement of other body parts), in the absence of endogenous or exogenous triggers or other neurological signs.

The typical patient becomes aware of a barely perceptible postural or action tremor, usually in the distal arms and hands. The head and lower limbs are less commonly affected. Head tremor (*titubation*) is milder than limb tremor and is predominantly of a side-to-side, "no-no" type. Tremor of the face, trunk, and voice are rarely seen. The kinetic tremor is higher in amplitude than the postural tremor and is the major determinant of disability. Handwriting is particularly troublesome. A striking improvement after ingestion of a small amount of ethanol is seen in 50% of patients and may be helpful in diagnosis. Over time, the tremor worsens, causing increasing functional disability. Only a fraction of affected persons seek medical attention, and there is often a long latency from onset to presentation for care. ET is thought to be a monosymptomatic illness without changes in cognition, strength, coordination, or muscle tone, and the results of the neurological examination are usually normal.

As many as two thirds of patients give a positive family history of tremor, and first-degree relatives of patients with ET are 5 to 10 times more likely to have ET than first-degree relatives of control subjects.

Patients with mild ET whose main source of disability is tremor during meals and whose tremors respond to ethanol often benefit from a cocktail before meals. The two most commonly used pharmacological treatments are beta-adrenergic blockers and primidone.

Stereotactic thalamotomy has been reported to suppress contralateral tremor as much as 75% in up to 90% of cases. The effect appears to be long lasting. Side effects of this procedure are relatively common, although most are transient, and bilateral thalamotomy may cause speech difficulty, so it should be avoided. Thalamic deep brain stimulation has shown very good efficacy in controlling ET. Tremor improves as much as 80% contralateral to the implantation, and bilateral stimulation can be performed safely with long-lasting benefits. DBS should be considered for cognitively intact, otherwise healthy patients with disabling medication-resistant tremor.

Neurology

B&D Ch. 75

Question 27. E. In the "communication stage" from 55 months onward, a child can use language to tell a story, share ideas, and discuss alternatives. They can understand concepts such as number, speed, time, space, and left vs. right. Their speech at this stage is 100% intelligible.

Human Development

K&S Ch. 2

Question 28. B. Wernicke's encephalopathy is due to thiamine deficiency. Although the most common clinical setting for this disorder is chronic alcoholism, a large number of cases occur in other conditions, with the only prerequisite being a poor nutritional state, either from inadequate intake, malabsorption, or increased metabolic requirement. Wernicke's encephalopathy may be precipitated acutely in at-risk patients by intravenous glucose administration or carbohydrate loading.

Wernicke's original description of the clinical triad of confusion, ophthalmoplegia, and ataxia is still valid. The confusional state develops over days or weeks and is characterized by inattention, apathy, disorientation, and memory loss. Stupor or coma is rare. Ophthalmoplegia, when present, commonly involves both lateral recti, either in isolation or together with palsies of other extraocular muscles. Patients may have horizontal nystagmus on lateral gaze, and many also have vertical nystagmus on upgaze. Sluggish reaction to light, light-near dissociation, and other pupillary abnormalities are sometimes seen. Truncal ataxia is common, but limb ataxia is not, findings similar to those seen in alcoholic cerebellar degeneration.

The clinical findings reflect the localization of pathological abnormalities in this disease; namely, the prominent involvement of periventricular structures at the level of the third and fourth ventricles. Lesions of the nuclei of cranial nerves III, VI, and VIII are responsible for the eye findings. The truncal ataxia is probably caused by the vestibular dysfunction and involvement of the superior cerebellar vermis.

Wernicke's encephalopathy is a clinical diagnosis, although brain MRI can be helpful. MRI may show signal abnormalities on T2-weighted, fluid-attenuated inversion recovery, and diffusion-weighted images in the periaqueductal regions, medial thalami, and bilateral mammillary bodies.

Patients suspected of Wernicke's encephalopathy should receive thiamine before administration of glucose to avoid precipitation of acute symptom worsening. Thiamine is the only treatment known to alter the outcome. A dose of 50 to 100 mg should be given parenterally in the acute stage because intestinal absorption is unreliable in debilitated and alcoholic patients. Thiamine can then be continued daily through the acute period.

If left untreated, Wernicke's encephalopathy is progressive. The mortality, even with thiamine treatment, was 10 to 20% in the early studies. With treatment, the majority of ocular signs resolve within hours, although a fine horizontal nystagmus persists in approximately 60% of patients.

In Korsakoff's syndrome, memory is impaired out of proportion to other cognitive functions. This is due to the selective localization of the lesions in the diencephalon and temporal lobes. Injury to these regions regardless of cause (e.g., infarction, trauma, tumors, or herpes encephalitis) can produce a syndrome indistinguishable from the amnesia syndrome seen in alcoholic patients.

The memory impairment is characterized by the presence of both anterograde and retrograde amnesia. Confabulation can be a prominent feature, especially in the early stages, although it may be absent in some patients.

Despite treatment with thiamine, improvement in memory function is slow and may be incomplete. Those who improve usually do so after a 1-month delay or longer. Occasionally, patients may not achieve maximal improvement for more than a year.

In 1903, Marchiafava and Bignami, two Italian pathologists, described a syndrome of selective demyelination of the corpus callosum in alcoholic Italians who indulged in large quantities of red wine. The disease seems to affect severe and chronic alcoholics in their middle or late adult life, with a peak incidence between ages 40 and 60. Because of the background history of alcohol abuse, a nutritional cause has been invoked, but no nutritional factor has been identified. A toxic cause, such as direct toxicity of ethanol or other constituents, seems equally plausible. The neurological presentation is that of a variable combination of mental and motor slowing, personality and behavior changes, incontinence, dysarthria, seizures, and hemiparesis. Occasionally patients present with coma. The most common is a frontal lobe or dementing syndrome. Sucking, grasping, and gegenhalten may be prominent. Pathologically, there is selective involvement of the central portion of the corpus callosum; the dorsal and ventral portions are spared or affected to a much lesser degree. There also may be symmetrical involvement of other white matter tracts. MRI is valuable for premortem visualization of these white matter lesions. Treatment should be directed at nutritional support and rehabilitation from alcoholism. In those patients who recovered, it is not clear whether improvement was a result of vitamin supplementation or merely a reflection of the disease's natural history.

Neurology

B&D Ch. 57

Question 29. D. The Judgment of Line Orientation Test is useful in detecting right hemisphere disease. This test involves matching lines of the same slope. A patient with right hemisphere disease will have a very hard time with this, whereas a patient with only left hemisphere disease can complete the task without difficulty. The Boston diagnostic aphasia examination is just that...an exam for aphasia. The sentence completion test is used to test the patient's associations with areas of interest by having the patient complete sentences. Responses that are particularly emotional or are repeated are noted by the examiner. The Thematic Apperception Test has patients create a story based on pictures they are presented with. The stories the patient generates tell the examiner about their thoughts, feelings, organization, assumptions etc.

Psychological Theory and Psychometric Testing

K&S Ch. 5

Question 30. D. First described in 1964 by Steele, Richardson, and Olszewski as a progressive illness characterized by vertical supranuclear ophthalmoplegia, axial rigidity, pseudobulbar palsy, and mild dementia, progressive supranuclear palsy (PSP) is the second most common form of neurodegenerative atypical parkinsonism. PSP typically begins in the sixth to seventh decades of life with gait disorder and falling. Patients develop an akinetic-rigid state with symmetrical signs and prominent axial rigidity. In contrast to the flexed posture of patients with PD, those with PSP may have an extended trunk or retrocolic neck posture. A characteristic facial appearance with a wide-eyed stare, furrowing of the forehead, and deepening of other facial creases allows experienced clinicians to make an instant diagnosis. Pseudobulbar palsy with dysarthria and dysphagia lend the patient a characteristic dysarthria with spasticity, hypokinesia, and ataxia and often "silent" aspiration. Frontal lobe features are common. There is striking executive dysfunction early in the disease course; concrete thought, difficulty shifting set, decreased verbal fluency, and personality changes such as impulsivity and poor judgment are nearly universal. Although considered a clinical hallmark of PSP, supranuclear vertical gaze palsy may not appear until later in the disease course, and some patients may never develop gaze palsy. Abnormal vertical saccades, best demonstrated by examination for opticokinetic nystagmus, compared to horizontal saccades, is one of the earliest ophthalmological signs of PSP. PSP almost always occurs sporadically, yet an increasing number of familial cases suggest a genetic etiology in some cases. There is growing support for the notion of altered regulation of tau gene expression in PSP. No toxic, viral, or other environmental risk factors have been described.

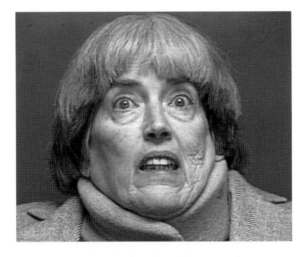

Typical facial expression of a patient with progressive supranuclear palsy, illustrating worried or surprised appearance, with furrowed brow and fixed expression of lower face.

Dopaminergic agents, particularly levodopa (LD), may provide temporary improvement in bradykinesia in approximately 40% of patients, but LD usually does not improve dysarthria, gait, or balance problems. The prognosis of PSP is poor, with serious impact on quality of life and a median duration of survival of approximately 8 years.

Pseudobulbar palsy (or spastic bulbar palsy) develops when there is disease involvement of the corticobulbar tracts that exert supranuclear control over those motor nuclei that control speech, mastication, and deglutition. The prefix "pseudo-" is used to distinguish this condition from "true" bulbar palsy that results from pure LMN involvement in brainstem motor nuclei. Articulation, mastication, and deglutition are affected in both pseudobulbar and bulbar palsies, but the degree of impairment in pseudobulbar palsy is generally milder. Spontaneous or unmotivated crying and laughter uniquely characterize pseudobulbar palsy. This is also termed *emotional lability*, *hyperemotionality*, *labile affect*, or *emotional incontinence* and is often a source of great embarrassment to the patient. A patient advocacy group has suggested a new term, involuntary emotional expression disorder, to prevent the possible misconception that the "pseudo" in pseudobulbar palsy implies that it is not a true disorder.

Neurology

B&D Chs 71&74

Question 31. B.   Of all the answer choices, only introjection is an immature defense. All other choices in this question are mature. Other immature defenses include acting out, blocking, hypochondriasis, regression, passive–aggressive behavior, somatization, projection, and schizoid fantasy. We will not take the space to define all 12 defenses listed in this question and answer explanation, but suffice it to say they are all fair game for a standardized exam and you should take the time to learn any that are unfamiliar to you. You may also see questions on several of them elsewhere throughout this book.

Psychological Theory and Psychometric Testing

K&S Ch. 6

Question 32. C.   The prevalence of adult-onset primary focal or segmental dystonia is 12.9 per 100 000. Cervical dystonia and blepharospasm are most commonly represented. The focal and segmental primary dystonias generally begin in adulthood with dystonic movements in the hand and arm, neck, or face. When spread occurs, the ultimate distribution tends to maintain a segmental pattern. Cervical dystonia is the most frequently diagnosed form of focal dystonia, accounting for about half of focal dystonia cases. Patients with cervical dystonia present with neck pain, difficulty maintaining a normal head position, and sometimes tremor. Dystonic tremor, which may be present not only in patients with cervical dystonia, but also in those with limb dystonia, is usually an irregular oscillatory movement that stops when the patient is allowed to place the head or limb in the position of the dystonic pulling, the so-called *null point*. There is a directional preponderance to dystonia movements, which is usually maintained throughout the course of the disease. Many studies have suggested that focal and segmental dystonia might have a genetic basis. Approximately 25% of adult-onset focal or segmental dystonia patients have a positive family history of dystonia, which would be consistent with an autosomal dominant condition with low penetrance. The locus has been mapped to chromosome 18. Medical treatment of adult-onset primary focal and segmental dystonia is difficult and employs those agents typically used in generalized dystonia. Adults are less able to tolerate effective doses of these agents, so the response to therapy is somewhat more disappointing than that seen in children. Botulinum toxin injections, on the other hand, are very helpful in the treatment of focal and segmental dystonia. Botulinum toxin is injected subcutaneously over the facial muscles or directly into larger deeper muscles that underlie pain and inappropriate movement in other focal dystonias. Many, though not all, clinicians use EMG to help guide toxin injection. Botulinum toxin injections have been proven effective in the treatment of blepharospasm and other facial dystonias, as well as cervical dystonia. Clinical experience suggests they are useful in the treatment of oromandibular, laryngeal, truncal, and limb dystonia. Overall, more than 75% of treated patients report moderate to marked improvement in dystonic pain or posture. The procedure is generally well tolerated, with excessive weakness of injected muscles or occasionally neighboring muscles the most often reported side effect. The mechanism of action of botulinum toxin appears complex.

Neurology

B&D Ch. 75

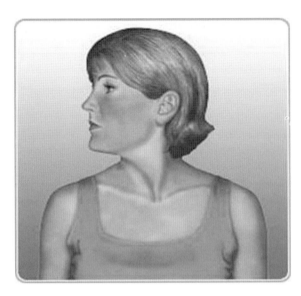

A patient with cervical dystonia (torticollis) with head rotation to the right demonstrating marked hypertrophy of the left sternocleidomastoid muscle.

Question 33. E. This question is really about orgasmic disorder. In order to properly diagnose orgasmic disorder you must rule out possible medical causes including medications. Some common causes of anorgasmia include alcohol, marijuana, SSRIs, TCAs, benzodiazepines, diabetes, spinal cord damage, hormones, pelvic injury, cardiac problems, liver disease or kidney disease.

Orgasmic disorder is defined as a recurrent delay in or absence of orgasm following a normal excitement phase. It must cause marked distress. The DSM divides the diagnosis into male and female orgasmic disorder. It occurs more frequently in women than in men.

Sexual Dysfunction

K&S Ch. 21

Question 34. A. Juvenile myoclonic epilepsy (JME) accounts for 4–10% of all cases of epilepsy, but the diagnosis often is delayed and the prevalence is underestimated because symptoms are not recognized. Other names for JME are *impulsive petit mal*, *jerk epilepsy*, and *myoclonic epilepsy of adolescence*. Age at onset usually is between 12 and 18 years, but onset may occur from 8 to 30 years. The characteristic feature is sudden, mild to moderate myoclonic jerks of the shoulders and arms that usually occur after awakening. Generalized tonic–clonic seizures develop in 90% of cases, and approximately one third of the patients have absence seizures. Myoclonic seizures precede generalized tonic–clonic seizures in approximately one half of the patients. Initially, myoclonic jerks are mild and explained as nervousness, clumsiness, or tics. They may be unrecognized as seizures until a generalized tonic–clonic seizure brings the patient to medical attention. Sleep deprivation, alcohol intake, and fatigue precipitate seizures. Affected persons are of normal intelligence, and neurological deterioration does not occur. A seizure disorder with onset between ages 1 and 5 years has been recognized that may represent a bridge between benign myoclonic epilepsy of infancy and JME. Development and intelligence are normal. Even though JME manifests as a clinically well-defined disorder with some variation, different genetic and pathophysiological mechanisms seem to be responsible for the condition. Multiple different genetic abnormalities and mechanisms may be responsible for influencing neuronal excitability in JME.

The interictal EEG in JME consists of bilateral, symmetrical spike and polyspike-and-wave discharges of 3 to 5 Hz, usually maximal in the frontocentral regions. The EEG correlate of the myoclonic jerks is a burst of high-voltage, 10–16-Hz polyspikes followed by irregular 1-Hz slow waves and single spikes or polyspike discharges. Focal EEG abnormalities occur in a significant number of patients with JME.

Valproic acid controls the seizures, but lifetime treatment is necessary. Lamotrigine, levetiracetam, topiramate, and zonisamide may be considered in patients who do not tolerate valproic acid. In some situations, lamotrigine may exacerbate myoclonus. Ethosuximide is useful to treat uncontrolled absence seizures.

Benign childhood epilepsy with centrotemporal spikes (BECTS) also is referred to as benign rolandic epilepsy. Seizures begin between 3 and 13 years of age with a peak onset at 9 to 10 years of age. The typical seizure characteristics are somatosensory disturbance of the mouth, preservation of consciousness, excessive pooling of saliva and tonic or tonic–clonic activity of the face, and speech arrest when the dominant hemisphere is affected. The somatosensory or motor activity may spread to the arm. Secondary generalization may occur, especially when the seizures are nocturnal. Seizures typically occur shortly after sleep onset, just before awakening, and with naps. Seizures can occur during the day. Headache and vomiting may be associated. Development, neurological examinations, and neuroradiological studies at the time of diagnosis typically are normal. Seizures usually stop in adolescence, and the outcome is favorable. Some children with BECTS have cognitive or behavioral problems, particularly difficulty with sustained attention, reading, and language processing. A family history of epilepsy is present in approximately 10% of cases.

The EEG consists of a normal background with midtemporal and central, high-amplitude, often diphasic spikes and sharp waves with increased frequency during sleep. The spikes and sharp waves are usually unilateral, but they may be bilateral. Because the overall prognosis for benign childhood epilepsy is good, treatment is not required after the first or even the second seizure, and some children never require treatment. Most anticonvulsant drugs are effective as monotherapy.

Neurology

B&D Ch. 67

Question 35. B. The practice described in the question is called "fee splitting" and is considered unethical. As a physician you cannot receive financial compensation for referring patients to other doctors, nor can you pay for such referrals. Such an arrangement puts the doctor's interests (the financial incentive to refer) over the best interests of the patient and leads to inappropriate referrals.

Ethics

K&S Ch. 58

Question 36. B. Advances in medical and surgical techniques in liver transplantation have improved long-term post-transplantation survival, with reported 5-year survival rates of 80–90%. Liver transplantation has become the accepted standard of care in children with end-stage liver disease. Congenital biliary atresia is the most common reason for liver transplantation in children. Other causes are biliary micronodular cirrhosis, viral hepatitis, Alagille syndrome, and several rare genetic disorders.

Neurological problems occur in 48% of pediatric orthotopic liver transplant recipients. A majority involve seizures, mental status changes, or coma. Three fourths of comatose patients had significant intracerebral hemorrhage on brain imaging. Neurological complications constitute a significant source of mortality and morbidity in these patients. A recent study reviewed data for 41 adults and pediatric patients who underwent liver transplantation. Encephalopathy occurred in 62% with either immediate or delayed onset. Seizures (multifocal myoclonus, focal, or status epilepticus) occurred in 11% and were associated with the presence of encephalopathy. Three patients had neuropathy. Other complications were headache, tremor, fatigue, restlessness, enuresis, dizziness, critical illness myopathy, and detached retina. Brain imaging revealed atrophy, subarachnoid hemorrhage, intracerebral hemorrhage, and infections.

Neurology

B&D Ch. 49B

Question 37. A. Erikson developed the concept of the epigenetic principle. The epigenetic principle states that human development occurs in sequential, clearly defined stages, and that each stage must be properly resolved for development to proceed normally. Other famous therapists listed in this question are the subject of their own questions elsewhere in this text.

Human Development

K&S Ch. 4

Question 38. C. An isolated, painful abducens palsy may represent microvascular ischemia, especially in older patients with vascular risk factors. Spontaneous resolution over 8 to 12 weeks is typical. In the absence of complete, spontaneous resolution, neuroimaging is essential. Head trauma, even if mild, is another relatively common cause of abducens palsy. Impaired ability to abduct the eye past midline or bilateral presentation predicts poor spontaneous recovery. The abducens nerve is the cranial nerve most commonly affected bilaterally in isolation. This occurs most often from trauma and increased intracranial pressure.

A third-nerve palsy is the most commonly encountered diabetic cranial mononeuropathy. Pupillary sparing, the hallmark of diabetic third-nerve palsy, results from ischemic infarction of the centrifascicular oculomotor axons due to diabetic vasculopathy of the vasa nervorum. The peripherally located pupillary motor fibers are spared as a result of collateral circulation from the circumferential arteries. With decreasing frequency, the fourth, sixth, and seventh nerves are also affected. Patients with Bell's palsy have a significantly higher frequency of diabetes than an age-matched population. Most make a full recovery in 3 to 5 months.

Neurology

B&D Chs 70&76

Question 39. E. Appropriate specifiers for substance induced anxiety disorder include "with generalized anxiety", "with panic attacks", "with obsessive–compulsive symptoms", and "with phobic symptoms". Other specifiers include "with onset during intoxication" and "with onset during withdrawal". "With delayed onset" is not appropriate to use with this diagnosis. Though some may think this question is picky or unfair, the details of the DSM are indeed fair game for a test of general psychiatric knowledge. The small details of the DSM give the test writer ample opportunity to form tricky questions. Know your DSM well!

Anxiety Disorders

K&S Ch. 16

Question 40. D. Herpes simplex virus-1 encephalitis (HSE) is the most common cause of sporadic, fatal encephalitis in the United States, accounting for approximately 10% of all cases of encephalitis and occurring with a frequency of about 1 case/250 000 population/year. Early recognition is important because the antiviral drug acyclovir (ACV) is effective in reducing morbidity and mortality. HSV-1 strains are causal agents in over 90% of cases of HSE in adults. Type 2 strains are more commonly isolated in monophasic or recurrent meningitis and congenitally acquired neonatal HSV meningoencephalitis. Fever is present in approximately 90% and headache in about 80% of patients with biopsy or polymerase chain reaction (PCR)-proven HSE. Other common features include disorientation (70%), personality change (70–85%), focal or generalized seizures (40–67%), memory disturbance (25–45%), motor deficit (30–40%), and aphasia (33%). The presence of olfactory hallucinations should also suggest the possibility of HSE.

Examination of CSF is the single most important diagnostic test in suspected cases of HSE. CSF is usually under increased pressure, with a lymphocytic pleocytosis of 10 to 1000 white blood cell count (WBC) per microliter. More than 95% of PCR- or biopsy-proven cases of HSE have a CSF pleocytosis, although rare cases with an initial acellular CSF have been reported. HSE is often hemorrhagic, and both red blood cells and xanthochromia can occur in the CSF, although neither feature occurs with significantly greater frequency in HSE than with other causes of focal encephalitis. CSF protein is usually moderately elevated, and glucose is normal in more than 90% of cases. Virus cannot be cultured from CSF in more than 95% of cases of HSE; however, HSV DNA can be detected in the CSF with PCR techniques. Amplification of HSV DNA from CSF by PCR testing has a sensitivity and specificity of greater than 95% for the diagnosis of HSE compared with brain biopsy and is the diagnostic procedure of choice for HSE. MRI is significantly more sensitive than CT and is the neuroimaging procedure of choice in patients with suspected HSE. Approximately 90% of patients with PCR-proven HSE will have MRI abnormalities involving the temporal lobes. The electroencephalogram (EEG) may be abnormal early in the course of disease, demonstrating diffuse slowing, focal abnormalities in the temporal regions, or periodic lateralizing epileptiform discharges (PLEDs). EEG abnormalities involving the temporal lobes are seen in approximately 75% of patients with PCR-proven HSE. Because of its safety, empiric therapy with ACV should be started immediately in cases of suspected focal encephalitis. The mortality rate in untreated cases of HSE is about 70%, which is reduced to 19–28% in patients treated with ACV.

Neurology

B&D Ch. 53B

Question 41. E. This question is really asking why pain disorder is a psychiatric condition rather than a medical one. And the answer, of course, is that in pain disorder the pain is thought to be mediated by psychological factors. In chronic pain syndromes, which are in the domain of medicine and not psychiatry, there is thought to be a physical cause for the pain even if that cause cannot be identified. In pain disorder there is believed to be no medical cause or the pain is grossly disproportionate to any pathological findings. In pain disorder psychological factors are felt to play a major role in the precipitation, maintenance or exacerbation of the pain. Any of the other choices could be true for either condition and are not the key difference used to differentiate the two.

Somatic Symptom Disorders

K&S Ch. 17

Question 42. B. Inclusion body myositis (IBM) is the most common myopathy in patients over the age of 50 years. Only rarely does it occur in people less than 50 years of age. Unlike dermatomyositis, polymyositis, and other autoimmune disorders, inclusion body myositis is much more common in men than in women. The disease weakens the distal muscles of the arms and legs. The deep finger flexors, including the flexor pollicis longus, and wrist flexors are involved early. They are usually more involved than the wrist and finger extensors. In the legs, early involvement of the quadriceps and anterior tibial muscles occurs. Profound atrophy is appreciable in the flexor forearms and quadriceps. The disease generally has a chronic progressive course and is considered unresponsive to prednisone and other immunosuppressive (e.g., methotrexate) and immunomodulating (e.g., IVIG) therapies. The clinical history and examination are the basis for suspecting the diagnosis of IBM. Muscle biopsy is confirmatory. The CK concentration may be normal or only mildly elevated (<10 times the upper limit of normal). The EMG demonstrates fibrillation potentials and positive sharp waves. The muscle biopsy demonstrates endomysial inflammation and invasion of non-necrotic muscle fibers similar to polymyositis. In addition, characteristic "rimmed" vacuoles may be profuse.

Dermatomyositis is an illness in which weakness is associated with a characteristic skin rash. It is the common form of myositis occurring in childhood through middle adult life. The rash usually occurs with onset of muscle weakness, although it may develop during the course of the disease. It is characteristically a purplish discoloration of the skin over the cheeks and eyelids. It often has a butterfly distribution and blanches on pressure. The weakness is symmetrical and affects the proximal more than distal muscles of the arms and legs. Muscle pain is noted, but not in all patients. The serum CK concentrations are usually elevated in dermatomyositis but can be normal earlier in the course or in patients with a very indolent course. Serum CK levels do not necessarily reflect activity of the disease. The characteristic histological feature on muscle biopsy is perifascicular atrophy (a crust of small fibers surrounding a core of more normal-sized fibers deeper in the fascicle).

Polymyositis is an acute or subacute illness that occurs in adults. Cases of polymyositis in infants and children probably represent muscular dystrophies with inflammation. It is more frequent in women than in men, as are other autoimmune diseases. As in dermatomyositis, weakness is symmetrical and affects the proximal more than distal muscles of the arms and legs. Systemic symptoms are common at onset, such as malaise, fever, and anorexia. A viral prodrome sometimes precedes the illness, but such events are sufficiently common enough that the association may be coincidental. The diagnostic studies in polymyositis are similar to those in dermatomyositis and include serum CK concentrations, serum autoantibodies, EMG, and muscle biopsy. Serum CK concentration should always be elevated in polymyositis, unlike dermatomyositis or inclusion body myositis, in which the CK concentration may be normal.

Neurology

B&D Ch. 79

Question 43. D. This question tests the four most commonly asked neural pathways on standardized psych exams. The tuberoinfundibular pathway goes from the hypothalamus to the anterior pituitary. It is important in the regulation of prolactin secretion. The nigrostriatal pathway goes from the substantia nigra to the basal ganglia. It is important in the development of extrapyramidal symptoms. The mesocortical pathway goes from the ventral tegmental area to the frontal cortex and is involved in the negative symptoms of schizophrenia. The mesolimbic pathway goes from the ventral tegmental area to the nucleus accumbens and is involved in positive psychotic symptoms. The ventral amygdalofugal pathways are a distracter. They are not commonly asked on exams and are part of the limbic system, running from the amygdala to the thalamus and hypothalamus.

Basic Neuroscience

K&S Ch. 3

Question 44. C. Mitochondrial encephalomyopathy, lactic acidosis, and stroke-like episodes (MELAS) is a maternally inherited encephalomyopathy clinically characterized by stroke-like episodes, vascular headaches, vomiting, seizures, and lactic acidosis. The stroke deficits are sometimes transient but can be permanent and cause progressive encephalopathy with dementia. Unusual clinical patterns include focal seizures, sometimes prolonged, which can herald a stroke. The unique radiological feature is that the stroke involves the cerebral cortex, sparing the white matter, mostly in the parietal and occipital regions. Neuroimaging may show additional lesions that have no clinical correlates. The onset is generally in childhood or early adult life. Most patients have RRF on muscle biopsy, but only rarely is there clinical weakness or exercise intolerance. The finding of excessive mutation load in the endothelium and smooth muscle of cerebral vessels has been suggested as the likely cause of stroke episodes and migraine headaches in these patients.

Myoclonic epilepsy with ragged-red fiber myopathy (MERRF) is another maternally inherited encephalomyopathy characterized by myoclonus, epilepsy, cerebellar ataxia, and myopathy with RRF. Onset is usually in childhood or early adulthood. The syndrome begins generally with myoclonic epilepsy in childhood, and other seizure patterns are added soon thereafter. Worsening ataxia and mental retardation is seen in later childhood.

The clinical deficit in Leber's hereditary optic neuropathy (LHON) is usually an isolated bilateral optic neuropathy. LHON is expressed predominantly in males of the maternal lineage, but the greater susceptibility of males to vision loss in LHON remains unexplained. The age of onset is typically between 15 and 35 years, and the vision loss is painless, central, and usually occurs in one eye weeks or months before involvement of the other eye. Funduscopic abnormalities may be seen in patients with LHON and in their asymptomatic relatives. Especially during the acute phase of vision loss, there may be hyperemia of the optic nerve head, dilatation and tortuosity of peripapillary vessels, circumpapillary telangiectasia, nerve fiber edema, and focal hemorrhage. Vision loss in LHON affects central or centrocecal fields and is usually permanent. A minority of patients show objective improvement, sometimes to a dramatic degree. In most LHON patients, vision loss is the only manifestation of the disease. Some families have additional members with associated cardiac conduction abnormalities, especially pre-excitation syndromes. There may also be a movement disorder or other minor neurological or skeletal abnormalities.

Kearns–Sayre syndrome (KSS) is defined by the triad of progressive external ophthalmoplegia (PEO), onset before age 20, and at least one of the following: short stature, pigmentary retinopathy, cerebellar ataxia, heart block, and elevated CSF protein (>100 mg/dL). Many patients with KSS are physically or mentally subnormal. Some clinical features of MELAS and MERRF may overlap with KSS. The clinical course in KSS is progressive, and most patients with associated mental retardation die in the third or fourth decade.

Neurology

B&D Ch. 63

Question 45. E.   This question covers the paraphilias. Sexual masochism is a preoccupation with fantasies or urges of being beaten, bound or humiliated. Fetishism is being sexually fixated on and aroused by inanimate objects like shoes or pantyhose. Voyeurism is preoccupation with fantasies of observing an unsuspecting person who is naked or involved in sexual activity. Transvestic fetishism involves fantasies and sexual urges to dress in clothing of the opposite gender in order to obtain sexual arousal. Frotteurism involves rubbing ones genitals against a nonconsenting person in order to obtain sexual arousal.

Paraphilias

K&S Ch. 21

Question 46. A.   Botulinum toxin blocks acetylcholine release at peripheral synapses, leading to the paralytic and autonomic clinical manifestations of botulism. Botulinum toxin causes irreversible blockade at peripheral cholinergic synapses. Recovery requires sprouting of new nerve terminals, accounting for the protracted clinical course of botulism.

Neurology

B&D Ch. 53C

Question 47. C.   Signs of nicotine withdrawal include depressed mood, insomnia, irritability, anxiety, poor concentration, restlessness, decreased heart rate, and increased appetite. To meet DSM criteria for nicotine withdrawal four of the above symptoms must be present within 24 hours of cessation of nicotine.

Substance Abuse and Addictive Disorders

K&S Ch. 12

Question 48. E. If stroke patients meet appropriate criteria, thrombolytic therapy may be administered. Thrombolytic therapy is able to recanalize acute intracranial occlusions, but the question remains whether thrombolytic therapy can recanalize occlusions of large extracranial or other large intracranial vessels (e.g., carotid terminus). A strong correlation has been shown between arterial recanalization and neurological improvement in acute cerebral ischemia.

In June 1996, the Food and Drug Administration (FDA) approved the use of intravenous tissue plasminogen activator (t-PA) for ischemic stroke within 3 hours of symptom onset. Intravenous t-PA administration requires close adherence to protocol guidelines. The management of patients following t-PA administration requires close neurologic and blood pressure monitoring as well as capabilities to handle potential hemorrhagic complications associated with thrombolytic therapy by physicians experienced in the management of cerebrovascular disease. Centers that do not have these capabilities can still administer intravenous t-PA in partnership with tertiary care facilities by starting the drug and transferring the patient. Successful centers have treated up to 15–20% of ischemic strokes with thrombolytic therapy, although nationally only a few percent of patients are likely to be treated with thrombolytic therapies. The most recent operational change in stroke care is formal certification of stroke centers, and a model that mirrors the trauma system with primary and comprehensive designated stroke centers is under development in the United States. Inclusion criteria for administration of t-PA in the NINDS t-PA trial were acute ischemic stroke with a clearly defined time of onset (<3 hours), neurological deficit measurable on the NIH Stroke Scale, and CT scan without evidence of intracranial hemorrhage. Patients who awoke from sleep had symptom onset defined as "when last seen awake and normal." Exclusion criteria for administration of t-PA were rapidly improving or isolated minor neurological deficits, seizure at the onset of stroke, prior intracranial hemorrhage, symptoms suggestive of subarachnoid hemorrhage, blood glucose level less than 50 mg/dL (2.7 mM) or greater than 400 mg/dL (22.2 mM), gastrointestinal or genitourinary bleeding within the 3 weeks before stroke, recent MI, current use of oral anticoagulants (PT>15 seconds or INR>1.5), a prolonged aPTT or use of heparin in the previous 48 hours, platelet count less than 100 000/μL, another stroke or serious head injury in the previous 3 months, major surgery within the previous 14 days, arterial puncture at a noncompressible site within the previous 7 days, or pretreatment SBP greater than 185 mmHg or DBP greater than 110 mmHg.

Neurology

B&D Ch. 51A

Question 49. D. In hypochondriasis the patient is convinced that they have a serious disease based on misinterpretation of bodily symptoms and despite assurance that they are not ill. In somatization disorder the patient presents with multiple physical complaints involving several organ systems that are not explained by any medical disorder. In malingering the patient is intentionally feigning symptoms for external incentives. In factitious disorder the patient is intentionally feigning symptoms for the benefits of the sick role. This patient does not have Lou Gehrig's disease or he would not have had several negative workups.

Somatic Symptom Disorders

K&S Ch. 17

Question 50. C. The cervical spinal column includes 37 joints that are continually in motion throughout life. Cervical osteoarthritis and spondylosis are ubiquitous with increasing age. Myelopathy caused by compression of the cervical spinal cord by the changes of spondylosis and osteoarthritis usually develops insidiously, but it may be precipitated by trauma or progress in stepwise fashion. Typical findings are a combination of leg spasticity, upper extremity weakness or clumsiness, and sensory changes in the arms, legs, or trunk. Either spinothalamic tract-mediated or posterior column-mediated sensory modalities may be impaired. Sphincter dysfunction, if it occurs, usually is preceded by motor or sensory findings. Neck pain is often not a prominent symptom, and neck range of motion may or may not be impaired. Some patients experience leg or trunk paresthesia induced by neck flexion (Lhermitte's sign).

The anterior–posterior diameter of the cervical spinal cord is usually 10 mm or less. Patients rarely develop cervical spondylotic myelopathy if the congenital diameter of their spinal canal exceeds 16 mm. In congenitally narrow canals, disk protrusion, osteophytes, hypertrophy of the ligamentum flavum, ossification of the posterior longitudinal ligament, and vertebral body subluxations can combine to compress the spinal cord. MRI or CT myelography provide excellent images of the relation between the spinal canal and the spinal cord. MRI provides more intramedullary detail such as secondary cord edema or gliosis. CT provides better images of calcified tissues. The natural history of cervical spondylotic myelopathy is variable. Some patients have stable neurological deficit for many years without specific therapy, whereas other patients have gradual or stepwise deterioration. Some patients improve with treatments such as bed rest, soft collars, or immobilizing collars, but these treatments have not been assessed in controlled trials. Many patients with cervical spondylotic myelopathy are treated by surgical decompression with variable surgical results. Surgical and nonsurgical treatment results are best when the neurological deficit is mild and present for less than 6 months and when the patient is younger than 70 years. Anterior cervical diskectomies are generally performed for spondylotic lesions at a limited number of levels, whereas posterior laminectomy, sometimes with an expanding "open-door" laminoplasty, is generally performed for congenital spinal canal stenosis.

Neurology

B&D Ch. 73

Question 51. B. Female sexual arousal disorder involves inability to attain an adequate lubrication–swelling response of normal sexual excitement. In sexual aversion disorder the patient has extreme aversion to or avoidance of sexual contact with a partner. In female orgasmic disorder there is a delay in or absence of orgasm following a normal excitement phase. Vaginismus is involuntary muscle spasm of the outer third of the vagina which interferes with sexual intercourse. Dyspareunia is recurrent genital pain associated with intercourse in either a male or female.

Sexual Dysfunction

K&S Ch. 21

Question 52. E. Nonarteritic anterior ischemic optic neuropathy (AION) is the most common cause of unilateral optic nerve swelling in adults older than 50 and commonly is associated with vascular risk factors such as diabetes or hypertension. Other risk factors include a crowded optic nerve head and nocturnal hypotension, possibly precipitated by antihypertensive therapy. Prognostically, many patients will have a stable deficit, although some may experience progression over a month, and the expected rate of spontaneous improvement is high. In 30–40% of patients, subsequent involvement of the fellow eye occurs, and this rate is increased by the presence of vascular risk factors. Recurrence in an affected eye, however, is very rare. There does not appear to be a significantly higher rate of stroke in patients with nonarteritic ischemic optic neuropathy. Posterior (retrobulbar) ischemic optic neuropathy is rare, but is often a sign of giant cell arteritis. The workup should therefore include an evaluation for arteritis, as well as for inflammatory and infiltrative conditions. Sometimes ischemic optic neuropathy without significant disk edema can occur after severe blood loss and shock. Arteritic anterior ischemic optic neuropathy usually is related to temporal arteritis and always associated with disk swelling. Rarely, this entity can affect the nerve only proximal to the lamina cribrosa and manifest without disk swelling; this situation is termed *arteritic posterior ischemic optic neuropathy*. The prevalence of temporal arteritis increases with age, and most patients are older than 70 years of age. Acute vision loss is the presenting symptom in 7–60% of cases and generally is significantly more severe than in nonarteritic AION. In approximately 25% of cases, vision is limited to perception of hand motion only, or light perception is absent.

Neurology

B&D Ch. 15

Question 53. E. Phencyclidine, inhalants, sedative hypnotics, and alcohol can all cause nystagmus during intoxication.

Substance Abuse and Addictive Disorders

K&S Ch. 12

Question 54. B. A thorough knowledge of the criteria for brain death is essential for the physician whose responsibilities include evaluation of comatose patients. Despite differences in state laws, the criteria for the establishment of brain death are fairly standard within the medical community. These criteria include the following:

Coma. The patient should exhibit an unarousable unresponsiveness. There should be no meaningful response to noxious, externally applied stimuli. The patient should not obey commands or demonstrate any verbal response, either reflexively or spontaneously. Spinal reflexes, however, may be retained.

No spontaneous respirations. The patient should be removed from ventilatory assistance and carbon dioxide should be allowed to build up because of the respiratory drive that hypercapnia produces. The diagnosis of absolute apnea requires the absence of spontaneous respiration at a carbon dioxide tension of at least 60 mmHg. A safe means of obtaining this degree of carbon dioxide retention involves the technique of apneic oxygenation, in which 100% oxygen is delivered endotracheally through a thin sterile catheter for 10 minutes. Arterial blood gas levels should be obtained to confirm the arterial carbon dioxide pressure.

Absence of brainstem reflexes. Pupillary, oculocephalic, corneal, and gag reflexes all must be absent, and there should not be any vestibulo-ocular responses to cold calorics.

Electrocerebral silence. An isoelectric EEG should denote the absence of cerebrocortical function. Some authorities do not regard the performance of an EEG as mandatory in assessing brain death and instances of preserved cortical function, despite irreversible and complete brainstem disruption, have been reported.

Absence of cerebral blood flow. Cerebral contrast angiography or radionuclide angiography can substantiate the absence of cerebral blood flow, which is expected in brain death. These tests are considered confirmatory rather than mandatory. On rare occasions, in the presence of supratentorial lesions with preserved blood flow to the brainstem and cerebellum, findings on cerebral radionuclide angiography may be misleading.

Absence of any potentially reversible causes of marked CNS depression. Such causes include hypothermia (temperature 32°C [89.6°F] or less), drug intoxication (particularly barbiturate overdose), and severe metabolic disturbance.

The American Academy of neurology has determined that a positive apnea test is an absolute necessity for the declaration of brain death.

Neurology

B&D Ch. 5

Question 55. C. To get this question right you must know the difference between an inhibitor and an inducer of the CYP450 system. An inhibitor decreases the enzyme activity leading to an increase in the plasma concentration of the drug. An inducer increases the enzyme activity leading to a decrease in the plasma concentration.

The question also touches on some other important concepts. For example there are some patients or ethnic groups who because of a genetic polymorphism in the CYP450 genes will have either increased or decreased enzyme activity. This can change them into slow or rapid metabolizers.

Paroxetine and fluoxetine are potent CYP2D6 inhibitors. Great caution must be shown mixing them with TCAs, Mellaril, codeine, beta blockers, Risperdal, clozapine, and aripiprazole. Thioridazine is contraindicated with CYP2D6 inhibitors.

The most important CYP450 enzymes for the psychiatrist to understand are CYP2D6, CYP1A2 and CYP3A4. You will no doubt see more questions about them all throughout this book and on your exam.

Psychopharmacology

K&S Ch. 36

Question 56. D. Amyotrophic lateral sclerosis (ALS) is a neurodegenerative disorder of undetermined etiology that primarily affects the motor neuron cell populations in the motor cortex, brainstem, and spinal cord. It is progressive and most patients eventually succumb to respiratory failure. Between 5 and 10% of ALS is familial rather than sporadic, the most common inheritance pattern being autosomal dominant. The incidence and prevalence rates for non–Western Pacific ALS are surprisingly uniform throughout the world. The incidence is estimated at 0.86 to 2.4 per 100 000 (~2 per 100 000 in the United States) and the prevalence is about 6 per 100 000. Perhaps the most significant breakthrough in understanding the cause of ALS (be it sporadic or familial) came in 1993, when Rosen and colleagues identified mutations in the gene encoding an enzyme called copper/zinc superoxide dismutase (*SOD1*) in patients with familial ALS. *SOD1* mutations are identified in up to 20% of all patients with familial ALS. A significant body of basic and clinical research lends strong support to a theory of ALS pathogenesis, which proposes selective motor neuron damage from a complex chain of injurious events involving excitotoxins, oxidative stress, neurofilament dysfunction, altered calcium homeostasis, mitochondrial dysfunction, enhanced motor neuron apoptosis, and proinflammatory cytokines. Onset of muscle weakness is more common in the upper than the lower extremities (classic, spinal ALS), but in approximately 25% of patients, weakness begins in bulbar-innervated muscles (bulbar-onset ALS). Pseudobulbar palsy may present with inappropriate or forced crying or laughter, which is often a source of great emotional distress for patients. The median duration of ALS from clinical onset ranges from 22 to 52 months, and the mean duration from 23 to 43 months, with an average 5-year survival rate of 22% (roughly 1 in 5) and a 10-year survival rate of 9.4% (roughly 1 in 10). The diagnosis of clinically definite ALS can sometimes be reached based on the history and clinical examination alone, but, owing to the seriousness of the diagnosis, ancillary investigations are necessary to exclude other possibilities. The EMG examination characteristically reveals a combination of acute (positive sharp waves and fibrillation potentials) and chronic (reduced neurogenic firing pattern with evidence of increased amplitude and duration, polyphasic motor unit potentials) changes in a widespread distribution that is not in keeping with any single root or peripheral nerve distribution. Fasciculation potentials are usually identified; their absence should prompt an investigation for another disorder. In 1996, riluzole (Rilutek) was approved by the US Food and Drug Administration as the first specific drug for the treatment of ALS. It is believed to principally function as an antiglutamate agent, although its mechanism of action is not yet fully understood. The care of patients with ALS has become increasingly complex. As a consequence, many patients receive the care of a multidisciplinary team in a specialized ALS center, rather than by a single treating physician. Explanations of the other answer choices to this question can be found in other question explanations in this volume.

Neurology

B&D Ch. 74

Question 57. E.   Females develop tardive dyskinesia more commonly than males. Patients over the age of 50 are more likely to develop tardive dyskinesia than those younger. Patients with brain damage and young children are more likely to develop tardive dyskinesia than older healthier counterparts.

Psychopharmacology

K&S Ch. 36

Question 58. B.   Brain tumors account for approximately 4% of epilepsy cases. Seizures are a common presenting symptom of brain tumors. The incidence of seizures is greater in primary low-grade brain tumors than in brain metastases or high-grade primary tumors. A study of 132 adult patients with newly diagnosed glioblastoma reported that seizures were the presenting symptom in 31% of patients. In a series of patients with low-grade supratentorial gliomas, seizures occurred in association with 75.5% of astrocytomas, 60.8% of mixed gliomas, and 62.5% of oligodendrogliomas. Seizures are sometimes focal, reflecting tumor location, but many become secondarily generalized at onset. Patients with temporal lobe tumors frequently describe auras: epigastric sensations and psychological phenomena such as déjà vu and depersonalization are common. Complex partial seizures and secondarily generalized tonic–clonic seizures are common.

Neurology

B&D Ch. 52C

Question 59. B.   Valproic acid will increase lamotrigine levels. Oral contraceptives will decrease lamotrigine levels. Phenobarbital and Phenytoin will decrease lamotrigine levels.

Psychopharmacology

K&S Ch. 36

Question 60. D.   Positron emission tomography (PET), like SPECT, depends on detection of emitted radioactivity (derived from injection of a radiolabeled tracer). Positrons are highly unstable particles and travel only a short distance in space before colliding with an electron. The resulting annihilation reaction results in the formation of two gamma rays of 511 keV traveling at 180° to each other. PET is based on the detection of these coincident gamma rays. PET utilizes the selective binding or uptake and retention of a variety of radiopharmaceuticals. These tracers may provide general information about physiological function, such as regional cerebral blood flow (usually assessed with $H_2^{15}O$) or cerebral glucose metabolism, assessed with [^{18}F]fluoro-2-deoxyglucose (FDG). FDG undergoes phosphorylation but, because of the 2-deoxy modification, cannot proceed further along the glycolytic pathway; as a result, glucose uptake is physiologically trapped. Brain glucose metabolism is correlated with synaptic activity, and FDG PET therefore provides a good measure of neural activity, but without specifying the particular neuronal subtype involved. The other major application of PET is in the labeling of pharmaceuticals that are substrates for specific enzymes, such as those involved in neurotransmitter synthesis or breakdown – examples are 6-[^{18}F]fluoro-L-dopa as a measure of dopamine synthesis and N-[^{11}C]methylpiperdin-4-yl propionate ([^{11}C]PMP) to measure acetylcholinesterase activity – or that bind to specific neurotransmitter receptors or transporters. It is this capacity of PET to study specific neurochemical processes that is its unique strength. Other advantages of PET include the generally preferable spatial resolution and quantifiability over those of SPECT (although some more recent SPECT cameras have vastly improved resolution).

SPECT is the nuclear medicine equivalent of computed tomography, similarly combining a series of two-dimensional images obtained by moving the gamma camera on a gantry in a circular or elliptical orbit around the patient. The information from this series of images is then combined into a three-dimensional volume. Unlike PET, SPECT is based on the detection of single gamma rays, rather than coincident detection of simultaneously emitted photons. Like PET, brain SPECT can be used to study general physiological functions such as perfusion, as well as in labeling neurotransmitter receptors and transporters. Brain perfusion often is measured using SPECT with ^{99m}Tc-hexamethylpropyleneamine oxime (HMPAO).

In addition to its superior spatial resolution, MRI takes advantage of changes in the paramagnetic properties of deoxyhemoglobin compared with oxygenated hemoglobin to deduce the degree of blood oxygenation (the so-called blood oxygenation level-dependent [BOLD] technique). As blood flow increases, oxygen extraction decreases, so the levels of deoxyhemoglobin decline and MRI signal intensity increases. This effect has been widely exploited in a large number of research settings in order to examine regional activation associated with a variety of cognitive processes, including language, reward processing, decision making, fear, and altruistic behavior and empathy, as well as motor and sensory processing. Functional MRI can provide valuable insights into brain plasticity and reorganization after injury such as trauma or stroke. Functional MRI has vastly superior temporal resolution compared with PET or SPECT and is widely available—most current commercial scanners have the capacity to perform such studies. The spatial resolution also is favorable, although not as good as with structural MRI, and comparable to that achieved with the best PET scanners. In contrast with PET, which permits a quantifiable absolute measure (e.g., blood flow, metabolic rate, ligand-binding potential), fMRI allows estimation of only the relative change in regional blood flow.

Neurology

B&D Ch. 33C

Question 61. A. The random movements of chorea are accentuated and often most noticeable during walking. The superimposition of chorea on the trunk and leg movements of the walking cycle gives the gait a dancing quality, and there is an exaggerated motion of the legs and arm swing. Chorea can also interrupt the walking pattern, leading to a hesitant gait. Additional voluntary compensatory movements appear in response to perturbations from the chorea. Chorea in Sydenham's chorea or chorea gravidarum may be sufficiently violent to throw patients off their feet; severe chorea of the trunk may render walking impossible. The chorea of Huntington's disease usually causes a lurching or stumbling and stuttering gait with frequent steps forward, backward, or to the side. Walking is slow, the stance is wide-based, the trunk sways excessively, and steps are variable in length and timing. Spontaneous knee flexion and leg-raising movements are common. Haloperidol reduces chorea but does not improve gait in Huntington's disease. Balance and equilibrium usually are maintained until the terminal stages of Huntington's disease, when an akinetic-rigid syndrome may supervene. Stereotactic thalamotomy is of course a neurosurgical technique designed to alleviate symptoms of Parkinson's disease. Pramipexole and benztropine are antiparkinsonian medications. Lioresal (Baclofen) is a potent muscle relaxant used in the treatment of muscle spasticity, for example in stroke and multiple sclerosis patients.

Neurology

B&D Ch. 22

Question 62. C. The most common akinetic-rigid gait disturbance is that encountered in Parkinson's disease. The posture is stooped with flexion of the shoulders, neck, and trunk. During walking, there is little associated or synergistic body movement. Arm swing is reduced or absent, and the arms are held immobile at the sides or slightly forward of the trunk. Tremor of the upper limbs frequently increases when walking (but parkinsonian tremor of the legs rarely affects walking). The gait is slow and shuffling, with small, shallow steps on a narrow base. The posture of generalized flexion of the patient with Parkinson's disease exaggerates the normal tendency to lean forward when walking. To maintain balance when walking and avoid falling forward, the patient may advance with a series of rapid, small steps (*festination*). Retropulsion and propulsion are similar manifestations of a flurry of small, shuffling steps made in an effort to preserve equilibrium. Instead of a single large step, a series of small steps are taken to maintain balance. Falls occur in Parkinson's disease when festinating steps are too small to restore balance.

Astasia–abasia refers to the inability to either stand or walk in a normal manner. Patients exhibit an unusual and dramatic gait disturbance, lurching wildly in various directions and falling only when a nearby physician, family member, or soft object will catch them. Astasia refers to the inability to maintain station (stand upright) unassisted. Abasia refers to lack of motor coordination in walking. The term literally means that the base of gait (the lateral distance between the two feet) is inconstant or unmeasurable. When seen in conversion disorder, the gait is bizarre and is not suggestive of a specific organic lesion: often the patient sways wildly and nearly falls, recovering at the last moment. However, an acquired total inability to stand and walk can be seen in true neurological diseases, including stroke, Parkinson disease, damage to the cerebellum, Guillain–Barré syndrome, normal pressure hydrocephalus and many others. In normal pressure hydrocephalus for example, when the condition remains untreated, the patient's gait becomes shortened, with frequent shuffling and falls; eventually standing, sitting, and even rolling over in bed become impossible. This advanced state is referred to as "hydrocephalic astasia–abasia".

Neurology

B&D Ch. 22

Question 63. E. Bacterial meningitis may be defined as an inflammatory response to bacterial infection of the pia-arachnoid and cerebrospinal fluid (CSF) in the subarachnoid space. Because the subarachnoid space is continuous over the brain, spinal cord, nerves, and nerve roots, infection in this space generally extends throughout the cerebrospinal axis. The incidence of bacterial meningitis is between 2 and 4 per 100 000 people per year in the United States. More than 1500 deaths due to bacterial meningitis are reported annually in the United States. Worldwide, three main pathogens, *Haemophilus influenzae*, *Streptococcus pneumoniae*, and *Neisseria meningitidis*, account for 75–80% of cases after the neonatal period. Group B streptococci, *Escherichia coli* and other enteric bacilli, and *Listeria monocytogenes* are major pathogens in neonatal meningitis. The most common bacteria that cause meningitis, *S. pneumoniae* and *N. meningitides*, initially colonize the nasopharynx by attaching to nasopharyngeal mucosa. At any time, *S. pneumoniae* can be isolated from 5–10% healthy adults and from 20–40% healthy children. Bacterial meningitis occurs when pathogens colonizing the nasopharynx cause bacteremia and breach the blood–brain barrier to reach into the brain.

The classical clinical presentation of adults with bacterial meningitis comprises headache, fever, and neck stiffness, often with signs of cerebral dysfunction; these manifestations are found in more than 85% of patients. Nausea, vomiting, myalgia, and photophobia are also common. The neck stiffness may be subtle or marked, accompanied by Kernig's or Brudzinski's signs (or both). These signs are elicited in over half of adults, but less in neonates and elderly; absence of clinical meningeal signs does not rule out the diagnosis of bacterial meningitis. Cerebral dysfunction is manifested by confusion, delirium, and a declining level of consciousness that ranges from lethargy to coma. Seizures occur in approximately 40% of cases. Cranial nerve palsies involving cranial nerves III, VI, and VII are found in 10–20% of cases and result from direct damage to the nerve by the surrounding infection or endarteritis of the vasa nervorum.

Neurology

B&D Ch. 53C

Question 64. A. In 1916, Guillain, Barré, and Strohl emphasized the main clinical features of GBS: motor weakness, areflexia, paresthesias with minor sensory loss, and increased protein in CSF without pleocytosis (albuminocytological dissociation). The frequent finding of motor conduction block and reduced nerve conduction velocities provided further electrophysiological confirmation of the widespread demyelination. Approximately two thirds of patients report a preceding event, most frequently an upper respiratory or gastrointestinal infection, surgery, or immunization 1 to 4 weeks before the onset of neurological symptoms. The agent responsible for the prodromal illness often remains unidentified. Specific infectious agents linked to GBS include cytomegalovirus (CMV), Epstein–Barr virus, varicella zoster virus, hepatitis A and B, HIV, *Mycoplasma pneumoniae*, and *Haemophilus influenzae*. The most common identifiable bacterial organism linked to GBS and particularly its axonal forms is *Campylobacter jejuni*, a curved Gram-negative rod that is a common cause of bacterial enteritis worldwide. Patients with classic GBS may initially present with weakness, with or without paresthetic sensory symptoms. The fairly symmetrical weakness of the lower limbs ascends proximally over hours to several days and may subsequently involve arm, facial, and oropharyngeal muscles, and, in severe cases, respiratory muscles. Hyporeflexia or areflexia are the invariable features of GBS but may be absent early in the course of the disease. Cranial nerve involvement has occurred in 45–75% of cases in different series. Facial paresis, usually bilateral, is found in at least one half of patients. In the first week of neurological symptoms the CSF protein may be normal but then becomes elevated on subsequent examinations. In approximately 10% of cases, the CSF protein remains normal throughout the illness. Abnormalities of electrophysiological studies are found in approximately 90% of established cases and reflect an evolving picture of multifocal demyelination associated with secondary axonal degeneration. The most common electrophysiological abnormalities include prolonged distal motor and F-wave latencies, absent or impersistent F waves, conduction block, reduction in distal CMAP amplitudes with or without temporal dispersion, and slowing of motor conduction velocities. Conduction block of motor axons is the electrophysiological correlate of clinical weakness and is recognized by a decrease of greater than 50% in CMAP amplitude from distal to proximal stimulation in the absence of temporal dispersion. Among specific therapeutic interventions aimed at mitigating the harmful effects of autoantibodies, plasma exchange and high-dose intravenous immune globulin (IVIG) infusions have been shown to be equally effective.

Neurology

B&D Ch. 76

Question 65. E. The clinical presentation of intracerebral hemorrhage (ICH) has two main elements: symptoms that reflect the effects of intracranial hypertension and those that are specific for the location of the hematoma. The general clinical manifestations of ICH related to increased intracranial pressure (ICP) (headache, vomiting, and depressed level of consciousness) vary in their frequency at onset of ICH. CT is sensitive to the high-density fresh blood in the brain parenchyma, along with associated features of local mass effect and ventricular extension. MRI adds further precision, especially in determining the time elapsed between onset and time of MRI examination. Cerebellar hemorrhage represents approximately 5–10% of the cases. Its clinical presentation is characteristic, with abrupt onset of vertigo, headache, vomiting, and inability to stand and walk, with absence of hemiparesis or hemiplegia. The physical findings that allow its clinical diagnosis are the triad of appendicular ataxia, horizontal gaze palsy, and peripheral facial palsy, all ipsilateral to the hemorrhage. The clinical course in cerebellar hemorrhage can be difficult to predict at onset. There is a notorious tendency for abrupt deterioration to coma and death after a period of clinical stability under hospital observation. The neurologist must be able to recognize when neurosurgical intervention, which is frequently life saving and function restoring for these patients, is indicated. To this effect, it is convenient to classify the clinical stages seen in this condition: (1) an initial "cerebellar" stage, in which the only clinical deficits detected are referable to the cerebellum; (2) an intermediate stage, in which, in addition to cerebellar signs, there are signs and symptoms referrable to hydrocephalus; and (3) the final stage, brainstem compression. Neurosurgical intervention is indicated when the first signs and symptoms of hydrocephalus develop. The prognosis for good functional recovery is excellent in patients with cerebellar hemorrhage who have had a timely suboccipital decompression before they have lapsed into coma. Even comatose patients, however, can make an excellent functional recovery, provided that the decompression is carried out expeditiously and soon after the onset of coma.

Neurology

B&D Chs 46&51B

Question 66. C. Stiff-person syndrome (SPS) is rare and no information is available about its epidemiology. SPS is a syndrome of progressive rigidity of axial and proximal appendicular muscles with muscle hypertrophy and extreme lumbar lordosis. Intense spasms are superimposed on a background of continuous muscle contraction. Gait is slow and stiff legged. Spasms and stiffness improve with sleep and are eliminated by general anesthesia and neuromuscular blocking agents. Clinical criteria for diagnosis include insidious development of limb and axial (thoracolumbar and abdominal) stiffness, clinical and electrophysiological confirmation of co-contraction of agonist and antagonist muscles, episodic spasms superimposed on chronic stiffness, and no other underlying illness that would explain the symptoms. EMG examination shows continuous firing of normal motor units. SPS is associated with autoimmune disorders, such as type I diabetes, thyroiditis, myasthenia gravis, pernicious anemia, and vitiligo. High titers of antibodies to the 65-kD fraction of glutamic acid decarboxylase and to other antigens are present. It is thought that SPS results from dysfunction of descending suprasegmental pathways possibly secondary to immune-mediated inhibition of GABA synthesis. Paraneoplastic SPS has been reported with breast and lung cancers and Hodgkin's disease. Untreated, SPS progresses to extreme disability. Diazepam at doses of 20 to 400 mg/day is the most effective symptomatic treatment. Clonazepam, baclofen, valproic acid, clonidine, vigabatrin, and tiagabine have also been reported to be effective. Intrathecal baclofen and local intramuscular injections of botulinum toxin have been helpful in some cases. Plasmapheresis, IVIg, and immunosuppression have been reported to have variable effects on the condition.

Neurology

B&D Chs 52G&71

Question 67. D.   Simple partial seizures of temporal lobe origin often are difficult to recognize as epileptic events. The report of symptoms by the patient may be the only clear evidence of the event. Complex partial temporal lobe seizures may begin with impairment of consciousness, or by a simple partial seizure, or an aura. Auras vary in duration from seconds to several minutes before impairment of consciousness. Most complex partial seizures last longer than 30 seconds, usually up to 1 to 2 minutes; few last less than 10 seconds, which is a distinguishing characteristic from absence seizures. Postictal recovery usually is slow, with significant confusion that may last for several minutes or longer. Some have suggested that clinical symptomatology at the very onset of the seizure occasionally provides clues about the site of ictal onset in the temporal lobe. These may include auditory or olfactory hallucinations, emotional or psychic symptoms, sensations of movement or rotation, or autonomic symptoms. The focus usually is in the superior temporal gyrus. The cause of olfactory seizures (*uncinate fits*), usually an unpleasant odor, is discharges in the medial temporal lobe. The cause of gustatory seizures is discharges deep in the sylvian fissure or the operculum. Epigastric sensations of nausea, "butterflies," emptiness, or tightness usually are caused by temporal lobe activity. Emotional changes and psychic phenomena, often attributed to simple partial seizures of temporal lobe origin, more commonly are associated with complex partial seizures.

Neurology

B&D Ch. 67

Question 68. A.   Carotid artery dissection commonly manifests with neck, face, and head pain ipsilateral to the dissection, frequently is associated with an ipsilateral Horner's syndrome, and often follows head or neck trauma. A dissection is produced by subintimal penetration of blood in a cervicocephalic vessel with subsequent longitudinal extension of the intramural hematoma between its layers. Most dissections involve the extracranial segment of the internal carotid artery or extracranial vertebral arteries. Intracranial dissections are usually subintimal and may follow trivial trauma, closed head trauma, basilar skull fracture, or penetrating injuries. Diagnosis is based on arteriographic findings, although high-resolution MRI and magnetic resonance angiography (MRA), computed tomographic angiography (CTA), and extracranial and transcranial Doppler ultrasound are rapidly replacing contrast angiography for the diagnosis of cervicocephalic arterial dissections, particularly in cases of carotid artery involvement. Features on arteriography include the presence of a pearl and string sign; double-lumen sign; short, smooth, tapered occlusion; or pseudoaneurysm formation. Therapeutic interventions have included immediate anticoagulation with heparin followed by a 3–6-month course of warfarin, and platelet antiaggregants instead of, or following, warfarin.

Neurology

B&D Chs 18&51A

Question 69. B.   Tolosa–Hunt syndrome (THS) is a painful syndrome of idiopathic, self-limited inflammation of the cavernous sinus, typically responsive to corticosteroids. Inflammation associated with systemic rheumatologic disease, metastatic or nasopharyngeal neoplastic infiltration, carotid–cavernous fistulas, and compression from an intracavernous internal artery aneurysm or meningioma may also cause a cavernous sinus syndrome. Pituitary apoplexy should be considered in the differential diagnosis for sudden onset, painful unilateral or bilateral oculomotor palsies, with or without accompanying visual loss. THS is a rare disorder characterized by severe and unilateral headaches with extraocular palsies, usually involving the third, fourth, fifth, and sixth cranial nerves, and pain around the sides and back of the eye, along with weakness and paralysis (ophthalmoplegia) of certain eye muscles. Symptoms are usually limited to one side of the head, and in most cases the individual affected will experience intense, sharp pain and paralysis of muscles around the eye. Symptoms may subside without medical intervention, yet recur without a noticeable pattern. In addition, affected individuals may experience paralysis of various facial nerves and drooping of the upper eyelid (ptosis). Other signs include double vision, fever, chronic fatigue, vertigo or arthralgia. Occasionally the patient may present with a feeling of protrusion of one or both eyeballs (exophthalmos). MRI scans of the brain and orbit with and without contrast, magnetic resonance angiography or digital subtraction angiography and a CT scan of the brain and orbit with and without contrast may all be useful in detecting inflammatory changes in the cavernous sinus, superior orbital fissure and/or orbital apex. Treatment of THS is usually completed using corticosteroids (often prednisone) and immunosuppressive agents (such as methotrexate or azathioprine). Corticosteroids act as analgesia and reduce pain (usually within 24–72hours), as well as reducing the inflammatory mass, whereas immunosuppressive agents help reduce the autoimmune response. Treatment is then continued in the same dosages for a further 7–10 days and then tapered slowly. The prognosis of THS is usually considered good. Patients usually respond to corticosteroids, and spontaneous remission can occur, although movement of ocular muscles may remain damaged. Roughly 30–40% of patients who are treated for THS experience a relapse.

Neurology

B&D Ch. 70

Question 70. A. Lorazepam (initially marketed under the brand names Ativan and Temesta) is a high-potency short-to-intermediate-acting 3-hydroxy benzodiazepine drug that has all six intrinsic benzodiazepine effects: anxiolytic, amnesic, sedative/hypnotic, anticonvulsant, antiemetic and muscle relaxant. Lorazepam is used for the short-term treatment of anxiety, insomnia, acute seizures including statusepilepticus and sedation of hospitalized patients, as well as sedation of aggressive patients. Lorazepam is considered to be a short-acting drug which, similar to other benzodiazepines, exerts its therapeutic as well as adverse effects via its interaction at benzodiazepine binding sites, which are located on GABA receptors in the central nervous system. After its introduction in 1977, lorazepam's principal use was in treating anxiety. Among benzodiazepines, lorazepam has a relatively high addictive potential. Lorazepam also has abuse potential; the main types of misuse are for recreational purposes or continued use against medical advice. Lorazepam may be safer than most benzodiazepines in patients with impaired liver function. Like oxazepam, it does not require hepatic oxidation, but only hepatic glucuronidation into lorazepam-glucuronide. Therefore, impaired liver function is unlikely to result in lorazepam accumulation to an extent causing adverse reactions. Similarly renal disease has minimal effects on lorazepam levels. The three benzodiazepines that are metabolized via glucuronidation are lorazepam, oxazepam, and temazepam and these come up often in this context on standardized examinations in psychiatry (mnemonic LOT).

Psychopharmacology

K&S Ch. 36

Question 71. C. Most of the body's serotonin is in the gastrointestinal (GI) tract. This is why serotonergic drugs typically cause varying degrees of stomach pain, nausea, vomiting, flatulence and diarrhea. These side effects are mediated mostly through effects on the serotonin 5HT-3 receptor. Sertraline and fluvoxamine produce the most intense GI symptoms. In most cases these side effects are transient, but in a small percentage of individuals, these effects never abate and a switch to another class of antidepressant must be made. The most effective way to offset these side effects is to use initial low doses of these agents or to use delayed-release preparations. Up to one-third of patients taking SSRIs will gain weight. This effect is mediated through a metabolic mechanism, increase in appetite, or both. It happens slowly over time and is resistant to diet and exercise regimens.

Psychopharmacology

K&S Ch. 36

Question 72. E. The standard and classic treatment for obsessive–compulsive disorder (OCD) is via pharmacotherapy, behavior therapy, or a combination of the two. SSRIs and clomipramine (Anafranil) are the pharmacologic agents of choice in OCD. Behavioral therapy techniques have been shown to be effective for OCD. These include exposure and response prevention, desensitization, thought-stopping, flooding, implosion therapy, and aversive conditioning. In behavior therapy, patients have to be truly committed to their own improvement. Family and group therapy are often helpful in supporting the family and improving relationships in patients with OCD. For extreme cases that are unresponsive to all these therapies, electroconvulsive shock therapy (ECT) and psychosurgery are considerations. ECT is not as effective as psychosurgery, but it should still be tried before psychosurgery. Cingulotomy is a common psychosurgical procedure for extreme OCD and is effective in 25–30% of otherwise treatment-unresponsive patients. Another surgical procedure that may also help intractable OCD is subcaudate tractotomy, also known as capsulotomy. The most common complication of psychosurgery is the development of seizures. Some patients who do not respond to psychosurgery following failure of prior pharmacotherapy and/or behavior therapy, may respond to these interventions after the psychosurgery is done.

Anxiety Disorders

K&S Ch. 16

Question 73. B. Lithium has myriad side effects that crop up in multiple choice questions on psychiatry examinations. Among its neurologic side effects, Lithium can cause dysphoria, lack of spontaneity, slowed reaction time and memory difficulties. Patients often complain of "altered creativity" and this is a well-described adverse effect of lithium. These are usually benign side effects that can occur even when the serum lithium level is below the toxic range. Lithium can also cause tremor, peripheral neuropathy, benign intracranial hypertension, lowered seizure threshold and a myasthenia gravis-like syndrome. Other common non-neurologic side effects of lithium include: weight gain, fluid retention, appetite loss, nausea, vomiting, diarrhea, nephrogenic diabetes insipidus (polyuria/polydipsia), hypothyroidism, hyperparathyroidism, benign T-wave changes, acne, rash, psoriasis, and hair loss.

Psychopharmacology

K&S Ch. 36

Question 74. D. Affective disorders (MDD + Bipolar) accounts for 50% of completed suicides. The other potentially tricky choice listed was personality disorders, which only account for 5% of completed suicides despite their many attempts and gestures. Of the personality disorders, 4 to 10% of borderlines commit suicide, and 5% of antisocial personality disorders commit suicide. Mixing the personality disorder with major depression or substance abuse greatly increases the risk. The risk of completed suicide in affective disorders is 30 times greater than that for the general population. Drug and alcohol abuse account for 25% of completed suicides and 5–10% of patients with schizophrenia complete suicide.

Management in Psychiatry

K&S Ch. 34

Question 75. E. The therapist's tasks in a group therapy setting include determining the size and setting of the group, choosing frequency and length of sessions, deciding on an open vs. closed group, formulating appropriate goals, selecting patients and building a therapeutic environment for the group that can identify and deal with problems within the group. We do not want to suppress catharsis, we want patients to speak about their feelings and emotions and feel relief after doing so.

Psychological Theory and Psychometric Testing

K&S Ch. 35

Question 76. C. Carbamazepine, in its extended-release form (Equetro), was finally FDA-approved in the US for treatment of bipolar disorder in 2004. It was first used to treat partial and generalized-onset epilepsy and trigeminal neuralgia. Carbamazepine is structurally similar to the tricyclic antidepressants. Carbamazepine is believed to cause blockade of type 2 sodium channels and have activity at A1 adenosine receptors. Carbamazepine absorption is slow and unpredictable. This results, at least partially, from autoinduction of its own metabolism via hepatic CYP450 3A4 enzymes. Carbamazepine has numerous side effects. Those that are dose-dependant include blurred vision, vertigo, gastrointestinal disturbances, and task-performance impairment. Idiosyncratic adverse effects (which are not dose-dependant) include agranulocytosis, Stevens–Johnson syndrome, aplastic anemia, hepatic failure, rash and pancreatitis. The drug's hematologic effects are not dose-dependant. Severe blood dyscrasias (aplastic anemia and agranulocytosis) occur in about 1 in 125 000 persons treated with carbamazepine. Patients should be warned that symptoms such as fever, rash, petechiae, sore throat, bruising and easy bleeding, may herald serious blood dyscrasia and they should be urged to seek medical attention immediately. Routine blood monitoring of the complete blood count is recommended at 3, 6, 9, and 12 months. If no evidence of bone marrow suppression is noted at 12 months, most clinicians would reduce the interval of monitoring.

Psychopharmacology

K&S Ch. 36

Question 77. E.   The grammar development stage is 36–54 months. At around 40 months children can use a wide range of grammatical forms such as plurals, past tense, negatives and questions. Children of this age can also understand prepositions, cause and effect, and know up to 5500 words.

Human Development

K&S Ch. 2

Question 78. A.   Clozapine should not be taken in conjunction with any other drug that is associated with the development of agranulocytosis or bone marrow suppression. Such agents include carbamazepine, phenytoin, propylthiouracil, sulfonamides, and captopril. Lithium combined with clozapine can increase risk of seizures, confusion and movement disorders. Lithium should not be taken with clozapine in patients who have previously experienced an episode of neuroleptic malignant syndrome. Clomipramine can increase the seizure risk by lowering the seizure threshold and by increasing clozapine plasma concentrations. Fluoxetine, paroxetine, risperidone and fluvoxamine can all increase the serum levels of clozapine. Also, paroxetine may trigger clozapine-associated neutropenia.

Psychopharmacology

K&S Ch. 36

Question 79. D.   Memantine is a low to moderate affinity NMDA receptor antagonist. It is FDA-approved in the USA for treatment of moderate to severe Alzheimer's disease. It is purported that overexcitation of NMDA receptors by the neurotransmitter glutamate may play a role in Alzheimer's disease, because glutamate plays an integral part in the neural pathways associated with learning and memory. Excess glutamate overstimulates NMDA receptors to allow too much calcium into nerve cells, leading to cell death that is observed in Alzheimer's disease. Memantine is believed to have neuroprotective effects by partially blocking NMDA receptors associated with abnormal transmission of glutamate, while allowing for physiologic transmission associated with normal cell functioning. Galantamine, donepezil, tacrine, and rivastigmine are all inhibitors of acetylcholinesterase.

Psychopharmacology

K&S Ch. 36

Question 80. E.   Organophosphorus poisoning mnemonics:

DUMBELS

D = Diarrhea

U = Urination

M = Miosis

B = Bradycardia

E = Emesis

L = Lacrimation

S = Salivation/ Sweating / Secretion

Organophosphates are used mainly as pesticides and herbicides but are also used as petroleum additives, lubricants, antioxidants, flame retardants, and plastic modifiers. Most cases of organophosphate toxicity result from exposure in an agricultural setting, not only among those mixing or spraying the pesticide or herbicide but also among workers returning prematurely to sprayed fields. Absorption may occur through the skin, by inhalation, or through the gastrointestinal tract. Organophosphates inhibit acetylcholinesterase by phosphorylation, with resultant acute cholinergic symptoms, with both central and neuromuscular manifestations. Symptoms include nausea, salivation, lacrimation, headache, weakness, and bronchospasm in mild instances and bradycardia, tremor, chest pain, diarrhea, pulmonary edema, cyanosis, convulsions, and even coma in more severe cases. Death may result from respiratory or heart failure. Treatment involves intravenous administration of pralidoxime (1 g) together with atropine (1 mg) given subcutaneously every 30 minutes until sweating and salivation are controlled. Pralidoxime accelerates reactivation of the inhibited acetylcholinesterase, and atropine is effective in counteracting muscarinic effects, although it has no effect on the nicotinic effects such as neuromuscular cholinergic blockade with weakness or respiratory depression. It is important to ensure adequate ventilatory support before atropine is given.

Poisoning

B&D Ch. 58

Question 81. B. *Clostridium tetani* secretes tetanospasmin, also known as tetanus toxin, and tetanolysin. The toxicity of tetanolysin is uncertain; tetanospasmin blocks release of inhibitory neurotransmitters by spinal interneurons, causing the dramatic muscle contractions that characterize tetanus. Tetanospasmin inhibits release of gamma-aminobutyric acid and glycine, which are inhibitory neurotransmitters in the brainstem and spinal cord. A single type of tetanus neurotoxin exists, in contrast to the multiple serotypes of botulinum toxin. The typical incubation period is 2 weeks but can range from hours to a month or more. Cardinal features include muscle rigidity and spasms, which may be accompanied by autonomic hyperactivity. Local tetanus, in which symptoms remain limited to a limb, is a rare form. Far more common is generalized tetanus, also called lockjaw, as trismus heralds the disorder in over 75% of cases. Sustained contraction of facial muscles causes a sneering grimace known as risus sardonicus. Other early symptoms include dysphagia and axial muscle involvement, such as neck stiffness, abdominal rigidity, and back pain. Early involvement of face, neck, and trunk muscles has been ascribed to the shorter axons of motor neurons supplying cranial and axial muscles, as compared with the limbs. Laryngospasm compromises ventilation and makes intubation extremely difficult. Sustained contraction of back muscles causes opisthotonos, an arching posture of the back. As tetanus progresses, reflex muscle spasms develop, triggered by sensory stimuli, movement, or emotion. Examination can be difficult, as it may prompt spasms. Therapeutic goals include protecting the airway, neutralizing circulating tetanospasmin and preventing its further production, managing spasms and dysautonomia, and general supportive care. Initial treatment of most patients with generalized tetanus includes endotracheal intubation, because laryngospasm may appear abruptly even in mild cases. Human tetanus immune globulin, given as a single dose of at least 500 IU intramuscularly, neutralizes circulating toxin. Infected wounds should be debrided after human tetanus-immune globulin administration, because the procedure may release further toxin. Metronidazole or penicillin should be given to eradicate *C. tetani*.

Poisonings

B&D Ch. 53C

Question 82. B. Sleep is composed of five distinct phases or stages: non-REM (NREM) sleep, which is divided into Stages I through IV and REM sleep. Each phase has its own unique characteristics when measured in three ways: electroencephalogram (EEG), electrooculogram (EOG) and electromyogram (EMG). The following table breaks down these phases into their distinct characteristics.

STAGE	EEG	EOG	EMG
Stage I	Low voltage, mixed frequency Theta (3-7 cps); vertex sharp waves	Slow	Decreased from awake
Stage II	Sleep spindles and K complexes	None	Decreased from awake
Stage III	Sleep spindles and slow waves	None	Decreased from awake
Stage IV	Mostly slow waves	None	Decreased from awake
REM sleep	Low voltage, mixed frequency saw-tooth waves, Theta activity, slow Alpha	Rapid	Nearly absent

Sleep Wake Disorders

K&S Ch. 24

Question 83. D. In the neonatal period, REM represents more than 50% of total sleep time and the EEG goes directly into REM phase without passing first through stages I through IV. Newborns sleep about 16 hours a day. By about 4 months of age, the sleep pattern shifts. Infants now pass through NREM sleep before their first REM episode and REM sleep drops to less than 40% of total sleep time. By young adulthood, NREM makes up about 75% of total sleep time. This 75% is divided as follows: Stage I 5%; Stage II 45%; Stage III 12%; Stage IV 13%. Thus, in adulthood, REM makes up about 25% of total sleep time. This distribution remains relatively constant into older age, although there is usually a reduction in both slow-wave sleep and REM sleep in the elderly.

Sleep Wake Disorders

K&S Ch. 24

Question 84. C. Phentolamine is a parenteral medication usually reserved for hospital use in intensive care unit or cardiac care unit settings. Its primary action is vasodilation due to α_1 blockade. It also can lead to reflex tachycardia because of hypotension and α_2 inhibition, which increases sympathetic tone. The primary application for phentolamine is for the control of hypertensive emergencies, most notably due to pheochromocytoma. It also has usefulness in the treatment of cocaine induced hypertension, where one would generally avoid beta blockers and where calcium channel blockers are not effective. Beta blockers (e.g., metoprolol) or combined alpha and beta adrenergic blocking agents (e.g., labetalol) should be avoided in patients with a history of cocaine abuse. They can cause an unopposed alpha-adrenergic mediated coronary vasoconstriction, causing the worsening of myocardial ischemia and hypertension. It is also used in the treatment of pheochromocytoma prior to the administration of beta blockers to avoid unopposed alpha-stimulation. In this context it is probably most safely given by infusion since bolus doses have a propensity towards causing precipitous falls in blood pressure. When given by injection it causes blood vessels to expand, thereby increasing blood flow. Phentolamine has a very short half-life of approximately 20-minutes duration. Monoamine oxidase inhibitor (MAOI) induced hypertensive crisis should be treated with alpha-adrenergic antagonists, such as phentolamine or chlorpromazine. These agents lower blood pressure within five minutes. Intravenous furosemide (Lasix) can be used to reduce the fluid load and beta-adrenergic receptor antagonists can be used for controlling tachycardia. A sublingual dose of nifedipine (Procardia) can be given and repeated in 20 minutes. MAOIs should not be taken by patients with pheochromocytoma or thyrotoxicosis. Bromocriptine and dantrolene are dopamine agonists and are used in the treatment of neuroleptic malignant syndrome. They have no place in the treatment of MAOI-induced hypertensive crisis and in fact bromocriptine should be used with extreme caution in patients on MAOIs, as it can interact adversely with MAOIs, worsening hypertensive crisis. Sedative-hypnotic agents, like diazepam, should also be used with caution in patients taking MAOIs.

Diagnostic and Treatment Procedures in Psychiatry

K&S Ch. 36

Question 85. D. Concurrent administration of an SSRI with an MAOI antidepressant or Lithium can raise plasma serotonin to toxic levels, producing a serotonin syndrome. Serotonin syndrome is serious and can, in some cases, be fatal. Symptoms tend to occur in the following order as the condition worsens: (1) diarrhea; (2) restlessness; (3) extreme agitation, hyperreflexia and autonomic instability, with possible rapid fluctuations in vital signs; (4) myoclonus, seizures, hyperthermia, uncontrollable shivering, and rigidity; and (5) delirium, coma, status epilepticus, cardiovascular collapse, and death. Treatment consists of promptly removing the offending agents and immediately instituting comprehensive supportive care with nitroglycerine, cyproheptadine, methysergide, cooling blankets, chlorpromazine, dantrolene, benzodiazepines, anticonvulsants, mechanical ventilation, and paralytic agents.

Management in Psychiatry

K&S Ch. 36

Question 86. A. The overwhelming factor that correlates with childhood physical abuse is poverty and psychosocial stress, especially financial stress. Abuse and neglect of children also correlates with less parental education, underemployment, poor housing, single parenting and welfare reliance. Risk of child abuse increases in families with many children and is also increased by other risk factors, such as physical handicap, mental retardation, and prematurity. Parental mental illness, parental substance abuse (in particular alcoholism), social isolation, and domestic violence also correlate with childhood abuse and neglect. Families in which there are many of these problems coexisting tend to be more prone to child abuse and neglect.

Public Policy

K&S Chs 32&55

Question 87. B. Interpersonal therapy (IPT) is a time-limited (acutely, 12–16 weeks) treatment with three phases: a beginning (1–3 sessions), middle, and end (3 sessions). The initial phase requires the therapist to identify the target diagnosis (MDD) and the interpersonal context in which it presents. In diagnosing major depression, the therapist follows DSM-IV criteria and employs severity measures such as the Hamilton Depression Rating Scale (Ham-D) or Beck Depression Inventory (BDI) to reify the problem as an illness rather than the patient's idiosyncratic defect. The therapist also elicits an "interpersonal inventory", a review of the patient's patterns in relationships, capacity for intimacy, and particularly an evaluation of current relationships. A focus for treatment emerges from the last: someone important may have died (*complicated bereavement*), there may be a struggle with a significant other (*role dispute*), or the patient may have gone through some other important life change (*role transition*); in the relatively infrequent absence of any of these, the default focus is on *interpersonal deficits*, a confusing term that really denotes the absence of a current life event.

The therapist links the target diagnosis to the interpersonal focus. This formulation defines the remainder of the therapy. The connection between mood and life events is practical, not etiological: there is no pretense that this is what "causes" depression. With the patient's agreement on this focus, treatment moves into the middle phase.

Other facets of the opening phase include giving the patient the "sick role", a temporary status recognizing that depressive illness keeps the patient from functioning at full capacity, and setting treatment parameters such as the time limit and the expectation that therapy will focus on recent interpersonal interactions.

In the middle phase of treatment, the therapist uses specific strategies to deal with whichever of the four potential problem areas is the focus. This might involve appropriate mourning in *complicated bereavement*, resolving an interpersonal struggle in a *role dispute*, helping a patient to mourn the loss of an old role and assume a new one in a *role transition*, or decreasing social isolation for *interpersonal deficits*. Whatever the focus, the therapy is likely to address the patient's ability to assert his or her needs and wishes in interpersonal encounters, to validate the patient's anger as a normal interpersonal signal and to encourage its efficient expression, and to encourage taking appropriate social risks. In the last few sessions, the therapist reminds the patient that termination is nearing, helps the patient to feel more capable and independent by reviewing his or her often considerable accomplishments during the treatment, and notes that ending therapy is itself a role transition, with inevitable good and painful aspects. Since IPT has also demonstrated efficacy as a maintenance treatment for recurrent MDD, and since patients who have had multiple episodes are very likely to have more, therapist and patient may decide to end acute treatment as scheduled and then to recontract for ongoing treatment, perhaps of less intensive dosage: e.g., monthly rather than weekly sessions.

The IPT therapist's stance is relaxed and supportive. The goal is to be the patient's ally. The acute time limit pressures the patient to take action. No formal homework is assigned, but the goal of solving the focal interpersonal problem area provides an overall task. Treatment centers on the patient's outside environment, not on the therapy itself. The scheduling of sessions once weekly accentuates that the emphasis is on the patient's real life, not the office. In sessions therapist and patient review the past week's events. When the patient succeeds in an interpersonal situation, the therapist acts as a cheerleader, reinforcing healthy interpersonal skills. When the outcome is adverse, the therapist offers sympathy, helps the patient to analyze what went wrong in the situation, brainstorms new interpersonal options, and role plays them with the patient in rehearsal for real life. The patient then tests them out. Given this emphasis on interpersonal interaction, it is not surprising that depressed patients learn new interpersonal skills from IPT that they have not seen with pharmacotherapy. Note that psychotherapy questions come up frequently on psychiatry examinations and candidates often find themselves underprepared for these important questions. Do make it a point to look up IPT along with other psychotherapy modalities, to maximize your understanding of them.

Psychotherapy

K&S Ch. 35

Question 88. E. The "dialectical" in dialectical behavioral therapy (DBT) refers to the way in which it uses a broad way of thinking that emphasizes the limitations of linear ideas about causation. It substitutes "both/and" for "either/or" and sees truth as an evolving product of the opposition of different views. The use of dialectical ideas in DBT arises largely from the clinical observation of the mixed and shifting nature of human emotion and experience in general and in patients with borderline personality disorder (BPD) in particular. Interaction with such a patient is unlikely to have the characteristics of a logical argument or even an orderly conversation. It is more likely to be akin to a dance to rapidly changing music. The person with BPD is seen as having difficulties in being detached from his or her experience and is often overwhelmed by it. Developing the capacity for being mindful and living in the moment allows a greater potential for feeling appropriately in charge of the self. A related concept is the balance between acceptance and change. The most difficult idea for some is that the world is as it is. But again there is some paradox in the notion that acceptance – for instance, of unchangeable traumatic events in the past – may be necessary for change to be possible.

Psychotherapy

K&S Ch. 35

Question 89. E. Most patients with obsessive–compulsive disorder (OCD) have both obsessions and compulsions – up to 75% according to some studies. Some psychiatrists feel that this statistic is closer to 100%, if the patient is properly assessed for both mental and behavioral compulsions. Nevertheless, as per DSM-IV-TR, a patient need not have both obsessions and compulsions to meet criteria for OCD; one or the other is sufficient. Obsessions are intrusive thoughts and compulsions are intrusive behaviors. In OCD, an idea or impulse intrudes insistently and persistently into a person's conscious awareness. Remember that by DSM diagnostic standards, compulsions are defined as repetitive behaviors or mental acts that the person feels driven to perform in response to an obsession, or according to rules that must be applied rigidly. These behaviors (or mental acts) are targeted at reducing distress or anxiety, and are clearly excessive in their nature. In this particular question, the patient presents with compulsive orderliness, alphabetizing and color-coding behaviors. There is no mention of obsessions, though the criteria for OCD are met without that stipulation in this case.

Obsessive Compulsive and Related Disorders

K&S Ch. 16

Question 90. B. By DSM-IV-TR criteria, pedophilia is defined as recurrent, intense sexually arousing fantasies, sexual urges, or behaviors involving sexual activity with a prepubescent child or children, generally 13 years of age or younger, persisting over at least 6 months. The perpetrator either has acted on these sexual urges, or the urges or fantasies must cause significant distress or interpersonal difficulty. The perpetrator must be at least 16 years of age and at least 5 years older than the victim. When a perpetrator is a late adolescent involved with a 12- or 13-year-old, the pedophilia diagnosis does not apply. Ninety-five percent of pedophiles are heterosexual and 50% are found to be using alcohol at the time of the incident.

Paraphilias

K&S Ch. 21

Question 91. D. The mainstay of pharmacologic treatment of childhood ADHD is the stimulant medication class of agents. Methylphenidate and amphetamine preparations are dopamine agonists. Methylphenidate has been shown to be effective in about 75% of all children with ADHD. Common side effects of the stimulants are: headaches, GI discomfort, nausea and insomnia. Of course stimulants also suppress appetite and can induce weight loss. Some children experience a rebound effect following the wearing-off of the stimulant, during which period they become irritable and hyperactive. Motor tics can also be exacerbated by the use of stimulants, which warrants caution when the medications are given in this specific population of children. Methylphenidate is also associated with growth stunting or suppression. This effect seems to be offset when children are given drug holidays during the summer months when they are not in school. About 75% of students on stimulant medications demonstrate improvement in attention as measured by objective tests of their academic performance. Dextroamphetamine and dextroamphetamine/amphetamine salt combinations (Adderall) are generally the second choice when methylphenidate fails.

Disruptive, Impulse Control, Conduct Disorders, and ADHD

K&S Chs 43&54

Question 92. B.   The predominant disturbance in dissociative fugue is sudden, unexpected travel away from home or one's customary place of work, with inability to recall one's past. There is also confusion about one's personal identity or the assumption of a new identity. The symptoms must cause significant distress or impairment in social, occupational, or other important areas of functioning. The fugue state must not occur during a period of substance abuse or as part of dissociative identity disorder, or as a consequence of a medical condition. These fugue episodes can last from minutes to months in duration. Traumatic circumstances leading to an altered state of consciousness with a wish to flee, are generally the underlying cause of most fugue states. The disorder is seen more commonly during natural disasters, wartime, or during times of terrorism or social upheaval. Dissociative fugue is usually treated with psychodynamic psychotherapy, attempting to help the patient recover lost memory of their identity and recent experiences. Hypnotherapy is at times also helpful in the process of recovery following fugue states.

Dissociative Disorders

K&S Ch. 20

Question 93. C.   Eating disorders occur in about 4% of adolescents and young adults. Anorexia nervosa has its most common age of onset in the mid-teenage years, but up to 5% of cases begin in the twenties. The most common age of onset is between 14 and 18 years of age. Anorexia nervosa is estimated to occur in about 0.5 to 1% of adolescent girls. The disorder occurs about 10 to 20 times more frequently in women than in men. It is most frequent in developed countries and it is seen with highest frequency in women whose profession requires thinness, such as acting and modeling and dance. Anorexia is associated with depression in about 65% of cases.

Feeding and Eating Disorders

K&S Ch. 23

Question 94. A.   Encopresis is defined by DSM as the repeated passage of feces into inappropriate places, such as clothes or the floor, whether intentionally or involuntarily. The child must be 4 years of age, or older. The episodes must occur at least monthly for 3 months or more. Encopresis is not due to a general medical condition. The behavior must cause the child significant distress or social or academic impairment. Males are found to have encopresis six times more frequently than females. Encopresis has been shown to develop with much greater frequency in children with a known history of sexual abuse. Some studies have associated encopresis with measures of maternal hostility and punitive and harsh parenting.

Elimination Disorders

K&S Ch. 47

Question 95. E.   The defining feature of the paranoid subtype of schizophrenia is the presence of auditory hallucinations or prominent delusional thoughts about persecution or conspiracy. However, people with this subtype may be more functional in their ability to work and engage in relationships than people with other subtypes of schizophrenia. The reasons are not entirely clear, but may partly reflect that people suffering from this subtype often do not exhibit symptoms until later in life and have achieved a higher level of functioning before the onset of their illness. People with the paranoid subtype may appear to lead fairly normal lives by successful management of their disorder. People diagnosed with the paranoid subtype may not appear odd or unusual and may not readily discuss the symptoms of their illness. Typically, the hallucinations and delusions revolve around some characteristic theme, and this theme often remains fairly consistent over time. A person's temperaments and general behaviors often are related to the content of the disturbance of thought. For example, people who believe that they are being persecuted unjustly may be easily angered and become hostile. Do review the five subtypes of schizophrenia thoroughly, as questions about them do appear with regularity on standardized tests. Also be sure to review the good and poor prognosticating factors of schizophrenia. These too are often tested on psychiatry examinations.

Psychotic Disorders

K&S Ch. 13

Question 96. D.   In order to be diagnosed with pathological gambling, an individual must present with persistent and recurrent maladaptive gambling that causes economic problems and significant disturbances in personal, social, or occupational functioning with at least five of the following symptoms:

1. Preoccupation. The subject has frequent thoughts about gambling experiences, whether past, future, or fantasy.

2. Tolerance. As with drug tolerance, the subject requires larger or more frequent wagers to experience the same "rush".

3. Withdrawal. Restlessness or irritability associated with attempts to cease or reduce gambling.

4. Escape. The subject gambles to improve mood or escape problems.

5. Chasing. The subject tries to win back gambling losses with more gambling.

6. Lying. The subject tries to hide the extent of his or her gambling by lying to family, friends, or therapists.

7. Loss of control. The person has unsuccessfully attempted to reduce gambling.

8. Illegal acts. The person has broken the law in order to obtain gambling money or recover gambling losses. This may include acts of theft, embezzlement, fraud, or forgery.

9. Risked significant relationship. The person gambles despite risking or losing a relationship, job, or other significant opportunity.

10. Bailout. The person turns to family, friends, or another third party for financial assistance as a result of gambling.

Studies have pointed towards a neurobiological determinant in pathological gamblers' risk-taking behaviors. Theories have focused on both serotonergic and noradrenergic receptor systems. Evidence supports the probability that male pathological gamblers have low plasma MHPG concentrations, as well as increased CSF MHPG concentrations and increased urinary output of norepinephrine. Chronic gamblers also have decreased platelet MAO activity, which is a marker of serotonergic dysfunction, which is linked to difficulties with inhibition and impulse control. Epidemiologic studies point to a prevalence rate of about 3 to 5% of problem gamblers in the general population at large and about 1% who meet criteria for pathological gambling.

Disruptive, Impulse Control, Conduct Disorders, and ADHD
K&S Ch. 25

Question 97. C.   Conduct disorder is defined, as per DSM-IV-TR, as a repetitive and persistent pattern of behavior in which the basic rights of others or major age-appropriate societal norms or rules are violated, as manifested by the presence of three (or more) of the following criteria in the past 12 months, with at least one criterion present in the past 6 months:

Aggression to people and animals:

- often bullies, threatens, or intimidates others

- often initiates physical fights

- has used a weapon that can cause serious physical harm to others (e.g., a bat, brick, broken bottle, knife, gun)

- has been physically cruel to people

- has been physically cruel to animals

- has stolen while confronting a victim (e.g., mugging, purse snatching, extortion, armed robbery)

- has forced someone into sexual activity

Destruction of property:

- has deliberately engaged in fire setting with the intention of causing serious damage

- has deliberately destroyed others' property (other than by fire setting)

Deceitfulness or theft:

- has broken into someone else's house, building, or car

- often lies to obtain goods or favors or to avoid obligations (i.e., "cons" others)

- has stolen items of nontrivial value without confronting a victim (e.g., shoplifting, but without breaking and entering; forgery)

Serious violations of rules:

- often stays out at night despite parental prohibitions, beginning before age 13 years
- has run away from home overnight at least twice while living in a parental or parental surrogate home (or once without returning for a lengthy period)
- is often truant from school, beginning before age of 13 years

The disturbance of behavior causes clinically significant impairment in social, academic, or occupational functioning. Many biopsychosocial factors contribute to the manifestation of childhood conduct disorder. Some of these factors include harsh, punitive parenting; family discord; low socioeconomic status; lack of proper parental supervision; and lack of social competence. The problems must begin to manifest before 13 years of age. In some children with conduct disorder, low plasma levels of dopamine-beta-hydroxylase have been found. This finding supports the notion of decreased noradrenergic functioning in conduct disorder. Also, a recent Canadian study demonstrated greater right frontal EEG activity at rest correlated with violent and aggressive behavior in children. There is also little doubt that children chronically exposed to violence and abuse have a higher risk for being violent themselves.

Disruptive, Impulse Control, Conduct Disorders, and ADHD

K&S Ch. 44

Question 98. E. Rett's disorder presents with normal development up until 5 months of age. Then the child experiences a loss of previously acquired motor, social, and language skills as well as deceleration of head growth. Rett's disorder is always seen in girls. Childhood disintegrative disorder has a similar loss of skills but the decline starts later (around 2 years of age), it can occur in both genders and there is no change in head circumference. In autism the child has severe deficits in social interactions, communication, and develops stereotyped patterns of behavior. The autistic child never develops appropriate verbal and social skills unlike Rett's and childhood disintegrative disorder where those skills are developed then lost. Asperger's disorder is an autism-like picture where the child has normal language development. Autistic children do not have normal language development. In pervasive developmental disorder NOS there is a clear disturbance of normal development and deficits in motor, social, communication or other areas, but the picture does not meet criteria for one of the other developmental disorders.

Neurodevelopmental Disorders

K&S Ch. 42

Question 99. D. Carl Jung expanded on Freud's work with concepts such as archetypes, the collective unconscious, complexes, introverts, extroverts, anima and animus, the persona, and individuation. Erich Fromm defined five personality types that he felt were common to and determined by Western society. Kurt Goldstein gave us the term self-actualization which refers to people using their creative powers to fulfill their potential. Edith Jacobson proposed theories regarding an infant's experience of pleasure or lack of pleasure and its impact on the mother–infant relationship. Otto Kernberg did a great deal of work concerning object relations and borderline personality organization.

Psychological Theory and Psychometric Testing

K&S Ch. 6

Question 100. E. Only opium and organophosphorus insecticides out of the options cause miosis. Organophosphate poisons irreversibly inhibit acetylcholinesterase and cause accumulation of acetylcholine at muscarinic and nicotinic receptors. Muscarinic effects of organosphosphorus poisons are :

- miosis and blurred vision
- increased sweating, salivation, lacrimation
- increased bronchial secretions, bronchoconstriction
- abdominal cramps, diarrhea, nausea, vomiting
- urinary frequency and incontinence

Nicotinic effects of organophosphorus poisons are :

- on striated muscles – twitching, fasciculations, cramps and muscle paralysis
- on sympathetic ganglia – hypertension and tachycardia

CNS effects of organophosphorus poisons are:

- anxiety, restlessness and confusion
- seizures and coma

This child presents with tachycardia and hypertension which are nicotinic manifestations. Sometimes the presentation can vary due to the muscarinic effect on cardiovascular system which causes bradycardia and hypotension, but this occurs due to severe organophosphorus poisoning.

n-Hexane is used as a solvent in paints, lacquers, and printing inks and is used especially in the rubber industry and in certain glues. Workers involved in the manufacturing of footwear, laminating processes, and cabinetry, especially in confined, unventilated spaces, may be exposed to excessive concentrations of this substance. Exposure to this chemical by inhalation or skin contact leads to a progressive distal sensorimotor axonal polyneuropathy; partial conduction block may also occur. Optic neuropathy or maculopathy and facial numbness also have followed *n*-hexane exposure.

The major symptoms of botulism are blurred vision, dysphagia and dysarthria. Pupillary responses to light are impaired, and reduction of tendon reflex responses is variable. Weakness progresses for several days and then reaches a plateau. Fatal respiratory paralysis may occur rapidly. Most patients have symptoms of autonomic dysfunction, such as dry mouth, constipation, or urinary retention. The edrophonium test is positive in approximately one third of patients and does not distinguish botulism from other causes of neuromuscular blockade. Wound cultures and serum assay for botulinum toxin confirm the diagnosis of wound botulism. Treatment consists of bivalent (type A and B) or trivalent (A, B, and E) antitoxin. Antibiotic therapy is not effective because the cause of symptoms (in all but infantile botulism) is the ingestion of toxin rather than organisms. Otherwise, treatment is supportive; the need for respiratory assistance is unusual. Acetylcholinesterase inhibitors are not beneficial. Recovery takes many months but usually is complete.

Poisoning

B&D Chs 58&78

Question 101. C. Oxazepam, lorazepam, and temazepam are only phase II metabolized (via glucoronidation) and as such have no active metabolites prior to excretion. The other benzos first undergo phase I metabolism (oxidation via the Cytochrome P450 system) which generates active metabolites that then go on to be phase II metabolized and excreted.

Psychopharmacology

K&S Ch. 36

Question 102. D. Benzodiazepines are pregnancy category D. Category D indicates positive evidence of human fetal risk. Weigh risk and benefit of using medication in a pregnant patient.

Psychopharmacology

K&S Ch. 36

Question 103. C. Some of the most common reasons for psychiatric malpractice suits include suicide attempt or completion by a patient, incorrect or negligent treatment, medication error or drug reaction, and incorrect diagnosis. Though other choices in this question are causes for malpractice suits suicide is the most common.

Forensic Psychiatry

K&S Ch. 57

Question 104. A. SSRIs delay ejaculation. Yohimbine, alprostadil and sildenafil can be used for impotence. Testosterone can increase sexual desire but is masculinizing.

Sexual Dysfunction

K&S Ch. 21

Question 105. B. Obsessive–compulsive disorder occurs in equal rates in men and women. All other choices listed in this question occur more in males. Don't forget this important fact for your exam.

Statistics

K&S Ch. 16

Question 106. B. Here are commonly asked forensics terms. You must know them all.

A socially harmful act is not enough to have committed a crime. To be found guilty the accused must also have *mens rea* (evil intent) and *actus reus* (voluntary conduct). In the case of many mentally ill patients that commit socially harmful acts they lack one of these elements.

Parens patriae is a doctrine that allows the state to intervene and act as a surrogate parent for those who are unable to care for themselves.

Respondeat superior holds that a person occupying a high position in a hierarchy is responsible for those in lower positions.

Substituted judgment is when a surrogate makes a decision on the basis of what the patient would have wanted, taking into account their wishes and values.

Justice is the equitable distribution of social resources and benefits.

Forensic Psychiatry

K&S Ch. 57

Question 107. E. Studies support CBT as the best therapy for panic disorder. SSRIs are also considered first line because of their effectiveness, safety, and low side effect profile. Studies also support the fact that CBT plus an SSRI will deliver better results than either treatment given alone.

Anxiety Disorders

K&S Ch. 16

Question 108. B. Disorders that are frequently comorbid with social phobia include other anxiety disorders, affective disorders and substance abuse disorders. About 1/3 of patients with social phobia will meet criteria for major depressive disorder. There is no significant comorbidity with the somatoform disorders in general and conversion disorder in particular.

K&S Ch. 16

Anxiety Disorders

Question 109. E. The addition of a benzodiazepine to a patient on an SSRI for panic disorder will lead to a more rapid resolution of the anxiety. The SSRI will take 2 to 4 weeks to work in most cases. The benzodiazepine can effectively control the patient's symptoms until the SSRI is fully working. The other choices will take longer to titrate or become effective and are not good choices for rapid resolution of panic symptoms. Propranolol is only indicated for performance anxiety and should not be used in other anxiety disorders.

Anxiety Disorders

K&S Ch. 16

Question 110. C. Carbamazepine acts like a vasopressin agonist and has antidiuretic actions. As such it can cause hyponatremia, especially in the elderly. The other choices are not known for this particular side effect.

Psychopharmacology/Lab Tests in Psychiatry

K&S Ch. 36

Question 111. D. Risperidone does not affect thyroid function tests but may alter the other choices listed as part of a metabolic syndrome. In addition the clinician may wish to consider an EKG if the patient has significant cardiac risk factors, as well as HbA1c.

Psychopharmacology/Lab Tests in Psychiatry

K&S Ch. 36

Question 112. D. The psychotherapist should maintain neutrality with his or her patients. Personal information should be limited and only given if it is to help the patient in some way. In this case his telling the patients is more about his grief than about the needs of the patients. It is therefore a boundary violation. Whenever revealing personal information the therapist should ask him or herself if they are doing it for the patient or themselves. Choices A and B are too much of a black and white statement to be true. There may be situations where a therapist can reveal personal information, but must examine why they are doing it first. Choice E misses the central issue in the ethical dilemma.

Ethics

K&S Ch. 58

Question 113. D. Kappa is a number that is used for binary data and tells us whether a given procedure or test produces reliable or reproducible results. It is often used to measure the degree of agreement between raters in a study. Correlation coefficient indicates reliability for non-binary data such as continuous measurements. Point prevalence is the number of cases at a specific point in time divided by the population at the same time. Period prevalence looks at the number of cases both existing and new during a specific time period. Lifetime prevalence reflects the proportion of people who have ever had a specific condition during their lifetimes.

Statistics

K&S Ch. 4

Question 114. C. This is a common case of countertransference which is expected to develop in the course of psychodynamic psychotherapy. The patient is reenacting her relationship with her mother with the therapist. The therapist is not rejecting the patient, her schedule does not allow her to meet three times per week. Nor is there evidence to suggest that countertransference on the part of the therapist is the issue here. There is no evidence of psychosis, or delusion, or of an erotomanic theme to the therapy. We have no evidence that the patient is stalking the therapist nor would it be reasonable to assume that this is the case given the information provided. Displacement is taking the emotional energy from one object and placing it onto another unrelated object. The patient is not doing that in this question.

Psychotherapy

K&S Ch. 1

Question 115. E. Neuroimaging is not considered standard of care for mania. It should be considered in all of the other scenarios listed in this question as well as before initial ECT treatments, with acute mental status change following head trauma, and in dementia of unknown etiology.

Lab Tests in Psychiatry

K&S Ch. 7

Question 116. A. Exposure with response prevention is considered the "gold standard" for treatment of OCD. Make sure you know this fact before you sit for your exam!

Anxiety Disorders

K&S Ch. 16

Question 117. B. The abnormal formation of the tricuspid valve you should be concerned with here is Ebstein's anomaly. It is the result of giving lithium during pregnancy, especially during the first trimester. Also worth noting is that valproic acid given during pregnancy causes neural tube defects in the fetus.

Psychopharmacology

K&S Ch. 36

Question 118. D. For many women libido increases during pregnancy and it is incorrect to say that most women experience absence of sexual desire during pregnancy. The other choices are part of normal adjustment to pregnancy. Many women experience pregnancy as a means of self realization, project hope onto the child, are afraid of inadequate mothering or have unconscious fears and ambivalence regarding the impact of the relationship with the child's father.

Human Development

K&S Ch. 2

Question 119. E. Competence is decided by the court. Capacity is decided by the psychiatrist. The four standards of capacity are:

1. Ability to communicate a choice

2. Ability to understand the information presented

3. Ability to understand how information applies to ones own circumstances

4. Ability to reason in a logical manner (even if most people wouldn't agree with the final decision)

Forensic Psychiatry

K&S Ch. 57

Question 120. A. The Benton visual retention test is one in which a patient is presented with geometric figures for 10 seconds then asked to draw them from memory. It is a test of short term memory. The Weschler Memory Scale is the most widely used memory test for adults. The Bender visual motor gestalt test is a test of visuomotor coordination and is useful in testing maturational levels in children. The Wisconsin Card Sorting Test assesses abstract reasoning and difficulty in problem solving.

Psychological Theory and Psychometric Testing

K&S Ch. 5

Question 121. B. Schizoid fantasy is indulging in autistic-like retreat to resolve conflict. Interpersonal intimacy is avoided and others are driven away by eccentricity. It is an immature defense. Anticipation is planning for future inner discomfort, and is mature. Altruism is using service to others to undergo an internally gratifying experience, and is mature. Humor is using comedy to express feelings without becoming uncomfortable or causing discomfort in others, and is mature. Suppression is consciously postponing attention to an impulse or conflict, and is mature.

Psychological Theory and Psychometric Testing

K&S Ch. 6

Question 122. B. Lithium has been associated with hyperplasia and adenomas of the parathyroid glands leading to hyperparathyroidism and hypercalcemia. Neutropenia is associated with clozapine. Pancreatitis is a rare but potentially deadly side effect of valproic acid. Hepatic failure is associated with valproic acid, hence the black box warning in the PDR. Eosinophilic colitis is associated with clozapine. Though these drugs are certainly not the only causes of these conditions these associations would be useful for the prudent student to know.

Psychopharmacology

K&S Ch. 36

Question 123. E. In order to be a good candidate for brief psychodynamic therapy the patient must be able to identify and discuss their feelings. The best candidates are highly motivated, have an area of focus for the therapy, and have at least one solid relationship. You are looking for psychological-mindedness and the ability to learn through relationships. Patients who are too concrete, regressed, and have no meaningful relationships are usually not good candidates. The ability to take a daily medication is not particularly relevant.

Psychotherapy

K&S Ch. 35

Question 124. A. Object relations theory is best represented by the work of Melanie Klein. Object relations theory is known for the schizoid, paranoid and depressive positions as well as tension between the true and false self. The other notable therapists listed in this question will undoubtedly be the subject of other questions throughout this book.

Psychotherapy

K&S Ch. 4

Question 125. C. Motivational enhancement therapy is a treatment that has proven successful at treating drug addiction, especially in cases where there is denial and ambivalence on the part of the substance abuser. The patient does not suffer from depression or anxiety so fluoxetine is not appropriate. There is no evidence that Joe is a borderline so dialectical behavior therapy is not warranted. ECT is used for depression, psychosis, and mania, not crack addiction. We don't have adequate information to make a judgment call about involuntary hospitalization.

Substance Abuse and Addictive Disorders/Psychotherapy

K&S Chs 12&35

Question 126. B. It is considered unethical to have any business involvement with patients or former patients. It is unethical to get patients to leave you anything in their will or to solicit them to leave anything to anyone in their will. As such the answer here is that you will not ask any of your current or former patients to make donations in any way.

Ethics

K&S Ch. 58

Question 127. C. In its most basic form interpretation is making something that was unconscious conscious. It is an explanatory statement that links a feeling thought, behavior or symptom to its unconscious meaning. Confrontation is addressing something the patient does not want to accept. Clarification is reformulating what the patient has said to create a coherent view of what has been communicated. Empathic validation is a demonstration of the therapist's empathic understanding of the patient's internal state. Affirmation is giving succinct comments in support of the patient's statements or feelings.

Psychological Theory and Psychometric Testing

K&S Ch. 35

Question 128. B. This is a common ethical situation encountered by physicians. Accepting gifts from a drug representative is a conflict of interest and is ethically questionable. There is evidence that gifts influence physician behavior, which is why drug companies try to give you things! They're not just giving you things to be nice. They know it will influence prescribing habits. The monetary value of the gift is not the determining factor in whether it is unethical. Physicians have done very poorly at self-regulating with regard to this issue. Doctors are just as influenced by gifts as anyone else in the office.

Ethics

K&S Ch. 57

Question 129. B. The proper way to work with an interpreter is to look at and direct questions to the patient. The interpreter should then translate the discussion for both sides. Don't look at the interpreter. She is not your patient. Having the family in the room is problematic because they may misinterpret or answer the questions without asking the patient and their involvement may pose a problem in terms of patient confidentiality. Shouting at people who do not speak English is common but unsuccessful. They're not deaf, they can't speak English no matter how slowly or loudly you say it!

Psychotherapy

K&S Ch. 1

Question 130. B. Epigenetic is a term used to describe Erikson's stages of development. Each stage contains a psychological crisis which must be negotiated before moving on to the next phase. Levinson's theories divided adult development up into four stages, each lasting about 25 years. Vaillant found that a happy childhood correlated with positive traits in middle life and that adaptive styles mature over time. He postulated that this maturation was dependant on internal development rather than changes in the environment. Neurodevelopmemtal theory concerns itself with physical brain development, formation and connection of neurons and brain plasticity. In normality-as-process, changes in personality over time are an essential part of the developmental process. Emphasis is placed on the changes one undergoes over time rather than labeling where a person should be at a given age.

Human Development

K&S Ch. 2

Question 131. C.   Routine monitoring for patients on lithium includes all of the choices except urine for creatinine and protein. However, this test should be considered in patients who have renal disease and are on lithium. Additional tests one might consider include pregnancy tests for women of childbearing age.

Psychopharmacology/Lab Tests in Psychiatry

K&S Ch. 36

Question 132. C.   DSM criteria for panic disorder state that the patient must have either recurrent attacks or one attack followed by 1 month or more of persistent concern about having more attacks, or worry about the implications of the attack or its consequences, or a significant change in behavior related to the attacks.

Anxiety Disorders

K&S Ch. 16

Question 133. C.   The DSM states that a diagnosis of major depression should not be made following a death unless a patient's symptoms are severe and persist for 2 months following the loss. Sadness, sleep disturbance, and appetite disturbance are part of normal grief. The clinician should be on the lookout for MDD when presented with feelings of excessive guilt unrelated to the deceased, suicidality, morbid preoccupation with worthlessness, or psychomotor retardation. Psychosis is also not part of the normal bereavement process.

Depressive Disorders

K&S Ch. 15

Question 134. D.   Methylenedioxymethamphetamine (ecstasy) is known for a hyperthermic syndrome that can progress to disseminated intravascular coagulation, rhabdomyolysis, liver and kidney failure, and death. Adverse effects of ecstasy are not dose related so this syndrome can occur at any dose. This is one of those facts that you must know for your exam and need to just memorize. Just in case you weren't sure flunitrazepam is Rohypnol. The other drugs mentioned are found in questions throughout this book.

Substance Abuse and Addictive Disorders

K&S Ch. 12

Question 135. D.   When treating social anxiety disorder combining CBT and pharmacotherapy does not show a clear benefit over using just one or the other for most initial treatment. There is evidence however, that there are some refractory cases that do respond better to a combination of both.

Anxiety Disorders

K&S Ch. 16

Question 136. D.   When considering the choices given, hopefully lamotrigine jumped out at you. The other choices are all very well known for causing significant weight gain. Clozapine and olanzapine cause some of the most weight gain of all the antipsychotics and carry high rates of metabolic syndrome. Valproic acid and lithium are both known to cause significant weight gain, amongst other troublesome side effects. Lamictal however, is relatively weight neutral and significant weight gain is rare.

Psychopharmacology

K&S Ch. 36

Question 137. D.   Skills training is part of a cognitive behavioral approach to substance abuse. Patients are helped to change beliefs, improve interpersonal communication, resist social pressure, increase assertiveness, and better manage stress. Unconscious symbolism is part of a psychodynamic approach to therapy, not part of a cognitive behavioral approach.

Substance Abuse and Addictive Disorders

K&S Ch. 12

Question 138. B.   Only MDs can order the start of a new seclusion once the previous seclusion order has ended. The nurse cannot extend the time on her own. All other answer choices are correct.

Forensic Psychiatry

K&S Ch. 54

Question 139. D. The lowest effective methadone dose for most patients is 50 mg per day. The average methadone dose for opiate addiction is 80 mg per day. Doses of 80 mg per day are twice as likely to lead to successful outcomes as doses of 50 mg or less.

Substance Abuse and Addictive Disorders

K&S Ch. 12

Question 140. E. Patients who have a high likelihood to go into the delirium tremens based on history should be detoxified inpatient. This is a major safety concern as the delirium tremens can be life threatening. As such this takes precedence over other considerations.

Substance Abuse and Addictive Disorders

K&S Ch. 12

Question 141. E. The best medication for this patient would be an SSRI to control the OCD symptoms and a dopamine blocker to control the tics. When we look at the choices the one that fits is choice E. Fluvoxamine is an SSRI with proven efficacy in treating OCD. Haloperidol is a strong dopamine blocker that can effectively control tics. Benzos, buspirone, and naltrexone are not used for tics.

Psychopharmacology

K&S Ch. 36

Question 142. B. The DSM criteria for hypomania specifically state that there are no psychotic features. If psychosis exists then the mood episode would be considered mania. Major depression, mania, mixed episodes and delirium can all involve psychosis. In addition it should be noted that dementia can also present with psychosis.

Bipolar Disorders

K&S Ch. 15

Question 143. E. In order to meet criteria for Bipolar I one must have at least one manic episode. So Bipolar I is out in this case. For Bipolar II one must have one hypomanic episode and one episode of major depressive disorder. So Bipolar II is out in this case because we have no depressive symptoms. To meet Cyclothymic disorder one must have hypomanic symptoms as well as depressive symptoms which do not meet criteria for major depression that go on for at least 2 years. This patient has no depressive symptoms so Cyclothymic disorder is out. There is no evidence of any substance abuse in the question stem so substance induced mood disorder is out. The correct answer is Bipolar disorder NOS which includes patients with clear bipolar symptoms who do not meet criteria for any specific bipolar disorder.

Bipolar Disorders

K&S Ch. 15

Question 144. E. Symptoms of pheochromocytoma can include anxiety, panic, tremulousness, flushing, feeling of impending doom, hypertension, and tachycardia. It can be mistaken for panic disorder. Hyperparathyroidism presents as constipation, polydipsia, nausea, depression, paranoia and confusion. Hypothyroidism presents with cold intolerance, weight gain, brittle hair, goiter, constipation, dry skin, lethargy, depressed affect, hallucinations, and paranoia. Raynaud's phenomenon presents with idiopathic paroxysmal bilateral cyanosis of the digits and can be exacerbated or triggered by stress. Crohn's disease does not have psychiatric manifestations.

Somatic Symptom Disorders

K&S Ch. 28

Question 145. D. When compared to the general population patients with social phobia tend to have fewer friendships, lower levels of education, higher rates of suicide, and less success in career advancement. They also have poorer marital function.

Anxiety Disorders

K&S Ch. 16

Question 146. C. Regularly scheduled primary care appointments are a crucial and standard part of treating hypochondriasis. In hypochondriasis the patient is convinced that they have an illness that they don't have. If they are not followed closely by their primary care physician they will go doctor shopping. While regularly following with the primary care doctor they should also be engaged in psychotherapy to work on the underlying psychological causes of the condition. None of the other disorders listed require regular follow-up by the primary care doctor. That is not to say these patients should not regularly follow up for routine medical care, but that it is not a crucial component of the treatment for the psychiatric condition.

Somatic Symptom Disorders

K&S Ch. 17

Question 147. C. Alcohol dependence, being widowed, being unemployed, and being socially isolated are all factors which increase chances of suicide in the elderly. Add to that list male gender, chronic illness, depression, irritation, rage, violence, and affective instability.

Management in Psychiatry

K&S Ch. 34

Question 148. B. For a patient on clozapine who develops a white count between 2000 and 3000 the correct action is to stop the clozapine. The clozapine may be tried again when the patient's white count improves. Monitor the WBC daily until it is over 3000. For a patient whose WBC count is between 3000 and 3500 you can switch to twice weekly monitoring until it is back above 3500. If the WBC count is lower than 2000 the patient can not be re-challenged on clozapine.

Psychopharmacology

K&S Ch. 36

Question 149. E. QTc interval is normally less than 450 milliseconds. Prolongation of the QTc interval longer than 500 milliseconds increases the risk for torsade de pointes. Under these circumstances any medication which may be increasing the QTc must be considered carefully and possibly discontinued, changed, or decreased.

Psychopharmacology

K&S Ch. 36

Question 150. A. Interferon is well known to exacerbate depression. Side effects include depressed mood, suicidality, suicidal ideation, insomnia, fatigue, and cognitive inefficiency. The other medications listed are not known to cause the exacerbation of depressive symptoms listed in this question.

Psychopharmacology

K&S Ch. 36

Vignettes

Vignette One

Gabriel Matthews is a 42-year-old construction worker who comes to you for help. Six months ago he was working with a chainsaw on a construction site and didn't realize that the gas cap on the saw was loose. The cap came off spilling gasoline all over his clothes and the saw. The heat from the engine ignited the gas setting his clothes on fire. He ran around the construction site ablaze until three other workers came to his aid and extinguished the fire by smothering it with clothing and dirt. He suffered severe burns and spent a significant amount of time in a burn unit.

Five weeks following the accident you are called to consult on him in the burn unit because he is having psychiatric symptoms which started 2 days after the fire and are progressively getting worse. He is having distressing nightmares about being on fire that wake him from sleep. His mood is low and he feels unable to be happy about anything. He is hopeless about the future and feels he has nothing to look forward to. He is getting more and more upset as his days in the unit go on and he has a short temper with the nurses. He keeps sending visitors away who come from his job and who were there the day that the accident happened. He has had several incidents of yelling at various family members when they came to visit. You meet his sister while on the unit who cries as she tells you how hostile Gabriel has been towards the family lately.

1.   Gabriel's most accurate diagnosis is:

   A. *Major depressive disorder*

   B. *Adjustment disorder with depressed mood*

   C. *Post-traumatic stress disorder*

   D. *Mood disorder secondary to a medical condition*

 Full test available online – see inside front cover for details.

2. Gabriel inquires about treatment available for his condition. Which treatments would you consider? (choose 3 of 5)

   A. *Family therapy*

   B. *SSRIs*

   C. *Benzodiazepines*

   D. *Cognitive behavioral therapy*

   E. *Dialectical behavior therapy*

3. Which of the following factors would be predictive of a poor prognosis for Gabriel? (choose 2 of 5)

   A. *Rapid onset of symptoms*

   B. *Strong social supports*

   C. *Absence of other axis I disorders*

   D. *Duration of symptoms greater than 6 months*

   E. *Borderline personality disorder*

4. Which one of the following symptoms is commonly found in patients with Gabriel's disorder?

   A. *Tactile hallucinations*

   B. *Thyroid abnormalities*

   C. *Decreased norepinephrine turnover in the locus coeruleus*

   D. *Alexithymia*

5. In addition to medication, which of the following would be considered appropriate treatment approaches for this disorder? (choose 4 of 5)

   A. *Overcome the patient's denial of the traumatic event*

   B. *Use of imaginal techniques or in vivo exposure*

   C. *Encourage proper sleep providing medication if necessary*

   D. *Promote full discharge of aggression as a cathartic exercise to relieve irritability*

   E. *Teach the patient cognitive approaches to dealing with stress*

6. Which of the following symptoms can be found in both schizophrenia and PTSD? (choose 2 of 4)

   A. *Hallucinations*

   B. *Restricted affect*

   C. *Decreased need for sleep*

   D. *Sense of foreshortened future*

7. Which of the following illnesses can present with decreased sleep? (choose 3 of 4)

   A. *Bipolar I disorder*

   B. *Generalized anxiety disorder*

   C. *Post-traumatic stress disorder*

   D. *Obsessive–compulsive disorder*

8. In Gabriel's case he associated the trauma of the fire with chainsaws. For years afterwards he would have severe anxiety whenever he saw a chainsaw. He would avoid going near the outdoor power equipment whenever he was in a hardware store. This is a good example of which one of the following?

   A. *Operant conditioning*

   B. *Learned helplessness*

   C. *Classical conditioning*

   D. *Premack's principle*

9. Which one of the following is not considered a symptom of increased arousal when diagnosing PTSD?

   A. *Poor concentration*

   B. *Outbursts of anger*

   C. *Feelings of detachment from others*

   D. *Difficulty falling asleep*

10. Which of the following should be considered in the differential for post-traumatic stress disorder? (choose 4 of 5)

    A. *Panic disorder*

    B. *Substance abuse*

    C. *Major depressive disorder*

    D. *Borderline personality disorder*

    E. *Schizotypal personality disorder*

Vignette Two

A 65-year-old woman presents to your office with a complaint of longstanding symptoms that have plagued her since her adolescence. She reports chronic suicidal ideation, low mood, inability to focus or concentrate. Her memory is fairly good, but she doesn't enjoy anything that she used to do. She used to play cards with friends, drive herself to the mall to go shopping, take trips to visit her children and grandchildren in various cities. She denies hearing voices or having paranoid or suspicious thoughts about people. Her sleep is very broken and she only gets about 4 hours each night. She has no motivation to shop, cook or clean for herself and she admits it to you. Her appetite is poor and she has already lost twenty pounds over the past year from not eating properly.

Her eldest daughter, age 42, accompanies her to your office. Her daughter is quite concerned for her mother because she has been on "every antidepressant you can imagine." As a nurse, her daughter is able to rattle off a list of medications that her mother has tried in the past: imipramine, doxepin, phenelzine, fluoxetine, paroxetine, venlafaxine, duloxetine. None of these improved her back to her baseline. She has also had trials of several of these medications with other augmenting agents such as: methylphenidate, lorazepam, aripiprazole, lithium, and buspirone.

On examination in your office, the patient is conversant and coherent, but very slow to speak and her affect is blunted and speech is quiet and monotonous with marked alogia. She denies suicidal or homicidal thoughts or intentions at this time.

1. Your immediate clinical thoughts after interviewing this patient should be focused on:

    A. *Sending her home with a trial of bupropion and desvenlafaxine at high doses along with L-methylfolate for augmentation, since she has never been on these agents*

    B. *Admitting her to the psychiatric hospital voluntarily for inpatient electroshock therapy*

    C. *Getting her a bed in a local skilled nursing facility because she cannot manage her activities of daily living appropriately*

    D. *Considering reporting her daughter to the authorities for elder abuse*

    E. *Enlisting a local ACT team (assertive community treatment team) to pick up her care and service her needs in her home instead of in a clinic setting*

2. You decide to admit her to the hospital and she agrees to go on a voluntary basis. Before considering electroshock therapy, which of the following would be appropriate to do as a pretreatment evaluation? (pick 3 of 6)

    A. *Bloodwork for blood count and comprehensive chemistry (CBC and chem-20)*

    B. *Head CT scan or MRI*

    C. *Thyroid function tests*

    D. *Electrocardiogram*

    E. *Electroencephalogram*

    F. *Neck and spine radiography*

3. Which of the following is a contraindication to electroshock therapy?

    A. *Pregnancy*

    B. *Space-occupying brain lesion*

    C. *Recent myocardial infarction within the past month*

    D. *Hypertension*

    E. *There are no absolute contraindications to electroshock therapy*

4. In order for a seizure to be deemed effective in electroshock therapy sessions, its duration must be at least:

    A. *5 seconds*

    B. *15 seconds*

    C. *25 seconds*

    D. *45 seconds*

    E. *60 seconds*

5. Which of the following are not generally considered to be adverse effects of electroshock therapy? (pick 2 of 6)

    A. *Death*

    B. *Headache*

    C. *Nausea and vomiting*

    D. *Dizziness and lightheadedness*

    E. *Hypertension*

    F. *Delirium*

6. Which of the following situations is an indication for maintenance electroshock therapy after an initial successful group of treatments? (pick 3 of 6)

    A. *Severe medication side effects and intolerance*

    B. *Profound memory loss following the initial treatment sessions*

    C. *Psychotic or severe symptoms*

    D. *Rapid relapse after successful initial treatment sessions*

    E. *Delirium resulting from initial treatment sessions*

    F. *Pregnancy*

7. Which of the following medications should be discontinued prior to electroshock therapy administration? (pick 3 of 6)

    A. *Venlafaxine*

    B. *Phenelzine*

    C. *Clozapine*

    D. *Fluoxetine*

    E. *Bupropion*

    F. *Alprazolam*

8. Which of the following agents is not generally used as an anesthetic agent in electroshock therapy because of its strong anticonvulsant properties?

    A. *Methohexital (Brevital)*

    B. *Ketamine (Ketalar)*

    C. *Etomidate (Amidate)*

    D. *Propofol (Diprivan)*

    E. *Alfentanil (Alfenta)*

9. Which of the following is the typical course of electrode placement in electroshock therapy that is followed by most practitioners?

    A. *Start with bilateral electrode placement always, as this is more effective*

    B. *Start with bilateral electrode placement, but move to unilateral placement if persistent memory loss occurs after 6 sessions*

    C. *Start with unilateral electrode placement, but move to bilateral placement if no improvement is seen after four to six unilateral treatments*

    D. *Start with unilateral electrode placement always, as this is safer and causes fewer side effects*

    E. *Start with unilateral electrode placement always, making sure placement is over the nondominant hemisphere to avoid language and cognitive deficits*

Vignette Three

Cathy Kelly is a 31-year-old computer programmer who works for a website design company. She comes to your office with reports of decreased mood, poor appetite, poor concentration, and feelings of worthlessness. She states, "I haven't gotten a good night's sleep in weeks and I've lost about 10 pounds recently." These symptoms have been present for the past 5 weeks. On further questioning she describes a period 2 years ago when she "had some trouble" around her sister's wedding. In the 4 days leading up to the wedding she was only sleeping 2 hours per night. She tells you, "I wasn't tired and had enough energy to make pastries and gifts for the wedding guests. I was up working almost all night." She recalls that "brilliant ideas for new projects" were running through her mind at that time. She continued going to work at her computer programming job during those 4 days and felt that she was very productive. When the wedding came she drank excessively and used her position as a bridesmaid to meet single friends of the groom. She took several men into a secluded bathroom and had sex with them during the wedding reception. When asked about substance abuse she reports using both cocaine and alcohol in the past to "make me feel better." She denies any cocaine use around the time of her sister's wedding however.

1. Which one of the following would be the most appropriate diagnosis for Cathy?

    A. *Bipolar I disorder*

    B. *Major depressive disorder*

    C. *Bipolar II disorder*

    D. *Cyclothymic disorder*

    E. *Substance induced mood disorder*

2. Which one of the following is a key differentiating factor between mania and hypomania?

    A. *Irritable mood*

    B. *Decreased need for sleep*

    C. *Marked impairment in social or occupational functioning*

    D. *Flight of ideas*

3. Which of the following factors should impact your choice of medications for Cathy? (choose 4 of 5)

    A. *The presence of psychosis*

    B. *The presence of rapid cycling*

    C. *The severity of symptoms*

    D. *Pregnancy*

    E. *Age*

4. In which of the following scenarios would you consider ECT for Cathy? (choose 2 of 4)

    A. *Cathy is pregnant and currently manic*

    B. *Cathy has severe mania and psychosis that has responded poorly to medication*

    C. *Cathy has mania secondary to a medical condition*

    D. *Cathy has substance induced mania*

5. Which of the following medical conditions can be associated with mania? (choose 3 of 4)

    A. *Glioma*

    B. *Cushing's disease*

    C. *Multiple sclerosis*

    D. *Thiamine deficiency*

6. Which of the following medications can cause a manic episode? (choose 4 of 5)

    A. *Isoniazid*

    B. *Cimetidine*

    C. *Metoclopramide*

    D. *Steroids*

    E. *Oxazepam*

7. During the periods when Cathy used cocaine which of the following were true concerning her brain? (choose 3 or 4)

    A. *Dopamine activity increased in the corpus striatum*

    B. *Dopamine activity decreased in the mesocortical pathway*

    C. *Dopamine activity increased in the mesolimbic pathway*

    D. *There was both dopamine and norepinephrine reuptake inhibition*

8. Which one of the following is not a potential sequelae of cocaine use?

    A. *Onset of hallucinations and paranoia*

    B. *A significant appearance of lights in the central visual field*

    C. *Hypersexuality*

    D. *Itching and respiratory depression*

9. Which of the following have a role in the treatment of cocaine overdose? (choose 3 of 4)

    A. *IV diazepam*

    B. *Haloperidol*

    C. *IV phentolamine*

    D. *Clonidine*

10. What percentage of patients with bipolar disorder have a co-occurring substance disorder like Cathy?

    A. *10%*

    B. *30%*

    C. *60%*

    D. *80%*

Vignette Four

Susan Walton is a 20-year-old college student. You interview her in the emergency room following an overdose of Tylenol. She reports that she was happily shopping with her boyfriend when he spotted an attractive woman on the other side of the street. "He's such an asshole," she tells you. She says he watched the woman closely as she walked away and Susan was certain that he was attracted to her. "I could tell by the way he was looking at her. She was such a whore. Is that what he wants? A whore like that?" she screams at you. According to her boyfriend Susan then reached into her purse, pulled out a bottle of Tylenol and swallowed as many pills as she could before her boyfriend wrestled the bottle from her hands. He became panicked and brought her to the emergency room. On the drive in she scratched up and down her arms using her fingernails, breaking the skin. She then began biting her forearms until they bled. He tried to pull the car over and stop her but she scratched his face when he tried to intervene. When she arrived in the emergency room she was crying hysterically and cursing at her boyfriend. When he attempted to comfort her she spat on him and smacked him in the face, scratching him again with her nails. She called him a "piece of trash" and insisted that he wants to cheat on her "with that whore" which he denied.

When she is calmer you take some further history from her. She tells you "I was severely sexually abused as a small child. But I didn't tell anyone until I was a teenager. I started having sex at the age of 15. I used cocaine. I smoked. I really didn't care. I was extremely self-abusive and it got to the point where I wanted to kill myself to rid myself of the anger, the hurt, the pain, the confusion." She admits that she has made prior suicide attempts. She tells you "When I was seventeen I looked forward to getting my drivers license so I could run the car into a support column on the highway, or into a semi truck. I drove very recklessly; I didn't want it to be an obvious suicide." She informs you that when she was 18 she had a very severe car accident and ended up in the intensive care unit.

1. Which one of the following is Susan's most likely diagnosis?

    A. *Major depressive disorder*

    B. *Borderline personality disorder*

    C. *Bipolar I disorder*

    D. *Histrionic personality disorder*

    E. *Social anxiety disorder*

2. Which of the following are criteria for Susan's diagnosis? (choose 4 of 5)

    A. *Chronic feelings of emptiness*

    B. *Intense episodic dysphoria*

    C. *Grandiosity*

    D. *Severe dissociative symptoms*

    E. *Transient stress related paranoia*

3. Susan's suicide attempt could best be attributed to which one of the following?

    A. *Severe depressed mood*

    B. *Overwhelming anxiety*

    C. *Perceived rejection*

    D. *Grandiose self-importance*

4. What is the treatment of choice for Susan's condition?

   A. *Psychoanalysis*

   B. *Family therapy*

   C. *Dialectical behavior therapy*

   D. *Supportive psychotherapy*

5. Which of the following choices apply to patients with Susan's condition? (choose 3 of 4)

   A. *They are in touch with reality only on a basic level*

   B. *They have limited capacity for insight*

   C. *They use many primitive defenses*

   D. *They have an integrated sense of self*

6. Which of the following defense mechanisms is Susan most likely to use based on her diagnosis? (choose 2 of 5)

   A. *Suppression*

   B. *Sublimation*

   C. *Humor*

   D. *Acting Out*

   E. *Splitting*

7. Which of the following are legitimate reasons why borderline patients commit acts of self-mutilation? (choose 3 of 4)

   A. *To obtain social isolation*

   B. *To express anger*

   C. *To elicit help from others*

   D. *To numb themselves to overwhelming affect*

8. Susan takes intolerable aspects of herself and exports them onto her boyfriend leading him over time to accept and play that role. This phenomenon is known as which one of the following?

   A. *Displacement*

   B. *Rationalization*

   C. *Splitting*

   D. *Projective identification*

9. Which of the following are not considered part of Susan's disorder? (choose 3 of 4)

   A. *Prolonged psychotic episodes*

   B. *Marked peculiarity of thinking*

   C. *Extreme suspiciousness*

   D. *Impulsive behaviors*

10. Which of the following medications may play a role in treating Susan's condition? (choose 4 of 5)

    A. *Antipsychotics*

    B. *SSRIs*

    C. *Anticonvulsants*

    D. *MAOIs*

    E. *Stimulants*

Vignette Five

Cathy Allen comes to Dr. Rupert Smith's office for an initial appointment. Dr. Smith is a psychiatrist who comes highly recommended. With Cathy is her husband Bob. Dr. Smith meets them in the waiting area. Cathy introduces herself and asks if her husband Bob can come in to the appointment with her.

1. The most therapeutically appropriate response to Cathy's request would be:

    A. *"No. I only want to meet with you because you're the patient."*

    B. *"Nice to meet you Cathy. I'm Dr. Smith. Of course your husband can come in if you want him to."*

    C. *"I'm Dr. Smith. Cathy, you come in."*

    D. *"Sure your husband can come in."*

2. Following this interchange Dr. Smith is now about to start the interview. Which of the following would be the most appropriate way to begin? (Choose 2 of 4)

    A. *"Tell me about the problems you've been having."*

    B. *"You look depressed to me. What's going on?"*

    C. *"Where would you like to begin?"*

    D. *"You're very thin. Is this your normal weight? How is your appetite?"*

Cathy gives a short sentence or two in response to Dr. Smith's initial question. She then sits silently and says no more. He tries to get her to speak more but is unsuccessful. Her body language indicates that she is anxious and uncomfortable. She gives very little information in response to follow-up questions.

3. How should Dr. Smith proceed?

    A. *"You obviously don't want to be here. Maybe we should stop the interview."*

    B. *"Bob, if she doesn't tell me what's wrong I can't help her."*

    C. *"Do you have any pets? Tell me about them."*

    D. *"I can't help but notice that you're uncomfortable talking to me. Is there anything I could do to make you more comfortable?"*

4. Following Dr. Smith's intervention Cathy opens up and tells him more about the problems she's been having. Being an astute psychiatrist, Dr. Smith pays attention to both the content and process of the interview. Which of the following would be considered process? (choose 3 of 4)

    A. *Cathy nervously tears a piece of paper into pieces*

    B. *Cathy describes poor sleep for the past two weeks*

    C. *Cathy changes the subject whenever the topic of her job comes up*

    D. *Cathy's body becomes tense and rigid while discussing her work*

5. The interview moves forward and Cathy describes some feelings of depression she's been having. Dr. Smith says "you say you haven't been sleeping. How many hours per night are you getting?" This question is an example of:

   A. *Confrontation*

   B. *Facilitation*

   C. *Clarification*

   D. *Explanation*

6. After discussing current symptoms of Cathy's illness Dr. Smith says "I think I understand your current symptoms pretty well. Now let's talk about your medical history." This comment is an example of:

   A. *Reassurance*

   B. *Transition*

   C. *Positive reinforcement*

   D. *Advice*

7. Following an hour long interview Dr. Smith seeks to wrap up. Which of the following are important steps he should keep in mind while concluding the session? (choose 4 of 5)

   A. *Give Cathy a chance to ask questions*

   B. *Thank the patient for sharing information*

   C. *Review any prescriptions to make sure the patient understands why she is to take them and how to take them*

   D. *Be clear about what the next step in the treatment will be*

   E. *Discourage Cathy from calling with questions between sessions*

8. Which of the following are essential elements in order for Dr. Smith to develop rapport with Cathy during the interview? (choose 4 of 5)

   A. *Putting the patient at ease*

   B. *Expressing compassion for pain*

   C. *Showing expertise*

   D. *Establishing authority as a physician*

   E. *Know the answer to almost every question the patient asks*

9. Which of the following variables are proven to be associated with decreased rates of patient compliance with treatment? (choose 2 of 4)

   A. *Intelligence*

   B. *Increased complexity of treatment regimen*

   C. *Increased number of behavioral changes*

   D. *Socioeconomic status*

10. In which one of the following models of the doctor–patient relationship does the physician behave in a paternalistic fashion?

    A. *Active–passive model*

    B. *Teacher–student model*

    C. *Mutual participation model*

    D. *Friendship model*

Vignette Six

You are asked to see a patient at your outpatient clinic. "Pearl" Probst comes to see you on a Monday morning. You quickly realize that "Pearl" is not a woman. She is a preoperative trans-sexual of 24 years of age. Her real name is Peter Probst and she lives alone in an apartment in the city where you work. Pearl tells you that she has felt like a woman trapped in a man's body since her pre-teenage years. She began dressing as a woman in college and has begun the pre-operative transition from male to female by taking female sex hormones. She plans on following this up with sex-change surgery at some point in the future.

Pearl tells you that she and her girlfriend engage in sexual acts involving bondage, inflicting pain on each other and stepping and spitting on each other. She asks you if you have any concerns about this behavior. She also reveals that she and her partner enjoy taking showers together and urinating on each other.

You ask if Pearl considers herself to be heterosexual or homosexual and she states "I am a gay woman of course!"

1. Pearl probably meets criteria for which of the following DSM disorders? (Pick 3 of 6)

    A. *Transvestic fetishism*

    B. *Gender identity disorder*

    C. *Urophilia*

    D. *Partialism*

    E. *Sexual sadomasochism*

    F. *Fetishism*

2. Which of the following is not a poor prognostic factor in the paraphilias?

    A. *Onset of symptoms in middle-age*

    B. *Frequent recurrent acts*

    C. *Concomitant substance abuse*

    D. *Lack of guilt or shame about the acts*

    E. *The act of intercourse does not occur with the paraphilia*

3. Which of the following are good prognostic factors in the treatment dynamic of paraphilias? (pick 3 of 6)

    A. *Substance abuse*

    B. *Successful relationships and adult attachments*

    C. *Normal intelligence*

    D. *The presence of multiple paraphilias*

    E. *The presence of concomitant axis one mental disorders*

    F. *The absence of a personality disorder*

4. Which of the following are not typically interventions that are used to treat paraphilias? (Pick 2 of 6)

    A. *Prison*

    B. *Insight-oriented psychotherapy*

    C. *Cognitive-behavioral therapy*

    D. *Interpersonal psychotherapy*

    E. *Twelve-step programs*

    F. *Antiandrogen therapy*

5. Which of the following factors, that is atypical of gender identity disorder, puts Pearl's case among the minority of patients with this disorder?

    A. *The fact that she is an adult trans-sexual who wants gender-reassignment surgery*

    B. *The fact that she is taking feminizing hormone therapy*

    C. *The fact that she has felt like a woman trapped in a man's body for years*

    D. *The fact that she is a biological male wanting to become a female*

    E. *The fact that she considers herself a "gay woman" and has a girlfriend*

6. Which of the following facts is not true about gender identity disorder (GID)?

    A. *There is no evidence that psychological or psychiatric intervention for children with GID can affect the direction of later sexual orientation*

    B. *There are well-established hormonal and psychopharmacologic protocols for GID in childhood*

    C. *When patient gender dysphoria is severe, sex-reassignment surgery may be the best solution*

    D. *No drug therapy has been shown to reduce cross-gender desires in adult patients with GID*

    E. *Treatment of adolescents with GID may involve giving cross-sex hormones to slow down or stop pubertal changes of the birth sex and implement cross-sex body changes*

Vignette Seven

You are a forensic psychiatrist working in private practice. You are faced with the evaluation of a fellow psychiatrist Dr. Dean Daniels, who is alleged to have had sexual relations with a former patient of his, Selena Victor. Dr. Daniels has already been arrested and charged and he is now out of jail on a 1 million dollar bond posted by his high-profile attorney, L. Lloyd Wolff Esq. As per his lawyer, he is charged with one count of rape and two counts of sexual assault. His lawyer informs you that Dr. Daniels has a history of depression and alcoholism and has been hospitalized psychiatrically in the past. Dr. Daniels has never had a malpractice case brought against him and his medical license has never been sanctioned in any way. Dr. Daniels is now back in his office practicing as usual until his first court date comes up next month.

1. If you agree to take this case on as an expert witness for the defense, what should be your next thoughts and maneuvers? (pick 3 of 7)

    A. *The defendant needs a thorough psychiatric evaluation*

    B. *Neuropsychological testing is not necessary, as it is unlikely to reveal deficits, given that he was practicing his profession actively at the time of the alleged crimes*

    C. *Dr. Daniels should not be practicing his profession now until his court appearance because he may incriminate himself further and ruin any chance at a proper defense at trial*

    D. *Dr. Daniels should have a brain PET and functional MRI to see if brain damage can be used as a mitigating factor in his defense*

    E. *Collateral information will be key in determining Dr. Daniels' mental status at the time the alleged acts were committed*

    F. *Competency to stand trial is an essential function of your evaluation as an expert witness for the defense*

    G. *Ethically, you cannot defend Dr. Daniels because he is a member of your own profession and there is a conflict of interest in this regard*

2. The legal components that will dictate if Dr. Daniels can or should be declared not guilty by reason of insanity by a jury are: (pick 3 of 6)

   A. *Duty to warn and protect*

   B. *"Mens rea"*

   C. *Competency to stand trial*

   D. *"Actus reus"*

   E. *The matter of Ford v. Wainwright*

   F. *M'Naghten Rule*

3. In order for you to declare him competent to stand trial, you must find Dr. Daniels able to: (pick 3 of 6)

   A. *Take the stand on trial in his own defense under the guidance of his attorney*

   B. *Recognize and identify the persons involved in his case*

   C. *Recall the various events surrounding the alleged crimes with accuracy*

   D. *Collaborate with his attorney with a reasonable degree of rational understanding*

   E. *Understand the charges that are being brought against him*

   F. *State whether he would prefer a psychiatric plea or a regular plea of guilty versus not guilty*

4. What role will alleged victim Selena Victor play in your defense of Dr. Daniels?

   A. *You will interview and examine her to destroy her credibility as a witness and support Dr. Daniels' defense*

   B. *The defense attorney can subpoena Selena for a psychiatric evaluation by you*

   C. *The prosecution can protect Selena as a witness and can prevent you from examining her for the defense*

   D. *If the prosecution obtains their own psychiatric expert to examine Selena, the defense team will be allowed to have you examine Selena as well. Barring that, the defense team will have the opportunity to have you review the report and write a critique of it and/or testify at trial in opposition to that report if the defense team deems it best to do so*

   E. *The judge has the ultimate discretion and final word to determine Selena's role in the judicial process*

5. In a case such as Dr. Daniels', what would be the possible sanctions if he were to go to trial and be found "not guilty by reason of insanity" by the jury on all three charges? (pick 3 of 6)

   A. *He could continue to practice psychiatry as before*

   B. *He could lose his medical license and be remanded to outpatient treatment by the court*

   C. *He could be allowed to retain his medical license and be remanded by the court to an intensive outpatient psychiatric day program for treatment*

   D. *He could eventually practice psychiatry again after completion of appropriate treatment of his disorder, based on mandated future psychiatric evaluation*

   E. *His name would be inscribed on a computer-based list of sex offenders if his state maintains such a list*

   F. *He could continue to practice psychiatry as before, but not with female patients*

Vignette Eight

Steven Geller is a 30-year-old male with paranoid schizophrenia. He stopped his medications 3 weeks ago. In response to the voices that followed, he then stopped eating and drinking. The voices have been telling him that his food is poisoned. "They put rat poison in your food" the voices told him. His mother became concerned when he wouldn't eat for two days. She made him several of his favorite foods and tried to convince him to eat but he barricaded himself in his room and would not come out for 24 hours. His mother then called EMS. You interview him in the emergency room after he is brought into the hospital.

1. Which of the following statements would you include in Steven's mental status exam given what you know at this point?

    A. *Thought content includes paranoid delusions*

    B. *Thought content includes auditory hallucinations*

    C. *Thought process includes flight of ideas*

    D. *Perceptions include auditory hallucinations*

On further interview Steven screams at you that he is "God's chosen one" and further states that people are trying to poison him to prevent him from revealing his identity to the world. He states that he will be "raised into the heavens on clouds." You question the veracity of this statement and he insists that it is true. He does not believe that it is a creation of his mind and is certain that those who doubt him are wrong. "I will burn the disbelievers" he tells you.

2. Where should this new information be included in the mental status exam?

    A. *Thought content*

    B. *Perceptions*

    C. *Attitude*

    D. *Thought process*

3. During your exam you notice that Steven is malodorous and is wearing dirty clothes. You note a rancid odor in the room and observe brown streaks on his pant legs. On closer inspection it appears to be feces. His family verifies that he has been failing to maintain hygiene since stopping his medication. Which of the following would be an accurate GAF score for Steven on Axis V?

    A. *20*

    B. *10*

    C. *40*

    D. *60*

You begin to perform a mini-mental status exam on Steven. You ask him to count backwards from 100 by 7s. He replies "93, 89, 81, 74." You ask him if he can go further and he replies "Go to hell. I am the chosen one. I won't do anything I don't want to."

4. How would you document this exchange? (choose 2 of 4)

   A. *Memory is intact*

   B. *Concentration is impaired*

   C. *Abstract thinking is intact*

   D. *Attitude is hostile*

5. Steven's belief about being the chosen one would best be described as:

   A. *Pseudologia phantastica*

   B. *Delusion of grandeur*

   C. *Algophobia*

   D. *Nihilistic delusion*

6. The mesocortical pathway which is responsible for the _____ symptoms of schizophrenia begins at the _____.

   A. *Positive; ventral tegmental area*

   B. *Negative; nucleus accumbens*

   C. *Positive; nucleus accumbens*

   D. *Negative; ventral tegmental area*

7. Which of the following are correct concerning schizophrenia? (choose 3 of 4)

   A. *Positive symptoms are associated with frequency of hospitalization*

   B. *Cognitive symptoms are directly related to long-term functional outcome*

   C. *Positive symptoms are directly related to long-term functional outcome*

   D. *Schizophrenia is associated with a 10% suicide rate.*

8. Which of the following would be consistent with a diagnosis of residual schizophrenia? (choose 3 of 4)

   A. *Command auditory hallucinations*

   B. *Absence of prominent delusions*

   C. *Unusual perceptual experiences in attenuated form*

   D. *Absence of disorganized behavior*

9. Which of the following are common aspects of appearance for schizophrenic patients? (choose 4 of 5)

   A. *Lack of spontaneous movement*

   B. *Echopraxia*

   C. *Agitation*

   D. *Bizarre posture*

   E. *Bright clothing*

10. Which of the following are often found as part of thought form for schizophrenic patients? (choose 3 of 4)

   A. *Verbigeration*

   B. *Ideas of reference*

   C. *Word salad*

   D. *Mutism*

Vignette Nine

Judy Albanese, a local college student, is brought into the emergency room when her roommate called EMS after she collapsed at the gym. She appears malnourished and emaciated. Her roommate told EMS that she hadn't been eating recently. She had cut down to one meal per day in order to lose weight. Yesterday the only thing she ate all day was a cereal bar. She has been spending 3 hours each day at the gym after classes in an effort to lose weight. Despite being emaciated she believes that she is overweight. She recently told her roommate "I'm so gross! I don't know how anyone stands to look at me. All the skinny girls get the boyfriends, the attention, and what do I get?" When you ask her more questions she admits to you "I feel cold all the time. I have terrible headaches, and when I shower big clumps of hair fall out of my head." She goes on to tell you "During class, instead of listening to lectures or taking notes, I think about what I have eaten that day, when I will eat again, what I will eat. I like to bake and bring the treats to school the next day, to give to my friends. I watch them eat. I'm really jealous of them when they eat. I read cookbooks for fun and have collected hundreds of recipes. I never look in the mirror without thinking, *Fat*.

1. Which of the following factors would you consider essential to make a diagnosis of anorexia nervosa? (choose 3 of 4)

    A. *Body weight less than 85% of expected for height and age*

    B. *A disturbance in how body weight is experienced*

    C. *Amenorrhea*

    D. *Binge eating and purging behavior*

2. Based on diagnostic criteria you determine that Judy has anorexia. Which of the following medical complications are likely to be associated with the diagnosis? (choose 5 of 6)

    A. *Bradycardia*

    B. *Pancytopenia*

    C. *Lanugo*

    D. *Osteopenia*

    E. *Metabolic encephalopathy*

    F. *Ulcerative colitis*

3. Which of the following would be considered indications that Judy should be admitted to a hospital? (choose 3 of 4)

    A. *Significant hypokalemia*

    B. *Weight less than 75% of expected for height and age*

    C. *Growth arrest*

    D. *Osteopenia*

4. As part of your evaluation of Judy you wish to calculate her BMI. How do you do that?

    A. *100 lbs for the first 5 ft in height + 5 lbs/inch over 5 feet ± 10%*

    B. *Height(m²)/weight(kg)*

    C. *[Age(y) × .375 + height (m)] × 0.093/0.09[daily caloric intake(Cal)]*

    D. *Weight(kg)/height(m)*

5. You consider treatment options for Judy. Which of the following have proven efficacy in patients with anorexia? (choose 4 of 5)

   A. *Cognitive behavioral therapy*

   B. *Family therapy*

   C. *Fluoxetine*

   D. *Olanzapine*

   E. *Bupropion*

6. Which of the following are possible complications of self-induced vomiting? (choose 3 of 4)

   A. *Russell's sign*

   B. *Mallory–Weiss syndrome*

   C. *Spontaneous abortion*

   D. *Atonic colon*

7. Which of the following are possible complications of ipecac abuse? (choose 3 of 4)

   A. *Skeletal muscle atrophy*

   B. *Rectal prolapse*

   C. *Cardiomyopathy*

   D. *Prolonged QTc interval*

8. Which of the following statements are correct concerning anorexia? (choose 2 of 3)

   A. *Risk of anorexia increases when family members have anorexia*

   B. *Patients with anorexia often demonstrate traits of paranoid personality disorder*

   C. *Patients with anorexia are characterized by emotional flexibility*

   D. *Adolescence is a time of increased risk for anorexia*

9. Which of the following should be included in the differential diagnosis for anorexia? (choose 4 of 5)

   A. *Major depressive disorder*

   B. *Anxiety disorders*

   C. *Bulimia nervosa*

   D. *Substance abuse*

   E. *Brief psychotic disorder*

10. Medical treatment for anorexia should include which of the following? (choose 3 of 4)

   A. *Combination estrogen and progesterone*

   B. *Dental follow-up*

   C. *Electrocardiogram*

   D. *Correction of hypokalemia*

Vignette Ten

Lisa is a 22-year-old barista at a local coffee shop who comes to your office seeking help after feeling that she did not get any better with her primary care physician. She gives a long history of anxiety around other people dating back to childhood. At one point while in high school her mother pressured her to become a camp councilor in order to "overcome shyness." Lisa was able to force herself to do it for a few weeks but then became overwhelmed by the anxiety and quit. She also went through a period of time during her school years when she wouldn't use public restrooms or would only use them if they were completely empty. She got into trouble for leaving class to go to the restroom all of the time. When the restroom was empty during classes she felt the most comfortable using it.

Now she reports being very anxious at work and at parties. She snuck out of the holiday party for her job because she was so uncomfortable. She worries that other people are judging her and won't like her. She says that she feels stupid interacting with others, especially at work. She had quit a previous job because there were weekly meetings which she had to attend and speak in front of 30 people. Her anxiety about these meetings led her to quit the job. When you ask about her personal life she tells you "I've gone on dates once or twice but have never had any long-term relationships. Dates are excruciating for me. Making conversation with new people makes me so uncomfortable and anxious."

Lisa's primary care physician had tried her on sertraline in the past. She comes to you to see if there is anything else you can offer her.

1. Which of the following should be included in Lisa's differential diagnosis? (choose 3 of 4)

    A. *Panic disorder*

    B. *Schizoaffective disorder*

    C. *Social phobia*

    D. *Generalized anxiety disorder*

2. Given Lisa's medication history which other medications may be worth trying? (Choose 3 of 4)

    A. *Paroxetine*

    B. *Clonazepam*

    C. *Citalopram*

    D. *Bupropion*

3. Which of the following has the best evidence to support its use in Lisa's condition?

    A. *Cognitive behavioral therapy*

    B. *Supportive psychotherapy*

    C. *Motivational interviewing*

    D. *Psychodynamic psychotherapy*

4. Lisa is most likely to be misdiagnosed with which of the following? (choose 2 of 4)

    A. *Schizoid personality disorder*

    B. *Avoidant personality disorder*

    C. *Schizotypal personality disorder*

    D. *Dependent personality disorder*

5. Which diagnosis best explains Lisa's avoidance of public restrooms during her school years?

    A. *Specific phobia*

    B. *Panic disorder*

    C. *Social phobia*

    D. *Agoraphobia*

6. The non-generalized subtype of social phobia is most successfully treated by which one of the following?

    A. *Benztropine*

    B. *Olanzapine*

    C. *Propranolol*

    D. *Lorazepam*

7. The major concern of patients with social phobia is which one of the following?

    A. *Avoidance of relationships*

    B. *The need for someone to be with them in stressful situations*

    C. *Fear of rejection*

    D. *Fear of embarrassment*

8. If we changed Lisa's age to 16 years old in the vignette above, how long would she need to have symptoms in order to meet DSM criteria for social phobia?

    A. *2 weeks*

    B. *2 months*

    C. *6 weeks*

    D. *6 months*

9. Which of the following are common side effects of Lisa's condition? (choose 3 of 4)

    A. *Blushing*

    B. *Dry mouth*

    C. *Sweating*

    D. *Fear of dying*

10. As many as one third of patients with Lisa's condition also meet criteria for which one of the following disorders?

    A. *Major depressive disorder*

    B. *Agoraphobia*

    C. *Cocaine abuse*

    D. *Body dysmorphic disorder*

Vignette Eleven

Carl Freeman is an obese 59-year-old male who is referred to you by his primary care physician for complaints of depression. Carl lives with his girlfriend Heidi Schmitz and her three children Blair, Denny, and Rao. He works as a customer service representative at a health insurance company. He tells you that "my co-workers resent me because I keep falling asleep at my desk during the day. I've even fallen asleep in the middle of phone calls with customers." Because he has had difficulty at work he was referred for a medical evaluation. He reports decreased energy, fatigue, and poor sleep. He states that he had difficulty concentrating at work. He tells you "I've been irritable and fatigued. I'm having terrible headaches. I've been gaining weight recently and I can't concentrate. Basically everything is going wrong right now." He tried to sleep more at night but this did not make him feel any better. He tried taking naps in his car during his lunch hour but this didn't help. His primary care physician felt that he was depressed and referred him to you. When you interview him on his sleep habits he reports that his wife stopped sleeping in the same room as him due to his snoring. He tells you that she calls him a "water buffalo" because of the noises he makes while he sleeps.

1. Which of the following should be included in the differential diagnosis for Carl? (choose 2 of 3)

    A. *Major depressive disorder*

    B. *Sleep apnea*

    C. *Klein–Levin syndrome*

    D. *Narcolepsy*

2. Which of the following would you include in a workup for this patient? (choose 2 of 3)

    A. *TSH*

    B. *Periodic limb movements of sleep test*

    C. *CPAP*

    D. *Nocturnal polysomnography*

3. Which of the following are possible complications of Carl's condition? (choose 3 of 4)

    A. *Increased risk of cardiovascular complications*

    B. *Decreased mood*

    C. *Increased neck girth*

    D. *Decreased cognition*

4. Which one of the following statements is correct concerning Carl's condition?

    A. *Carl has a parasomnia*

    B. *Carl has a dyssomnia*

    C. *Modafinil would be the treatment of choice for Carl*

    D. *Carl's condition places him at increased risk for Parkinson's disease*

5. Which one of the following is Carl most likely to be misdiagnosed with?

   A. *Pavor nocturnus*

   B. *Somnambulism*

   C. *Jactatio capitis nocturna*

   D. *Gastroesophageal reflux*

6. Which of the following choices are true concerning obstructive sleep apnea? (choose 2 of 3)

   A. *Airflow ceases during apnic episodes*

   B. *Respiratory effort decreases during apnic episodes*

   C. *Patients need at least 3 apnic episodes per hour to meet criteria*

   D. *Respiratory effort increases during apnic episodes*

7. Which of the following complications are common with obstructive sleep apnea? (choose 3 of 4)

   A. *Arrhythmias*

   B. *Changes in blood pressure during apnic episodes*

   C. *Pulmonary hypotension*

   D. *Chronic increase in systemic blood pressure*

8. Which of the following are true concerning REM sleep behavior disorder? (choose 2 of 4)

   A. *It occurs primarily in females*

   B. *Loss of atonia during REM is a major component*

   C. *Violent behavior can be a complication*

   D. *Symptoms improve following treatment with stimulants or fluoxetine*

9. Which of the following are symptoms of sleep-related gastroesophageal reflux? (choose 3 of 4)

   A. *Awakening from sleep*

   B. *Cough*

   C. *Chest tightness*

   D. *Cessation of airflow*

10. Which of the following would be considered sleep hygiene measures? (choose 3 of 4)

    A. *Avoid daytime naps*

    B. *Exercise during the day*

    C. *Use of zolpidem*

    D. *Arise at the same time each morning*

Vignette Twelve

Ryan Huang is a 35-year-old male who is unemployed and lives with his mother. He comes to your clinic with compliant of voices telling him to kill his mother because "She is the fiend. She is the devil." He reports sleeping in his car for the past few days because he is trying to stay away from his mother so that he doesn't hurt her. "I don't want to go to jail" he tells you.

Ryan has a history of violence towards his mother. When he was in his 20s she took out an order of protection against him following an incident where he choked her in response to command auditory hallucinations. When the order of protection expired she did not renew it. In subsequent years he began to do better. Eventually she allowed him to move back into the home.

Ryan reported that the voices began when he was 16 years old. He doesn't like them because they tell him to harm others as well as himself. During his first psychiatric hospitalization he developed oculogyric crisis from multiple PRN Haldol injections. Since this experience he has demonstrated an unwillingness to maintain compliance with medications. He is currently prescribed ziprasidone but has only intermittent compliance.

Ryan's mother also tells you that he has a significant alcohol problem. She says he drinks daily. Ryan himself admits to periods of "the shakes" and previous blackouts. His drinking tends to get worse at certain points. He will go on binges and drink excessively for up to a week at a time.

Ryan's trauma history includes being raped repeatedly by an older male cousin between the ages of 13 and 16. He admits that this has impacted him but has difficulty explaining how. He denies current flashbacks.

Medical history is significant for smoking 1 pack per day of cigarettes, hypertension, high cholesterol and poorly controlled diabetes. He endorses a head injury which happened when he was 13. When he tried to resist a rape attempt by his cousin, his cousin beat him until he was unconscious. On exam he recalls 1 out of 3 objects after 5 minutes. He is oriented to person, place, and time.

1. Which of the following should be considered in Ryan's differential diagnosis? (choose 4 of 5)

    A. *Schizophrenia*

    B. *Substance induced psychotic disorder*

    C. *Post-traumatic stress disorder*

    D. *Generalized anxiety disorder*

    E. *Dementia NOS*

2. Which of the following would you include in a medical workup for Ryan? (choose 5 of 6)

    A. *Thyroid function tests*

    B. *Thiamine level*

    C. *Head CT*

    D. *EKG*

    E. *Urine toxicology*

    F. *Prolactin level*

3. Which of the following are the most likely side effects Ryan will experience from treatment with ziprasidone? (choose 2 of 4)

    A. *Weight gain*

    B. *Extrapyramidal symptoms*

    C. *Sedation*

    D. *Cardiac effects*

4. Ryan's history includes significant substance abuse. Heavy use of which one of the following drugs before the age of 16 has been correlated with an increased relative risk of schizophrenia?

    A. *Phencyclidine*

    B. *Alcohol*

    C. *LSD*

    D. *Cannabis*

5. If a patient presents with psychosis for more than one month but does not meet criteria A for schizophrenia what diagnoses are possible? (choose 2 of 4)

    A. *Schizoaffective disorder*

    B. *Delusional disorder*

    C. *Schizotypal disorder*

    D. *Psychosis NOS*

6. Which one of the following medications are not antagonists at the 5HT2A receptor?

    A. *Haloperidol*

    B. *Aripiprazole*

    C. *Olanzapine*

    D. *Ziprasidone*

7. Which of the following choices are true concerning delusional disorder? (choose 2 of 4)

    A. *Auditory hallucinations may be present*

    B. *Memory impairment may be seen*

    C. *Tactile hallucinations may be present*

    D. *Unnecessary medical interventions may be part of the picture*

8. Which one of the following is correct concerning brief psychotic disorder?

    A. *The patient will not return to normal functioning*

    B. *Primary preventative measures can involve treatment with low dose risperidone*

    C. *Hallucinations may be present but delusions are not*

    D. *Symptoms last between one day and one month*

9. Which of the following are true concerning psychotic symptoms? (choose 4 of 5)

    A. *Tactile hallucinations are more common in medical and neurologic conditions than in schizophrenia*

    B. *Illusions are sensory misperceptions of actual stimuli*

    C. *Delusions are fixed false beliefs which are not supported by cultural norms*

    D. *Word salad is the violation of basic rules of grammar seen in severe thought disorder*

    E. *Cataplexy is synonymous with waxy flexibility*

10. A differential diagnosis for new onset psychosis may include which of the following medical conditions? (choose 4 of 5)

   A. *Systemic lupus erythematosus*

   B. *Temporal lobe epilepsy*

   C. *Neurosyphilis*

   D. *Wilson's disease*

   E. *Phymatous rosacea*

Vignette Thirteen

John Jameson, a 42-year-old man, is brought by ambulance, accompanied by police to your emergency room at 2:00am in the morning. Upon arrival, he is agitated and the police and emergency medical technicians cannot manage his aggression. He refuses to answer your questions and gives you a verbal tongue lashing when you try to approach him. Nobody else accompanies him and there are no collaterals present from whom you can obtain information. You discover he has never been to your hospital before, as there is no medical record at your facility in his name. Mental status examination is impossible at this time, as he is completely uncooperative with you. He shouts obscenities at you and yells out that his mother should be shot for what she has done to him.

1. What are your very next steps in management with respect to this patient? (pick 2 of 6)

   A. *Draw blood for basic labs and obtain a CT scan of the head to rule out organic causes for his agitation*

   B. *Ask the police and emergency technicians why they brought him*

   C. *Admit him to the psychiatry unit on an involuntary basis*

   D. *Do your best to obtain his mother's contact information and call her as soon as possible to find out what "she has done to him"*

   E. *Have him restrained by police and/or hospital security so you can administer him an intramuscular injection of haloperidol and lorazepam to help calm him*

   F. *Obtain medical consultation and clearance from the emergency room physician*

2. Which of the following is not a predictor of dangerousness to others in violent patients, such as in the patient scenario depicted in this vignette? (pick 2 of 6)

   A. *Prior violent acts*

   B. *Chronic anger, hostility, or resentment*

   C. *Female gender*

   D. *Numerous medical problems*

   E. *Childhood brutality or deprivation*

   F. *Access to weapons or instruments of violence*

3. When attempting to interview this violent and agitated patient, the psychiatrist should do which of the following? (pick 3 of 6)

   A. *Conduct the interview in a quiet, nonstimulating area of the emergency room*

   B. *Avoid asking the patient if he has weapons on him to avoid further anger and agitation.*

   C. *Request that security personnel give their assistance during the interview, if needed.*

   D. *Avoid any behavior that could be misconstrued by the patient as menacing, such as standing over the patient.*

   E. *Explain to the patient that any refusal to answer questions will result in him being medicated and admitted to hospital over his objection.*

   F. *Interview the patient in an enclosed locked room to prevent the patient from fleeing.*

4. Once the patient is sedated, the emergency room medical physician completes a workup on the patient. The workup, including drug screen and head CT, is negative and the patient is cleared from a medical and surgical perspective. If you are unable to obtain any further history on this patient, your disposition for him should be to: (pick 3 of 6)

   A. *Discharge him home with outpatient psychiatric follow-up*

   B. *Admit him to the psychiatric inpatient unit on an involuntary basis*

   C. *Start him on aripiprazole and divalproex sodium in the emergency room*

   D. *Contact police to return to the emergency room to arrest the patient*

   E. *Obtain a social work consultation after holding him overnight in the emergency room pending further information*

   F. *Attempt to call his mother and tell her about his feelings towards her*

5. Once admitted to the psychiatric unit, it is discovered that the patient has a lengthy history of schizophrenia, paranoid type, since 17 years of age, and has been hospitalized in this fashion no less than 25 times since the onset of his illness began. These recurrent hospitalizations have mostly been due to his refusal to take medications upon discharge. Currently, he is refusing to take medication on the unit, when it is offered to him by nursing staff.

   Which of the following would currently be good choices of medication for this patient, on the inpatient unit? (pick 2 of 6)

   A. *Risperidone*

   B. *Olanzapine*

   C. *Asenapine*

   D. *Ziprasidone*

   E. *Quetiapine*

   F. *Lurasidone*

6. If the patient is given Risperidone (Risperdal Consta) biweekly intramuscular injection and is well stabilized in the hospital on this agent, which of the following would be the best discharge disposition for him for ongoing treatment and care once he is ready to leave the acute inpatient psychiatry unit? (choose 3 of 7)

   A. *State psychiatric inpatient facility (long-term admission)*

   B. *Assertive community treatment team (ACT team) home visits*

   C. *Partial hospital program*

   D. *Continuing day treatment program*

   E. *Outpatient mental health department of a university/teaching hospital*

   F. *Outpatient freestanding mental health clinic*

   G. *Mental health practitioner in the patient's primary care physician's group practice*

Vignette Fourteen

Robert Bradbury is a 30-year-old male with a history of chronic paranoid schizophrenia who is being treated with clozapine. He goes to an outpatient psychiatry appointment and has the following discussion with his psychiatrist.

Doctor: How are things going Robert?

Robert: Fine. I've been working in the afternoons following my program and it's going very well. I'm continuing to drool a lot, like I told you last time, but its manageable.

Doctor: How are your symptoms? Are you hearing any voices?

Robert: No. I haven't heard voices in about a year now. I'm really glad about that (smiles).

Doctor: Good. Good. Tell me about this job you've been doing.

Robert: Well I'm doing a patient work program through the hospital. We move furniture, run errands, deliver mail within the hospital. Stuff like that.

Doctor: Do you like it?

Robert: I do, but there is this one woman that I work with who is so nasty (frowns). She talks down to the patient workers like she's better than us or as if we're not as good as other people. It gets me upset sometimes.

Doctor: How do you handle it?

Robert: My boss tells me just to ignore her, that it's her problem, not mine, and that she's not worth getting upset over.

Doctor: Are you able to do that?

Robert: Yeah. If she says something nasty I just walk away. I try not to let it bother me as much as it used to. There are plenty of people at work who are friendly so it doesn't matter.

Doctor: Good. I like your attitude about this. Sounds like you're handling it well.

Robert: Thanks. Oh, before we finish I need a refill on my clozapine. I went for bloodwork two days ago.

The next seven questions are regarding Robert's mental status exam:

1. Robert's attitude is best described as: (choose 2 of 6)

    A. *Guarded*

    B. *Hostile*

    C. *Apathetic*

    D. *Cooperative*

    E. *Friendly*

    F. *Ingratiating*

2. Robert's affect is best described as:

    A. *Incongruent*

    B. *Within normal range*

    C. *Constricted*

    D. *Blunted*

    E. *Flat*

3. Robert's thought process is best described as: (choose 2 of 6)

   A. *Flight of ideas*

   B. *Tangentiality*

   C. *Circumstantiality*

   D. *Linear*

   E. *Goal directed*

   F. *Thought blocking*

4. Robert's impulse control is best described as:

   A. *Good*

   B. *Fair*

   C. *Poor*

5. Robert's insight is best described as:

   A. *Good*

   B. *Fair*

   C. *Poor*

6. Robert's judgment is best described as:

   A. *Good*

   B. *Fair*

   C. *Poor*

7. Robert's perceptions are best described as:

   A. *No auditory hallucinations*

   B. *No visual hallucinations*

   C. *No olfactory hallucinations*

   D. *No tactile hallucinations*

   E. *No gustatory hallucinations*

8. What is the best feedback the doctor can give Robert about his excessive drooling?

   A. *It is expected. We should continue to follow it.*

   B. *It will go away once his dose of clozapine is increased*

   C. *It is a clear indication to stop the medication*

   D. *It is most likely unrelated to his medications*

9. If Robert is on clozapine for 8 months, how often should he have his WBC/ANC drawn?

   A. *Every month*

   B. *Every week*

   C. *Every two weeks*

   D. *Every two months*

10. In addition to monitoring Robert's WBC/ANC which other tests would be appropriate to monitor on Robert over time? (choose 7 of 8)

    A. EKG

    B. Liver function tests

    C. Clozapine level

    D. Fasting glucose

    E. Weight

    F. Waist circumference

    G. Triglycerides and cholesterol

    H. Echocardiogram

Vignette Fifteen

A woman of 35 years of age presents to the emergency room in a state of acute anxiety and agitation. After administration of an intramuscular injection of 2 mg of lorazepam, she calms down a bit and is able to give you more of her history. For the past 10 years, she has been functioning as a bank teller and lives alone in a studio apartment and is self-sufficient. She reports that for the past decade she has felt that she is not one person, but three different persons. She feels that her self-states take over her being whenever she is in an extremely stressful situation. When asked about her parents and youth, she closes her eyes and begins to talk in a more youthful voice stating "I have to run away. I can't be home when papa gets here." She seems distant as if in a trance. When she finally comes to her senses, she admits that she was repeatedly beaten and raped from ages 5 to 11 years by her step-father. She admits to flashbacks and excessive easiness to startle and these symptoms persist even now in her. She states that this child-like voice is that of "Melanie" one of her self-states, who comes out when she is under stress at work or in her relationships with men. She denies suicidal or homicidal ideation. She denies experiencing auditory or visual hallucinations, past or present. No delusions or ideas of reference are noted. She is much calmer now in the emergency room after your intervention with her.

1. Which of the following clinical features of this patient's disorder are correct? (pick 2 of 6)

    A. Clinical studies report female to male ratios of up to 10 to 1 in diagnosed cases

    B. Fifteen percent of cases are associated with childhood trauma and maltreatment

    C. Psychotherapies of choice include dynamic, cognitive and hypnotherapy

    D. Studies have shown a strong genetic component to the disorder

    E. Inability to recall important personal information is not part of this disorder

    F. About 10% of patients also meet criteria for somatization disorder

2. Which of the following would be expected to worsen the prognosis of this patient's disorder?

    A. Concomitant diabetes and hypertension

    B. Concomitant eating disorder

    C. Recommending clonazepam for anxiety symptoms

    D. The patient forcing herself to maintain a high level of daily functioning despite having serious symptoms

    E. Group therapy for patients with the same disorder only

    F. Past traumatic brain injury from a motor vehicle accident

3. Which one of the following is not a recommended pharmacologic choice for this patient's disorder?

    A. Quetiapine

    B. Fluoxetine

    C. Divalproex sodium

    D. Lithium carbonate

    E. Zolpidem

4. Which of the following symptoms is not typically seen in this patient's disorder?

    A. Seizure-like episodes

    B. Survivor guilt

    C. Suicidal thoughts

    D. Asthma and breathing problems

    E. Manic episodes

5. Which of the following would help you rule out a factitious or malingered disorder in this patient's case? (pick 2 of 6)

    A. Marked inconsistencies in her story and symptom presentation

    B. The patient prevents you from speaking to collaterals

    C. Marked dysphoria about her symptoms

    D. A significant history of legal problems

    E. Feeling confused and ashamed about her symptoms

    F. A history of poor work performance by the patient

Vignette Sixteen

Kevin Moran is a 75-year-old man who is brought to your office by his 38-year-old daughter Susan for a consultation. Mr. Moran has not been himself for at least a year his daughter states. He lost his wife to cancer 18 months ago and they were married for 50 years. Susan tells you that her father cannot live on his own anymore and she had to take him into her home where she has a spare bedroom for him. The reason for his inability to live independently is because he gets easily confused, forgetful, loses his sense of direction and starts to wander alone in the street with no purpose. The police brought him home once after they found him wandering in his neighborhood late at night and the poor man couldn't find his way home. Luckily he was able to remember his own name and his daughter's name, which helped police to trace him back to her home. Susan says her father cannot really cook or clean for himself because he forgets that he leaves the stove on and burns pots and pans which could result in a severe fire hazard. He can eat, but he forgets the names of common household items like forks and cups, and sometimes even forgets what they are used for.

His medical history is significant for coronary artery disease since age 68, hypertension controlled on medication, type II diabetes for which he takes oral medications only and a small stroke a few years ago for which he has been given aspirin. He also has high serum cholesterol and elevated serum triglycerides.

1. Given his history, the most likely diagnosis is: (pick 2 of 6)

    A. *Major depressive disorder*

    B. *Generalized anxiety disorder*

    C. *Vascular dementia*

    D. *Diffuse Lewy body disease*

    E. *Alzheimer's dementia*

    F. *Pick's disease*

2. What would be your next maneuver with respect to this patient in the outpatient setting? (pick 3 of 7)

    A. *Start sertraline 25 mg daily*

    B. *Start trazodone 50 mg at bedtime*

    C. *Start donepezil 5 mg daily*

    D. *Obtain an electroencephalogram*

    E. *Start risperidone 0.25 mg at bedtime*

    F. *Obtain an outpatient brain MRI*

    G. *Obtain neuropsychological consultation*

3. His daughter is concerned that she cannot manage her father properly in the home. What suggestions can you make to help her with this situation? (pick 3 of 6)

    A. *Refer him to an ACT team for ongoing management*

    B. *Obtain a visiting-nurse consultation*

    C. *Refer her to caregiver support programming and groups*

    D. *Convince her to get family members to provide coverage in the home to monitor the patient more closely*

    E. *Consult a physiatrist to have the patient placed in a subacute rehabilitation facility*

    F. *Seek skilled nursing facility or assisted-living facility placement for the patient*

4. If the patient has a dementia of the Alzheimer type, what would be his expected prognosis if he were to remain untreated?

    A. *1 to 3 years*

    B. *4 to 6 years*

    C. *7 to 10 years*

    D. *11 to 15 years*

    E. *15 to 20 years*

5. The treatment of choice for a case of dementia believed to have features of both Alzheimer and vascular type would be: (pick 3 of 7)

    A. *An antiplatelet aggregant agent*

    B. *An atypical antipsychotic agent*

    C. *A sedative–hypnotic anxiolytic agent*

    D. *A cholinesterase inhibiting agent*

    E. *Vitamin B complex supplementation*

    F. *An antidepressant agent*

    G. *An antihypertensive agent*

6.   Which of the following is not typically a complication of this man's illness?

   A.   *Agitation and sundowning*

   B.   *Personality changes*

   C.   *Aggression*

   D.   *Hallucinations and delusions*

   E.   *Depression*

   F.   *Mania*

7.   Which of the following drugs should be avoided in this patient? (pick 2 of 7)

   A.   *Rivastigmine*

   B.   *Aspirin*

   C.   *Memantine*

   D.   *Benztropine*

   E.   *Diphenhydramine*

   F.   *Fluoxetine*

   G.   *Galantamine*

Vignette Seventeen

Wanda Reardon is a 55-year-old woman who is hospitalized for acute relapse of a multiple sclerosis flare up. She has had the disease for 25 years and it has been classified as relapsing and remitting in variety. You are called to her bedside because she is in an acute confusional state. Upon admission to the hospital yesterday, her neurologist started her on intravenous methylprednisolone and omeprazole for the MS exacerbation. Her history reveals that she is a former cigarette smoker who quit 10 years ago. She also has a history of hypertension and gastritis. Her medications at home include enalapril, lansoprazole and interferon β1A (Avonex) weekly injections for her multiple sclerosis.

When you arrive at the bedside to examine Wanda after reviewing her chart, you find that she is unable to attend to you or your questions. She is talkative, but what she says makes no grammatical or logical sense. Her eyes are rolling back in her head and her eyelids are drooping frequently during your interaction with her. She is rocking side to side in her bed in a hyperactive manner. She is unable to engage you or answer any of your questions appropriately. She is disoriented to time, place and person. When you call her name, she is able to look at you briefly, but her attention wanes and in a brief moment she looks away and is unable to respond further to you. Her rocking behavior is quite severe and you fear that she may fall out of her bed, despite the fact that her bed rails are up.

1.   Which of the following symptoms are not generally characteristic of Wanda's present syndrome? (pick 2 of 6)

   A.   *Mood stability*

   B.   *Irritability*

   C.   *Sleep–wake cycle disturbance*

   D.   *Language disturbance*

   E.   *Gradual onset over weeks to months*

   F.   *Memory impairment*

2. Which of the following risk factors predispose this patient to the current condition you now find her in? (Pick 3 of 6)

   A. *Smoking history*

   B. *Female gender*

   C. *Her age*

   D. *Her current medications*

   E. *Her multiple sclerosis*

   F. *Hypertension*

3. The CNS area(s) believed to be most closely implicated in this patient's present condition is (are) the:

   A. *Cerebellum*

   B. *Frontal and parietal lobes*

   C. *Midbrain and nigrostriatal pathway*

   D. *Reticular formation and dorsal tegmental pathway*

   E. *Hippocampus and amygdala*

4. Which of the following neurotransmitters is probably the least likely to be implicated in the pathophysiology of delirium?

   A. *Norepinephrine*

   B. *Dopamine*

   C. *Serotonin*

   D. *Acetylcholine*

   E. *Glutamate*

5. Which of the following electroencephalography findings would you expect to find in this patient?

   A. *Temporal lobe spikes*

   B. *Hypsarrhythmia*

   C. *Generalized background slowing*

   D. *Triphasic waves*

   E. *Periodic lateralizing epileptiform discharges (PLEDS)*

6. Which of the following agents would not be appropriate treatment for Wanda's current condition? (pick 2 of 6)

   A. *Haloperidol*

   B. *Risperidone*

   C. *Diphenhydramine*

   D. *Quetiapine*

   E. *Benztropine*

   F. *Olanzapine*

7. Which of the following are true about the course and prognosis of delirium? (pick 3 of 6)

   A. *Prodromal symptoms can occur months prior to onset of florid symptoms*

   B. *Symptoms usually persist as long as causally relevant factors are present*

   C. *Delirium usually progresses to dementia according to longitudinal studies*

   D. *Delirium does not adversely affect mortality in patients who develop it*

   E. *Prognosis of delirium worsens with increased patient age and longer duration of the episode*

   F. *Periods of delirium are sometimes followed by depression or post-traumatic stress disorder*

Vignette Eighteen

Allan Newbold is a 30-year-old man who consults you at your private office for anxiety. He describes his anxiety as an excessive preoccupation with his appearance. He is always worried that he isn't attractive enough to the opposite sex. He has no medical or surgical history at all. He has never seen a psychiatrist before. He denies depression, but he is very upset because he always feels his body could be better. He exercises twice a day and has a physique that is similar to most fit models or competitive bodybuilders. You ask him to identify his specific shortcomings and he tells you that his skin doesn't tan evenly so he has to resort to artificial spray-on tans which "look fake" he says. He also feels that his body has hair in the "wrong places" and "I always have to go to the laser hair removal salon or get it waxed off. Even then, there's always some left over." He also feels that because he is a natural bodybuilder who doesn't use artificial means of building muscle, like steroids, that his muscles are unable to develop evenly and symmetrically. He opens his shirt and shows you his bare chest pointing out to you how his abdominal muscles are uneven and lumpy and asymmetrical. To your eye and superficial glance, they look perfectly normal and you tell him so. He replies: "Of course you think they're normal! Everyone I ask tells me they're normal, but I know they're just lying to me."

Allan tells you he is actually a physical therapist by training, "I love my job because I work with kids mostly and help them in ways that no one else really can." He also reveals that he does TV and magazine modeling on the side and has even posed nude in Playgirl magazine. He was named "man of the year" for that publication a few years back. He tells you he is heterosexual and has a girlfriend, Eve Chandler, who is a 24-year-old fitness model and hedge fund associate. He tells you that his sex life and sexual functioning "are fantastic! No problems there!" When you ask if Eve thinks his body has imperfections, he says "She tells me it's all in my head and that my body rocks, but I know she's only saying it to be kind to me!" He spends a huge amount of time and effort at esthetic salons, tanning salons, and with the dermatologist, looking for creams, lotions, injectables, and any other procedures that he feels might enhance his appearance. He spends at least $2000 a month on such products and services.

1. The basic pathophysiology of the disorder that Allan is suffering from is believed to be related to:

   A. *Dopamine*

   B. *Norepinephrine*

   C. *Epinephrine*

   D. *Serotonin*

   E. *Glutamate*

2. The psychodynamic explanation of Allan's disorder and behavior is best described as:

   A. *Early parental losses that lead to a self-focused neurosis*

   B. *Acting out behavior due to poor impulse control and poor frustration tolerance*

   C. *The displacement of a sexual or emotional conflict onto nonrelated body parts*

   D. *Arrested development in the anal phase of psychosexual development*

   E. *An unresolved oedipal complex*

3. Which of the following factors are atypical of Allan's most likely diagnosis? (pick 2 of 6)

   A. *The fact that he is man*

   B. *The fact that the onset of his disorder presented prior to 30 years of age*

   C. *The fact that Allan has never suffered a major depressive episode in the past*

   D. *The fact that Allan is unmarried*

   E. *The fact that Allan is a professional and is high-functioning*

   F. *The fact that Allan spends an extraordinary amount of money on himself*

4. Which of the following are considered appropriate treatments for Allan's primary disorder? (pick 3 of 6)

    A. *Clomipramine*

    B. *Bupropion*

    C. *Fluoxetine*

    D. *Modafinil*

    E. *Phenelzine*

    F. *Carbamazepine*

5. Which of the following is typically true about the course and prognosis of Allan's primary disorder?

    A. *It is usually gradual and insidious in onset*

    B. *It is usually of short duration and self-limited*

    C. *It has an undulating course with few symptom-free intervals*

    D. *The part of the body on which concern is focused typically remains the same over time*

    E. *The preoccupation with imagined defects is not usually associated with significant distress or impairment*

Vignette Nineteen

Grace Hanover is a 50-year-old woman who is referred to you by her primary care physician. He has no clue what's going on with Grace medically, because she comes for follow-up every single month with a new physical complaint despite the fact that he has told her so many times that there is nothing that he can find that's wrong with her. Her physician tells you that Grace indeed does suffer from hypertension and hyperlipidemia for the past 3 years, but that she has been taking enalapril and simvastatin daily since then, which have normalized her blood pressure and serum lipid levels quite nicely. He tells you that her many complaints have been going on since he has known her, which is 20 years now, but he knows that these complaints predated her being his patient.

You ask her physician what symptoms she presents with and he runs off a ridiculously long shopping list that is overwhelming and implausible. Her biggest (and longest complaint) is sexual dysfunction on the order of low libido, poor sexual arousal, inability to orgasm either through masturbation or intercourse. This has been going on for 20 years, or even more. Gynecologic consultations have been multiple over the years and testing has never revealed any organic cause to these problems.

Over the years she has complained of gastrointestinal discomfort after eating, though not all the time, periodic dizziness and feeling weak in her legs for no particular reason, generalized body aches and pains, particularly in her neck, lower back, arms and legs, and chronic constipation despite drinking plenty of water every day and eating a very well-balanced diet.

Her physician says: "She's just weird, and I never know what she's going to come up with next when she comes to the office. I think it's all in her head, but I'm not sure. I think her insurance company must hate her, because with all the tests she's undergone over the past 20 years (and all of them were negative!), it must have cost them hundreds of thousands of dollars!"

Grace works in public relations and has a six-figure salary job. She is rarely absent from work, despite her many physical problems. She has never been married and has no children. She was an only child and was doted on by her father, while her mother was actually the breadwinner in the household and was more distant with Grace. Grace has no psychiatric history to speak of. She denies depression, mania, and psychosis. She does have some anxiety, but denies panic attacks or social phobia.

1. Which of the following symptoms would push your differential diagnosis away from a conversion disorder in Grace's case? (pick 3 of 7)

    A. *Backaches*

    B. *Headaches*

    C. *Anorgasmia*

    D. *Dizziness*

    E. *Constipation*

    F. *Gastrointestinal discomfort*

    G. *Arm and leg pain*

2. Which of the following etiological theories are believed to be possible contributors to Grace's primary problem? (pick 3 of 6)

    A. *Abnormal regulation of the cytokine system*

    B. *Only personality disordered patients have Grace's disorder*

    C. *Decreased metabolism in the frontal lobes and nondominant hemisphere*

    D. *Apoptosis and gliosis of brainstem neurons*

    E. *Catecholaminergic deficits or imbalance in the central nervous system*

    F. *Genetic predisposition of the disorder in first-degree female relatives of probands of patients with Grace's disorder*

3. Which of the following statements about the epidemiology of Grace's primary disorder are not true? (pick 3 of 6)

    A. *Men outnumber women with the disorder about 5 to 20 times*

    B. *The lifetime prevalence of somatization disorder among woman is about 1 to 2%*

    C. *The disorder occurs more frequently in patients of upper class and higher socioeconomic status*

    D. *The disorder usually begins in adulthood after the age of 30*

    E. *Concomitant personality traits associated with somatization disorder include obsessive–compulsive, paranoid and avoidant features*

    F. *Bipolar I disorder and substance abuse occur no more frequently in somatization disorder patients than in the general population at large*

4. Which of the following facts are true about the course and prognosis of Grace's primary disorder? (pick 3 of 6)

    A. *The course of the disorder is typical acute and static in its presentation*

    B. *Patients with the disorder have a 20% chance of being diagnosed with this disorder 5 years later*

    C. *Patients with the disorder are no more likely to develop another medical illness in the next 20 years than people without the disorder*

    D. *The disease rarely remits completely*

    E. *It is unusual for a patient with the disorder to be free of symptoms for greater than one year*

    F. *The overall prognosis of the disorder is good to excellent in most cases*

5. The only treatment maneuver for Grace's primary disorder that seems to be able to decrease personal health care expenditure by about 50% is:

    A. *Atypical antipsychotics*

    B. *Antidepressant medications*

    C. *Electroshock therapy*

    D. *Group and individual psychotherapy*

    E. *Mood stabilizers like lithium and divalproex sodium*

    F. *Opioid antagonists like naltrexone*

Vignette Twenty

Kerry Fields is a 26-year-old man who comes to you because he is an extreme athlete and is addicted to opioid pain-killers. He skis, snowboards, drives motocross motorcycles and all-terrain vehicles, and knows only too well how to abuse his body from all this physical activity. He has had a shoulder surgery for severe rotator cuff tear, and at least three knee surgeries on each knee for meniscal tears and repairs. He also has spinal scoliosis and has herniated two cervical and three lumbar intervertebral disks in the past. He has never undergone back surgery, though he has been used to living with chronic pain.

He tells you his problem is balancing pain with narcotic overuse. He is currently taking Roxicodone 30 mg daily two tablets QID and they are barely keeping him stable. He confesses to you that he also drinks every night, at least two or three vodkas with soda and sometimes more. He also smokes cannabis about an ounce a week on average. He tells you his back pain, neck pain, and knee pain is typically a 7 out of 10 most days, unless he is doing some extreme sporting activity or other, when his pain can climb to 9 out of 10, after the activity is over. He wants help from you and your honest recommendations.

1. Which of the following would be good recommendations for treating Kerry's problems? (pick 3of 6)

    A. *Go to an inpatient facility for alcohol, narcotic and cannabis detoxification*

    B. *Do an outpatient narcotic taper and switch Kerry to a Vivitrol (naltrexone) monthly injection*

    C. *Send Kerry to a specialized pain clinic for appropriate recommendations and management*

    D. *Continue the Roxicodone as prescribed for pain and give Kerry disulfiram (Antabuse) for alcohol relapse prevention*

    E. *Send Kerry for orthopedic and neurologic consultation to determine the etiology of his pain*

    F. *Consider a switch from Roxicodone to oral methadone to address both pain and narcotic dependence, along with acamprosate calcium to address alcohol relapse prevention*

2. What is the correct dosing strategy if Kerry is going to begin taking disulfiram?

    A. *500 mg once daily*

    B. *250 mg once daily*

    C. *Start 500 mg once daily for 1 to 2 weeks, then reduce to 250 mg daily for maintenance*

    D. *Start 250 mg once daily for 1 to 2 weeks, then increase to 500 mg daily for maintenance*

    E. *500 mg twice a day*

3. What are the disadvantages of buprenorphine/naloxone tablets for opioid relapse prevention in Kerry's case? (pick 3 of 6)

    A. *The naloxone content of the tablet may trigger a precipitated withdrawal on its own*

    B. *Buprenorphine/naloxone tablets cannot be taken with full opioid agonist painkillers*

    C. *Buprenorphine/naloxone tablets are generally not as effective as full opioid agonist painkillers for the management of moderate to severe chronic pain*

    D. *Buprenorphine/naloxone tablets can easily be diverted and injected for recreational purposes by intravenous drug users*

    E. *Buprenorphine/naloxone tablets must be taken under the tongue and patients frequently complain that they have a bad taste*

    F. *Buprenorphine/naloxone tablets can be abused and overused for its euphoric effects by recreational narcotic users who take excessive quantities of this medication*

4. Which of the following agents decrease serum methadone levels?

    A. *Phenytoin*
    B. *St. John's Wort (hypericum)*
    C. *Dextromethorphan*
    D. *Erythromycin*
    E. *Verapamil*
    F. *Disulfiram*

5. Which of the following substances of abuse causes a withdrawal syndrome when stopped abruptly that manifests with insomnia, irritability, drug craving, restlessness, nervousness, depressed mood, tremor, malaise, myalgia, and increased sweating?

    A. *Cocaine*
    B. *Opiates*
    C. *Phencyclidine (PCP)*
    D. *Cannabis*
    E. *Alcohol*

Vignettes

Answer Key

Vignette One

1. C
2. ABD
3. DE
4. D
5. ABCE
6. AB
7. ABC
8. C
9. C
10. ABCD

Vignette Two

1. B
2. ABD
3. E
4. C
5. DE
6. ACD

7. CEF
8. D
9. C

Vignette Three

1. C
2. C
3. ABCD
4. AB
5. ABC
6. ABCD
7. ACD
8. D
9. ABC
10. C

Vignette Four

1. B
2. ABDE
3. C

4. C
5. ABC
6. DE
7. BCD
8. D
9. ABC
10. ABCD

Vignette Five

1. B
2. AC
3. D
4. ACD
5. C
6. B
7. ABCD
8. ABCD
9. BC
10. B

Vignette Six

1. BCE
2. A
3. BCF
4. AD
5. E
6. B

Vignette Seven

1. AEF
2. BDF
3. BDE
4. E
5. BCD

Vignette Eight

1. D
2. A
3. B
4. BD

5. B

6. D

7. ABD

8. BCD

9. ABCD

10. ACD

Vignette Nine

1. ABC

2. ABCDE

3. ABC

4. B

5. ABCD

6. ABC

7. ACD

8. AD

9. ABCD

10. BCD

Vignette Ten

1. ACD

2. ABC

3. A

4. AB

5. C

6. C

7. D

8. D

9. ABC

10. A

Vignette Eleven

1. AB

2. AD

3. ABD

4. B

5. D

6. AD

7. ABD

8. BC

9. ABC

10. ABD

Vignette Twelve

1. ABCE

2. ABCDE

3. CD

4. D

5. BD

6. A

7. CD

8. D

9. ABCD

10. ABCD

Vignette Thirteen

1. BE

2. CD

3. ACD

4. BEF

5. AB

6. BCD

Vignette Fourteen

1. DE

2. B

3. DE

4. A

5. A

6. A

7. A

8. A

9. C

10. ABCDEFG

Vignette Fifteen

1. AC

2. BF

3. D

4. E

5. CE

Vignette Sixteen

1. CE

2. CFG

3. BCF

4. C

5. ADG

6. F

7. DE

Vignette Seventeen

1. AE

2. ADE

3. D

4. B

5. C

6. CE

7. BEF

Vignette Eighteen

1. D

2. C

3. AC

4. ACE

5. C

Vignette Nineteen

1. CEF

2. ACF

3. ACD

4. BCD

5. D

Vignette Twenty

1. ACF

2. C

3. BCE

4. ABC

5. D

Vignettes

Explanations

Vignette One

1. C. Post-traumatic stress disorder is the best explanation for the scenario in this vignette. In PTSD the person experienced or witnessed an event which involved actual or threatened death or serious injury and they responded with fear, helplessness, or horror. They then need at least one symptom of reexperiencing, three symptoms of avoidance and two symptoms of increased arousal to meet DSM criteria. In this case the nightmares are a symptom of reexperiencing. The restricted range of affect (low mood, unable to be happy), sense of foreshortened future, and avoiding people associated with the trauma all count as avoidance symptoms. Irritability and outbursts of anger with his family and the nurses, and difficulty staying asleep are considered symptoms of increased arousal.

Although he may have some symptoms of depression he does not meet MDD criteria and the overall picture is better explained by PTSD. There is more going on symptom wise than would be explained by an adjustment disorder with depressed mood. Although he no doubt has several medical issues at this point mood disorder secondary to a medical condition does not fully account for the full picture we are seeing. The most comprehensive explanation is found with PTSD.

K&S Ch. 16

2. ABD. Most patients with PTSD receive both medication and therapy. SSRIs and SNRIs are first line for PTSD. CBT is the type of therapy with the most evidence of effectiveness for PTSD. Psychodynamic psychotherapy does not have significant evidence of effectiveness in PTSD. Dialectical behavior therapy is first line for borderline personality disorder, not PTSD. Benzodiazepines should be avoided in PTSD both because of the high risk for potential addiction and because some studies have shown that benzodiazepines slow recovery rates for PTSD. Patients take longer to recover when they are on benzodiazepines so they are not a good choice. In this vignette, family therapy is certainly a good idea given the stress the family is under and the patient's reaction to them.

K&S Ch. 16

3. DE. Rapid onset of symptoms, strong social supports, absence of other psychopathology or substance abuse, short duration of symptoms (less than 6 months), and good premorbid functioning would all be considered good prognostic factors for PTSD. The opposite of any of these would be considered poor prognostic factors. As a general rule, the very old and very young have the highest likelihood of developing PTSD with those in the middle of life faring best.

K&S Ch. 16

4. D. Alexithymia is an inability to describe feeling states and can be a symptom of PTSD. Tactile hallucinations and thyroid abnormalities are not usually associated with PTSD. We see increased norepinephrine turnover in the locus coeruleus in PTSD, not decreased.

K&S Ch. 16

5. **ABCE.** Overcoming denial, use of imaginal techniques or in vivo exposure, encouragement and help for proper sleep, and learning cognitive approaches to stress can all be helpful to patients with PTSD as part of a successful therapeutic approach. Cathartic expression of aggression is not a common component of PTSD treatment and patients are encouraged to verbalize feelings rather that act them out aggressively.

K&S Ch. 16

6. **AB.** Hallucinations and restriction of affect can occur in both schizophrenia and PTSD. Restricted affect would be considered a symptom of avoidance in PTSD. Decreased need for sleep is characteristic of mania. A sense of foreshortened future is a symptom of avoidance seen in PTSD.

K&S Ch. 16

7. **ABC.** Decreased sleep and most importantly decreased need for sleep can be seen in bipolar I disorder. Generalized anxiety disorder may present with sleep disturbance as one of the physical symptoms (the others are muscle tension and fatigue). PTSD can present with difficulty falling or staying asleep as part of the increased arousal symptoms. OCD does not have a sleep disturbance as part of its DSM criteria.

K&S Ch. 16

8. **C.** This is an example of classical conditioning. Classical conditioning is when a neutral (conditioned) stimulus is paired with a stimulus that evokes a response (unconditioned stimulus) such that over time the neutral stimulus eventually elicits the same response as the unconditioned stimulus. In this case the unconditioned stimulus was the fire and the reaction was fear and horror. In time the neutral stimulus of the chainsaw takes on the power to generate the fear originally caused by the fire. Classical conditioning is part of the behavioral model for PTSD.

In operant conditioning voluntary behavior is modified as the patient actively tries different behaviors to see which will deliver a desired reward. Learned helplessness is a model of depression in which a patient repetitively fails at a task and eventually stops trying, adopting a hopeless apathetic position. Premack's principle states that behavior engaged in at a high frequency can be used to reinforce behavior that occurs at a low frequency.

K&S Chs 4&16

9. **C.** Feelings of detachment from others is considered a symptom of avoidance when diagnosing PTSD. All other choices in the question are symptoms of increased arousal.

K&S Ch. 16

10. **ABCD.** The differential diagnosis for PTSD should include all of the choices mentioned in this question except schizotypal personality disorder. Panic disorder can present with symptoms which could be considered in line with avoidance and hyperarousal. Substance abuse can mimic anxiety symptoms and there is a high overlap between PTSD and substance abuse, especially alcohol. Major depressive disorder presents with symptoms similar to the avoidance symptoms of PTSD (restricted affect, diminished interest in activities, feelings of detachment). Borderline personality disorder may present with mood lability, irritability and angry outbursts which could be mistaken for hyperarousal symptoms in PTSD.

K&S Ch. 16

Vignette Two

1. **B.** This question asks you to focus on the most clinically appropriate maneuver in this case. You could certainly send the patient home with yet another medication trial, but the fact that she has already failed multiple medication trails makes the prognosis for success very poor. Clearly, her daughter has done the patient no harm so there is no question here of reporting her to state authorities as a case of possible elder abuse. ACT teams are an excellent treatment modality principally for patients who have poor insight into their mental disorder and, as a result, are poorly adherent to medication regimens that would prevent decompensation. ACT teams, because of their mobility and their high staff to patient ratio, are able to service such patients in their home environment and at the same time ensure that the medications are filled and taken appropriately. ACT teams are not a substitute for skilled nursing care or skilled nursing facility placement. Such teams are unable to handle and manage patients at home who have multiple

medical problems and need structure and help with basic activities of daily living, such as shopping, cooking, and cleaning. Such patients are much better served by skilled nursing facility placement, or if less severe, by visiting nurse services complemented by home healthcare assistance. In this particular case though, placing the patient in a skilled nursing facility is not the best immediate maneuver. The patient is profoundly depressed and in need of intensive psychiatric care prior to nursing home placement. If placed in such a facility in her present mental state, the patient will surely not be able to be managed by a nursing home consulting psychiatrist, given the profound severity of her depression and disintegration of her activities of daily living. The best maneuver in this case would be to convince the patient and her daughter that a voluntary psychiatry inpatient admission would be best for the patient. Consideration of electroshock therapy, once admitted, is quite appropriate, given the patient's failure to improve with numerous trials of antidepressant medications. The most common indication for ECT is major depressive disorder, for which ECT is the fastest and most effective available therapy. ECT should be given consideration when patients have failed multiple medication trials, are acutely suicidal, homicidal, or psychotic, or have severe symptoms of stupor or agitation.

K&S Ch. 36

2. ABD. The pretreatment evaluation for ECT includes physical examination, neurological examination, anesthesia consultation, and complete medical and surgical history. Laboratory testing should include blood and urine chemistries, chest radiography, and an electrocardiogram. A dental exam is advisable, particularly in the elderly who may have poor dentition or poor dental hygiene. Spine radiography should be done only if there is history or suspicion of preexisting spinal disorder. Brain CT or MRI scan should be done if there is history or suspicion of a seizure disorder or a space-occupying lesion. In this particular vignette, the patient may well have a brain tumor of some sort that is causing her refractory depression. Even though a brain tumor is not an absolute contraindication to ECT, a brain scan should be performed in this case to rule out that possibility. Thyroid function tests and routine electroencephalogram are not needed for pretreatment ECT evaluation.

K&S Ch. 36

3. E. Electroshock therapy has no absolute contraindications. Patients with situations that put them at increased risk merely need closer and more careful monitoring before, during, and after the procedure. Pregnancy is not a contraindication for ECT. Patients with space-occupying brain lesions are at risk for brain edema and herniation following the procedure. Those patients with smaller mass lesions can be premedicated with dexamethasone (Decadron), which reduces the risks following the procedure. Patients with recent myocardial infarction are a high-risk group, but the risk is diminished two weeks after the myocardial infarction and even further diminished 3 months following the infarction. Patients with hypertension should be well-stabilized on their antihypertensive medications prior to ECT being administered.

K&S Ch. 36

4. C. For a seizure to be effective in the course of ECT, it should last at least 25 seconds. Proper objective seizure monitoring must be undertaken by the physician conducting the ECT. There must be evidence that a bilateral generalized seizure has taken place after the electrical stimulation has been applied. The EEG and electromyogram enable this to be monitored objectively.

K&S Ch. 36

5. DE. The most worrisome side effect of ECT is memory loss. About 75% of patients given ECT complain that memory impairment is the worst adverse effect. Most patients with memory impairment report a return to baseline within 6 months following treatment. Fractures and muscle or back soreness are possible with ECT, but with routine use of muscle relaxants, fractures of long bones do not generally occur. A minority of patients experience nausea, vomiting and headache following ECT. Mortality rate with ECT is about 0.002% per treatment and 0.01% for each patient. Hypertension can occur during the seizure, but can be controlled by antihypertensive agents administered at that time. Hypertension is not typically a long-term adverse effect of ECT.

K&S Ch. 36

6. **ACD.** The indications for maintenance ECT treatments are: severe medication side effects and intolerance, psychotic or severe symptoms, and rapid relapse after a successful initial round of treatments. Maintenance ECT should always be considered after a remission of symptoms from a first round of treatment, because initial positive response is rarely maintained and relapses often occur despite an initial response to a first round of treatments.

K&S Ch. 36

7. **CEF.** Benzodiazepines should be tapered and withdrawn prior to ECT because of their anticonvulsant properties. Lithium must be withdrawn prior to ECT because it can cause a postictal delirium and can prolong seizure activity. Clozapine and bupropion should also be withdrawn prior to ECT, because they are known to be associated with late-appearing seizures. Antidepressants in the class of the SSRIs, SNRIs, tricyclics and MAO inhibitors are *not* contraindicated with ECT.

K&S Ch. 36

8. **D.** Methohexital (Brevital) is the most commonly used anesthetic agent for ECT because of its shorter duration of action and lower association with postictal arrhythmias. Etomidate (Amidate) is sometimes used in elderly patients, because it does not increase the seizure threshold and it is well understood that seizure threshold increases as patient's age. Ketamine (Ketalar) is sometimes used because it doesn't raise the seizure threshold. It is however associated with the emergence of psychotic symptoms following anesthesia. Alfentanil (Alfenta) is used concomitantly with barbiturates in some cases, because it allows for lower dosing of the barbiturates which lowers the seizure threshold further. It is however associated with an increased incidence of nausea. Propofol (Diprivan) is less useful as an anesthetic agent in ECT because it raises the seizure threshold.

K&S Ch. 36

9. **C.** Electrode placement for ECT can either be unilateral or bilateral. Bilateral placement leads to a more rapid therapeutic response in most cases, but it also results in a higher frequency of memory impairment. Most practitioners will begin treatment with unilateral ECT because of its more favorable adverse effect profile. If the patient does not improve after four to six unilateral treatments, most clinicians will strongly consider moving to bilateral electrode placement thereafter. Initial bilateral electrode placement is considered in cases of severe depressive symptoms, with catatonic stupor, acute suicide risk, manic symptoms, treatment-resistant schizophrenia and in cases of marked agitation.

K&S Ch. 36

Vignette Three

1. **C.** Cathy would best be described as having bipolar II disorder. To meet criteria for bipolar II requires at least 1 MDD episode and 1 hypomanic episode. Cathy clearly meets MDD criteria. Hypomania is defined by a clear period of irritable, expansive, or elevated mood lasting for at least 4 days but does not cause marked impairment in functioning. In addition there must be at least 3 of the same symptoms which define manic episodes (pressured speech, decreased need for sleep, grandiosity, flight of ideas, distractability, increased goal directed activity, excess involvement in behaviors with high potential for harmful consequences). Cathy fits this profile. If she were to have mania her symptoms would continue for 1 week or more and/or she would have marked impairment in functioning, neither of which are true in this case. Major depressive disorder is incorrect because it does not explain the entire picture we are seeing. Cyclothymic disorder is defined as hypomania plus subthreshold depressive symptoms for a period of 2 years or longer. This doesn't fit Cathy's case. Substance induced mood disorder would certainly be included in a differential for Cathy, but would not be the best choice because we have given you no data on the connection between substance abuse and mood changes. She also denies the use of substances, which would likely precipitate a manic episode around the time of her sister's wedding (cocaine).

K&S Ch. 15

2. **C.** Key differentiating factors between hypomania and mania would include the time period (4–6 days for hypomania vs. 7+ days for mania) and the presence or absence of marked impairment in social or

occupational functioning. Irritable mood, decreased need for sleep and flight of ideas could be present in either.

K&S Ch. 15

3. **ABCD.** Psychosis, rapid cycling, severity of symptoms and pregnancy are all valid concerns which would impact the choice of medications in the bipolar patient. For a patient in their 30s age wouldn't be a major factor.

K&S Chs 15&36

4. **AB.** ECT for bipolar has been proven very effective in severe mania with psychosis and in pregnancy. Mania secondary to a medical condition or substance abuse would not necessarily lead to ECT and would most likely be treated with medications.

K&S Chs 15&36

5. **ABC.** Glioma, Cushing's disease, and multiple sclerosis have all been associated with mania. Thiamine deficiency is not associated with mania but is a crucial component of Wernicke–Korsakoff syndrome seen in alcoholics.

K&S Ch. 15

6. **ABCD.** Isoniazid, cimetidine, metoclopramide and steroids can all cause a manic episode. Of course there are others such as bronchodilators, antidepressants, anticonvulsants, stimulants, barbiturates and several drugs of abuse. Benzodiazepines would tend to lessen mania, not cause it.

K&S Ch. 15

7. **ACD.** Cocaine use causes rapid dopamine and norepinephrine reuptake inhibition. It increases dopamine in the mesolimbic and mesocortical pathways and decreases dopamine in the corpus striatum.

K&S Ch. 12

8. **D.** Sequelae of cocaine use include hallucinations, paranoia, euphoria, increased energy, hypersexuality, and irritability. With heavy cocaine use patients can experience a shower of lights in their central vision, as well as visual hallucination of black dots on their skin and in the environment (coke bugs). Itching and respiratory depression come from opiate abuse, not cocaine.

K&S Ch. 12

9. **ABC.** Treatment for cocaine overdose can include cold blankets and ice packs for hyperthermia, IV diazepam for seizures, IV phentolamine for malignant hypertension and both haloperidol and lorazepam for agitation. Clonidine is useful in treating the autonomic effects of opiate withdrawal, but is not used in cocaine overdose.

K&S Ch. 12

10. **C.** Sixty percent of patients with bipolar disorder have a co-occurring substance abuse disorder. As such Cathy is not unusual in this regard. It means that it is very important to screen for substance abuse in any bipolar patients.

K&S Ch. 15

Vignette Four

1. **B.** Susan has borderline personality disorder. Characteristics of the disorder include frantic efforts to avoid abandonment, unstable and intense interpersonal relationships, idealization and devaluation, unstable self image, impulsivity in self damaging ways, affective instability, chronic feelings of emptiness, intense inappropriate anger, and transient stress related paranoia or dissociation. In Susan's case we see impulsivity in self damaging ways, unstable interpersonal relationships, intense inappropriate anger, efforts to avoid abandonment, affective instability, and unstable self image.

K&S Ch. 27

2. **ABDE.** Characteristics of Susan's diagnosis are frantic efforts to avoid abandonment, unstable and intense interpersonal relationships, idealization and devaluation, unstable self-image, impulsivity in self-damaging ways, affective instability, chronic feelings of emptiness, intense inappropriate anger, transient stress related paranoia or dissociation. Grandiosity is not a characteristic of borderline personality disorder but can be seen in bipolar disorder and psychotic disorders.
K&S Ch. 27

3. **C.** Perceived rejection is the centerpiece of many borderline suicide attempts and is certainly the precipitating factor in Susan's case.
K&S Ch. 27

4. **C.** The treatment of choice for borderline personality disorder is dialectical behavior therapy.
K&S Ch. 27

5. **ABC.** Borderline patients may only be in touch with reality on a basic level, have limited capacity for insight, and use primitive defenses such as splitting. They do not have an integrated sense of self. Their unstable sense of self is an important part of the disorder.
K&S Ch. 27

6. **DE.** Acting out and splitting are two of the defenses most commonly associated with borderline personality disorder. The others have no particular association with borderline personality disorder.
K&S Ch. 27

7. **BCD.** Patients with borderline personality self-harm in order to express anger, elicit help from others, and numb themselves to overwhelming affect. Their goal is not to socially isolate themselves and they may feel quite dependent on others, despite the fact that they eventually do drive others away by their extreme behavior.
K&S Ch. 27

8. **D.** Projective identification is a defense mechanism used by borderline patients which was first described by Otto Kernberg. Intolerable aspects of the self are projected onto another person. The other person is then induced to play the projected role. This is of particular concern for psychiatrists working with borderline patients as they can be pulled into this dynamic if they lose their neutral stance. Displacement is a defense mechanism where emotional energy is taken from one object and placed onto another unrelated object. Rationalization is using rational explanations to justify beliefs and attitudes that would otherwise be socially unacceptable. Splitting is seeing other people or situations as either all good or all bad. It is a commonly used defense of the borderline patient.
K&S Chs 6&27

9. **ABC.** Impulsive behaviors are certainly part of the borderline picture. Prolonged psychotic episodes are not. Borderline patients may have brief episodes of psychosis when under significant stress but prolonged psychosis is something seen on Axis I. Marked peculiarity of thinking is more a descriptor of schizotypal personality disorder than of borderline. Extreme suspiciousness is more a descriptor of paranoid personality disorder than of borderline. That is not to say that a borderline patient may never be suspicious, but extreme suspiciousness is not one of the defining DSM criteria.
K&S Ch. 27

10. **ABCD.** All of the choices except stimulants may have a role in treating Susan's condition. Antipsychotics have been used for anger, hostility, and brief psychotic episodes. SSRIs have been used for depressive features and aggression. Anticonvulsants are helpful for mood lability and aggression. MAOIs have been helpful in modulating impulsive behavior in some patients. Stimulants are not considered effective treatment for borderline personality disorder.
K&S Ch. 27

Vignette Five

1. B.   During the initial contact the doctor wishes to establish rapport quickly, put the patient at ease, and show respect. If the patient wishes to have someone else in the initial session with them then that should be respected. Patients have a right to know the position and professional status of the people involved in their care. As such introducing yourself is important. The answer choice which best addresses all of these issues is choice B.

K&S Ch. 1

2. AC.   Starting the interview with an open ended question is best. It allows the patient to describe what has brought them in and signals to them that you are interested in hearing what they have to say. Choices A and C are open ended and allow the patient to tell Dr. Smith what is wrong in her own words. Choices B and D are too closed ended and specific for an opening question. They are both phrased so directly the patient may interpret them as rude.

K&S Ch. 1

3. D.   A patient may be frightened or anxious at the beginning of an interview. The first step in addressing this is by acknowledging the patient's anxiety and offering reassurance. Of the choices given the one that does this best is choice D. Choices A and B have an accusatory tone which may make the patient shut down more. Choice C is ignoring the dynamic in the room and talking about a completely unrelated subject that does not address the patient's underlying discomfort.

K&S Ch.1

4. ACD.   The content of an interview is what gets said between doctor and patient, such as subjects discussed and topics mentioned. The process of the interview is what happens nonverbally, such as body language, behaviors, or avoidance of difficult topics. Choices A, C, and D are all behaviors, body language, or avoidance of difficult topics. Choice B is a topic which was spoken about in the session and as such is content.

K&S Ch. 1

5. C.   In clarification the therapist tries to get more details about what the patient has already said. That is what Dr. Smith is doing in this question. Confrontation is pointing out something that the patient is missing or denying. Facilitation is using both verbal and nonverbal cues to encourage a patient to keep talking. Explanation is when the doctor describes the treatment to the patient in clear understandable language and gives them opportunity to ask questions.

K&S Ch. 1

6. B.   In transition the doctor lets the patient know that they have gathered enough information on one subject and encourage them to move on to another subject. In reassurance the patient informs them of their condition in a way that leads to increased trust and compliance and is experienced by the patient as empathic and caring. In positive reinforcement the doctor makes the patient feel as if they are not upset no matter what the patient says so as to facilitate an open exchange of information. In advice the doctor recommends a course of action to the patient. This should always be done after the patient has had time to speak freely about their problems. If done before this it can be received as inappropriate or intrusive.

K&S Ch. 1

7. ABCD.   In ending the session it is important to give patients a chance to ask questions and explain future plans and next steps. You should thank the patient for sharing information. Any prescriptions should be reviewed and the patient should understand why they are being given medication and how to take it. Patients should be encouraged to call with questions if they need clarification of their treatment, if anything emergent arises, or if they have side effects to medications and need guidance.

K&S Ch. 1

8. ABCD.   Putting the patient at ease, expressing compassion for pain, showing expertise, and establishing authority as a physician are all necessary parts of developing rapport with a patient. To do this well the doctor must balance the roles of empathic listener, expert, and authority. Doctors are not expected to be all knowing and should be honest with the patient when they do not know the answer to a patient's question.

K&S Ch. 1

9. BC.   Decreased rates of patient compliance have been proven to be associated with increased complexity of the treatment regimen and an increased number of behavioral changes required for the treatment to succeed. Intelligence, gender, marital status, race, religion, socioeconomic status, and education level have not been proven to correlate with compliance rates.

K&S Ch. 1

10. B.   All of these answer choices represent different models of the doctor–patient relationship. In the teacher–student model the physician's dominance is emphasized. The physician is paternalistic and controlling. The patient's role is one of dependence and acceptance. In the active–passive model patients assume no responsibility for their care and take no part in their treatment. This is appropriate for patients who are unconscious or delirious. In the mutual participation model there is equality between both parties and each depends on the other for cooperation and input. Long-term management of chronic diseases often leads to this model. In the friendship model patient and doctor become friends. This is an arrangement that is considered unethical and dysfunctional. It often reflects psychological problems on the part of the physician.

K&S Ch. 1

Vignette Six

1. BCE.   Gender identity disorder is defined as a strong and persistent cross-gender identification. In adolescents and adults, the disturbance is manifested by symptoms such as a stated desire to be the other sex, frequent passing as the other sex, desire to live or be treated as the other sex, or the conviction that he or she has the typical feelings and reactions of the other sex. There is a persistent discomfort with his or her sex or sense of inappropriateness in the gender role of that sex. In adolescents and adults, the disturbance is manifested by symptoms such as preoccupation with getting rid of primary sex characteristics or belief that he or she was born the wrong sex.

Transvestic fetishism is a disorder in a heterosexual male who, over at least a 6-month period, has recurrent, intense sexually arousing fantasies, sexual urges, or behaviors involving cross-dressing. Pearl would not be considered a heterosexual male in this case and so does not meet criteria for this disorder. Partialism, also called *oralism*, is categorized under paraphilias not otherwise specified. People with this disorder concentrate their sexual activity on one part of the body to the exclusion of all others. The typical presentation involves preference for oral sex without intercourse. Urophilia is also a paraphilia not otherwise specified. Pearl does meet criteria for urophilia as it involves the intense desire to urinate on a partner or be urinated on. In both men and women, this may also be associated with sexual arousal via the insertion of foreign objects into the urethra for the purpose of sexual stimulation.

Sexual sadism and sexual masochism are two different paraphilias, but they are related. The former involves at least 6 months of recurrent, intense sexually arousing fantasies, sexual urges, or behaviors involving acts in which psychological or physical suffering of the victim is sexually exciting to the person. The latter involves at least 6 months of similar fantasies, urges or behaviors involving acts of being humiliated, beaten, bound, or otherwise made to suffer. It would seem that Pearl and her partner meet criteria for these paraphilias. Fetishism is again a paraphilia of at least 6 months' duration, during which time the person has recurrent, intense sexually arousing fantasies, urges, or behaviors involving the use of nonliving objects (for example, female undergarments, or fake rubber penises). Pearl does not seem to have a fetishistic paraphilia.

K&S Ch. 21

2. A.   Poor prognosis for paraphilias is associated with early age of onset, a lack of guilt or shame about the act, a high frequency of acts, and concomitant substance abuse. The prognosis is also better when there is a history of the act of coitus with the paraphilia and when the patient is self-referred rather than referred by a legal agency.

K&S Ch. 21

3. BCF.   Good prognostic indicators for paraphilias include normal intelligence, the absence of substance abuse, the absence of personality disorders, the presence of normal adult attachments and relationships, the absence of concomitant axis one mental disorders, and the presence of only one paraphilia.

K&S Ch. 21

4. AD.   There are essentially five types of psychiatric intervention used to treat paraphilias. These include reduction of sexual drives, external control, treatment of comorbid conditions, dynamic therapy and cognitive-behavioral therapy. Prison is an external control mechanism to prevent sexual crimes, but it does not usually involve a treatment element. Interpersonal psychotherapy is not usually useful in helping prevent paraphiliac behaviors, urges and fantasies. Sex therapy can be effective and is considered an adjunctive modality to dynamic therapy. Twelve-step programs based on the Alcoholics Anonymous model are of course useful in supporting individuals with sexual addiction and troublesome behaviors. Antiandrogen therapy may reduce sex drive and aberrant sexual behavior by decreasing serum testosterone levels to subnormal concentrations.

K&S Ch. 21

5. E.   Most patients with gender identity disorder (GID) are males. Men present with the disorder at a rate of about 1 in 30 000 and women present with disorder at a rate of about 1 in 100 000. Prospective studies of children with GID indicate that few become transsexuals and want to change their sex. Adult transsexuals typically complain of being uncomfortable wearing the clothes of their assigned sex and so they prefer to wear clothes of the opposite sex and act in ways compatible with the opposite sex. They find their own genitals to be repugnant, which may lead to their repeated requests for gender-reassignment surgery and hormone therapy. About two-thirds of adult men with GID are sexually attracted to men only. Therefore, Pearl would be counted among the minority one-third of male patients with GID who are exclusively attracted to female partners.

K&S Ch. 22

6. B.   At this time, there is no evidence that indicates that psychological or psychiatric intervention for children with GID can change their future sexual orientation. Also, there are no particular hormonal or psycho-pharmacological treatments for GID in childhood. Adolescents with GID can now be given cross-sex hormones in pre-pubescence to slow down or arrest pubertal development and begin the cross-over to the opposite gender at that time. No drug therapy has been shown to reduce cross-gender desires in adult patients with GID. When adult patients suffer from severe gender dysphoria, sex-reassignment surgery may be the best solution.

K&S Ch. 22

Vignette Seven

1. AEF.   This is a classic, though complex, case scenario. It comes up frequently in day-to-day practice for the forensic psychiatric consultant. As a psychiatric expert witness for the defense, you are engaged by the defense lawyer to help the accused in his defense. You must act within the scope and expertise of your profession and practice. You must evaluate the defendant and any pertinent collaterals, as well as examine the circumstances surrounding the alleged acts, and then produce a written report that supports the defense attorney's stance in his defense of his client. You cannot skew the facts or perjure yourself in an attempt to help the defense team and their client.

Note that ethically there is no reason that you cannot participate as an expert witness in this case. The fact that the defendant is also a psychiatrist has no bearing on the experts who may be brought forth to defend him. The only conflict of interest that may arise would stem from a situation in which Dr. Daniels and you were best friends, relatives, business partners, or had other past or present collaborations or combined interests that would render your judgment in the case unnecessarily biased in his favor. In such a case, you would have to decline the case and refuse to participate in it.

Your job begins with a thorough consultation with the defense attorney to discuss the facts of the case, as well as the defense team's stance and approach to the defense. Is the defense seeking a psychiatric defense: i.e. applying the M'Naghten Rule looking for a "not guilty by reason of insanity" plea on any or all of the charges? Is the defense seeking mitigation of the charges on the basis of psychiatric incapacitation or deficits? Does the defense attorney feel that there are mitigating circumstances in the defendant's behavior that reflect a mental status that was not sound at the time the alleged events took place? Who are the collateral people that can be interviewed who might lend weight in evidence to the desired defense? Are there facts in the defendant's psychiatric and/or medical history that may help in establishing mitigation of guilt? Does the attorney himself feel that his client is competent to stand trial and has this issue been brought to bear by the defense, the prosecution, or the judge?

All of these (and many more) questions need to be answered before you can begin to approach this case. Once you are satisfied that you have enough background data and information to begin work on the case, your next step is to interview and examine Dr. Daniels thoroughly. This may need to take place over several different sessions held over a period of time, in order for you to gather as complete details as you can, and also to establish his recollection and redaction of the facts as he sees them. You may feel that medical and neurologic assessment should be part of the defense investigation and suggest this to the defense attorney, if you think it would be helpful to the client's defense. Part of your interview and assessment (and part of your function in this case) is to assess the defendant's current competency to stand trial. The defense attorney may not ask you to do this formally, because he may have no doubts about the fact that the good doctor has full capacity to stand trial. Even so, you must ask the classic questions of the defendant to be sure that you as a consultant have no doubts about his ability to stand trial. The defendant must demonstrate knowledge of the charges brought to bear against him, knowledge of the circumstances on which the charges are based, knowledge of the important persons involved in the playing out of the case, knowledge of the possible outcomes of the various types of pleas that the defense may enter in his behalf. Above all, the defendant must demonstrate an ability to collaborate with his lawyer in his own defense. Note that the defendant's current mental status is what is assessed in competency to stand trial, and not his mental status at the time the alleged acts were committed.

In order to assess for mitigation of responsibility or for a "not guilty by reason of insanity" plea, you must evaluate Dr. Daniels mental status at the time the alleged incidents occurred. You must establish (if you can) intent to harm versus lack of such intent, as this will mitigate or implicate his responsibility if it is deemed that the alleged acts were committed. Obtaining information from collateral persons who may have been involved around these events may be a crucial maneuver in trying to piece together the defendant's mental status at that time.

Should you recommend functional brain imaging studies to help in the client's defense? This type of recommendation and evidence is extremely controversial and very new to the process. Generally speaking, such evidence is not really contemplated unless there are some clear-cut facts in the neurologic or medical history that would warrant such studies to be done. Neuropsychological testing may also reveal deficits that might warrant such imaging, depending on the history. Brain injury, stroke, brain tumor, seizure history, severe and chronic substance use, are but some of the historical factors that may trigger an expert witness to suggest that brain imaging might be helpful. Even if such imaging is conducted on the defendant, and even if the results show brain abnormalities, the evidence, as it is presented to prosecutors, the judge and perhaps eventually a jury, may not be helpful because of its complexity and the lack of good precedents in the law annals to help support the data as a mitigating factor to the defendant's guilt.

There is no case scenario (expect perhaps in the case of a mute or profoundly mentally retarded defendant) in which neuropsychological testing should not be conducted. Even if the testing reveals nothing to help the defendant (i.e., a thorough battery shows he has an above-average intelligence with no dangerous personality characteristics, nor any deficits in executive functioning or reasoning), this will not necessarily hurt the defense. How is this possible? Once the testing is complete, the consulting neuropsychologist must colleague with the defense team verbally before writing up a final report. If upon discussion, the defense attorney feels that the testing results would not be helpful (or may even be a hindrance) to the defense, he can certainly request that a report not be written at that time. Certainly, the prosecution team must be told of the neuropsychological testing, and they can subpoena the neuropsychologist to testify at trial, if the case goes that far, but a noncontributory report need not be immediately presented, because it certainly can then be used by the prosecution against the defendant. This is indeed a legal "game" that is often played out between defense and prosecution, in order to spin or skew the evidence in one direction or another. Most of these cases never get to trial and wind up either being dropped by prosecutors if evidence if too weak, or even thrown out by the judge before moving forward to pre-trial, if the judge feels the charges and allegations are frivolous or unsubstantiated! If the charges are neither dropped nor thrown out of court, a trial may still never come to pass, as many cases are settled as a plea bargain by both sides before the case can go further.

Should Dr. Daniels be practicing his profession (if the state permits him to do so) between now and his future court date? This is a matter that falls between him and his defense attorney, who will no doubt advise and guide him. In certain situations, it is deemed best for the defendant to continue "business as usual" in the interim, as it points to a professional who is currently unimpaired and who can carry on working without a problem in his chosen profession. In other circumstances, his defense attorney may feel it best for him not to continue practicing, because it may help the defense mount a psychiatric plea that points more towards impairment and the need for mitigation of responsibility. Again, these are lawyers' tactics that are outside the purview of the psychiatric expert witness. Of course, you are entitled to your opinion as an expert witness, based on your findings, and you should impart this opinion to the defense team, but they are the ones who will finally advise and guide their client accordingly.

K&S Chs 58&59

2. BDF. The commission of a criminal act has two components: voluntary conduct (actus reus) and evil intent (mens rea). Evil intent cannot be present if the offender's mental status is so impaired or diseased as to have deprived the offender of the rational intent to commit the act. The law can only be invoked in the presence of evil or malicious intent. Intent to do harm is not sufficient on its own as grounds for criminal action. The M'Naghten Rule is the statute derived from the 1843 case of Daniel M'Naghten in the British courts. This is known as the right–wrong rule or test. The question brought to bear in this rule is "did the defendant understand the nature and quality of the act and the difference between right and wrong with respect to the act" at the time the act was committed. If a mental illness causes the defendant to be unaware of the consequences of his/her acts, or if he/she was incapable of understanding that these acts were wrong, the person could then be absolved of criminal responsibility for the acts. *Ford v. Wainwright* is a landmark case in the matter of competence to be executed and has nothing to do with the case in this vignette. The duty to warn and protect derives from the case of *Tarasoff v. Regents of the University of California*, which was the landmark case setting the precedent for clinicians to be responsible for warning and protecting intended victims of patients expressing intent to harm others.

K&S Ch. 58

3. BDE. The standard for competence to stand trial is set quite low to enable as many defendants to have their day in court as possible. This standard was set by the US Supreme Court in the landmark case of *Dusky v. United States*. The defendant must be able to demonstrate knowledge of the charges brought against him. He must demonstrate knowledge of the penalties associated with being found guilty of each of these charges. He must demonstrate a knowledge and recognition of the various persons involved in his case: his attorneys, the prosecuting attorneys, the judge, the witnesses who will be called, the jury. He must be able to collaborate with his attorney with a reasonable degree of rational understanding of the proceedings against him. Note that the defendant's current mental status (and not his mental status at the time the alleged acts were committed) is what is brought to bear in determining his competency to stand trial. The defendant does not have to recall every minute detail of the acts that he is alleged to have committed. The defendant does not have to be able to take the stand as a witness in his own defense. The defendant does not have to have an opinion on what kind of plea his defense team should enter on his behalf. Defense and prosecuting attorneys usually have the discretion to hire and appoint their own psychiatric expert witness to attest to the defendant's competency to stand trial. The judge has the final word on which, if any of these opinions, he/she is willing to hear and entertain in the decision-making process on competency to stand trial. The judge also has the discretion to appoint his/her own psychiatric expert witness(es) to lend further weight to the decision in cases where the defendant's competency to stand trial may be difficult to determine.

K&S Ch. 58

4. E. This is a tough, tough question, particularly if you have little or no experience in the forensic arena. The answer, upon reflection, is simple. Judges have the final word on how anything will play out in their courtroom. In this vignette, as it is presented, both sides will undoubtedly want a crack at this all-important witness. Remember that she is not the one on trial here and she is not a plaintiff here either. She is merely the accuser in a criminal trial brought against Dr. Daniels by state prosecutors. So Selena can be a key witness for either side, and of course her testimony may be the most important factor in this case, but the judge is the only one who can dictate how that is to be conducted. Of course, prosecutors and judges work together to represent the best interests of "the people of the state" when trying criminal cases; the results are not always fair and unbiased, unfortunately. After all, judges and prosecutors are usually elected political officials in the US, and they seek to maintain popularity among their voters and constituents by winning high-profile criminal cases that demonstrate their keen abilities to serve and protect the people.

So, to get off the political soap-box and back to psychiatric test preparation, it would be ideal if you could interview Selena and thus lessen her credibility as a witness. This would help you defend your client, Dr. Daniels. It's unlikely that the prosecution will allow that to happen and they will certainly petition the judge to prevent this. They may ask the judge to let the prosecution first appoint their own psychiatric expert witness and have Selena be examined by that expert. The prosecution may try to block Selena from being examined all together, but again the judge will determine if that should be upheld or overruled. Mr. Wolff can certainly try to subpoena Selena to be psychiatrically examined for the defense, but prosecutors can ask the judge to block this for the reasons already mentioned. The prosecution can try to protect their case against Dr. Daniels by trying to petition the judge not to allow Selena to submit to an examination by a defense-appointed psychiatrist, but again, the judge decides. If the judge allows the prosecution to call a witness, in the interest of fairness and good judicial practice, he/she will usually allow the defense the opportunity to do the same. That said, judges can act and rule however they like (and have been known to do so in these cases) and their decisions are indemnified against any retaliation or accusation of wrongdoing or unprofessionalism for the most part.

K&S Ch. 58

5. BCD.   If Dr. Daniels' defense team has put in a psychiatric plea on all three charges and the prosecution has allowed this to go to trial before a jury, then there is almost certainly a psychiatric impediment in the good doctor's case. If the jury finds the good doctor not guilty by reason of insanity on all three counts, then there was certainly some compelling reason for the doctor's mental status to have been clouded during these events, given that the jury felt he did not know right from wrong at the time these acts were committed. With this knowledge alone, we know that Dr. Daniels needs psychiatric treatment of some kind. We don't know why his mental status was clouded, but a psychiatric disorder was likely the root cause at that time.

Based on these facts, there is little doubt that the judge will mandate Dr. Daniels to some sort of psychiatric treatment. Dr. Daniels is highly unlikely to be permitted to return to psychiatric practice immediately without some sort of treatment mandate. Dr. Daniels will not be classified as a sex-offender because he was found not guilty of these charges, albeit by reason of psychiatric incapacitation. The decision to remove or maintain the doctor's license comes not from the court, but from the state licensing department, who, upon reviewing the facts of the case, will determine the destiny of the doctor's practice privileges. It is absolutely possible (though it may come as a shock) that the state licensing department could allow the doctor to return to practice after treatment is successfully completed, despite the nature of these charges.

K&S Ch. 58

Vignette Eight

1. D.   Thought process refers to the form of the patient's thoughts. Descriptions of thought process would include the terms goal directed, linear, circumstantial, tangential, loosening of associations, flight of ideas, thought blocking, neologisms, racing thoughts, or word salad. Thought content includes delusions, preoccupations, obsessions, compulsions, phobias, hypochondriacal symptoms or antisocial urges. Perceptions primarily refers to hallucinations, be they auditory, visual, tactile, olfactory, or gustatory. In this case the only statement that is both correct and accurate is that the perceptions section of the mental status exam should include auditory hallucinations.

K&S Ch. 7

2. A.   The beliefs that Steven is having qualify as delusions. A delusion is a fixed false belief that is not supported by social norms. They are listed under the thought content section of the mental status exam.

K&S Ch. 7

3. B.   The GAF stands for global assessment of functioning. It is a 100 point scale of functioning which is included as Axis V in a full five axis diagnosis.This question is testing to see if you know some of the landmarks on the GAF. A GAF of 10 represents persistent danger of hurting self or others or persistent inability to maintain personal hygiene. A GAF of 20 represents some danger of hurting self or others or occasionally fails to maintain personal hygiene. A GAF of 40 represents some impairment in reality testing or communication or major impairment in several areas such as work or school. A GAF of 60 represents moderate symptoms or moderate difficulty in social or occupational functioning.

K&S Ch. 9

4. BD.   Concentration may be impaired in several psychiatric disorders. It is tested by asking the patient to start at 100 and count backwards by 7s or by asking them to spell the word world backwards and forward. Attitude in the mental status exam describes the patient's attitude towards the examiner. Words commonly used include cooperative, friendly, interested, seductive, defensive, hostile, evasive, apathetic, ingratiating, and guarded. Memory would be tested by giving the patient three words to remember then coming back to them in 5 minutes and see if he remembered them. Abstract thinking is tested through the use of proverbs. It is a reflection of the patient's ability to handle concepts.

K&S Ch. 7

5. B.   A delusion of grandeur is a person's exaggerated conception of his importance, identity, or power. Pseudologia phantastica is a type of lying in which a person appears to believe in the reality of their fantasies and acts on them. Algophobia is the dread of pain. A nihilistic delusion is a false feeling that self or others are nonexistent or that the world is coming to an end.

K&S Ch. 8

6. D.   The mesocortical pathway which is responsible for the negative symptoms of schizophrenia begins at the ventral tegmental area and extends to the frontal lobes.

K&S Ch. 3

7. ABD.   Positive symptoms in schizophrenia are most associated with frequency of hospitalization but are not good predictors of long-term functional outcome. Cognitive symptoms have the strongest correlation with long-term functional outcome. Schizophrenia is associated with a 10% suicide rate. Most schizophrenics who commit suicide do so in the first few years of their illness and are therefore young.

K&S Chs 13&34

8. BCD.   Residual schizophrenia is defined by the absence of prominent delusions, hallucinations, disorganized speech or grossly disorganized or catatonic behavior. It is possible for them to have negative symptoms or positive symptoms in an attenuated form such as odd beliefs or unusual perceptual experiences.

K&S Ch. 13

9. ABCD.   All of the choices given except bright clothing are commonly seen in schizophrenics. Lack of spontaneous movement, odd stiffness or clumsiness, echopraxia (imitation of posture or behavior of the examiner), agitation, and bizarre posture are all possible in addition to tics and stereotypies.

K&S Ch. 13

10. ACD.   Thought form (a.k.a. thought process) of schizophrenic patients can include verbigeration (meaningless repetition of specific words or phrases), word salad (incomprehensible connection of thoughts with loss of normal grammatical structure) and mutism (voicelessness without any physical impediments of speech). Ideas of reference are part of thought content, not thought form.

K&S Ch 8

Vignette Nine

1. ABC.   Anorexia nervosa can be divided into restricting type and binge-eating–purging type. Refusal to maintain body weight above 85% of the expected body weight for height and age is an essential criterion. In addition the anorexic patient has an intense fear of becoming fat, has a disturbance in the way their body is experienced, and presents with amenorrhea. Binge eating and purging can occur in either anorexia or bulimia.

K&S Ch. 23

2. **ABCDE.**   Medical complications associated with anorexia include but are not limited to bradycardia, pancytopenia, lanugo, osteopenia, metabolic encephalopathy, arrhythmias, elevated LFTs, elevated BUN, decreased T3 and T4, parotid gland enlargement, seizures, and peripheral neuropathy.

K&S Ch. 23

3. **ABC.**   Indications that anorexia should be managed inpatient include significant hypokalemia, weight loss to under 75% of expected weight for height and age, growth arrest, risk of self-harm or development of psychosis, rapid weight loss, or the failure of outpatient management.

K&S Ch. 23

4. **B.**   BMI (body mass index) is calculated as weight (kg)/height (m)^2. Other choices are just distractors and are nothing you should memorize.

K&S Ch. 23

5. **ABCD.**   Treatment for anorexia should address psychiatric, medical and nutritional issues. Weight restoration is a major goal. Psychopharmacology can include the use of both antipsychotics and antidepressants. Psychotherapy and family therapy are important and there is evidence for the use of cognitive behavioral therapy in all eating disorders, especially bulimia. The most effective psychotherapy focuses on helping the patient develop alternative coping strategies and defenses as well as changing problematic eating behaviors. Bupropion should be avoided in patients with eating disorders as it lowers the seizure threshold which can increase risk of seizures during periods of electrolyte disturbances which eating disorder patients are prone to.

K&S Ch. 23

6. **ABC.**   Complications of self-induced vomiting found in anorexia or bulimia can include esophagitis, scars and abrasions on the back of the hand (Russell's sign), Mallory–Weiss syndrome (bleeding from tears in the esophageal mucosa caused by repetitive retching), Barrett's esophagus, erosion of tooth enamel, parotid gland swelling, increased serum amylase, hypokalemia, and an increased rate of spontaneous abortion and low birth weight during pregnancy. Atonic colon can be found in anorexics but is a result of laxative abuse, not self-induced vomiting.

K&S Ch. 23

7. **ACD.**   Abuse of ipecac syrup can lead to skeletal muscle atrophy, prolonged QTc interval, cardiomyopathy, and tachycardia. Rectal prolapse can be seen in eating disorders following severe laxative abuse.

K&S Ch. 23

8. **AD.**   The risk of anorexia is higher in families that contain anorexics. Anorexia is unrelated to paranoid personality disorder. Eating disorder patients tend toward personality traits that are rigid and perfectionistic. They tend to be emotionally inflexible. Adolescence is a time of heightened risk. Patients may control eating as a reaction to other changes in their lives that are outside of their control.

K&S Ch. 23

9. **ABCD.**   Disorders which may be misdiagnosed as an eating disorder, or vice versa, include all listed in this question except brief psychotic disorder. In MDD weight loss often accompanies loss of appetite, sometimes severe weight loss. A thorough evaluation for symptoms of MDD should be done including an understanding of how the patient feels about the weight loss. In MDD the patient is not afraid of gaining weight. In anxiety disorders patients may lose weight due to changes in appetite due to anxiety, or issues surrounding obsessions. These patients should be screened carefully for areas in which anxiety may impede normal eating. Bulimia may be misdiagnosed as anorexia especially in cases of binge eating–purging anorexia. Keep the patient's body weight in mind as an important marker. Below 85% of expected body weight is considered anorexia whether they are purging or not. Substance abuse can often come along with severe weight loss

as patients do not eat properly and become malnourished. These patients do not fear gaining weight as an anorexic does.

K&S Ch. 23

10. **BCD.** There are a whole range of medical considerations which come along with anorexia. Combinations of estrogen and progesterone have not been shown to be successful at reversing osteopenia in anorexia. Dental follow-up is essential particularly for those who purge because the stomach acid eats away at tooth enamel over time and greatly increases risk of caries and tooth decay. Electrocardiogram is important as many anorexics develop hypokalemia leading to arrhythmias as well as changes in QTc interval. Correcting hypokalemia is necessary to prevent significant cardiac issues. Checking all electrolytes, administering vitamin supplementation, checking a CBC, and evaluation for severity of bone loss due to osteopenia are some of the other measures which should be considered.

K&S Ch. 23

Vignette Ten

1. **ACD.** Lisa clearly has some form of anxiety disorder based on the symptoms given in the vignette. As such, panic disorder, social phobia, and GAD should be included in a differential diagnosis and more questions should be asked to better determine the correct diagnosis. There is no mention of psychosis in the vignette, so schizoaffective disorder should not be included.

K&S Ch. 16

2. **ABC.** Based on Lisa's history the most likely diagnosis is social anxiety disorder. First line pharmacotherapy consists of SSRIs and SNRIs. Benzodiazepines can also be very effective at decreasing anxiety when the patient has to function in a specific social situation. Lisa has already been tried on sertraline with poor results. However we don't know what dosage was tried and for how long she was on the medication. She has also tried bupropion which tends to be very activating and can make anxiety worse. Our best bet would be to return to first line treatments and make sure they are given adequate therapeutic trials. Paroxetine and citalopram would both be considered first line. Clonazepam is a very reasonable add-on to one of these medications to control acute anxiety in specific social situations. Bupropion should be avoided for its potential to make anxiety worse.

K&S Ch. 16

3. **A.** Cognitive behavioral therapy has solid evidence behind its use in social anxiety disorder as well as other anxiety disorders. The other answer choices do not. CBT should be considered the first line psychotherapy for social anxiety disorder.

K&S Ch. 16

4. **AB.** Social anxiety disorder can overlap with or easily be misdiagnosed as schizoid personality disorder or avoidant personality disorder. Important to keep in mind is that in social phobia the patient fears embarrassment in social situations. In avoidant personality disorder the person fears rejection in relationships. In schizoid personality disorder the patient does not desire close relationships and is very happy without them.

K&S Ch. 16

5. **C.** Patients with social phobia can demonstrate avoidance of public restrooms and this is clearly mentioned in the DSM IV. Their fear is not a specific phobia of the sink, toilet, or room. Their fear is of being embarrassed if someone hears, sees, or smells them using the bathroom. As such it is a form of social phobia.

K&S Ch. 16

6. **C.** The non-generalized subtype of social phobia is performance anxiety. Successful treatment consists of beta adrenergic antagonists such as propranolol. These will decrease the physical manifestations of the anxiety. Always keep in mind that beta blockers are contraindicated in asthma due to their ability to cause bronchoconstriction. As such if given an asthmatic with performance anxiety one could choose a

low dose benzodiazepine or SSRI (which would be considered second line agents for social phobia) but don't give them a beta blocker. Also be careful with benzodiazepine doses if they have to speak publicly because of cognitive impairment.

K&S Ch. 16

7. **D.** Fear of embarrassment is the major fear of those with social phobia. It is present in all situations that they fear, whether it is using a public restroom or talking at a party. Fear of rejection is found most prominently in those with avoidant personality disorder. They often don't form relationships for fear of rejection. The need for someone to be with the patient in stressful or anxiety producing situations is a part of agoraphobia. The example is the person who won't leave their front gate without a friend or family member with them. Having someone with them doesn't help the avoidant or social phobia patient. Avoidance of relationships is most characteristic of the schizoid personality disorder patient, who neither has nor seeks close relationships. He is a loner and is happy that way. One could argue that avoiding relationships could also describe the avoidant patient, but the underlying motivation is different. The avoidant patient wants relationships but is afraid of rejection. The schizoid patient doesn't want them at all.

K&S Chs 16&17

8. **D.** According to DSM criteria, if the patient is under 18 years old the symptoms of social anxiety disorder must last for 6 months before the diagnosis is made. This makes sense as discomfort in social situations can be a normal part of adolescent development and we don't want to diagnose anyone prematurely or inappropriately.

K&S Ch. 16

9. **ABC.** Blushing, dry mouth, and sweating are all commonly seen in social phobia, as are muscle twitching and anxiety over scrutiny and embarrassment. Fear of dying is a more severe symptom which is seen in panic attacks, as would be dizziness and a sense of suffocation. Panic attacks can co-occur with social phobia but should be diagnosed as such if present. They are not a necessary part of the social phobia picture.

K&S Ch. 16

10. **A.** As many as one third of patients with social anxiety disorder also meet criteria for major depressive disorder. Many social phobia patients also have alcohol problems. This makes sense when you think about the availability of alcohol in social situations and its ability to take the edge off of their anxiety and allow them to better tolerate social interaction.

K&S Ch. 16

Vignette Eleven

1. **AB.** Of the choices given, the most likely to be in Carl's differential are sleep apnea and major depressive disorder. Carl is experiencing decreased energy, fatigue, decreased concentration and poor sleep. Sleeping longer hours is not making him feel rested or better. Both of these diagnoses can present this way. The warning signs suggesting sleep apnea are Carl's obesity and the snoring which drove his wife out of their bedroom. Sleep apnea can include morning headaches, long pauses without breathing during sleep, and waking up gasping for air. Because of the impact on mood and irritability it can masquerade as a psychiatric disorder and should be considered in overweight people who present looking depressed. Treatment for the disorder is a CPAP machine (continuous positive airway pressure).

Klein–Levin syndrome is a rare condition characterized by hypersomnia and hyperphagia. These patients can have mood changes but also show confusion, lack of sexual inhibitions, hallucinations, disorientation, memory impairment and incoherent speech. Periods of excessive sleeping can extend from days to months. This is not the picture we are seeing with Carl.

Narcolepsy is a pattern of excessive daytime sleepiness, sleep attacks, cataplexy, hypnagogic/hypnopompic hallucinations, and direct descent into REM sleep during sleep attacks. Sleep attacks are most common during heightened emotional states.

K&S Ch. 24

2. AD.   A workup for Carl should include thyroid function tests, as thyroid disorders can mimic mood disorders and must be ruled out. Nocturnal polysomnography (sleep study) is the test of choice to diagnose sleep apnea. A periodic limb movements of sleep test is not a real test. There is a periodic limb movements of sleep disorder (restless legs syndrome). It is diagnosed with nocturnal polysomnography, but there is not a special test with that name. CPAP is the machine used to treat sleep apnea. It does not diagnose sleep apnea. Therefore it would not be used as part of a workup.

K&S Ch. 24

3. ABD.   Possible complications of sleep apnea include decreased mood, increased risk of stroke, and cardiovascular complications. Patients with obstructive sleep apnea may have large necks but the sleep apnea doesn't cause their neck to get bigger. The big neck contributes to the collapse of airway when they're asleep.

K&S Ch. 24

4. B.   Sleep apnea is considered a dyssomnia. Dyssomnias are disorders relating to duration, quality, or timing of sleep. They can lead to too much sleep or too little sleep. Examples would be narcolepsy, sleep apnea, and circadian rhythm disorder. Parasomnias are disorders in which undesired behaviors occur during sleep or sleep transitions. Examples would be nightmare disorder, sleep terrors, or sleepwalking. Modafinil is used for narcolepsy, not sleep apnea. An increased risk for Parkinson's disease is seen in REM behavior disorder, not in sleep apnea.

K&S Ch. 24

5. D.   The differential diagnosis for sleep apnea should include insufficient sleep, gastroesophageal reflux, and nighttime panic attacks. Pavor nocturnus is another name for sleep terror disorder. It presents as sudden arousal from sleep with behavior indicative of extreme fear. The patient may be awake but disoriented. They won't remember the event the next day. Somnambulism is another name for sleepwalking disorder. It is more common in males. It can include retrograde amnesia as well as confusion. Treatment primarily involves maintaining safety for the patient. Jactatio capitis nocturna is a rhythmic movement disorder which includes head banging during sleep. Treatment involves preventing injury.

K&S Ch. 24

6. AD.   In obstructive sleep apnea airflow ceases during episodes and respiratory effort increases. This is in contrast to central sleep apnea where airflow stops and respiratory effort decreases. To be diagnosed with sleep apnea, the apnic episodes must last for 10 seconds or longer and occur a minimum of 30 times per night. In severe cases the patient may have as many as 300 episodes per night.

K&S Ch. 24

7. ABD.   Complications of obstructive sleep apnea include pulmonary and cardiovascular death, arrhythmias, transient alterations in blood pressure during each episode, pulmonary hypertension, and over time, an increase in systemic blood pressure which may be mistaken for essential hypertension.

K&S Ch. 24

8. BC.   REM sleep behavior disorder is a chronic progressive condition which is most often seen in men. There is a loss of atonia during REM sleep which leads to sometimes violent behaviors in which the patient acts out their dreams. Serious injury to the patient and those sleeping next to them is a risk. It tends to get worse with the use of stimulants, tricyclics and fluoxetine. Clonazepam and carbamazepine have proven effective in decreasing the symptoms.

K&S Ch. 24

9. ABC.   Sleep-related gastroesophageal reflux can cause awakening from sleep due to burning substernal pain or a sense of tightness in the chest. Coughing and choking sensations can occur repeatedly. Despite all of these symptoms airflow is not impeded as it is in sleep apnea. However given the symptoms, it is clear how this could be mistaken for sleep apnea.

K&S Ch. 24

10. ABD.   Sleep hygiene measures should be instituted in all patients with primary insomnia. They consist of arising at the same time each day, limit daily time in bed, discontinue any CNS activating drugs such as caffeine, avoid daytime naps, exercise, avoid evening stimulation, take hot baths before bed, avoid regular meals near bedtime, practice evening relaxation routines, and maintain comfortable sleeping conditions. The use of medication for sleep is considered treatment for insomnia but is not considered part of sleep hygiene.

K&S Ch. 24

Vignette Twelve

1. ABCE. Ryan is a complex case with a great deal of missing information. As such there are several diagnoses to be included on the differential. Schizophrenia should definitely be considered as a result of his command auditory hallucinations and aggression history. Substance-induced psychotic disorder should be included as he has a significant alcohol history and we don't have a urine toxicology on him so can't say for sure that he hasn't been using other drugs. Post-traumatic stress disorder needs to be explored because he has a very clear trauma history. He denies current flashbacks, but that is not enough data to rule out the diagnosis. Dementia NOS should be included because he only remembers one out of three objects on memory testing. This is clearly a poor result, but we have no idea what is causing it. He clearly had a concussion/head trauma in the past, he could have memory impairment due to chronic alcohol use or his poor performance on the exam could be a result of thought disorganization due to psychosis. His medical and cardiovascular risk factors place him at higher risk for vascular dementia. We don't have a clear understanding of his executive functioning. We just don't have enough information to know. As such, dementia NOS should be included until more information can be collected and we can clearly understand the pattern of symptoms we are seeing. The only disorder in the question that should not be included is generalized anxiety disorder. The vignette does not mention a single symptom of GAD.

K&S Chs 10,13&16

2. ABCDE. A workup for Ryan should include, but is not limited to the following items. Thyroid function tests to rule out a biological cause for a mood disorder which could be presenting with psychotic symptoms. (We don't have enough info in the vignette to rule this out as a possibility at this point.) Thiamine level should be included due to the possibility for Wernike–Korsakoff given the picture of heavy alcohol use and memory impairment. Head CT should be included to rule out possible organic cause of hallucinations and memory impairment, particularly with a history of head trauma. EKG should be included because of the need to treat CAH with antipsychotic medication and the need to monitor cardiac status during this process. In addition his hypertension, hypercholesterolemia, and diabetes put him at higher risk for heart disease. Urine toxicology should be included to rule out the possibility that other substances have been involved in this complex picture. The only one that should not be considered is prolactin level. The patient is not on any medication which would elevate prolactin at this point and as such there is no current need to monitor it.

K&S Chs 10,13&16

3. CD. If we were to treat Ryan with ziprasidone the most likely side effects would include sedation and cardiac effects. Ziprasidone does not cause significant weight gain or extrapyramidal symptoms like some of the other antipsychotics. The patient should be instructed to take ziprasidone with food for adequate absorption.

K&S Ch. 36

4. D. There is evidence that heavy cannabis use during early adolescence increases the relative risk of developing schizophrenia to as much as 6 times that of the general population.

K&S Ch. 13

5. BD. Criteria A for schizophrenia is defined as two or more of the following for 1 month: delusions, hallucinations, disorganized speech, disorganized behavior, and negative symptoms. Only one is needed if the initial psychotic symptom is a bizarre delusion, voices commenting directly on behavior, or two voices conversing. Psychosis lasting longer than a month that does not meet criteria A for schizophrenia can either be a delusional disorder or psychosis NOS. All of the other diagnostic options would meet criteria A. Schizotypal personality disorder is characterized by bizarre, odd, and magical thinking but florid psychosis is not part of the picture. As such it is not the right choice.

K&S Ch. 13

6. A. This question is important because it is antagonism at the 5HT2A receptor that makes the atypical antipsychotics atypical. It is through this mechanism that they help with negative symptoms rather than worsen them. Haloperidol is a typical neuroleptic and has no action on the 5HT2A receptor. Aripiprazole can be confusing because it is a partial agonist at D2 and 5HT1A but antagonizes 5HT2A.
K&S Ch. 36

7. CD. In delusional disorder auditory or visual hallucinations are not present but tactile, olfactory or gustatory hallucinations may be if related to the patient's delusions. Delusions are non-bizarre in delusional disorder. There is no memory impairment as in dementia (which may also present with psychosis). If the patient has delusional disorder somatic type then unnecessary medical interventions are quite likely.
K&S Ch. 14

8. D. In brief psychotic disorder symptoms last between one day and one month after which the patient returns to normal functioning. It may be characterized by hallucinations, delusions, paranoia, disorganized speech and behavior, even catatonia. Antipsychotics are used to treat the episode while it is ongoing. There are no known primary preventative measures.
K&S Ch. 14

9. ABCD. All of the following statements are true. Tactile hallucinations are more common in medical and neurologic conditions than in schizophrenia. Illusions are sensory misperceptions of actual stimuli. Delusions are fixed false beliefs which are not supported by cultural norms. Word salad is the violation of basic rules of grammar seen in severe thought disorder. Cataplexy is the sudden loss of muscle tone seen in narcolepsy attacks. Catalepsy is synonymous with waxy flexibility.
K&S Chs 13&14

10. ABCD. The differential diagnosis for new onset psychosis should include many medical conditions. Among them are systemic lupus erythematosus, temporal lobe epilepsy, neurosyphilis, Wilson's disease, AIDS, B12 deficiency, heavy metal poisoning, delirium, dementia, Huntington's disease, pellagra, tumor, stroke, or bleed, herpes encephalitis, or autism. Phymatous rosacea is a skin disorder that has nothing to do with psychosis.
K&S Chs 13&14

Vignette Thirteen

1. BE. This is a straightforward case with respect to initial early management. The predominant determinant of your actions as an emergency room psychiatrist is based on the principles of maintaining staff and patient safety and collecting more data, before approaching more complex workup and disposition decisions. As an emergency room psychiatrist it is imperative to collect as much history and collateral information as possible. The primary source of that information in this case is from police and emergency medical technicians, because there are no identified family members or collaterals from whom one might obtain information. Once a proper history of events is obtained, further workup, management and disposition planning can be made.

Even before obtaining a history though, the psychiatrist must ensure that the patient and staff in the emergency room are safe. Safety of patient and others comes before all in an acute or emergency room setting. To this end, the psychiatrist's first maneuver should be to have the agitated or aggressive patient restrained and medicated so that no acute harm comes to the patient or the staff that are attending to him. Haloperidol, with or without lorazepam, when given intramuscularly, is an excellent choice of management. The initial dosage depends upon the age and body size of the individual, as well as the severity of the agitation. An initial dose of haloperidol 5 mg intramuscularly can be repeated every 20–30 minutes (with or without addition of lorazepam) until sedation ensues. With the advent of short-acting, atypical antipsychotic agents, such as aripiprazole, ziprasidone and olanzapine, strong consideration should be given to these agents, given their superior safety and tolerability profile.
K&S Ch. 4

2. CD. There are many well-described risk factors for aggressive behavior in patients. Many major mental illnesses predispose the patient to potential acting out and acts of violence directed against others. These conditions include: mental retardation; ADHD; conduct disorder; delirium; dementia; psychotic disorders; mood disorders; intermittent explosive disorder; adjustment disorder with disturbance of conduct and cluster B personality disorders. The likelihood of violence to others increases during periods of decompensation in major mental disorders. Acute use of alcohol or other substances of abuse can also trigger acute dangerousness to others. The frequency of violence among males outweighs that in females, when it comes to homicide, assault and battery, or rape. With respect to domestic violence episodes, the rates of outward violence are about equal in both sexes. The most tell-tale predictor of violence is, of course, a history of prior violent behavior. Being a battered, underprivileged child predisposes the individual to a future likelihood of violent behavior. Low educational level, having poor family supports, unstable housing, unemployment, and poor coping skills or a lack of resources for help, can all be contributors to homicidality and violence. Medical problems, unless they involve acute or chronic physical pain, do not typically predict violent acts of aggression in individuals.

K&S Ch. 4

3. **ACD.** The psychiatrist should attempt to conduct an assessment with a potentially violent patient in a way that promotes containment of the behavior and limits the potential for harm. There are several steps that a psychiatrist can take to try to minimize the patient's agitation and potential risk. The interview should be conducted in a calm, quiet and nonstimulating area. Sufficient physical space should be available for both patient and psychiatrist, with no physical barrier to leaving the room for either one. The psychiatrist should avoid any kind of behavior that might be misconstrued by the patient as threatening, such as standing over the patient, touching the patient, or staring at the patient. The psychiatrist should ask whether the patient is carrying weapons, but should not ask the patient to hand over any weapons. Assistance from security personnel, as well as physical or chemical restraints, may be helpful if the psychiatrist deems these to be appropriate.

K&S Ch. 7

4. **BEF.** The patient is voicing homicidal ideation and perhaps even intention, directed at his mother. Psychiatrists can be sued for failing to protect society from the violent acts of their patients if it was reasonable for the psychiatrist to have known about the patient's violent tendencies and if the psychiatrist could have done something to safeguard the public. The landmark case of *Tarasoff v. Regents of the University of California*, resulted in the California Supreme Court ruling that mental health professionals have a duty to protect identifiable, endangered third parties from threats of imminent and serious harm made by their outpatients. In this case, the psychiatrist is certainly acting quite responsibly in wanting to contact the patient's mother to inform her of the patient's feelings and possible intentions of harm directed against her. Of course, the psychiatrist in this case, should not discharge the patient, particularly if the patient continues to voice these feelings and intentions.

In this case, the most conservative course of action would be to admit the patient to the psychiatry unit, most likely on an involuntary basis, given his lack of cooperation with you in the emergency room. This would enable safety, stabilization and further history taking to take place simultaneously in a confined clinical setting, with the highest level of care and clinical attention to the patient. It would not be wrong to detain the patient overnight in the emergency room so that a social work consultation can be obtained in the morning, focused on obtaining more detailed history and collateral information about the patient and also adding more weight to the disposition plan for the patient. There is no evidence in this vignette that the police have intentions to arrest and charge the patient with a crime once he is psychiatrically cleared in the emergency room. Typically, police officers will inform the psychiatrist or the triage nurse of this so that they can be contacted to pick the patient up upon discharge to bring the patient to the police station for booking. Starting aripiprazole and divalproex sodium is pre-emptive and presumptive of a psychotic or bipolar disorder that warrants ongoing medication management of this kind. There is no indication of any such diagnosis in this vignette given that too little symptomatic information is presented.

K&S Ch. 58

5. **AB.** Given the patient's refusal of oral medication, the psychiatrist should begin thinking about the need for a long-acting, injectable antipsychotic agent to ensure the patient's compliance and stability. Of the six agents listed in answers A through F, only olanzapine and risperidone have long-acting injectable formulations (Zyprexa Relprevv and Risperdal Consta). These would be the two agents of choice in this

case, given the current presentation of patient's refusal to take oral medications on a voluntary basis. Olanzapine and risperidone also come in oral disintegrating tablet formulation (Zydis and M-tabs, respectively). This may be an advantage to the psychiatrist, if the patient eventually agrees to take oral medication. The melting tablets can be given by nursing staff while the patient is directly observed. This formulation prevents the cheeking or spitting out of medication once it has been placed in the oral cavity. If the patient is not acutely agitated, but refuses oral medication, a court petition for medication-over-objection may need to be presented to a judge, depending on the state.

K&S Chs 36&58

6. BCD.   In this case, the patient needs a higher level of outpatient mental health care than a simple outpatient clinic setting. This stems from the fact that he has failed this level of care previously and has relapsed numerous times in the past. He also has a history of noncompliance with medication and very poor insight and judgment with respect to his mental illness and how to cope with it. The assertive community treatment team (ACT team) model exists in most states in the USA. It is truly the highest level of outpatient mental health care because the treatment team visits the patient at the patient's residence multiple times every month. The team helps the patient with medication monitoring and management and in many cases can prevent patient noncompliance that may result in an acute decompensation. The program was developed in the 1970s by researchers in Madison, Wisconsin. The patient is assigned to a treatment team that is composed of a psychiatrist, nurse, social workers, case managers and other possible interventionists. The team can provide care and clinical coverage virtually 24 hours a day, 7 days a week. The high staff-to-patient ratio (anywhere from 6 to 12 staff per patient) enables the ACT team to help the patient with a rich variety of case management modalities and options.

Partial hospital programs are useful for refractory patients who are discharged from the hospital. These programs are designed to be time-limited and are a step-down from the acute inpatient setting for the patient. These partial hospitals offer a less restrictive level of care for the chronic psychiatric patient, while maintaining a well-structured framework that is close to that offered on an inpatient hospital unit. The patient sleeps at home and comes to the partial hospital each day to attend programming and get physician and nursing care during the day, as well as case management and psychotherapy. Classically, patients can spend up to 12 to 16 weeks in these programs following an acute hospitalization. They should then be discharged to a less-restrictive outpatient level of care for ongoing maintenance care.

The continuing day treatment program for the chronically mentally ill is also an excellent choice for the patient presented in this vignette. These programs run 5 to 7 days a week and provide a less structured, though comprehensive, treatment modality for these patients. Patients sleep at home and attend the program during the day, where they receive a similar array of therapies to that which is available in the partial hospital setting. Key to this modality (and that of the partial hospital as well) is the fact that nursing staff can administer oral and injectable medication on site and while directly observing the patient. The census of a day program is usually greater than that of a partial hospital program, due to the fact that the psychiatrist will usually see and evaluate the patient less often in the day treatment program setting.

K&S Ch. 13

Vignette Fourteen

1. DE.   Attitude in the mental status exam describes the patient's attitude towards the examiner. Words commonly used include cooperative, friendly, interested, seductive, defensive, hostile, evasive, apathetic, ingratiating, and guarded. Based on the information in this vignette the patient is best described as cooperative and friendly.

K&S Ch. 7

2. B.   Affect is the patient's present emotional responsiveness based on facial expressions and expressive behavior. It may or may not be congruent with mood. Words used to describe affect include full range (within normal range), constricted, blunted, and flat. Full range would be considered normal. Flat would be used to describe a patient who is showing no signs of affective expression. A patient with constricted affect shows less emotion than someone who is full range but more than someone who is blunted. Someone who is blunted shows less emotion than someone who is constricted but more than someone who is flat.

K&S Ch. 7

3. **DE.**   Thought process refers to the form of the patient's thoughts. Examples of this would be goal directed, linear, circumstantial, tangential, loosening of associations, flight of ideas, thought blocking, neologisms, racing thoughts, or word salad. In this case Robert's thoughts are completely normal and as such the best description would be linear or goal directed.

K&S Ch. 7

4. **A.**   Impulse control refers to the patient's ability to control sexual, aggressive and other impulses. It may be determined based on recent history and the patient's behavior during the interview. It is often rated as good, fair, or poor.

K&S Ch. 7

5. **A.**   Insight is the patient's understanding and awareness of his or her own illness. It can be rated as good, fair, or poor.

K&S Ch. 7

6. **A.**   Judgment is reflection of the patient's capacity for good social judgment. What kind of decisions are they making? Do they understand the outcome of their behavior? Can they predict what they would do in imaginary situations? It can be rated as good, fair, or poor.

K&S Ch. 7

7. **A.**   Perceptions primarily refers to hallucinations, be they auditory, visual, tactile, olfactory, or gustatory. In Robert's case there are none present. Choices B, C, D, and E may be true for Robert but they were never asked about in the vignette and Robert never mentioned any of them. Therefore we have no evidence of whether he is experiencing them or not.

K&S Ch. 7

8. **A.**   Sialorrhea (excessive drooling) is a common and predictable side effect of clozapine. Robert and his doctor should keep an eye on it but it is not a reason to stop the medication if the patient can tolerate it. It may get worse with a dosage increase.

K&S Ch. 7

9. **C.**   The appropriate schedule for measuring WBC/ANC in a patient on Clozapine would include a baseline WBC/ANC, weekly WBC/ANC for the first 6 months, biweekly WBC/ANC for the next 6 months, and monthly WBC/ANC thereafter.

K&S Ch. 36

10. **ABCDEFG.**   All of the tests listed except an echocardiogram would be appropriate to monitor in Robert over time. EKG is important for anyone on antipsychotics, paying special attention to the QTc interval. Clozapine is metabolized through the liver so LFT's are important. A clozapine level to ensure a therapeutic dose is important. Fasting glucose, weights, waist circumference, triglycerides, and cholesterol are all important parts of monitoring for metabolic syndrome, which we know clozapine has a high likelihood to cause.

K&S Ch. 36

Vignette Fifteen

1. **AC.**   There are very few studies on dissociative identity disorder (DID), so very little epidemiological data exists on the subject. Studies have pointed towards a female to male ratio of diagnosed cases as somewhere between 5 and 10 to 1. The disorder is principally linked to severe early childhood trauma experiences, usually abuse, neglect, or maltreatment. The rates of reported trauma in adult sufferers of DID range from 85 to 97%. Physical and sexual abuse are most frequently reported as the type of childhood trauma sustained by sufferers of DID. Studies have not, up until now at any rate, demonstrated much in the way of a genetic component to the disorder. About 70% of DID patients also meet criteria for post-traumatic stress disorder (PTSD). A key DSM criterion for DID is the inability of the patient to recall important personal information that is too extensive to

be explained by ordinary forgetfulness. About 40 to 60% of DID patients also meet criteria for somatization disorder. Psychotherapy is a key component in the progress and recovery of the DID patient. Those modalities that have been seen to be useful to DID patients include supportive psychotherapy, dynamic psychotherapy, cognitive therapy and hypnotherapy.

K&S Ch. 20

2. BF.   Group psychotherapy can be very useful in DID, but it is better conducted only with patients with this disorder because of the tendency of other patients to be overly fascinated or frightened by these patients. Prognosis of DID is poorer in patients with comorbid organic mental disorders, psychotic disorders, and severe medical illnesses. Refractory substance abuse disorders and eating disorders are also thought to worsen the prognosis of patients with DID. As far as appropriate medication choices are concerned, patients with DID may benefit from a low-dose benzodiazepine, which may help to diminish anxiety, hyperarousal, panic, and intrusive symptoms suffered by these patients. A proper substance abuse history should be taken prior to starting any benzodiazepine of course. Patients that are able to maintain a high level of daily functioning tend to do better with this condition than those that are lower functioning.

K&S Ch. 20

3. D.   There are many valid choices of medication to address the myriad of symptoms that may accompany DID. Lithium is not one of them. It has no place as a mood stabilizer in DID, unless there is a concomitant diagnosis of bipolar disorder. On the other hand the anticonvulsant and antipsychotic mood stabilizing agents are excellent choices for DID patients. These include: divalproex sodium, lamotrigine, gabapentin, topiramate, carbamazepine, risperidone, quetiapine, olanzapine, and ziprasidone. The SSRI class of antidepressants also has been shown to be efficacious in reducing the symptoms associated with DID. These of course include fluoxetine, paroxetine, sertraline, citalopram, and escitalopram. These are useful for depressive symptoms and mood lability, but may be less effective for the intrusive hyperarousal symptoms of PTSD often associated with DID.

K&S Ch. 20

4. E.   Dissociative identity disorder is conceptualized as a trauma spectrum disorder. Many patients with DID, up to 70%, meet criteria for PTSD. About 40 to 60% of patients with DID also meet criteria for somatization disorder. Many DID patients also meet criteria for a mood disorder, in particular the depressive disorders. Frequent rapid mood swings are also seen commonly in DID patients. These mood swings are not believed to be bipolar in nature, but are believed to be post-traumatic and dissociative in nature and not true cyclic mood disorder.

K&S Ch. 20

5. CE.   Patients with dissociative identity disorder must be ruled out for malingering, factitious disorder, conversion disorder and somatoform disorders. The following indicators may point a clinician away from DID as a diagnosis and towards one of these psychosomatic disorders: increased symptoms when under observation, refusal to allow collateral contacts, symptom exaggeration, outright lies, using fabricated symptoms to excuse antisocial behavior, or a history of legal issues. Patients with veritable DID are generally conflicted, confused, ashamed and distressed by their symptoms. Patients with nongenuine DID often show little dysphoria about their disorder.

K&S Ch. 20

Vignette Sixteen

1. CE.   Mr. Moran is showing the signs and symptoms of progressive memory and executive function decline that are compatible with a dementia. Dementia is defined as a progressive loss of cognitive functioning in the presence of a clear sensorium. The basic faculties that are affected include memory, thinking, attention and comprehension. Dementia can be caused by different etiological factors, and can be multifactorial. About 15% of demented patients have reversible illness if treatment is rendered prior to the development of irreversible damage. Mr. Moran's presentation could well be that of a dementia of the Alzheimer type. He has been confused and forgetful, which are cardinal features of Alzheimer's dementia. He has also been wandering aimlessly and cannot remember his way around familiar territory. This is

essentially a visual agnosia; is presented with places that are familiar to him, but he does not remember them or recognize them and he cannot negotiate his way around them. Part of the essential criteria for Alzheimer's dementia are the classic cognitive disturbances of aphasia, apraxia, agnosia and disturbance in executive functioning. A patient must have at least one of these four deficits, with marked memory impairment, in order to meet criteria for dementia of the Alzheimer type. Mr. Moran also forgets the names of household items. This is both an agnosia (he cannot name/recognize objects) and an apraxia (he has forgotten how to use certain common items).

Now, Mr. Moran could certainly be suffering from a vascular dementia, or a combination of a vascular dementia with Alzheimer's dementia. The differential diagnosis of vascular dementia presents itself in this case by the patient's medical history. The patient, we are told, has a history of hypertension, diabetes, hyperlipidemia, and cardiovascular disease. He is a vasculopath and certainly these cardiovascular risk factors are also stroke risk factors. He could be having repeated silent strokes that eventually begin to compromise his cognitive functioning. The medical and neurological examination and work-up will help you clarify which type of dementia is the more likely to be the culprit of his decline in functioning in this case.

Note that there is no mention in this vignette of any manifestation of depression or anxiety, which make these two answers incorrect in this case. As for the possibility of a dementia due to diffuse Lewy-body disease or a frontotemporal dementia, these are very specific dementing entities that present with their own specific set of symptoms and signs, none of which are really mentioned in this vignette. We urge you to refer to other question explanations in this volume that elaborate on these two special types of dementias. They do appear frequently on standardized examinations and it is essential to know their features.

K&S Ch. 10

2. CFG.   A medical and neurological workup are essential for this patient to help you clarify your differential diagnosis. You should be thinking about a dementia of the Alzheimer type, a vascular dementia, or a dementia with features of both Alzheimer and vascular types. An outpatient brain imaging study is essential. The MRI is best, as it affords the most anatomic detail and its sensitivity to ischemic lesions is much greater than CT scan. A brain tumor is not completely out of the realm of possibility in this case, and the MRI can be performed with gadolinium contrast administration to see if there is a presence of any enhancing space-occupying lesion that could be responsible for this patient's cognitive impairment.

Neuropsychological consultation for a testing battery can be extremely valuable in a case such as this. A thorough battery includes testing for cognitive and executive functioning and is highly sensitive to subtle deficits in cognition, visuospatial abilities, and multitasking and reasoning skills. In the face of a negative or nonspecific medical workup, such a battery may lend weight to a subtle diagnosis of Alzheimer's dementia.

An electroencephalogram is not a high priority in this case. There is no evidence of seizure activity, or anything remotely resembling ictal events, from the history given in this vignette. For such a test to be useful, a picture of repeated discrete events that involve waxing and waning of attention and awareness should be a part of the presenting history, which it is not in this case.

Starting medication can be useful for this patient, but which one(s)? There is no evidence of depressive symptoms or sleep disturbance presented in this case history. Therefore, sertraline and trazodone would not be very helpful at this juncture. On the other hand, the case history points strongly in the direction of a dementia, and donepezil would be an excellent choice to start, even before a workup is conducted and a diagnosis solidified. Donepezil (Aricept) is FDA-approved for Alzheimer's dementia and it may have efficacy in vascular dementia as well, though the FDA did not approve the agent for this indication. The dosing is simple: 5 mg daily for the first month, increasing to 10 mg daily thereafter. New evidence suggests further titration to the new 23 mg daily dose may be more beneficial in maintaining cognition than the former 10 mg dosing. Donepezil can always be stopped if the diagnosis of Alzheimer's dementia is brought into question once a workup has been completed on this particular patient.

K&S Ch. 10

3. BCF.   This patient is getting to be too much to handle at home, without outside support, assistance and guidance. Soon, his daughter will become a patient herself, because her emotional and physical burden of caring for the patient will cause her caregiver burnout. Thus, referring the patient's daughter to caregiver support programming and groups is a wise thing to do. Obtaining a visiting nurse consultation in the

patient's home is also an excellent maneuver in this case. A homecare nurse can assess the patient's basic homecare needs and make appropriate recommendations to his physicians for these services. Ultimately, if around the clock homecare is not feasible for the patient and his family members, consideration will have to be given to skilled nursing facility placement, if his condition continues to deteriorate, which we might expect to happen in this particular case.

An ACT team referral is quite inappropriate in this case. Such teams are unable to provide the broad-based medical, nursing and homecare that this patient will eventually need. ACT teams are based on a psychiatric model and are charged with the responsibility of helping mental health patients to maintain their stability in the outpatient setting, despite a lack of insight and ability to do so themselves. Medical issues that are deeply complex, such as in this case, are far too burdensome for ACT teams, that have only a psychiatric nurse and a psychiatrist among their team members. Family members can certainly provide coverage at home for this patient, if he begins to become home-bound. This, however, is not ideal, as family members are not usually trained to this intense medical task and they generally have to sacrifice their own lives and well-being to tend to their relative. A subacute rehabilitation facility is hardly an appropriate placement for this patient. Such facilities are geared towards patients that need intensive physical therapy to restore their ambulatory functioning. These placements are deemed to be temporary and the expectation is that these patients will recover functional ability and eventually make their way home, whenever possible.

K&S Ch. 10

4. C.   Alzheimer type dementia has an average survival expectancy of about 8 years from the time of initial onset of the disease. Studies typically point to a range from about 5 to 10 years of survival for these patients. Note that more than 50% of nursing home beds in the USA are occupied by patients with Alzheimer's dementia.

K&S Ch.10

5. ADG.   Alzheimer's dementia is treated with either an acetylcholinesterase inhibitor, a NMDA antagonist, or both together. The three acetylcholinesterase inhibitors currently in use in the US include donepezil, rivastigmine and galantamine. The NMDA antagonist that is FDA-approved for Alzheimer's dementia is memantine.

With respect to the treatment and prevention of vascular dementia, the approach is to treat modifiable underlying risk factors for cerebrovascular disease. These measures include prescribing antiplatelet aggregants such as aspirin, clopidogrel, or aspirin/dipyridamole combination therapy (Aggrenox). Antihypertensive medication, antidiabetic medications and insulin, as well as lipid-lowering medications all have a place in the treatment and prevention of further worsening of cerebrovascular disease. Smoking cessation is ultimately a very important recommendation to patients in this regard as well.

The other agents mentioned in answer choices B, C, E and F have no real place in the treatment of dementia itself, though they may be useful in treatment associated comorbid symptoms and problems.

K&S Ch. 10

6. F.   Dementia is often accompanied by other devastating symptoms that are associated with cognitive decline. Patients can often be seen to exhibit subtle or gross personality changes that are uncharacteristic for them when at baseline. They may become depressed and unmotivated for self care, even if they still have the cognitive capacity to engage in this behavior. Aggression and violent verbal and physical outbursts can be seen in moderate to late-stage Alzheimer's dementia. Sundowner syndrome can also be seen, which occurs when day–night cycle is disrupted by a lack of external light or lack of cues as to the date, season and time of day. Patients in this instance can become delirious, aggressive, agitated and acutely more confused as the day proceeds and may need sedation to abort such episodes. Such episodes may also be accompanied by frank delusions and hallucinations. Mania, however, is not typically seen in dementing patients, unless they have a history of bipolar or schizoaffective disorder with such episodes in the past.

K&S Ch. 10

7. DE.   Benztropine (Cogentin) and diphenhydramine (Benadryl) are dangerous in the demented patient because their anticholinergic properties can worsen cognitive impairment and cause greater confusion in these

patients. Patients exposed to these agents may also develop an anticholinergic delirium and may require sedation due to agitation and disinhibition of their behavior. The rest of the medication choices listed are all viable therapies for the patient presented in this vignette.

K&S Ch. 10

Vignette Seventeen

1. **AE.** Wanda of course is suffering from a delirium. Delirium is characterized by a waxing and waning of level of consciousness and a cognitive impairment that evolves over a short period of time. Common associated psychiatric symptoms include mood disturbance, perceptual disturbance, and behavioral disturbance. Delirium usually evolves rapidly over a period of hours or days.Irritability, impulsivity, anger, and rage, can all be seen at times within the constellation of symptoms that make up a delirium. Cognitive deficits can manifest as memory and language impairment. There may be noted incoordination (apraxia) in certain cases of delirium as well. Patients with delirium often have disturbance of sleep and/or of the sleep-wake circadian cycle. Identification and reversal of underlying causes of delirium are the cornerstones of treatment of the disorder.

K&S Ch. 10

2. **ADE.** Wanda is of course suffering from an acute delirium. Delirium is defined as an acute onset of waxing and waning level of consciousness, with impairment in cognitive functioning. Recognizing a delirium is important so that identifying the underlying causes can be undertaken and appropriate measures taken to treat and prevent these causes. Delirium prevalence is highest in postcardiotomy patients. Some studies point to these rates as high as 90%. Advanced age is a risk factor for delirium, but generally in the over 70-year-old population. About 30 to 40% of hospitalized patients over age 65 have an episode of delirium. Preexisting brain damage or disease is a serious risk factor for delirium. This patient has multiple sclerosis and is in the midst of an acute exacerbation of that disease. This certainly predisposes her to an acute delirium. A history of alcohol abuse or tobacco smoking is also a risk factor for an acute delirium. Diabetes, cancer, blindness and malnutrition are also delirium risk factors. Hypertension, in and of itself, is not a risk factor for delirium. According to DSM-IV-TR, the male gender is an independent risk factor for delirium. Intoxication or withdrawal from pharmacologic or toxic agents is certainly a strong risk factor for delirium. The fact that Wanda is on interferon at home and methylprednisolone in the hospital, can predispose her to a delirium. Classic medications that can predispose patients to a delirium include narcotic painkillers, steroids, anesthetic agents, antineoplastic agents and anticholinergic agents and antibiotics, antifungals and antiviral agents.

K&S Ch. 10

3. **D.** The exact pathophysiology of delirium is not well-understood. The major neuroanatomical area implicated in delirium is the reticular formation. The reticular formation is the area of the brainstem responsible for regulation of attention and arousal. The major pathway implicated in the etiology of delirium is the dorsal tegmental pathway. This pathway projects from the mesencephalic reticular formation to the tectum and thalamus.

K&S Ch. 10

4. **B.** The complex pathophysiology of delirium is not well understood. Studies tend to point towards decreased acetylcholine activity in the brain as a causative factor in delirium. The delirium associated with alcohol withdrawal has been associated with hyperactivity of noradrenergic neurons in the locus ceruleus. Serotonin and glutamate have also been implicated in the pathophysiology of delirium.

K&S Ch. 10

5. **C.** The EEG characteristically shows generalized background slowing in delirium. Triphasic waves are mostly specific for a hepatic encephalopathy and not for delirium of other etiologies. PLEDS is the characteristic EEG finding in herpes simplex virus encephalitis. Temporal lobe spikes would be indicative of a seizure focus in the temporal lobe. Hypsarrhythmia is an EEG pattern of high amplitude waves and spikes on a chaotic disorganized background that is characteristic of infantile spasms.

K&S Ch. 10

6. **CE.** Psychosis and insomnia are the two major symptoms of delirium that are likely to warrant medication management. Haloperidol, a butyrophenone antipsychotic agent, is the most commonly used sedative agent used in cases of hospital-based delirium. It can be given orally, intramuscularly or intravenously, though the intravenous route of administration is not FDA-approved. Despite that fact, intravenous haloperidol is standard of care for this type of patient in an intensive care unit setting. Note that a monitored bed is essential when giving intravenous haloperidol because of the risk of torsades de pointes, a potentially fatal cardiac arrhythmia. Use of atypical antipsychotics such as risperidone, olanzapine, quetiapine and aripiprazole are felt to be effective in delirium management, though there is a dearth of studies to lend evidence to this management. Anticholinergic drugs like diphenhydramine and benztropine, along with phenothiazine antipsychotics such as chlorpromazine, are very poor choices in delirium management. Use of such drugs can prolong or even worsen the delirium, rather than improve it, and so they are to be avoided in delirium management. Insomnia can be treated with short or intermediate half-life benzodiazepines such as lorazepam. However, any benzodiazepine can have a paradoxically agitating effect on patients with delirium. Thus the use of these agents is generally reserved for patients with known alcohol-withdrawal delirium (delirium tremens).

K&S Ch. 10

7. **BEF.** Even though the onset of delirium is usually acute and sudden in nature, premonitory or prodromal symptoms can be seen in the days (not months!) preceding the onset of florid symptoms. The symptoms of delirium usually persist while causally relevant factors are present, though typical duration of episodes is usually about 1 week. The more advanced the age of the patient and the longer the delirium episode lasts, the longer the delirium usually takes to resolve. Delirium is known to increase patient mortality within the first year following an episode. This is due mostly to the serious nature of the concomitant medical problems that lead to the delirium. Controlled studies have not been conducted to demonstrate that delirium typically progresses to a dementia. Nevertheless, many clinicians believe this to be the case. It is however well understood that periods of delirium may lead to symptoms of depression or post-traumatic stress disorder in the aftermath of the episode.

K&S Ch. 10

Vignette Eighteen

1. **D.** Allan is of course suffering from body dysmorphic disorder (BDD). The cause of this disorder is unknown. There is a high comorbidity with depressive disorders. Patients with BDD often have family histories of mood disorders and obsessive-compulsive disorder. In many patients with BDD, the symptoms are responsive to serotonin-specific medications, which leads researchers to feel that the disorder itself is related to imbalances in serotonin.

K&S Ch. 17

2. **C.** All of the answers are valid psychodynamic explanations for adulthood neurosis. However, the most accurate explanation of BDD symptoms falls under the defense mechanism of a displacement of sexual or emotional conflict onto body parts unrelated to the issue. The defense mechanisms of repression, projection, distortion, dissociation and symbolization also are in play in this dynamic.

K&S Ch. 17

3. **AC.** Data indicate that BDD typically has its initial onset between the ages of 15 and 30 years. In this regard, Allan is quite typical. Women are more affected than men, though slightly. So in this regard, Allan would be considered atypical. Most sufferers of BDD are unmarried and in this regard Allan is among the majority. The fact that Allan has never suffered a major depressive episode in the past is quite atypical of BDD. There is a high comorbidity of BDD with mood and depressive disorders. One study found that 90% of BDD sufferers had experienced a major depressive episode in their lifetimes. The fact that Allan is high-functioning and spends a lot of money on himself and his appearance has no bearing on his BDD at all.

K&S Ch. 17

4. **ACE.** Pharmacotherapy for BDD is usually approached first-line with serotonergic agents such as SSRIs, MAOIs, or TCAs. These serotonergic agents are typically effective at reducing symptoms in about 50%

of patients. Augmentation with buspirone, lithium, methylphenidate, or an atypical antipsychotic is appropriate if first-line therapy is ineffective.

K&S Ch. 17

5. C.   BDD usually begins during the adolescent years. The onset can be gradual or abrupt. The disorder usually has an undulating course with few symptom-free intervals. The part of the body on which concern is focused may remain the same or it may change over time. The preoccupation with imagined defects is almost always associated with significant distress and impairment.

K&S Ch. 17

Vignette Nineteen

1. CEF.   Of course, Grace meets DSM criteria for a somatization disorder and not for a conversion disorder. Remember that a somatization disorder begins before age 30 and symptoms persist over a period of years. The somatization disorder diagnosis requires the presence of the specific list of symptoms from multiple systems at any time during the course of the disorder. Specifically, the patient must have at least four pain symptoms, two gastrointestinal symptoms, one sexual symptom and one pseudoneurological symptom. Conversion disorder differentiates from somatization disorder by manifesting as only a pseudoneurological symptom or symptoms, which typically involve motor or sensory functioning. Other bodily systems, gastrointestinal and sexual are not part of the clinical picture of conversion disorder. Note that pain symptoms fall in a nebulous category that encompasses both the physical and neurological and so could be a part of either a somatization or conversion disorder. Recall that conversion and somatization disorders are both disorders in which the patient's symptoms are not being voluntarily produced. They are manifested involuntarily as a product of psychological distress and interpersonal problems. Most often, these triggering conflicts are subconscious, though patients may at times be able to identify stressors and triggers when asked about them. Another classic difference between these two disorders is the way in which patients react emotionally to their symptoms. Somatization disorder patients often describe their symptoms in a more histrionic, emotional, and exaggerated fashion. Conversion disorder patients typically display la belle indifference, which is simply an inappropriately cavalier attitude towards serious symptoms and a marked unconcern regarding what may appear to be serious impairment.

K&S Ch. 17

2. ACF.   There are multiple etiological theories that attempt to explain the complexity of somatization disorder. Certainly, psychosocial factors can play a great role in the presentation of this disorder. Many such patients are found to originate from unstable homes, with histories of physical abuse. Psychodynamically, the symptom presentation may be conceptualized as a manifestation of repressed instinctual impulses. Biological factors seem to point to a neuropsychological relation of somatization disorder to attention deficit symptoms or disorders. Studies using evoked potentials have proposed a link between the somatic symptoms and those of excessive distractibility, inability to habituate to repetitive stimuli, and lack of stimulus selectivity. A small number of neuroimaging studies have demonstrated decreased frontal lobe and nondominant hemisphere metabolism.

Genetic factors may also play a role in the etiology of somatization disorder. The disorder tends to run in families and occurs in approximately 10 to 20% of the first degree female relatives of probands of patients with somatization disorder. One study demonstrated a 29% concordance rate of somatization disorder in monozygotic twins and 10% in dizygotic twins. Male relatives of women with somatization disorder show an increased risk of antisocial personality disorder and substance-related disorders. The other answer choices have no proven relationship to the etiology of somatization disorder and are merely nonsense distracters.

K&S Ch. 17

3. ACD.   Women with somatization disorder tend to outnumber men with the disorder by about 5 to 20 times. The lifetime prevalence of the disorder in the general population is about 1 or 2%. Among general primary care patients, patients with somatization disorder may number about 5 to 10%. The disorder is inversely related to social position and occurs most often in patients with low income and little education. Somatization disorder must begin before age 30 and typically begins in the teenage years. Two

disorders that are not more commonly seen in patients with somatization disorder include bipolar I disorder and substance abuse.

K&S Ch. 17

4. BCD.   Somatization disorder is a chronic, undulating and relapsing disorder that rarely remits completely. Patients with the disorder are no more likely to develop another medical illness in the next 20 years than patients who do not have somatization disorder. A patient with somatization disorder has about an 80% chance of being diagnosed with the disorder 5 years later. It is unusual for patients with somatization disorder to be symptom-free for more than a year. The prognosis of the disorder overall is poor to fair at best.

K&S Ch. 17

5. D.   Both individual and group psychotherapy seems to be the most useful strategy for somatization disorder, as these have been shown to reduce patients' personal health expenditure by 50%. This is so because psychotherapy helps to decrease rates of hospitalization in these patients. Giving psychotropic medications to these patients, even when somatization disorder is accompanied by a mood or anxiety disorder, is a risk. This is because these patients are notorious for marginal or poor compliance with such medications. There is very little data that exists to support the use of psychotropic medications in somatization disorder when it is not comorbid with other mental disorders.

K&S Ch. 17

Vignette Twenty

1. ACF.   Pain and opioid dependence, when they coexist, make up one of the most delicate and difficult disease combinations to treat effectively. This is even more complex when alcohol and cannabis abuse cloud and complicate the clinical scenario. Detoxification of the patient off of the painkillers, as well as alcohol and cannabis, on an inpatient basis is certainly an excellent maneuver. Once the patient comes out of the inpatient facility, a subsequent referral to pain management and perhaps physiatry would be ideal, because the patient will certainly need to have his pain addressed at that point. Outpatient narcotic tapers typically don't work well for a number of reasons. The patient is not being monitored and so is being asked to use his judgment and willpower to adjust the medication on his own. We already know that Kerry has a problem with abuse and dependence on a variety of substances. Asking him to monitor his own home-based taper off narcotics is a bit naïve on the part of any good clinician. There is no doubt that he will fail to manage such a taper appropriately, because of chronic pain and a lack of willpower and a predisposition to addictive behavior. Also, giving Kerry naltrexone long-acting monthly injections (Vivitrol) is a pipe-dream. This medication is FDA-approved for both alcohol and opioid relapse prevention, but it has no analgesic properties whatsoever. Naltrexone will certainly reduce the cravings for both narcotics and alcohol; however, one cannot take narcotics with Vivitrol because at best, they won't work because they will be blocked by the antagonistic effect of the Vivitrol and at worst, the combination of narcotics with Vivitrol could induce a precipitated withdrawal state. Guidelines dictate that at least 5 days must elapse between the last dose of a short-acting narcotic (or 10 days if a long-acting narcotic is being taken) and the first dose of naltrexone.

Sending Kerry to a specialized pain clinic is an outstanding option. Pain specialists, who are neurologists, psychiatrists, internists, anesthesiologists and physiatrists, are well-poised to put Kerry on a strict painkiller regimen that will be tailored to his abusive tendencies. Options for this include fentanyl transdermal patch therapy or methadone for chronic pain. They will also recommend ancillary services like physical therapy to help Kerry improve his condition and his pain.

Continuing Roxicodone is absolutely not an option in this case. Kerry will merely continue to overuse and abuse this medication, which is a short-acting opioid narcotic useful for only short-term, acute treatment of intense pain, such as post-operative pain. Disulfiram (Antabuse) cannot be given to Kerry until he abstains from alcohol for several days to at least a week. Recall that Antabuse blocks aldehyde dehydrogenase in the liver, which is the hepatic enzyme responsible for alcohol metabolism. Thus, levels of acetaldehyde build up in the bloodstream. As such, if alcohol is consumed while the patient is on Antabuse, an aversive reaction of nausea, vomiting, hypertension, headache, flushing, thirst, sweating and dyspnea is the result. For Antabuse to be started, Kerry must either be detoxed off the alcohol first, or be abstinent of his own accord in order to avoid this adverse reaction. The minimum safe duration off alcohol before starting to take disulfiram is 12 hours.

Orthopedic and neurologic consultations are useful, but they won't help Kerry in the immediate with his substance dependence and abuse issues, or with his pain management. These are more pressing issues in the moment and these consultations can take place after both pain and addiction are directly addressed.

Methadone and acamprosate calcium (Campral) are excellent choices for outpatient management of Kerry's problems with narcotic painkillers and alcohol. Methadone is along-acting synthetic narcotic that can be prescribed lawfully in an outpatient office when it is given for chronic pain. When methadone is prescribed only as opioid replacement therapy for narcotic addiction, it can only be given in a federally-licensed and regulated methadone clinic. Methadone is thought to be most effective for opioid relapse prevention at or above doses of 60 mg daily. Campral is a wonderful medication for alcohol relapse prevention. Campral effectively reduces cravings for alcohol consumption. Campral's mechanism of action is believed to involve the antagonism of glutamate and the NMDA receptor. In order for Campral to be effective, the patient must have already stopped drinking alcohol for a short period, perhaps about one week.

K&S Ch. 36

2. C. The correct dosing strategy for disulfiram (Antabuse) is to start the patient on 500 mg daily for the first 1-2 weeks, and then lower the maintenance dose to 250 mg daily. Disulfiram should not be administered until the person has abstained from alcohol for at least 12 hours.

K&S Ch. 36

3. BCE. Suboxone (buprenorphine/naloxone) is a sublingual tablet or disintegrating film strip that is rapidly absorbed under the tongue. It comes in two strengths: 8/4 mg and 2/0.5 mg. The first digit is the dose of buprenorphine and the second digit is the dose of naloxone. The unique property of buprenorphine is that is both an agonist and antagonist at the μ-opiate receptor site. This property makes buprenorphine a very modest painkiller and it also renders the medication very difficult to abuse. At doses above 40 mg daily, buprenorphine gates the μ-opiate receptor and no further agonistic effects occur. This essentially breaks up most of the medication's potential for building tolerance and inducing euphoria. Also, if full opioid agonists are consumed in conjunction with Suboxone, the user may well experience a disturbing precipitated withdrawal syndrome.

The naloxone content of Suboxone is a failsafe mechanism to prevent the diversion of the product by intravenous opiate users for the purposes of self-injection for recreational purposes. When absorbed by the two large veins under the tongue, the naloxone has no real clinical effect; however, if the product is emulsified and injected intravenously, the naloxone component of the medication acts as a potent and rapid opioid antagonist and abusers can experience a significant precipitated withdrawal if any attempt is made to inject it.

Suboxone tablets and film strips must be taken under the tongue in order to be fully effective. Typical maintenance doses for opioid relapse prevention range from 4 to 16 mg daily.

K&S Ch. 36

4. ABC. Among the agents that can decrease methadone blood levels are: phenytoin, hypericum, dextromethorphan, abacavir, carbamazepine, cocaine, dexamethasone, nevirapine, rifampin, spironolactone, and tobacco products. Among the agents that can increase methadone blood levels are: ciprofloxacin, erythromycin, disulfiram, verapamil, dihydroergotamine, grapefruit, moclobemide, Echinacea.

K&S Ch. 36

5. D. Cannabis intoxication produces memory impairment, perceptual distortions, decreased problem-solving ability, loss of coordination, increased heart rate, anxiety, and panic attacks. Abrupt cessation of cannabis after prolonged heavy use may cause a characteristic withdrawal syndrome that encompasses insomnia, irritability, drug craving, restlessness, depressed mood, nervousness and anxiety. This can be followed by anxiety, nausea, tremors, muscle twitches, sweating, myalgia, and general malaise. Typically, the withdrawal syndrome begins about 24 hours after the last use, peaks at about 2 to 4 days, and diminishes after about 2 weeks.

K&S Chs 36&52

Topic Index